Ventricular Arrhythmias and Sudden Cardiac Death

Ventricular Arrhythmias and Sudden Cardiac Death

EDITED BY

Paul J. Wang, MD

Cardiac Arrhythmia Service
Stanford University Medical Center
Stanford, CA
USA

Amin Al-Ahmad, MD

Cardiac Arrhythmia Service
Stanford University Medical Center
Stanford, CA
USA

Henry H. Hsia, MD

Cardiac Arrhythmia Service
Stanford University Medical Center
Stanford, CA
USA

Paul C. Zei, MD, PhD

Cardiac Arrhythmia Service
Stanford University Medical Center
Stanford, CA
USA

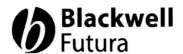

Blackwell Futura

© 2008 by Blackwell Publishing
Blackwell Futura is an imprint of Blackwell Publishing

Blackwell Publishing, Inc., 350 Main Street, Malden, Massachusetts 02148-5020, USA
Blackwell Publishing Ltd, 9600 Garsington Road, Oxford OX4 2DQ, UK
Blackwell Science Asia Pty Ltd, 550 Swanston Street, Carlton, Victoria 3053, Australia

First published 2008

1   2008

ISBN: 978-1-4051-6114-5

Library of Congress Cataloging-in-Publication Data
Ventricular arrhythmias and sudden cardiac death / edited by Paul J. Wang ... [et al.].
      p. ; cm.
Includes bibliographical references and index.
ISBN 978-1-4051-6114-5 (alk. paper)
1. Ventricular tachycardia.   2. Cardiac arrest.   3. Ventricular tachycardia–Treatment.   4. Cardiac arrest–Treatment.
I. Wang, Paul J.
[DNLM: 1. Tachycardia, Ventricular.   2. Death, Sudden, Cardiac.   3. Tachycardia, Ventricular–therapy.
WG 330 V4657   2008]
RC685.T33V43 2008
616.1′23025–dc22   2007031922

A catalogue record for this title is available from the British Library

Commissioning Editor: Gina Almond
Development Editor: Kate Newell and Fiona Pattison
Editorial Assistant: Victoria Pitman
Production Controller: Debbie Wyer

Set in 9.5/12pt Minion by Aptara Inc., New Delhi, India
Printed and bound in Singapore by Markono Print Media Pte Ltd.

For further information on Blackwell Publishing, visit our website:
www.blackwellcardiology.com

The publisher's policy is to use permanent paper from mills that operate a sustainable forestry policy, and which has been manufactured from pulp processed using acid-free and elementary chlorine-free practices. Furthermore, the publisher ensures that the text paper and cover board used have met acceptable environmental accreditation standards.

Contents

Contributors

Amin Al-Ahmad, MD
Cardiac Arrhythmia Service
Stanford University Medical Center
Stanford, CA
USA

Charles Antzelevitch, PhD
Masonic Medical Research Laboratory
Utica, NY
USA

Nitish Badhwar, MBBS, FACC
Section of Cardiac Electrophysiology
UCSF, Division of Cardiology
University of California
San Francisco, CA
USA

Marci S. Bailey, RN
Research Coordinator
Washington University School of Medicine
St. Louis, MO
USA

J. Thomas Bigger, MD
Columbia University College of Physicians and Surgeons
New York, NY
USA

J. David Burkhardt
Cardiac Pacing and Electrophysiology
Department of Cardiovascular Medicine
Cleveland Clinic Foundation
Cleveland, OH
USA

Hugh Calkins, MD
Professor of Medicine
Director of the Arrhythmia Service
Director of the Electrophysiology Laboratory
Director of the Johns Hopkins ARVD
   Program Johns Hopkins Medical Institutions
Baltimore, MD
USA

David J. Callans, MD
University of Pennsylvania Health System
Philadelphia, PA
USA

Lan S. Chen, MD
The Department of Neurology
Indiana University School of Medicine
Indianapolis, Indiana
USA

Peng-Sheng Chen, MD
The Krannert Institute of Cardiology
Division of Cardiology
Department of Medicine
Indiana University School of Medicine
Indianapolis, IN
USA

Ralph J. Damiano, Jr. MD
Chief of Cardiothoracic Surgery
John Shoenberg Professor of Surgery
Washington University School of Medicine
St. Louis, MO
USA

Jacques MT de Bakker, PhD
Head, Department of Experimental Cardiology Academic
   Medical Center; Amsterdam, The Netherlands

The Center of Heart Failure Research, Department of
   Experimental Cardiology, Academic Medical Center,
   Amsterdam, The Netherlands
The Heart Lung Center, University Medical Center Utrecht,
   The Netherlands
The Department of Medical Physiology, University Medical
   Center Utrecht, The Netherlands
The Interuniversity Cardiology Institute of the Netherlands,
   Utrecht
The Netherlands

Derek J. Dosdall, PhD
University of Alabama at Birmingham
Department of Biomedical Engineering
Birmingham, AL
USA

N.A. Mark Estes III, MD
Professor of Medicine
Director, Cardiac Arrhythmia Center
Tufts University School of Medicine
Boston, MA
USA

Ilan Goldenberg, MD
The Cardiology Division
Department of Medicine
University of Rochester Medical Center
Rochester, NY
USA

Jeffrey J. Goldberger, MD
The Division of Cardiology
Department of Medicine
Feinberg School of Medicine
Northwestern University
Chicago, IL
USA

Anurag Gupta, MD
Stanford University Medical Center
Stanford, CA
USA

Mark C. Haigney, MD
Uniformed Services University
Bethesda, MD
USA

Munther Homoud, MD
Tufts-New England Medical Center
Boston, MA
USA

Henry H. Hsia, MD
Cardiac Arrhythmia Service
Stanford University Medical Center
Stanford, CA
USA

Jian Huang, MD, PhD
University of Alabama at Birmingham
Departments of Medicine
Birmingham, AL
USA

Mathew D. Hutchinson, MD
University of Pennsylvania Health System
Philadelphia, PA
USA

Raymond E. Ideker, MD, PhD
University of Alabama at Birmingham
Departments of Physiology and Biomedical
    Engineering Medicine
Birmingham, AL
USA

Rahul Jain, MD
Division of Cardiology
The Johns Hopkins University School of
    Medicine
MD
USA

Robert E. Kleiger, MD
Washington University School of Medicine
St. Louis, MO
USA

Keane K. Lee, MD
Stanford University Medical Center
Stanford, CA
USA

Mark S. Link, MD
Tufts-New England Medical Center
Boston, MA
USA

Kevin J. Makati, MD
Tufts-New England Medical Center
Boston, MA
USA

Barry J. Maron, MD
Hypertrophic Cardiomyopathy Center
Minneapolis Heart Institute Foundation
MN
USA

Pirooz S. Mofrad, MD
Stanford University Medical Center
Standford, CA
USA

Robert J. Moraca, MD
Fellow in Cardiothoracic Surgery
Washington University School of Medicine
St. Louis, MO
USA

Arthur J. Moss, MD
Professor of Medicine (Cardiology)
Director, Heart Research Follow-Up
    Program
University of Rochester Medical Center
Rochester, NY
USA

Robert J. Myerburg, MD, FACC
Professor of Medicine and Physiology
Chief, Division of Cardiology
University of Miami
Miami, FL
USA

Andrea Natale, MD
Section Head, Electrophysiology and Pacing
Director of the Electrophysiology Laboratories
The Cleveland Clinic Foundation
Cleveland, OH
USA

Jeffrey Olgin, MD
Section of Cardiac Electrophysiology
Division of Cardiology
University of California, San Francisco
San Francisco, CA
USA

Marco Perez, MD
Stanford University
Stanford, CA
USA

Karen P. Phillips, MB, BS (Hons), FRACP
Clinical Cardiac Electrophysiology Fellow
Department of Cardiovascular Medicine
Cleveland Clinic Foundation
Cleveland, OH
USA

Walid I. Saliba, MD
Director, Electrophysiology Laboratories
Section of Cardiac Pacing and Electrophysiology
Department of Cardiovascular Medicine
Cleveland Clinic Foundation
Cleveland, OH
USA

Mauricio Scanavacca, MD
Heart Institute
University of Sao Paulo Medical School
Sao Paulo
Brasil

Melvin M. Scheinman, MD, FACC
Section of Cardiac Electrophysiology
University of California, San Francisco
San Francisco, CA
USA

Robert A. Schweikert, MD
Director, EP Clinical Operations
Section of Cardiac Electrophysiology and Pacing
Department of Cardiovascular Medicine
Cleveland Clinic Foundation
Cleveland, OH
USA

Kyoko Soejima, MD
Assistant Professor
Division of Cardiology
Keio University
Tokyo
Japan

Eduardo Sosa, MD
Heart Institute
University of Sao Paulo Medical School
Sao Paulo
Brazil

Moshe S, Swissa, MD
Division of Cardiology
Department of Medicine
Kaplan Medical Center, Rehovot
The Hebrew University, Jerusalem
Israel

William G. Stevenson, MD
Director, Clinical, Cardiac Electrophysiology, Program
Cardiovascular Division
Brigham and Women's Hospital
Boston, MA
USA

Usha Tedrow, MD
Associate Director, Clinical Cardiac,
    Electrophysiology, Program
Cardiovascular Division
Brigham and Women's Hospital
Boston, MA
USA

Zian H. Tseng, MD
Section of Cardiac Electrophysiology
Division of Cardiology
University of California, San Francisco
San Francisco, CA
USA

George F. Van Hare, MD

Professor of Pediatrics, Clinical Professor of Pediatrics;
   and Director, Pediatric Arrhythmia Center
Stanford University School of Medicine and UCSF
Palo Alto, CA
USa

Harold VM van Rijen

The Department of Medical Physiology
University Medical Center Utrecht
The Netherlands

Paul J. Wang, MD

Stanford University Medical Center
Stanford, CA
USA

Oussama Wazni, MD

Associate Director
Cleveland Clinic Center for Cardiovascular Research
Cleveland Clinic
Cleveland, OH
USA

Jonathan Weinstock, MD

Tufts-New England Medical Center
Boston, MA
USA

Bruce L. Wilkoff, MD

Professor of Medicine and Director, Cardiac Pacing and
Tachyarrhythmia Devices
Cleveland Clinic Foundation
Cleveland, OH
USA

Wojciech Zareba, MD, PhD

The Cardiology Division, Department of Medicine
University of Rochester Medical Center
Rochester, NY
USA

Paul C. Zei, MD, PhD

Cardiac Arrhythmia Service
Stanford University Medical Center
Stanford, CA
USA

Foreword

When, 40 years ago, intracardiac stimulation and activation studies were started for the analysis of cardiac arrhythmias, nobody could have predicted the advances that were going to be made in the years thereafter in our understanding and management of ventricular arrhythmias and sudden death.

Since then an enormous amount of information has become available, leading to our current understanding of mechanisms, etiology, epidemiology, risk stratification, and management of these, unfortunately too often occurring, life-threatening situations.

The best way to present that knowledge, and also the relation between those different areas, is to put it in the form of a book.

We live in a time when information spreads rapidly by way of the internet. However, tunnel vision is one of the dangers of that medium: the subspecialist, looking only for what is new in his or her specialized area, may lose sight of the complete picture with its inherent dangers.

Therefore one has to welcome this book for its coverage and time of publication. By selecting the contributors carefully, the editors have succeeded in bringing together, in one book, an excellent and complete overview of what the cardiologist should know for optimal management of the patient with a ventricular arrhythmia. Among the many in-depth presentations one will find how to select the candidate for catheter ablation, when to implant an ICD, and what measures have to be taken to reduce sudden death out of hospital.

Hein J. Wellens
Maastricht, The Netherlands
August 2007

CHAPTER 1

The role of spatial dispersion of repolarization and intramural reentry in inherited and acquired sudden cardiac death syndromes

Charles Antzelevitch

Abstract

The cellular basis for intramural reentry that develops secondary to the development of transmural dispersion of repolarization (TDR) is examined in this review. The hypothesis that amplification of spatial dispersion of repolarization underlies the development of intramural reentry and life-threatening ventricular arrhythmias associated with inherited ion channelopathies is probed. The roles of TDR in the long-QT, short-QT, and Brugada syndromes as well as catecholaminergic polymorphic ventricular tachycardia are critically examined. In the long-QT syndrome, amplification of TDR is generally secondary to preferential prolongation of the action potential duration (APD) of M cells, whereas in the Brugada syndrome, it is due to selective abbreviation of the APD of right ventricular epicardium. Preferential abbreviation of APD of either endocardium or epicardium appears to be responsible for amplification of TDR in the short-QT syndrome. The available data suggest that the long-QT, short-QT, and Brugada syndromes are pathologies with very different phenotypes and etiologies, but which share a common final pathway in causing sudden cardiac death.

Ventricular Arrhythmias and Sudden Cardiac Death, 1st edition. Edited by P.J. Wang, A. Al-Ahmad, H. Hsia, and P.C. Zei © 2008 Blackwell Publishing, ISBN: 978-1-4051-6114-5.

Keywords:

long QT syndrome; short QT syndrome; Brugada syndrome; polymorphic ventricular tachycardia; electrophysiology

Inherited sudden cardiac death secondary to the development of life-threatening ventricular arrhythmias have been associated with a variety of ion channelopathies such as the long-QT, short-QT, and Brugada syndromes. Table 1.1 lists the genetic defects thus far identified to be associated with these primary electrical diseases. These ion channel defects have been shown to amplify spatial dispersion of repolarization, in some cases with the assistance of pharmacologic agents that further exaggerate the gain or loss of function of ion channel activity. Before examining these interactions, we will review the basis for intrinsic electrical heterogeneity within the ventricular myocardium.

Intrinsic electrical heterogeneity within the ventricular myocardium

It is now well established that ventricular myocardium is comprised of at least three electrophysiologically as well as functionally distinct cell types: epicardial, M, and endocardial cells [1,2]. These three principal ventricular myocardial cell types differ with respect to phase 1 and phase 3 repolarization characteristics. Ventricular epicardial and M,

Table 1.1 Inherited disorders caused by ion channelopathies

		Rhythm	Inheritance	Locus	Ion channel	Gene
Long-QT syndrome	(RW)	TdP	AD			
	LQT1		AD	11p15	I_{Ks}	KCNQ1, KvLQT1
	LQT2		AD	7q35	I_{Kr}	KCNH2, HERG
	LQT3		AD	3p21	I_{Na}	SCN5A, Na_v1.5
	LQT4		AD	4q25		ANKB, ANK2
	LQT5		AD	21q22	I_{Ks}	KCNE1, minK
	LQT6		AD	21q22	I_{Kr}	KCNE2, MiRP1
	LQT7	(Anderson–Tawil syndrome)	AD	17q23	I_{K1}	KCNJ2, Kir 2.1
	LQT8	(Timothy syndrome)	AD	6q8A	I_{Ca}	CACNA1C, Ca_v1.2
	LQT9		AD	3p25	I_{Na}	CAV3, Caveolin-3
	LQT10		AD	11q23.3	I_{Na}	SCN4B, $Na_v b4$
LQT syndrome (JLN)		TdP	AR	11p15	I_{Ks}	KCNQ1, KvLQT1
				21q22	I_{Ks}	KCNE1, minK
Brugada syndrome	BrS1	PVT	AD	3p21	I_{Na}	SCN5A, Nav1.5
	BrS2	PVT	AD	3p24	I_{Na}	GPD1L
	BrS3	PVT	AD	12p13.3	I_{Ca}	CACNA1C, Ca_v1.2
	BrS4	PVT	AD	10p12.33	I_{Ca}	CACNB2b, $Ca_v B_{2b}$
Short-QT syndrome	SQT1	VT/VF	AD	7q35	I_{Kr}	KCNH2, HERG
	SQT2		AD	11p15	I_{Ks}	KCNQ1, KvLQT1
	SQT3		AD	17q23.1-24.2	I_{K1}	KCNJ2, Kir2.1
	SQT4		AD	12p13.3	I_{Ca}	CACNA1C, Ca_v1.2
	SQT5		AD	10p12.33	I_{Ca}	CACNB2b, $Ca_v \beta 2b$
Catecholaminergic VT	CVPT1	VT	AD	1q42-43		RyR2
	CPVT2	VT	AR	1p13-21		CASQ2

Abbreviations: AD, autosomal dominant; AR, autosomal recessive; JLN, Jervell and Lange-Nielsen; LQT, long QT; RW, Romano–Ward; TdP, Torsade de Pointes; VF, ventricular fibrillation; VT, ventricular tachycardia; PVT, polymorphic VT.

but not endocardial, cells generally display a prominent phase 1, due to a large 4-aminopyridine (4-AP)-sensitive transient outward current (I_{to}), giving the action potential either a spike-and-dome or a notched configuration. These regional differences in I_{to} were first suggested on the basis of action potential data [3] and subsequently demonstrated using patch clamp techniques in canine [4], feline [5], rabbit [6], rat [7], ferret [8], and human [9,10] ventricular myocytes.

The magnitude of the action potential notch and corresponding differences in I_{to} have also been shown to be different between right and left ventricular epicardium [11]. Similar interventricular differences in I_{to} have also been described for canine ventricular M cells [12]. This distinction is thought to form the basis for why the Brugada syndrome, a

channelopathy-mediated form of sudden death, is a right ventricular disease.

Wang and co-workers [13] reported a larger L-type calcium channel current (I_{Ca}) in canine endocardial versus epicardial ventricular myocytes, although other studies have failed to detect any difference in I_{Ca} among cells isolated from epicardium, M, and endocardial regions of the canine left ventricular wall [14,15]. Myocytes isolated from the epicardial region of the left ventricular wall of the rabbit show a higher density of cAMP-activated chloride current when compared to endocardial myocytes [16]. I_{to2}, initially ascribed to a K^+ current, is now thought to be caused primarily by the calcium-activated chloride current ($I_{Cl(Ca)}$); it is thought to also contribute to the action potential notch but it is not known whether this current differs among the three ventricular myocardial cell types [17].

Characteristics of the M cell

Residing in the deep structures of the ventricular wall between the epicardial and endocardial layers, are M cells and transitional cells. The M cell, masonic midmyocardial Moe cell, discovered in the early 1990s, was named in memory of Gordon K Moe [2,18,19]. The hallmark of the M cell is that its action potential can prolong more than that of epicardium or endocardium in response to a slowing of rate or in response to agents that prolong APD (Figure 1.1) [1,18,20]. Histologically, M cells are similar to epicardial and endocardial cells. Electrophysiologically and pharmacologically, they appear to be a hybrid between Purkinje and ventricular cells [21]. Like Purkinje fibers, M cells show a prominent APD prolongation and develop early afterdepolarizations (EAD) in response to I_{Kr} blockers, whereas epicardium and endocardium do not. Like Purkinje fibers, M cells develop delayed afterdepolarizations (DAD) more readily in response to agents that calcium load or overload the cardiac cell. α_1 Adrenoceptor stimulation produces APD prolongation in Purkinje fibers, but abbreviation in M cells, and little or no change in endocardium and epicardium [22].

Although transitional cells are found throughout much of the wall in the canine left ventricle, M cells displaying the longest action potentials (at basic cycle lengths (BCLs) ≥ 2000 ms) are often localized in the deep subendocardium to midmyocardium in the anterior wall [23], deep subepicardium to midmyocardium in the lateral wall [18], and throughout the wall in the region of the right ventricular (RV) outflow tracts [2]. M cells are also present in the deep cell layers of endocardial structures, including papillary muscles, trabeculae, and the interventricular septum [24]. Unlike Purkinje fibers, M cells are not found in discrete bundles or islets [24,25] although there is evidence that they may be localized in discrete muscle layers. Cells with the characteristics of M cells have been described in the canine, guinea pig, rabbit, pig, and human ventricles [4,18,20,23–44].

Isolated myocytes dissociated from discrete layers of the left ventricular wall display APD values

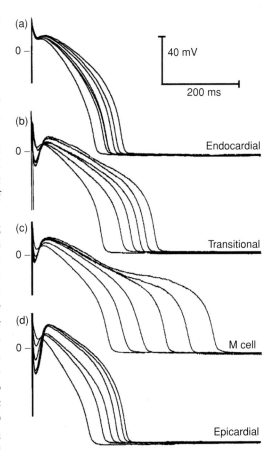

Figure 1.1 Transmembrane activity recorded from cells isolated from the epicardial, M, and endocardial regions of the canine left ventricle at basic cycle lengths (BCL) of 300–5000 milliseconds (steady-state conditions). The M and transitional cells were enzymatically dissociated from the midmyocardial region. Deceleration-induced prolongation of APD is much greater in M cells than in epicardial and endocardial cells. The spike-and-dome morphology is also more accentuated in the epicardial cell. From [4], with permission.

that differ by more than 200 milliseconds at relatively slow rates of stimulation. When the cells are in a functional syncytium that comprises the ventricular myocardium, electrotonic interactions among the different cells types lead to reduction of the APD dispersion to 25–55 milliseconds. The transmural increase in APD from epicardium to endocardium is relatively gradual, except between the epicardium and subepicardium where there is often a sharp increase in APD (Figure 1.2). This has been shown to be due to an increase in tissue

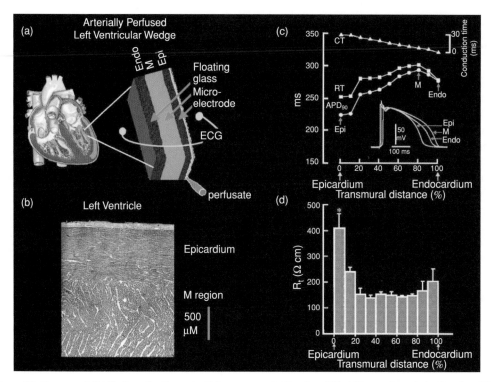

Figure 1.2 Transmural distribution of action potential duration and tissue resistivity across the ventricular wall. (a) Schematic diagram of the coronary-perfused canine LV wedge preparation. Transmembrane action potentials are recorded simultaneously from epicardial (Epi), M region (M), and endocardial (Endo) sites using three floating microelectrodes. A transmural ECG is recorded along the same transmural axis across the bath, registering the entire field of the wedge. (b) Histology of a transmural slice of the left ventricular wall near the epicardial border. The region of sharp transition of cell orientation coincides with the region of high tissue resistivity depicted in Panel (d) and the region of sharp transition of action potential duration illustrated in Panel (c). (c) Distribution of conduction time (CT), APD$_{90}$, and repolarization time (RT = APD$_{90}$+ CT) in a canine left ventricular wall wedge preparation paced at BCL of 2000 milliseconds. A sharp transition of APD$_{90}$ is present between epicardium and subepicardium. Epi: epicardium; M: M cell; Endo: endocardium. RT: repolarization time; CT: conduction time. (d) Distribution of total tissue resistivity (R_t) across the canine left ventricular wall. Transmural distances at 0% and 100% represent epicardium and endocardium, respectively. *$P < 0.01$ compared with R_t at mid-wall. Tissue resistivity increases most dramatically between deep subepicardium and epicardium. Error bars represent SEM ($n = 5$). From [21,23], with permission.

resistivity in this region [23], which may be related to the sharp transition in cell orientation in this region as well as to reduced expression of connexin43 [45,46], which is principally responsible for intracellular communication in ventricular myocardium. Moreover, LeGrice et al. [47] have shown that the density of collagen is heterogeneously distributed across the ventricular wall. A greater density of collagen in the deep subepicardium may also contribute to the resistive barrier in this region of the wall, limiting the degree of electrotonic interaction between myocardial layers. The degree of electrotonic coupling, together with the intrinsic differences APD, contribute to TDR in the ventricular myocardium [48].

The ionic bases for these features of the M cell include the presence of a smaller slowly activating delayed rectifier current (I_{Ks}) [30], a larger late sodium current (late I_{Na}) [49], and a larger Na–Ca exchange current (I_{Na-Ca}) [50]. In the canine heart, the rapidly activating delayed rectifier (I_{Kr}) and the inward rectifier (I_{K1}) currents are similar in the three transmural cell types. Transmural and apico-basal differences in the density of I_{Kr} channels have been described in the ferret heart [51]. I_{Kr} message and channel protein are much larger in the ferret epicardium. I_{Ks} is larger in M cells isolated from the right versus left ventricles of the dog [12]. These ionic distinctions sensitize the M cells to a variety of pharmacological agents. Agents that block the rapidly activating delayed rectifier current (I_{Kr}), I_{Ks}, or that increase calcium channel current (I_{Ca}) or late I_{Na}, generally produce a much greater prolongation of the APD of the M cell than of epicardial or endocardial cells leading to amplification of TDR.

Amplification of transmural heterogeneities normally present in the early and late phases of the action potential can lead to the development of a variety of arrhythmias, including Brugada, long-QT, and short-QT syndromes as well as catecholaminergic ventricular tachycardia (VT).

Brugada syndrome

The Brugada syndrome is an inherited primary electrical disease in which amplification of TDR is believed to lead to the development of polymorphic VT and sudden cardiac death [52]. The Brugada ECG is characterized by an elevated ST segment or J wave appearing in the right precordial leads (V1–V3), often followed by a negative T wave. First described in 1992, the syndrome is associated with a high incidence of sudden cardiac death secondary to a rapid polymorphic VT or ventricular fibrillation (VF) [53]. The ECG characteristics of the Brugada syndrome are dynamic and often concealed, but can be unmasked by potent sodium channel blockers such as ajmaline, flecainide, procainamide, disopyramide, propafenone, and pilsicainide [54–56].

The Brugada syndrome (BrS) is associated with mutations in SCN5A, the gene that encodes the α subunit of the cardiac sodium channel, in approximately 15% of probands [57]. Over one hundred mutations in SCN5A have been linked to the syndrome in recent years (see [58] for references; also see http://www.fsm.it/cardmoc). Only a fraction of these mutations have been studied in expression systems and shown to result in loss of function of sodium channel activity. Weiss et al. [59] described a second locus on chromosome 3, close to but distinct from SCN5A, linked to the syndrome in a large pedigree in which the syndrome is associated with progressive conduction disease, a low sensitivity to procainamide, and a relatively good prognosis. The

gene was recently identified in a preliminary report as the *Glycerol-3-Phosphate Dehydrogenase 1-Like (GPD1L)* gene and the mutation in *GPD1L* was shown to result in a reduction of I_{Na} [60].

The third and fourth genes associated with the Brugada syndrome were recently identified and shown to encode the α1 (*CACNA1C*) and β (*CACNB2b*) subunits of the L-type cardiac calcium channel. Mutations in the α and β subunits of the calcium channel also lead to a shorter than normal QT interval, in some cases creating a new clinical entity consisting of a combined Brugada/short-QT syndrome [61].

Several experimental models of the BrS have been developed using the right coronary-perfused right ventricular wedge preparation [62–66]. The available data point to amplification of heterogeneities intrinsic to the early phases (phase 1-mediated notch) of the action potential of cells residing in different layers of the right ventricular wall of the heart as the basis for the development of extrasystolic activity and polymorphic VT in BrS (Figure 1.3). Rebalancing of the currents active at the end of phase 1 can lead to accentuation of the action potential notch in right ventricular epicardium, which is responsible for the augmented J wave and ST segment elevation associated with the Brugada syndrome (see [52,67] for references). Under physiologic conditions, the ST segment is isoelectric due to the absence of major transmural voltage gradients at the level of the action potential plateau. Accentuation of the right ventricular action potential notch under pathophysiological conditions leads to exaggeration of transmural voltage gradients and thus to accentuation of the J wave or to an elevation of the J point (Figure 1.3). If the epicardial action potential continues to repolarize before that of endocardium, the T wave remains positive, giving rise to a saddleback configuration of the ST segment elevation. Further accentuation of the notch is accompanied by a prolongation of the epicardial action potential causing it to repolarize after endocardium, thus leading to inversion of the T wave [62,63]. Despite the appearance of a typical Brugada ECG, accentuation of the RV epicardial action potential (AP) notch alone does not give rise to an arrhythmogenic substrate. The arrhythmogenic substrate may develop with a further shift in the balance of current leading to loss of the action potential dome at some epicardial sites but not others. A steep gradient of TDR develops as a consequence, creating a vulnerable window, which when captured by a premature extrasystole can trigger a reentrant arrhythmia. Because loss of the action potential dome in epicardium is generally heterogeneous, epicardial dispersion of repolarization develops as well. Propagation of the action potential dome from sites at which it is maintained to sites at which it is lost causes local reexcitation via phase 2 reentry, leading to the development of a closely coupled extrasystole capable of capturing the vulnerable window across the ventricular wall, thus triggering a circus movement reentry in the form of VT/VF (Figures 1.3 and 1.4) [62,68,69]. The polymorphic VT may start in epicardium reentry, but quickly shifts to an intramural reentry before self-terminating or deteriorating to VF [69].

Evidence in support of these hypotheses derives from experiments involving the arterially perfused right ventricular wedge preparation [62,63,66,69, 70] and from studies in which monophasic action potential (MAP) electrodes were positioned on the epicardial and endocardial surfaces of the right ventricular outflow tract (RVOT) in patients with the Brugada syndrome [71,72].

Long-QT syndrome

The long-QT syndromes (LQTS) are phenotypically and genotypically diverse, but have in common the appearance of a long QT interval in the ECG, an atypical polymorphic VT known as Torsade de Pointes (TdP), and, in many but not all cases, a relatively high risk for sudden cardiac death [73–75]. Ten genotypes of the congenital LQTS have been identified. The identified syndromes are distinguished by mutations in at least eight different ion channel genes, a structural anchoring protein, and a caveolin protein located on chromosomes 3, 4, 6, 7, 11, 17, and 21 (Table 1.1) [76–81].

The most recent genes associated with LQTS are *CAV3* which encodes caveolin-3 and *SCN4B* which encodes $Na_V B4$, an auxiliary subunit of the cardiac sodium channel. Caveolin-3 spans the plasma membrane twice, forming a hairpin structure on the surface, and is the main constituent of caveolae, small invaginations in the plasma membrane. Mutations both in *CAV3* and in *SCNB4* produce a gain in function in late I_{Na}, causing an LQT3-like phenotype [82,83].

LQTS shows both autosomal recessive and autosomal dominant patterns of inheritance: (1) a rare autosomal recessive disease associated with deafness (Jervell and Lange-Nielsen), caused by two genes that encode for the slowly activating delayed rectifier potassium channel (*KCNQ1* and *KCNE1*); and (2) a much more common autosomal dominant form known as the Romano–Ward syndrome, caused by mutations in 10 different genes (Table 1.1). Eight of the 10 genes encode cardiac ion channels.

Acquired LQTS refers to a QT prolongation caused by exposure to drugs that prolong the duration of the ventricular action potential [84] or QT prolongation secondary to cardiomyopathies including dilated or hypertrophic cardiomyopathy, as well as to abnormal QT prolongation associated with bradycardia or electrolyte imbalance [85–89]. The acquired form of the disease is far more prevalent than the congenital form and in some cases may have a genetic predisposition [90].

Amplification of spatial dispersion of repolarization within the ventricular myocardium has been identified as the principal arrhythmogenic substrate in both acquired and congenital LQTS. The amplification of spatial dispersion of refractoriness can take the form of an increase in transmural, transseptal, or apico-basal dispersion of repolarization. This exaggerated intrinsic heterogeneity together with EAD- and DAD-induced triggered activity, both caused by reduction in net repolarizing current, underlie the substrate and trigger for the development of TdP arrhythmias observed under LQTS conditions [91,92]. Models of the LQT1, LQT2, and LQT3 forms of the LQTS have been developed using the canine arterially perfused left ventricular wedge preparation (Figure 1.5) [93]. These models suggest that in these three forms of LQTS, preferential prolongation of the M cell APD leads to an increase in the QT interval as well as an increase in TDR, which contributes to the development of spontaneous as well as stimulation-induced TdP via an intramural reentry mechanism (Figure 1.6) [35,40,94–97]. The spatial dispersion of repolarization is further exaggerated by sympathetic influences in LQT1 and LQT2, accounting for the great sensitivity of patients with these genotypes to adrenergic stimuli (Figures 1.5 and 1.6).

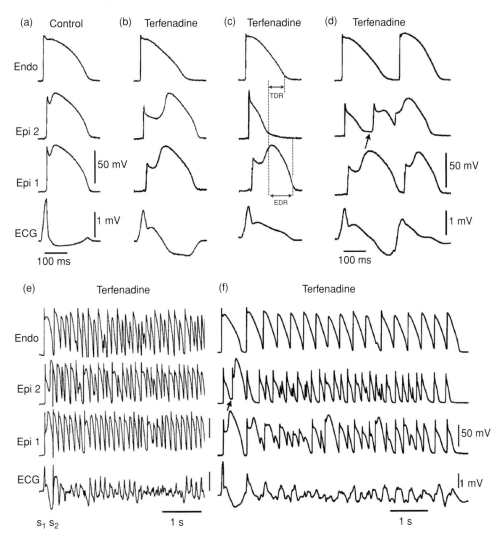

Figure 1.3 Cellular basis for electrocardiographic and arrhythmic manifestation of Brugada syndrome. Each panel shows transmembrane action potentials from one endocardial (top) and two epicardial sites together with a transmural ECG recorded from a canine coronary-perfused right ventricular wedge preparation. (a) Control (BCL 400 ms). (b) Combined sodium and calcium channel block with terfenadine (5 μM) accentuates the epicardial action potential notch, creating a transmural voltage gradient that manifests as an ST segment elevation or exaggerated J wave in the ECG. (c) Continued exposure to terfenadine results in all-or-none repolarization at the end of phase 1 at some epicardial sites but not others, creating a local epicardial dispersion of repolarization (EDR) as well as a transmural dispersion of repolarization (TDR). (d) Phase 2 reentry occurs when the epicardial action potential dome propagates from a site where it is maintained to regions where it has been lost, giving rise to a closely coupled extrasystole. (e) Extrastimulus (S1 – S2 = 250 ms) applied to epicardium triggers a polymorphic VT. (f) Phase 2 reentrant extrasystole triggers a brief episode of polymorphic VT. (Modified from Ref. [63], with permission).

Voltage gradients that develop as a result of the different time course of repolarization of phases 2 and 3 in the three cell types give rise to opposing voltage gradients on either side of the M region, which are in part responsible for the inscription of the T wave [44]. In the case of an upright T wave, the epicardial response is the earliest to repolarize and the M cell action potential is the latest. Full repolarization of the epicardial action potential coincides with the peak of the T wave and repolarization of

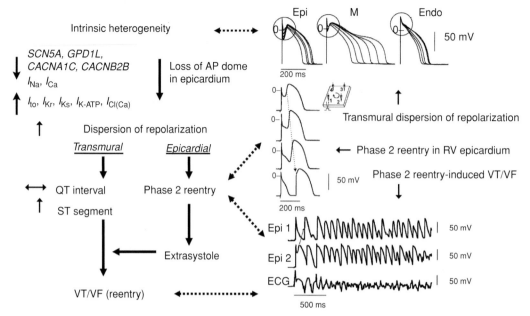

Figure 1.4 Proposed mechanism for the Brugada syndrome. A shift in the balance of currents serves to amplify existing heterogeneities by causing loss of the action potential dome at some epicardial, but not endocardial sites. A vulnerable window develops as a result of the dispersion of repolarization and refractoriness within epicardium as well as across the wall. Epicardial dispersion leads to the development of phase 2 reentry, which provides the extrasystole that captures the vulnerable window and initiates VT/VF via a circus movement reentry mechanism. Modified from [128], with permission.

the M cells is coincident with the end of the T wave. The duration of the M cell action potential therefore determines the QT interval, whereas the duration of the epicardial action potential determines the QT$_{peak}$ interval. The interval between the peak and end of the T wave (T$_{peak}$–T$_{end}$ interval) in precordial ECG leads is suggested to provide an index of TDR [2]. Recent studies provide guidelines for the estimation of TDR in the case of more complex T waves, including negative, biphasic, and triphasic T waves [98]. In these cases, the interval from the nadir of the first component of the T wave to the end of the T wave provides an approximation of TDR.

Because the precordial leads (V1–V6) are designed to view the electrical field across the ventricular wall, T$_{peak}$–T$_{end}$ is the most representative of TDR in these leads. T$_{peak}$–T$_{end}$ intervals measured in the limb leads are unlikely to provide an index of TDR, but may provide a measure of global dispersion within the heart [99,100]. Because TDR can vary dramatically in different regions of the heart, it is inadvisable to average T$_{peak}$–T$_{end}$ among all or several leads [100]. Because LQTS is principally a left ventricular disorder, TDR is likely to be greatest in the left ventricular wall or septum and thus be best reflected in left precordial leads or V3, respectively [101]. In contrast, because Brugada syndrome is a right ventricular disorder, TDR is greatest in the right ventricular free wall and thus is best reflected in the right precordial leads [102].

T$_{peak}$–T$_{end}$ interval does not provide an absolute measure of transmural dispersion *in vivo* [100], although changes in this parameter are thought to reflect changes in spatial dispersion of repolarization, including TDR, and thus may be prognostic of arrhythmic risk under a variety of conditions [103–108]. Takenaka et al. [107] recently demonstrated exercise-induced accentuation of the T$_{peak}$–T$_{end}$ interval in LQT1 patients, but not LQT2. These observations coupled with those of Schwartz et al. [109], demonstrating an association between exercise and risk for TdP in LQT1 but not LQT2 patients, once again point to the potential value of T$_{peak}$–T$_{end}$ in forecasting risk for the development of TdP. Direct evidence in support of T$_{peak}$–T$_{end}$ measured in V5 as an index to predict TdP in patients with LQTS was provided by Yamaguchi and co-workers [101]. These authors concluded that T$_{peak}$–T$_{end}$ is

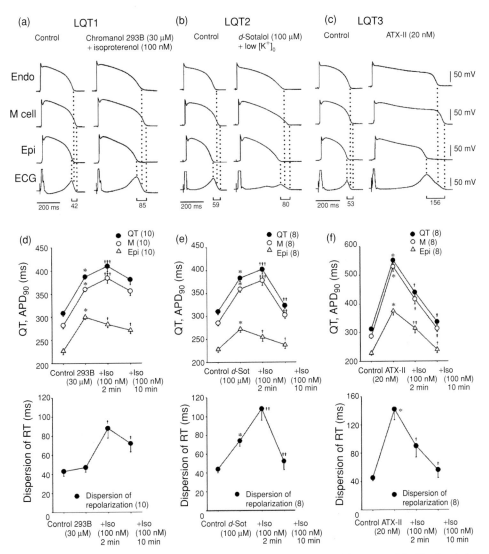

Figure 1.5 LQT1, LQT2, and LQT3 models of LQTS. Panels (a)–(c) show action potentials recorded simultaneously from endocardial (Endo), M, and epicardial (Epi) sites of arterially perfused canine left ventricular wedge preparations together with a transmural ECG. BCL = 2000 milliseconds. Transmural dispersion of repolarization across the ventricular wall, defined as the difference in the repolarization time between M and epicardial cells, is denoted below the ECG traces. LQT1 model was mimicked using Isoproterenol + chromanol 293B – an I_{Ks} blocker. LQT2 was created using the I_{Kr} blocker d-sotalol + low $[K^+]_o$. LQT3 was mimicked using the sea anemone toxin ATX-II to augment late I_{Na}. Panels (d)–(f): Effect of isoproterenol in the LQT1, LQT2, and LQT3 models. In LQT1, isoproterenol (Iso) produces a persistent prolongation both of the APD_{90} of the M cell and of the QT interval (at both 2 and 10 min), whereas the APD_{90} of the epicardial cell is always abbreviated, resulting in a persistent increase in TDR (d). In LQT2, isoproterenol initially prolongs (2 min) and then abbreviates the QT interval and the APD_{90} of the M cell to the control level (10 min), whereas the APD_{90} of epicardial cell is always abbreviated, resulting in a transient increase in TDR (e). In LQT3, isoproterenol produced a persistent abbreviation of the QT interval and the APD_{90} of both M and epicardial cells (at both 2 and 10 min), resulting in a persistent decrease in TDR (f). $*P < 0.0005$ versus Control; $\dagger P < 0.0005$, $\dagger\dagger P < 0.005$, $\dagger\dagger\dagger P < 0.05$, versus 293B, d-Sotalol (d-Sot), or ATX-II. (Modified from references [35,40,94] with permission).

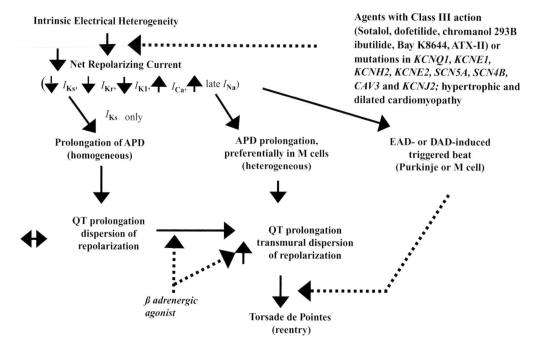

Figure 1.6 Proposed cellular mechanism for the development of Torsade de Pointes in the long-QT syndromes.

more valuable than QTc and QT dispersion as a predictor of TdP in patients with acquired LQTS. Shimizu et al. [106] demonstrated that T_{peak}–T_{end}, but not QTc, predicted sudden cardiac death in patients with hypertrophic cardiomyopathy. Most recently, Watanabe et al. [108] demonstrated that prolonged T_{peak}–T_{end} is associated with inducibility as well as spontaneous development of VT in high-risk patients with organic heart disease. Evidence in support of a significant correlation between T_{peak}–T_{end}, and T_{peak}–T_{end} dispersion and the occurrence of life-threatening arrhythmic events in patients with BrS was recently presented by Castro and co-workers [102].

The accumulated data support the hypothesis that TDR rather than QT prolongation underlies the principal substrate for the development of TdP [91,110–113]. Our working hypothesis for the development of LQTS-related TdP presumes the presence of electrical heterogeneity in the form of TDR under baseline conditions and the amplification of TDR by agents that reduce net repolarizing current via a reduction either in I_{Kr} or in I_{Ks} or augmentation either of I_{Ca} or of late I_{Na} (Figure 1.6). Conditions leading to a reduction in I_{Kr} or augmentation of late I_{Na} produce a preferential prolongation of the

M cell action potential. As a consequence, the QT interval prolongs and is accompanied by a dramatic increase in TDR, thus creating a vulnerable window for the development of reentry. The reduction in net repolarizing current also predisposes to the development of EAD-induced triggered activity in M and Purkinje cells, which provide the extrasystole that triggers TdP when it falls within the vulnerable period. β Adrenergic agonists further amplify transmural heterogeneity (transiently) in the case of I_{Kr} block, but reduce it in the case of sodium channel current (I_{Na}) agonists [33,94].

Agents that selectively block I_{Kr} for increase in late I_{Na} always produced a preferential prolongation of the M cell action potential and thus augment TDR. However, not all agents that prolong the QT interval increase TDR. Amiodarone, a potent antiarrhythmic agent used in the management of both atrial and ventricular arrhythmias, is rarely associated with TdP. Chronic administration of amiodarone produces a greater prolongation of APD in epicardium and endocardium, but less of an increase, or even a decrease at slow rates, in the M region, thereby reducing TDR [114]. In a dog model of chronic complete atrioventricular block and acquired LQTS, 6 weeks of amiodarone was shown to produce a major QT prolongation without producing TdP. In contrast, after 6 weeks of dronedarone, TdP occurred in 4 of 8 dogs with the highest spatial dispersion of repolarization (105 ± 20 ms) [115].

Another example of an agent that prolongs the QT interval but does increase TDR is sodium pentobarbital. Indeed, sodium pentobarbital has been shown to produce a dose-dependent prolongation of the QT interval, which is accompanied by a reduction in TDR [39]. TdP is not found to happen under these conditions nor can it be induced with programmed electrical stimulation. Amiodarone and pentobarbital have in common the ability to block I_{Ks}, I_{Kr}, and late I_{Na}. This combination produces a preferential prolongation of the APD of epicardium and endocardium so that the QT interval is prolonged, but TDR is actually reduced and TdP does not develop. Cisapride is another agent that blocks both inward and outward currents. In the canine left ventricular wedge preparation, cisapride produces a biphasic dose-dependent prolongation of the QT interval and TDR. TDR peaks at 0.2 μM, and it is only at this concentration that TdP is observed. Higher concentrations of cisapride lead to an abbreviation of TDR and elimination of TdP, even though QT is further prolonged [113]. This finding suggests that the spatial dispersion of repolarization is more important than the prolongation of the QT interval in determining the substrate for TdP.

Chromanol 293B, a blocker of I_{Ks}, also increases QT without augmenting TDR. Chromanol 293B prolongs APD of the three cell types homogeneously, neither increasing TDR nor widening the T wave. TdP is never observed under these conditions. The addition of β adrenergic agonist, however, abbreviates the APD of epicardial and endocardial cells but not that of the M cell, resulting in a marked accentuation of TDR and the development of TdP [94].

Short-QT syndrome

The short-QT syndrome (SQTS) is characterized by a QTc ≤360 milliseconds and high incidence of VT/VF in infants, children and young adults [116–118]. The first genetic defect responsible for this familial syndrome (*SQTS1*) involved two different missense mutations that resulted in the same amino

acid substitution of lysine for an asparagine in position 588 of *HERG* (*N588K*). The mutation caused a gain of function in the rapidly activating delayed rectifier channel, I_{Kr}[119]. A second gene, reported by Bellocq et al. [120] (*SQTS2*), involved a missense mutation in *KCNQ1* (*KvLQT1*), which caused a gain of function in I_{Ks}. A third gene (*SQTS3*) involved *KCNJ2*, the gene that encodes the inward rectifier channel. Mutations in *KCNJ2* caused a gain of function in I_{K1}, leading to an abbreviation of QT interval. SQT3 is associated with QTc interval of <330 milliseconds, not quite as short as SQT1, and SQT2. Two additional genes recently linked to SQTS encode the α1 (*CACNA1C*) and β (*CACNB2b*) subunits of the L-type cardiac calcium channel. SQT4, caused by mutations in the α subunit of calcium channel, have been shown to lead to the QT interval <360 milliseconds, whereas SQT5 caused by mutations in the β subunit of the calcium channel is characterized by QT intervals of 330–360 milliseconds [61]. Mutations in the α and β subunits of the calcium channel may also lead to ST segment elevation, creating a combined Brugada/ SQTS [61].

In SQT1, 2, and 3, the ECG commonly displays tall peaked symmetrical T waves secondary to acceleration of phase 3 repolarization. An augmented T_{peak}–T_{end} interval is associated with this electrocardiographic feature of the syndrome, suggesting that TDR is significantly increased (Figure 1.7). A left ventricular wedge model of the SQTS developed using the ATP-sensitive potassium channel (I_{K-ATP}) opener, pinacidil, to augment outward repolarizing current also demonstrated an increase in TDR due to a preferential abbreviation of endocardial/M cell action potential duration. The increase in TDR coupled with the abbreviation of QT and refractoriness permitted the development of intramural reentry, giving rise to a rapid polymorphic VT [121]. The increase in TDR was further accentuated by isoproterenol, leading to easier induction and more persistent VT/VF. Of note, an increase in TDR to values greater than 55 milliseconds was associated with inducibility of VT/VF. In LQTS models, a TDR of >90 milliseconds is required to induce TdP. The easier inducibility in SQTS is due to the reduction in the wavelength (refractory period × conduction velocity) of the reentrant circuit, which reduces the pathlength required for maintenance of reentry [121].

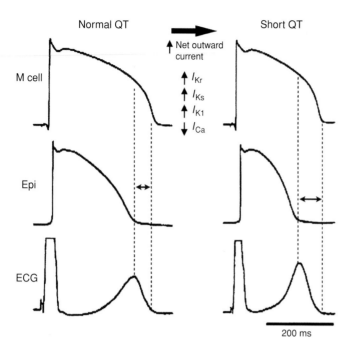

Normal QT

Short QT

M cell

Epi

ECG

↑ Net outward current

↑ I_{Kr}
↑ I_{Ks}
↑ I_{K1}
↓ I_{Ca}

200 ms

Figure 1.7 Proposed mechanism for arrhythmogenesis in the short-QT syndrome. An increase in net outward current due to a reduction in late inward current or augmentation of outward repolarizing current serves to abbreviate action potential duration heterogeneously leading to an amplification of transmural dispersion of repolarization and the creation of a vulnerable window for the development of reentry. Reentry is facilitated both by the increase in TDR and abbreviation of refractoriness.

Intramural reentry secondary to amplification of TDR as a common denominator in channelopathy-induced sudden cardiac death

The three inherited sudden cardiac death syndromes reviewed differ with respect to the characteristics of the QT interval (Figure 1.8). In LQTS, QT increases as a function of disease or drug concentration. In the Brugada syndrome it remains largely unchanged and in the SQTS QT interval decreases as a function of either disease or drug. What these three syndromes have in common is an amplification of TDR, which results in the development of polymorphic VT and fibrillation when dispersion of

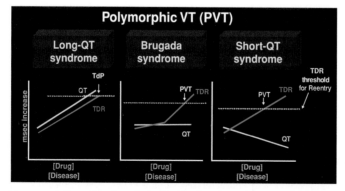

Figure 1.8 The role of transmural dispersion of repolarization (TDR) in channelopathy-induced sudden cardiac death. In the long-QT syndrome, QT increases as a function of disease or drug concentration. In the Brugada syndrome it remains largely unchanged and in the short-QT syndrome QT interval decreases as a function of disease or drug. The three syndromes have in common the ability to amplify TDR, which results in the development of TdP when dispersion reaches the threshold for reentry. The threshold for reentry decreases as APD and refractoriness are reduced. Modified from [129], with permission.

repolarization and refractoriness reaches the threshold for reentry. When polymorphic VT occurs in the setting of long QT, we refer to it as TdP. The threshold for reentry decreases as APD and refractoriness are reduced and the pathlength required for establishing a reentrant wave is progressively reduced.

Conclusion

Amplification of spatial dispersion of refractoriness in ventricular myocardium, particularly when due to augmentation of TDR, can predispose to the development of potentially lethal reentrant arrhythmias in a variety of ion channelopathies including long-QT, short-QT, and Brugada syndromes. These principles apply to arrhythmogenesis associated with both hypertrophic and dilated cardiomyopathies [122–125] as well as some arrhythmias associated with ischemia and reperfusion [126,127].

References

1 Antzelevitch C, Sicouri S, Litovsky SH, et al. Heterogeneity within the ventricular wall. Electrophysiology and pharmacology of epicardial, endocardial, and M cells. Circ Res 1991;69:1427–1449.

2 Antzelevitch C, Shimizu W, Yan GX, et al. The M cell: its contribution to the ECG and to normal and abnormal electrical function of the heart. J Cardiovasc Electrophysiol 1999;10:1124–1152.

3 Litovsky SH, Antzelevitch C. Transient outward current prominent in canine ventricular epicardium but not endocardium. Circ Res 1988;62:116–126.

4 Liu DW, Gintant GA, Antzelevitch C. Ionic bases for electrophysiological distinctions among epicardial, midmyocardial, and endocardial myocytes from the free wall of the canine left ventricle. Circ Res 1993;72:671–687.

5 Furukawa T, Myerburg RJ, Furukawa N, Bassett AL, Kimura S. Differences in transient outward currents of feline endocardial and epicardial myocytes. Circ Res 1990;67:1287–1291.

6 Fedida D, Giles WR. Regional variations in action potentials and transient outward current in myocytes isolated from rabbit left ventricle. J Physiol (Lond) 1991;442:191–209.

7 Clark RB, Bouchard RA, Salinas-Stefanon E, Sanchez-Chapula J, Giles WR. Heterogeneity of action potential waveforms and potassium currents in rat ventricle. Cardiovasc Res 1993;27:1795–1799.

8 Campbell DL, Rasmusson RL, Qu YH, Strauss HC. The calcium-independent transient outward potassium current in isolated ferret right ventricular myocytes. I. Basic characterization and kinetic analysis. J Gen Physiol 1993;101:571–601.

9 Wettwer E, Amos GJ, Posival H, Ravens U. Transient outward current in human ventricular myocytes of subepicardial and subendocardial origin. Circ Res 1994; 75:473–482.

10 Nabauer M, Beuckelmann DJ, Uberfuhr P, Steinbeck G. Regional differences in current density and rate-dependent properties of the transient outward current in subepicardial and subendocardial myocytes of human left ventricle. Circulation 1996;93:168–177.

11 Di Diego JM, Sun ZQ, Antzelevitch C. I_{to} and action potential notch are smaller in left vs. right canine ventricular epicardium. Am J Physiol 1996;271:H548–H561.

12 Volders PG, Sipido KR, Carmeliet E, Spatjens RL, Wellens HJ, Vos MA. Repolarizing K^+ currents ITO1 and IKs are larger in right than left canine ventricular midmyocardium. Circulation 1999;99:206–210.

13 Wang HS, Cohen IS. Calcium channel heterogeneity in canine left ventricular myocytes. J Physiol 2003;547:825–833.

14 Cordeiro JM, Greene L, Heilmann C, Antzelevitch D, Antzelevitch C. Transmural heterogeneity of calcium activity and mechanical function in the canine left ventricle. Am J Physiol Heart Circ Physiol 2004;286: H1471–H1479.

15 Banyasz T, Fulop L, Magyar J, Szentandrassy N, Varro A, Nanasi PP. Endocardial versus epicardial differences in L-type calcium current in canine ventricular myocytes studied by action potential voltage clamp. Cardiovasc Res 2003;58:66–75.

16 Takano M, Noma A. Distribution of the isoprenaline-induced chloride current in rabbit heart. Pflugers Arch 1992;420:223–226.

17 Zygmunt AC. Intracellular calcium activates chloride current in canine ventricular myocytes. Am J Physiol 1994;267:H1984–H1995.

18 Sicouri S, Antzelevitch C. A subpopulation of cells with unique electrophysiological properties in the deep subepicardium of the canine ventricle. The M cell. Circ Res 1991;68:1729–1741.

19 Anyukhovsky EP, Sosunov EA, Gainullin RZ, Rosen MR. The controversial M cell. J Cardiovasc Electrophysiol 1999;10:244–260.

20 Anyukhovsky EP, Sosunov EA, Rosen MR. Regional differences in electrophysiologic properties of epicardium, midmyocardium and endocardium: *In vitro* and *in vivo* correlations. Circulation 1996;94:1981–1988.

21 Antzelevitch C, Dumaine R. Electrical heterogeneity in the heart: physiological, pharmacological and clinical implications. In: Page E, Fozzard HA, Solaro RJ, eds. *Handbook of Physiology. Section 2: The Cardiovascular System*. New York: Oxford University Press; 2001:654–692.

22 Burashnikov A, Antzelevitch C. Differences in the electrophysiologic response of four canine ventricular cell types to a_1-adrenergic agonists. Cardiovasc Res 1999;43:901–908.

23 Yan GX, Shimizu W, Antzelevitch C. Characteristics and distribution of M cells in arterially-perfused

canine left ventricular wedge preparations. Circulation 1998;98:1921–1927.

24 Sicouri S, Antzelevitch C. Electrophysiologic characteristics of M cells in the canine left ventricular free wall. J Cardiovasc Electrophysiol 1995;6:591–603.

25 Sicouri S, Fish J, Antzelevitch C. Distribution of M cells in the canine ventricle. J Cardiovasc Electrophysiol 1994;5:824–837.

26 Antzelevitch C, Sicouri S. Clinical relevance of cardiac arrhythmias generated by afterdepolarizations. Role of M cells in the generation of U waves, triggered activity and torsade de pointes. J Am Coll Cardiol 1994;23:259–277.

27 Stankovicova T, Szilard M, De Scheerder I, Sipido KR. M cells and transmural heterogeneity of action potential configuration in myocytes from the left ventricular wall of the pig heart. Cardiovasc Res 2000;45:952–960.

28 Sicouri S, Antzelevitch C. Drug-induced afterdepolarizations and triggered activity occur in a discrete subpopulation of ventricular muscle cell (M cells) in the canine heart: Quinidine and Digitalis. J Cardiovasc Electrophysiol 1993;4:48–58.

29 Drouin E, Charpentier F, Gauthier C, Laurent K, Le Marec H. Electrophysiological characteristics of cells spanning the left ventricular wall of human heart: evidence for the presence of M cells. J Am Coll Cardiol 1995;26:185–192.

30 Liu DW, Antzelevitch C. Characteristics of the delayed rectifier current (IKr and IKs) in canine ventricular epicardial, midmyocardial, and endocardial myocytes. Circ Res 1995;76:351–365.

31 Weissenburger J, Nesterenko VV, Antzelevitch C. Transmural heterogeneity of ventricular repolarization under baseline and long QT conditions in the canine heart *in vivo*: Torsades de Pointes develops with halothane but not pentobarbital anesthesia. J Cardiovasc Electrophysiol 2000;11:290–304.

32 Sicouri S, Quist M, Antzelevitch C. Evidence for the presence of M cells in the guinea pig ventricle. J Cardiovasc Electrophysiol 1996;7:503–511.

33 Li GR, Feng J, Yue L, Carrier M. Transmural heterogeneity of action potentials and Ito1 in myocytes isolated from the human right ventricle. Am J Physiol 1998;275:H369–H377.

34 Rodriguez-Sinovas A, Cinca J, Tapias A, Armadans L, Tresanchez M, Soler-Soler J. Lack of evidence of M-cells in porcine left ventricular myocardium. Cardiovasc Res 1997;33:307–313.

35 Shimizu W, Antzelevitch C. Sodium channel block with mexiletine is effective in reducing dispersion of repolarization and preventing Torsade de Pointes in LQT2 and LQT3 models of the long-QT syndrome. Circulation 1997;96:2038–2047.

36 El-Sherif N, Caref EB, Yin H, Restivo M. The electrophysiological mechanism of ventricular arrhythmias in the long QT syndrome: tridimensional mapping of activation and recovery patterns. Circ Res 1996;79:474–492.

37 Weirich J, Bernhardt R, Loewen N, Wenzel W, Antoni H. Regional- and species-dependent effects of K^+-channel blocking agents on subendocardium and mid-wall slices of human, rabbit, and guinea pig myocardium [Abstract]. Pflugers Arch 1996;431:R 130.

38 Burashnikov A, Antzelevitch C. Acceleration-induced action potential prolongation and early afterdepolarizations. J Cardiovasc Electrophysiol 1998;9:934–948.

39 Shimizu W, McMahon B, Antzelevitch C. Sodium pentobarbital reduces transmural dispersion of repolarization and prevents torsade de pointes in models of acquired and congenital long QT syndrome. J Cardiovasc Electrophysiol 1999;10:156–164.

40 Shimizu W, Antzelevitch C. Cellular basis for the ECG features of the LQT1 form of the long QT syndrome: effects of b-adrenergic agonists and antagonists and sodium channel blockers on transmural dispersion of repolarization and Torsade de Pointes. Circulation 1998;98:2314–2322.

41 Shimizu W, Antzelevitch C. Cellular and ionic basis for T-wave alternans under Long QT conditions. Circulation 1999;99:1499–1507.

42 Balati B, Varro A, Papp JG. Comparison of the cellular electrophysiological characteristics of canine left ventricular epicardium, M cells, endocardium and Purkinje fibres. Acta Physiol Scand 1998;164:181–190.

43 McIntosh MA, Cobbe SM, Smith GL. Heterogeneous changes in action potential and intracellular Ca^{2+} in left ventricular myocyte sub-types from rabbits with heart failure. Cardiovasc Res 2000;45:397–409.

44 Yan GX, Antzelevitch C. Cellular basis for the normal T wave and the electrocardiographic manifestations of the long QT syndrome. Circulation 1998;98:1928–1936.

45 Poelzing S, Akar FG, Baron E, Rosenbaum DS. Heterogeneous connexin43 expression produces electrophysiological heterogeneities across ventricular wall. Am J Physiol Heart Circ Physiol 2004;286:H2001–H2009.

46 Yamada KA, Kanter EM, Green KG, Saffitz JE. Transmural distribution of connexins in rodent hearts. J Cardiovasc Electrophysiol 2004;15:710–715.

47 LeGrice IJ, Smaill BH, Chai LZ, Edgar SG, Gavin JB, Hunter PJ. Laminar structure of the heart 1: cellular organization and connective tissue architecture in ventricular myocardium. Am J Physiol 1996;269:H571–H582.

48 Viswanathan PC, Rudy Y. Cellular arrhythmogenic effects of the congenital and acquired long QT syndrome in the heterogeneous myocardium. Circulation 2000;101:1192–1198.

49 Zygmunt AC, Eddlestone GT, Thomas GP, Nesterenko VV, Antzelevitch C. Larger late sodium conductance in M cells contributes to electrical heterogeneity in canine ventricle. Am J Physiol 2001;281:H689–H697.

50 Zygmunt AC, Goodrow RJ, Antzelevitch C. I(NaCa) contributes to electrical heterogeneity within the canine ventricle. Am J Physiol Heart Circ Physiol 2000;278:H1671–H1678.

51 Brahmajothi MV, Morales MJ, Reimer KA, Strauss HC. Regional localization of ERG, the channel protein

responsible for the rapid component of the delayed rectifier, K$^+$ current in the ferret heart. Circ Res 1997;81:128–
135.

52 Antzelevitch C. Brugada syndrome. PACE 2006;29:
1130–1159.

53 Brugada P, Brugada J. Right bundle branch block, persistent ST segment elevation and sudden cardiac death:
a distinct clinical and electrocardiographic syndrome:
a multicenter report. J Am Coll Cardiol 1992;20:1391–
1396.

54 Brugada R, Brugada J, Antzelevitch C, et al. Sodium
channel blockers identify risk for sudden death in
patients with ST-segment elevation and right bundle
branch block but structurally normal hearts. Circulation 2000;101:510–515.

55 Shimizu W, Antzelevitch C, Suyama K, et al. Effect of
sodium channel blockers on ST segment, QRS duration,
and corrected QT interval in patients with Brugada syndrome. J Cardiovasc Electrophysiol 2000;11:1320–1329.

56 Priori SG, Napolitano C, Gasparini M, et al. Clinical and
genetic heterogeneity of right bundle branch block and
ST-segment elevation syndrome: a prospective evaluation of 52 families. Circulation 2000;102:2509–2515.

57 Chen Q, Kirsch GE, Zhang D, et al. Genetic basis and
molecular mechanisms for idiopathic ventricular fibrillation. Nature 1998;392:293–296.

58 Antzelevitch C, Brugada P, Brugada J, Brugada R. *The
Brugada Syndrome: From Bench to Bedside*. Oxford:
Blackwell Futura; 2005.

59 Weiss R, Barmada MM, Nguyen T, et al. Clinical
and molecular heterogeneity in the Brugada syndrome.
A novel gene locus on chromosome 3. Circulation
2002;105:707–713.

60 London B, Sanyal S, Michalec M, et al. AB16-1: a mutation in the glycerol-3-phosphate dehydrogenase 1-like
gene (GPD1L) causes Brugada syndrome [Abstract].
Heart Rhythm 2006;3:S32.

61 Antzelevitch C, Pollevick GD, Cordeiro JM, et al. Loss-
of-function mutations in the cardiac calcium channel underlie a new clinical entity characterized by
ST-segment elevation, short QT intervals, and sudden
cardiac death. Circulation 2007;115:442–449.

62 Yan GX, Antzelevitch C. Cellular basis for the Brugada
syndrome and other mechanisms of arrhythmogenesis associated with ST segment elevation. Circulation
1999;100:1660–1666.

63 Fish JM, Antzelevitch C. Role of sodium and calcium
channel block in unmasking the Brugada syndrome.
Heart Rhythm 2004;1:210–217.

64 Di Diego JM, Cordeiro JM, Goodrow RJ, et al. Ionic and
cellular basis for the predominance of the Brugada syndrome phenotype in males. Circulation 2002;106:2004–
2011.

65 Aiba T, Hidaka I, Shimizu W, et al. Steep repolarization
gradient is required for development of phase 2 reentry
and subsequent ventricular tachyarrhythmias in a model
of the Brugada syndrome: high-resolution optical mapping study [Abstract]. Circulation 2004;110:III-318.

66 Morita H, Zipes DP, Morita ST, Wu J. Temperature modulation of ventricular arrhythmogenicity in a canine
tissue model of Brugada syndrome. Heart Rhythm
2007;4:188–197.

67 Antzelevitch C. The Brugada syndrome: ionic basis and
arrhythmia mechanisms. J Cardiovasc Electrophysiol
2001;12:268–272.

68 Lukas A, Antzelevitch C. Phase 2 reentry as a mechanism
of initiation of circus movement reentry in canine epicardium exposed to simulated ischemia. Cardiovasc Res
1996;32:593–603.

69 Aiba T, Shimizu W, Hidaka I, et al. Cellular basis for
trigger and maintenance of ventricular fibrillation in the
Brugada syndrome model: high-resolution optical mapping study. J Am Coll Cardiol 2006;47:2074–2085.

70 Morita H, Zipes DP, Lopshire J, Morita ST, Wu J. T
wave alternans in an in vitro canine tissue model of
Brugada syndrome. Am J Physiol Heart Circ Physiol
2006;291:H421–H428.

71 Antzelevitch C, Brugada P, Brugada J, et al. Brugada syndrome. A decade of progress. Circ Res 2002;91:1114–
1119.

72 Kurita T, Shimizu W, Inagaki M, et al. The electrophysiologic mechanism of ST-segment elevation in Brugada
syndrome. J Am Coll Cardiol 2002;40:330–334.

73 Schwartz PJ. The idiopathic long QT syndrome: progress
and questions. Am Heart J 1985;109:399–411.

74 Moss AJ, Schwartz PJ, Crampton RS, et al. The long QT
syndrome: prospective longitudinal study of 328 families. Circulation 1991;84:1136–1144.

75 Zipes DP. The long QT interval syndrome: a Rosetta
stone for sympathetic related ventricular tachyarrhythmias. Circulation 1991;84:1414–1419.

76 Wang Q, Shen J, Splawski I, et al. *SCN5A* mutations
associated with an inherited cardiac arrhythmia, long
QT syndrome. Cell 1995;80:805–811.

77 Mohler PJ, Schott JJ, Gramolini AO, et al. Ankyrin-B
mutation causes type 4 long-QT cardiac arrhythmia and
sudden cardiac death. Nature 2003;421:634–639.

78 Plaster NM, Tawil R, Tristani-Firouzi M, et al. Mutations
in Kir2.1 cause the developmental and episodic electrical
phenotypes of Andersen's syndrome. Cell 2001;105:511–
519.

79 Curran ME, Splawski I, Timothy KW, Vincent GM,
Green ED, Keating MT. A molecular basis for cardiac
arrhythmia: *HERG* mutations cause long QT syndrome.
Cell 1995;80:795–803.

80 Wang Q, Curran ME, Splawski I, et al. Positional cloning
of a novel potassium channel gene: *KVLQT1* mutations
cause cardiac arrhythmias. Nat Genet 1996;12:17–23.

81 Splawski I, Tristani-Firouzi M, Lehmann MH, Sanguinetti MC, Keating MT. Mutations in the hminK gene
cause long QT syndrome and suppress I$_{Ks}$ function. Nat
Genet 1997;17:338–340.

82 Vatta M, Ackerman MJ, Ye B, et al. Mutant caveolin-3
induces persistent late sodium current and Is associated
with long-QT syndrome. Circulation 2006;114:2104–
2112.

83 Domingo AM, Kaku T, Tester DJ, et al. AB16-6: sodium channel β4 subunit mutation causes congenital long QT syndrome [Abstract]. Heart Rhythm 2006;3:S34.

84 Bednar MM, Harrigan EP, Anziano RJ, Camm AJ, Ruskin JN. The QT interval. Prog Cardiovasc Dis 2001;43:1–45.

85 Tomaselli GF, Marban E. Electrophysiological remodeling in hypertrophy and heart failure. Cardiovasc Res 1999;42:270–283.

86 Sipido KR, Volders PG, De Groot SH, et al. Enhanced Ca(2+) release and Na/Ca exchange activity in hypertrophied canine ventricular myocytes: potential link between contractile adaptation and arrhythmogenesis. Circulation 2000;102:2137–2144.

87 Volders PG, Sipido KR, Vos MA, et al. Downregulation of delayed rectifier K(+) currents in dogs with chronic complete atrioventricular block and acquired torsades de pointes. Circulation 1999;100:2455–2461.

88 Undrovinas AI, Maltsev VA, Sabbah HN. Repolarization abnormalities in cardiomyocytes of dogs with chronic heart failure: role of sustained inward current. Cell Mol Life Sci 1999;55:494–505.

89 Maltsev VA, Sabbah HN, Higgins RS, Silverman N, Lesch M, Undrovinas AI. Novel, ultraslow inactivating sodium current in human ventricular cardiomyocytes. Circulation 1998;98:2545–2552.

90 Roden DM. Long QT syndrome: reduced repolarization reserve and the genetic link. J Intern Med 2006;259:59–69.

91 Belardinelli L, Antzelevitch C, Vos MA. Assessing predictors of drug-induced Torsade de Pointes. Trends Pharmacol Sci 2003;24:619–625.

92 Antzelevitch C, Shimizu W. Cellular mechanisms underlying the long QT syndrome. Curr Opin Cardiol 2002;17:43–51.

93 Shimizu W, Antzelevitch C. Effects of a K(+) channel opener to reduce transmural dispersion of repolarization and prevent Torsade de Pointes in LQT1, LQT2, and LQT3 models of the long-QT syndrome. Circulation 2000;102:706–712.

94 Shimizu W, Antzelevitch C. Differential effects of beta-adrenergic agonists and antagonists in LQT1, LQT2 and LQT3 models of the long QT syndrome. J Am Coll Cardiol 2000;35:778–786.

95 Ueda N, Zipes DP, Wu J. Prior ischemia enhances arrhythmogenicity in isolated canine ventricular wedge model of long QT 3. Cardiovasc Res 2004;63:69–76.

96 Ueda N, Zipes DP, Wu J. Functional and transmural modulation of M cell behavior in canine ventricular wall. Am J Physiol Heart Circ Physiol 2004;287:H2569–H2575.

97 Akar FG, Yan GX, Antzelevitch C, Rosenbaum DS. Unique topographical distribution of M cells underlies reentrant mechanism of torsade de pointes in the long-QT syndrome. Circulation 2002;105:1247–1253.

98 Emori T, Antzelevitch C. Cellular basis for complex T waves and arrhythmic activity following combined I(Kr) and I(Ks) block. J Cardiovasc Electrophysiol 2001;12:1369–1378.

99 Opthof T, Coronel R, Wilms-Schopman FJ, et al. Dispersion of repolarization in canine ventricle and the electrocardiographic T wave: T(p–e) interval does not reflect transmural dispersion. Heart Rhythm 2007;4:341–348.

100 Yuan S, Kongstad O, Hertervig E, Holm M, Grins E, Olsson B. Global repolarization sequence of the ventricular endocardium: monophasic action potential mapping in swine and humans. PACE 2001;24:1479–1488.

101 Yamaguchi M, Shimizu M, Ino H, et al. T wave peak-to-end interval and QT dispersion in acquired long QT syndrome: a new index for arrhythmogenicity. Clin Sci (Lond) 2003;105:671–676.

102 Castro HJ, Antzelevitch C, Tornes BF, et al. Tpeak-Tend and Tpeak-Tend dispersion as risk factors for ventricular tachycardia/ventricular fibrillation in patients with the Brugada syndrome. J Am Coll Cardiol 2006;47:1828–1834.

103 Wolk R, Stec S, Kulakowski P. Extrasystolic beats affect transmural electrical dispersion during programmed electrical stimulation. Eur J Clin Invest 2001;31:293–301.

104 Tanabe Y, Inagaki M, Kurita T, et al. Sympathetic stimulation produces a greater increase in both transmural and spatial dispersion of repolarization in LQT1 than LQT2 forms of congenital long QT syndrome. J Am Coll Cardiol 2001;37:911–919.

105 Frederiks J, Swenne CA, Kors JA, et al. Within-subject electrocardiographic differences at equal heart rates: role of the autonomic nervous system. Pflugers Arch 2001;441:717–724.

106 Shimizu M, Ino H, Okeie K, et al. T-peak to T-end interval may be a better predictor of high-risk patients with hypertrophic cardiomyopathy associated with a cardiac troponin I mutation than QT dispersion. Clin Cardiol 2002;25:335–339.

107 Takenaka K, Ai T, Shimizu W, et al. Exercise stress test amplifies genotype-phenotype correlation in the LQT1 and LQT2 forms of the long-QT syndrome. Circulation 2003;107:838–844.

108 Watanabe N, Kobayashi Y, Tanno K, et al. Transmural dispersion of repolarization and ventricular tachyarrhythmias. J Electrocardiol 2004;37:191–200.

109 Schwartz PJ, Priori SG, Spazzolini C, et al. Genotype-phenotype correlation in the long-QT syndrome: gene-specific triggers for life-threatening arrhythmias. Circulation 2001;103:89–95.

110 Antzelevitch C, Belardinelli L, Zygmunt AC, et al. Electrophysiologic effects of ranolazine: a novel antianginal agent with antiarrhythmic properties. Circulation 2004;110:904–910.

111 Antzelevitch C. Drug-induced channelopathies. In: Zipes DP, Jalife J, eds. *Cardiac Electrophysiology. From Cell to Bedside*, 4th ed. New York: WB Saunders; 2004:151–157.

112 Fenichel RR, Malik M, Antzelevitch C, et al. Drug-induced torsade de pointes and implications for drug development. J Cardiovasc Electrophysiol 2004;15:475–495.

113 Di Diego JM, Belardinelli L, Antzelevitch C. Cisapride-induced transmural dispersion of repolarization and torsade de pointes in the canine left ventricular wedge preparation during epicardial stimulation. Circulation 2003;108:1027–1033.

114 Sicouri S, Moro S, Litovsky SH, Elizari MV, Antzelevitch C. Chronic amiodarone reduces transmural dispersion of repolarization in the canine heart. J Cardiovasc Electrophysiol 1997;8:1269–1279.

115 van Opstal JM, Schoenmakers M, Verduyn SC, et al. Chronic Amiodarone evokes no Torsade de Pointes arrhythmias despite QT lengthening in an animal model of acquired long-QT syndrome. Circulation 2001;104:2722–2727.

116 Gussak I, Brugada P, Brugada J, et al. Idiopathic short QT interval: a new clinical syndrome? Cardiology 2000;94:99–102.

117 Gussak I, Brugada P, Brugada J, Antzelevitch C, Osbakken M, Bjerregaard P. ECG phenomenon of idiopathic and paradoxical short QT intervals. Cardiac Electrophysiol Rev 2002;6:49–53.

118 Gaita F, Giustetto C, Bianchi F, et al. Short QT syndrome: a familial cause of sudden death. Circulation 2003;108:965–970.

119 Brugada R, Hong K, Dumaine R, et al. Sudden death associated with short QT-syndrome linked to mutations in HERG. Circulation 2003;109:30–35 .

120 Bellocq C, Van Ginneken AC, Bezzina CR, et al. Mutation in the KCNQ1 gene leading to the short QT-interval syndrome. Circulation 2004;109:2394–2397.

121 Extramiana F, Antzelevitch C. Amplified transmural dispersion of repolarization as the basis for arrhythmogenesis in a canine ventricular-wedge model of short-QT syndrome. Circulation 2004;110:3661–3666.

122 Akar FG, Rosenbaum DS. Transmural electrophysiological heterogeneities underlying arrhythmogenesis in heart failure. Circ Res 2003;93:638–645.

123 Akar FG, Tomaselli GF. Conduction abnormalities in nonischemic dilated cardiomyopathy: basic mechanisms and arrhythmic consequences. Trends Cardiovasc Med 2005;15:259–264.

124 Vos MA, Jungschleger JG. Transmural repolarization gradients in vivo: the flukes and falls of the endocardium. Cardiovasc Res 2001;50:423–425.

125 van Opstal JM, Verduyn SC, Leunissen HD, De Groot SH, Wellens HJ, Vos MA. Electrophysiological parameters indicative of sudden cardiac death in the dog with chronic complete AV-block. Cardiovasc Res 2001;50: 354–361.

126 Yan GX, Joshi A, Guo D, et al. Phase 2 reentry as a trigger to initiate ventricular fibrillation during early acute myocardial ischemia. Circulation 2004;110:1036–1041.

127 Di Diego JM, Antzelevitch C. Cellular basis for ST-segment changes observed during ischemia. J Electrocardiol 2003;36(Suppl):1–5.

128 Antzelevitch C. The Brugada syndrome: diagnostic criteria and cellular mechanisms. Eur Heart J 2001;22:356–363.

129 Antzelevitch C, Oliva A. Amplification of spatial dispersion of repolarization underlies sudden cardiac death associated with catecholaminergic polymorphic VT, long QT, short QT and Brugada syndromes. J Intern Med 2006;259:48–58.

CHAPTER 2

Mechanisms of ventricular tachycardia: underlying pathological and physiological abnormalities

Jacques MT de Bakker, & Harold VM van Rijen

Introduction

Cardiac excitation is mediated by interplay between various voltage- and time-dependent depolarizing and repolarizing membrane currents of heart cells and their electrical coupling. In cells of the working myocardium, the initial rapid depolarization is initiated by the voltage-gated sodium channel, which generates an inward current. In most cells, the upstroke is followed by an early repolarization phase, caused by an outward potassium current called I_{TO}. This early repolarization indirectly affects the action potential duration, because it controls the subsequent course of other voltage-gated conductances. The following plateau phase depends on a delicate balance between inward and outward currents of which the inward current is supported by the L-type calcium current. Several voltage-gated potassium channels that are active over different time frames contribute to the repolarization of the cardiac cells. Several other ion and exchanger channels maintain or modulate the resting membrane potential and action potential.

Considerable differences in the morphology of the action potentials are present in various areas of the heart and are caused by different expression levels of ion channels. In addition, the electrophysiologic substrate is changed by age, neurohormonal influences and, disease. Thus, physiological and pathophysiological abnormalities may affect the balance between the inward and outward currents and/or change the coupling between the cells—alterations that may finally result in tachycardias.

Mechanisms of tachycardia

The mechanisms of cardiac tachycardias are traditionally divided into those based on abnormalities of impulse generation and those based on abnormal impulse conduction (Table 2.1).

Automaticity

Abnormal impulse generation arises from changes in the balance between depolarizing and repolarizing membrane currents and may be expressed as automaticity or triggered activity. Automaticity is caused by a slow rise in the membrane potential during diastole and is a normal property of cells of the sinus and A-V node and the His–Purkinje system. Usually the frequency of subsidiary pacemakers, which have the capability for normal automaticity, is lower than that of the sinus node—the reason that they are usually suppressed. In addition, tight electrical coupling with surrounding quiescent cells may clamp the membrane potential of subsidiary pacemaker cells to a low value,

Ventricular Arrhythmias and Sudden Cardiac Death, 1st edition. Edited by P.J. Wang, A. Al-Ahmad, H. Hsia, and P.C. Zei © 2008 Blackwell Publishing, ISBN: 978-1-4051-6114-5.

Table 2.1 Mechanisms of cardiac arrhythmias

Abnormal impulse initiation

Automaticity
– Normal
– Abnormal

Triggered activity
– Early afterdepolarization
– Delayed afterdepolarization

Abnormal impulse conduction
– slowing of conduction
– unidirectional conduction block
– heterogeneity in conduction and refractoriness
– electrotonic coupling

---

preventing their manifestation. If, however, cell-to-cell coupling is reduced due to increased interstitial collagen deposition or reduced connexin expression, subsidiary pacemakers may reveal their occurrence. Other factors, such as sympathetic nerve activation, make the slope of diastolic depolarization of most pacemaker cells steeper and diminish the inhibitory effects of overdrive. Thus, sympathetic activation may enhance subsidiary pacemaker activity by enhancing Phase 4 depolarization and overrule sinus node activity. Ventricular and atrial cells from the working myocardium usually do not show spontaneous diastolic depolarization. If their resting membrane potential is so markedly reduced as to be less than -60 mV, however, spontaneous diastolic depolarization may arise and cause repetitive impulse initiation [1].

It is likely that at least some of the ionic currents causing abnormal automatic activity are different from those causing normal automaticity. Action potentials resulting from abnormal automaticity are mediated by slow inward calcium currents and deactivation of potassium currents [2]. Abnormal automaticity has been shown to arise in Purkinje fibers that survive on the subendocardium and cause ventricular tachycardia [3]. Abnormal automaticity has also been observed in diseased atrial and ventricular myocardium from human hearts. In these cases, the reduced membrane potential was most likely caused by electrotonic interaction with nonexcitable "ghost" cells that were still coupled to surrounding myocardial cells [4].

Triggered activity

Triggered activity is impulse generation caused by afterdepolarization. This is a second depolarization that occurs either during repolarization (early after depolarization, EAD) or following repolarization (delayed afterdepolarization, DAD).

Early afterdepolarization

EADs occur during normal repolarization of the action potential that has been initiated from a high level of membrane potential (-70 to -90 mV). An EAD may occur when the balance between inward and outward current is altered in favor of the inward current. Such a shift might be caused by factors that either decrease the outward current carried by K^+ channels or increase the inward current carried by Na^+ and Ca^{2+} channels. EADs preferentially occur when the rate is markedly slowed, reducing the outward current generated by the delayed rectifier K^+ current and the Na/K pump, especially when K^+ in the extracellular environment is lower than normal which also reduces the outward current [5]. EADs occur more readily in Purkinje than in ventricular myocardium. However, midmyocardial (M) cells are prone to the development of EADs as well, because of their prolonged action potential duration, and therefore may be important for triggered activity under various conditions [6]. Gene mutations on depolarizing or repolarizing membrane currents too may cause EADs and trigger polymorphic ventricular tachycardia [7]. Either a late sodium current or decreased outward potassium current may cause increased action potential duration. Both result in a net decrease in outward current that prolongs action potential duration.

Such changes may also arise under pathologic conditions, which may cause changes either in the biophysical characteristics of the ion channels or in ion channel protein synthesis. In the hypertrophied noninfarcted ventricular muscle of hearts with healed myocardial infarction prolongation of action potential duration (APD) has been found to be associated with a reduced transient outward current (I_{To}) [8]. A slowed heart rate favors the occurrence of EADs by reducing the outward current generated by the delayed rectifier K^+ current and the Na^+/K^+ pump, especially if the extracellular potassium concentration is reduced.

In addition, drugs may induce EADs and Torsade de pointes. Class III antiarrhythmic drugs prolong the time course for repolarization by reducing the delayed rectifier K^+ current and increasing the likelihood for EADs. However, sodium channel-blocking drugs may also increase repolarization time, thereby promoting the occurrence of EADs.

Delayed afterdepolarization

DADs are transient or oscillatory depolarizations that occur after repolarization of an action potential and that are induced by that action potential. They may be sub-threshold, but if they are large enough, they may generate a full action potential. DADs occur under conditions that there is an increase in Ca^{2+} in the myoplasm and the sarcoplasmic reticulum (calcium overload) [9]. A high level of intracellular Ca^{2+} or the presence of catecholamines or cAMP will enhance the uptake of calcium by the SR. The calcium uptake in the SR may rise during repolarization to a critical level at which a second spontaneous release of Ca^{2+} from the SR occurs after the action potential. This secondary release of calcium generates a transient inward current resulting in the DAD. DADs can also be caused by cardiac glycosides. They inhibit the Na^+/K^+ pump, which leads to an increase in intracellular Na^+. The increased Na^+ is extruded in exchange for Ca^{2+}, which finally results into an increase in intracellular Ca^{2+}.

DADs may also be associated with cardiac pathology. They have been observed in hypertrophic ventricular myocardium and in Purkinje fibers surviving at the subendocardial surface of canine infarcts. In some instances the membrane potentials of the myocardial cells were low and caused by the underlying disease. Heart failure has been shown to result in calcium overload and thus is a candidate for the initiation of DADs. DADs are influenced by action potential duration, longer durations favoring the occurrence of DADs. More calcium can enter the cell at longer action potentials. Stimulus rate has a profound effect on afterdepolarization amplitude. If DADs do not reach threshold, triggered activity does not occur. In fibers showing subthreshold afterdepolarizations, triggering may result if the rate at which the fiber is driven increases; the amplitude of the afterdepolarization increases. This may also occur after a premature stimulus. The increase in amplitude of DADs with increasing drive rate is most likely responsible for perpetuation of triggered activity.

Reentrant excitation

In the healthy heart, the electrical impulse dies out after complete activation of the myocardium because it is surrounded by refractory tissue that it has excited before. Under special conditions, the propagating impulse will not die out completely but excite the myocardium that has recovered from refractoriness. In that case activation would revolve around a zone of conduction block, which can be anatomically or functionally determined. Most evident is reentry, which may arise in patients with the Wolff Parkinson White (WPW) syndrome and where activation revolves around the atrioventricular groove via the atrium, the A-V node, the ventricle and the aberrant connection between the atrium and the ventricle. In this case the atrioventricular groove is the area of conduction block. For reentry to occur, the length of the circuit must be such that after one rotation of the activation front, the tissue ahead is excitable again. This implies that the wavelength, which is the product of conduction velocity and refractory period, must be less than the length of the reentrant circuit. It is evident that a short refractory period and a low conduction velocity will favor reentry.

Excitability and cell-to-cell coupling determine conduction velocity in myocardial tissue. Excitability is mediated by the sodium channel; a reduced sodium channel availability or changes in the biophysical characteristics of the channel may reduce conduction velocity. Altered sodium channel availability has been shown to occur in certain genetic channelopathies such as the Brugada syndrome, but has also been observed in heart failure and at the border zone of infarcted myocardium (Figure 2.1) [10]. Pharmacologically, Class I drugs reduce the sodium conductance. Earlier, these drugs were used to combat arrhythmias but results of the CAST (Cardiac Arrhythmia Suppression Trial) study have shown that these drugs are proarrhythmic [11]. CAST tested the hypothesis that suppression of ventricular ectopy by flecainide, encainide, and moricizine after a myocardial infarction would reduce the incidence of sudden death. The trial was discontinued because flecainide and encainide revealed a statistically higher incidence of death

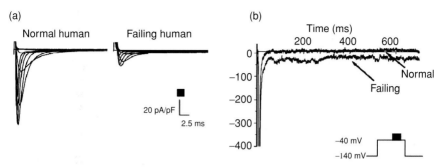

Figure 2.1 Reduced maximal sodium current (Panel a) and increased late sodium current (Panel b) in ventricular cardiomyocytes derived from a failing and a normal human heart. Adapted from Valdivia C *et al.*, J Mol Cell Cardiol, 2002.

or cardiac arrest compared to the placebo group. A short wavelength predisposing for reentrant arrhythmias also implies that a short refractory period promotes reentry. Shortening of action potential duration (and refractoriness) arises during acute ischemia where the extracellular potassium concentration increases because of leakage of potassium out of the cell. The increased extracellular potassium concentration shortens action potential duration and reduces the upstroke of the action potential because of the reduced membrane potential. Conduction of the electrical impulse not only depends on the sodium channel but also on cell-to-cell coupling. This is mediated by gap junction channel proteins, mainly connexin43 in the working myocardium of the ventricle. Not only the amount of connexins but also their distribution plays a crucial role in impulse propagation. In the normal myocardium more connexins are available for longitudinal than for transverse conduction. This together with the fact that myocardial cells are brick-like structures and longer than thick, results in a lower conduction velocity perpendicular to the fiber direction as compared to propagation in the fiber direction. The extracellular matrix, which is meant to give the heart its rigidity and mechanical integrity, too plays an important role in the electrical coupling between myocytes [12]. In the normal myocardium the matrix consists of thin collagen fibers, leaving enough room for gap-junctional side-to-side connection between the cells. Under hypertrophic conditions, however, the balance between collagen synthesis and degradation is disturbed and the amount of interstitial collagen increases, thereby separating the myocardial cells and reducing side-to-side electrical connections (Figure 2.2) [13]. This may have profound effect on the conduction of

the electrical impulse and increase vulnerability for reentry.

The presence of circuits fulfilling the requirements for reentry does not imply that reentry indeed occurs. For reentry to start, unidirectional conduction block—block of conduction in one direction of the reentrant circuit—must be present. Unidirectional conduction block may occur in several ways. One cause of unidirectional block that enables the initiation of reentry is a regional difference in recovery of excitability (see Dispersion of repolarization). Secondly, asymmetrical depression of excitability may result in unidirectional conduction block. This may occur when there is a gradient in high K^+ due to ischemia. An important factor for unidirectional block in infarcted myocardium is based on geometrical factors. The cause of unidirectional block in these cases is due to a mismatch between current supply and current demand at tissue discontinuities, sites where large and small bundles merge (Figure 2.3).

Dispersion of repolarization and conduction

An important cause of unidirectional conduction block that enables initiation of reentry is the regional difference in recovery of excitability. When differences in the refractory period exist in adjacent areas, conduction of a premature impulse may be blocked in the region with the longest refractory period, while continuing in regions with short refractory periods. Continuation of reentry induced by a premature impulse is facilitated because the premature action potential shortens refractory period. Under normal conditions, the differences between longest and shortest refractory period duration in

(a)   Normal

(b)   Hypertensive

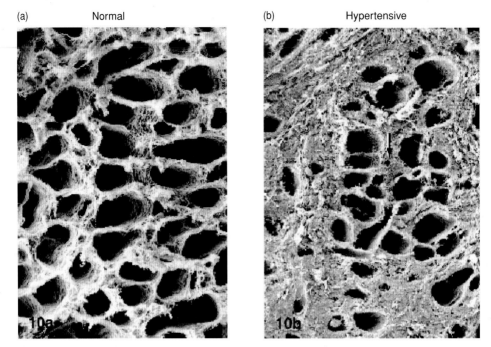

Figure 2.2 Extracellular matrix of a human papillary muscle. (a) normal heart, (b) hypertrophic heart. Adapted from Icardo JM *et al.*, Anat Rec, 1998.

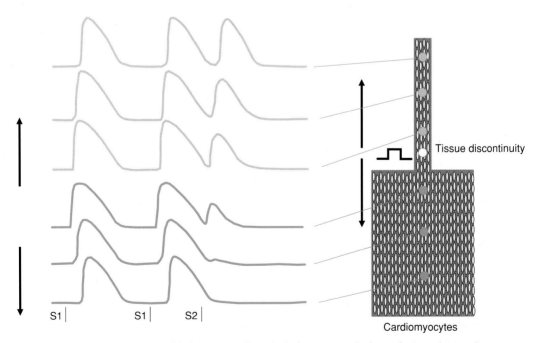

Figure 2.3 Unidirectional conduction block at a tissue discontinuity in a patterned culture of neonatal rat cardiomyocytes. The preparation was stimulated (marker) near the discontinuity. Activation provoked by the premature stimulus S2 only conducts toward the narrow channel. Tracings are action potentials recorded at the sites indicated.

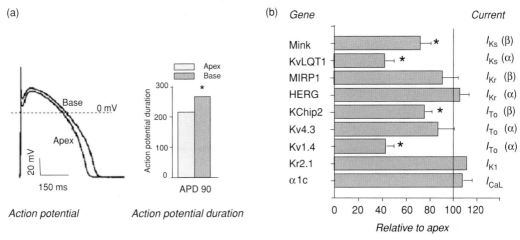

Figure 2.4 Base-to-apex gradient in action potential duration (Panels a) and related differences in ion channel expression (Panel b). Significant differences are indicated by asterisks. Adapted from Szentadrassya N et al., Cardiovasc Res, 2005.

the ventricles is in the order of 40 milliseconds. The intrinsic electrical heterogeneities in ventricular myocardium are responsible for the dispersion in repolarization. Both transmural and apico-basal gradients have been observed in the heart. The transmural gradient arises because of the different cell types involved; epicardial, midmyocardial, and endocardial myocytes reveal differences in the expression of the various potassium currents [14]. In addition, the effect of drugs on the various cell types differs, making M-cells more vulnerable to EAD-induced triggered activity.

The apico-basal inhomogeneity in distribution of ion channels has had less attention, but probably plays an equal or even more important role in arrhythmogenicity. Several studies in the mouse, dog, and human heart show that the action potential duration at the base is longer as compared to the apex. This has been confirmed in both—the intact heart and in isolated cardiomyocytes. The study of Szentadrassy et al. [15] showed that in basal cells Kv 1.4 (encoding the α-subunit of the ion channel for I_{TO}) and KvLQT1 (encoding the α-subunit for the ion channel for I_{KS}) are expressed to only 40% of the amount expressed in apical cells (Figure 2.4). London and co-workers [16] showed that in double transgenic mice that lack both the fast and slow component of the transient outward current have action potential prolongation and spontaneous ventricular arrhythmias. Conduction

velocity was similar to controls, but action potential duration was prolonged and dispersion of refractoriness between apex and base was enhanced compared to controls. A single premature pulse elicited a reentrant ventricular tachycardia. Burst pacing elicited VTs with alternating frequencies.

Although prolongation of APDs and refractory periods has been suggested to be antiarrhythmogenic, it has been shown to cause afterdepolarizations that may deteriorate into Torsades de pointes (TdP) [17]. In the I_{TO} knockout mice, reentrant arrhythmias were induced due to enhanced dispersion of repolarization. The role of APD heterogeneities as a substrate for unidirectional block and reentry has been supported by simulation studies by Viswanathan and Rudy [18].

Acquired ventricular arrhythmias

Action potential prolongation is often found in hypertrophic and failing hearts. Two mechanisms are most likely involved in this change in APD: a downregulation of potassium current and alteration in intracellular calcium handling. Downregulation of each of the major repolarizing K^+ currents has been reported [19]. The impact of changes in the various K^+ currents depends on the etiology of heart failure. Computer simulations show that a reduced I_{TO} impairs action potential duration rate adaptation, which may result in enhanced spatial

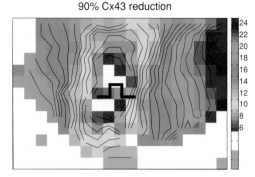

Figure 2.5 Effect of a 90% reduction of Cx43 expression (right panel) on epicardial activation of the right ventricle in a Langendorff perfused mouse heart. Crowding of isochronal lines indicates reduced conduction velocity. Numbers are in millisecond and indicate areas that are activated within the same time interval.

differences in APD [20]. Ventricular myocytes from failing human hearts show reduced I_{K1} density, which may enhance automaticity in the failing cells. Minor changes (pharmacologic agents) in depolarizing current during the plateau phase of the action potential may change the balance between inward and outward current in favor of the first and cause secondary depolarizations. Cells from failing human hearts show only a slight decrease in the L-type calcium current, but increased Na/Ca exchanger current density has been reported [21]. The increased exchanger activity was associated with increased incidence of DADs. In hypertrophic and dilated hearts, altered density and distribution of gap junction channel proteins have been observed [22]. In the infarct border zone and in surviving myocytes within the infarct area, Cx43 expression has been shown to be disrupted. A poor cell-to-cell coupling may contribute to regional inhomogeneities in APD, predispose to local activation block and reentry. Reduction of sodium current density has been observed in chronic infarcts and this reduction in sodium current expression may also contribute to slowing of conduction in the diseased heart.

Ventricular tachycardia in chronic cardiac disease

Cardiac disease is associated with structural and electrical remodeling of the myocardium. Structural remodeling involves increased interstitial collagen deposition, replacement fibrosis, changes in cell size, and myocyte disarray—factors that may affect the electrophysiological integrity of the myocardium. Electrical remodeling involves changes in gap junction and ion channel expression. In the healthy myocardium there is an abundance of connexins and sodium channels, which means that the heart has conduction reserve. Studies carried out in conditional Cx43 knockout mice have shown that a 50% reduction in Cx43 expression hardly affects conduction velocity (Figure 2.5) [23]. The reduction must be > 90% to obtain a 20% reduction in conduction velocity. A 50% reduction in sodium channel expression too reduces conduction velocity by approximately 20% [24]. One should realize, however, that several parameters are altered during a cardiac disease and it is the combination of these various factors, each of which alone might have only a minor effect, which may profoundly affect conduction. In this respect structural remodeling may play a crucial role. A large number of heart diseases are accompanied by a change in balance between collagen deposition and breakdown in favor of increased deposition.

Myocardial infarction

In response to myocardial infarction, the heart initiates a complex reparative process of ventricular healing and remodeling, where specific biochemical, morphological, and structural alterations occur in both the infarct and noninfarct zones.

Myocardial infarction is associated with loss of necrotic cardiomyocytes, which is followed by a reparative process that rebuilds infarcted

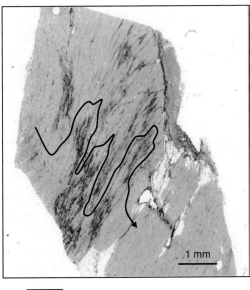

■	Fibrosis
▨	Myocardium

Figure 2.6 Suggested zigzag route activation has to travel from top to bottom in an infarcted area where myocardial fibers and fibrotic strands intermingle.

myocardium to maintain structural integrity of the myocardium. In the human heart it is only 6–8 weeks following the onset of myocardial infarction that the healing process is considered to be complete. Ventricular arrhythmias may arise in the remodeled phase of myocardial infarction and, although focal arrhythmias have been observed, the mechanism of most tachyarrhythmias is based on reentry. Most striking for remodeling is the formation of a stable scar, consisting of fibrosis. Although compact fibrosis may arise in infarct scar, it usually comprises patchy fibrosis exhibiting an intermingling of collagen and myocardial fibers [25]. This structure is eminently suited to cause conduction delay by increased pathways the electrical impulse has to follow within the labyrinth of surviving myocardial bundles composing the infarct scar (Figure 2.6). In addition, unidirectional conduction block may arise at sites with tissue discontinuities. Deposition of replacement fibrosis is, however, not the only process of remodeling in the myocardium. At the infarct border zone, connexin expression is reduced, whereas surviving myocytes within the scar area often reveal redistribution of the connexins

[13]. These changes in cell-to-cell coupling may contribute to the occurrence of reentrant tachycardias in the infarcted zone. Remodeling is, however, not restricted to the infarcted area and the border zone. Also regions remote from the infarct area are involved in the remodeling process. These areas often show gradual morphological changes indicative of hypertrophy to adapt the compromised heart to the increased workload. Ventricular hypertrophy is a strong risk factor for ventricular arrhythmias.

Action potential duration is typically prolonged in remote areas and results from downregulation of K^+ currents. I_{K1}, I_{To}, and I_{Ks} have been shown to decrease in cells from explanted human hearts. Downregulation of the potassium currents increases APD and favors the occurrence of EADs.

Several studies have shown that in the failing human heart SCN5A expression and peak I_{Na} density decrease. This represents a "loss of function" that could be arrhythmogenic by reducing conduction and promoting reentry. In addition, it has been shown that a late sodium current (I_{NaL}) is present in failing cardiac cells. This gain of function might result in EADs, arrhythmias that can be eliminated by the antiarrhythmic drug amiodarone that blocks I_{Na}[26].

Dilated and hypertrophic cardiomyopathy

Dilated cardiomyopathy (DCM) is the most common form of cardiomyopathy, but constitutes a heterogeneous group of disorders. DCM is a disease of the heart muscle in which ventricular dilation is accompanied by contractile dysfunction of the left and/or right ventricle. Intrinsic as well as extrinsic etiologies (hypertension, thyroid disease, viral infection, chronic alcohol abuse) may lead to DCM. About 35% of DCM patients have affected first-degree relatives, indicating a role of genetics in disease pathology. In DCM, histology is usually not specific but shows substantial myocyte hypertrophy. Mild focal and interstitial fibrosis as well as "ghost cells", myocytes without myofibrillary elements, and apoptosis are present. Right ventricular biopsies from patients with DCM reveal a heterogeneous reduction of Cx43 expression [27]. In DCM the voltage-gated sodium channel and the L-type calcium channel have been shown to be reduced to 30–50% of controls. In view of these changes it is not surprising that in DCM hearts cardiac conduction abnormalities may arise and that frequent ventricular ectopy and nonsustained ventricular tachycardia are prevalent. Conduction abnormalities are evidenced by fractionated electrograms that are frequently found. Monomorphic VT is uncommon, but if present it is based on bundle branch reentry in 20–40% of the patients. The majority of the monomorphic VTs seem to be caused by scar-related reentry similar to that in chronic infarction. Spontaneously and induced nonsustained (polymorphic) VTs and ectopic beats often reveal a focal origin [28].

Hypertrophic cardiomyopathy (HCM) is a genetic disorder happening in genes encoding sarcomeric proteins. Left ventricular wall thickening is characteristic of HCM and histopathology demonstrates hypertrophied cardiomyocytes. Characteristic of HCM is, however, myofiber disarray [29]. Disruption of the normal alignment of myocardial cells is only found sporadically in the other types of heart disease. The distribution of intercellular junctions is altered in HCM hearts featuring myofiber disarray. Connexin43 is randomly distributed rather than being confined to intercalated discs. Lateralization of connexins occurs between adjacent myocytes. In addition, the gap junction surface area is reduced despite a normal number of intercellular contact points. Ion channel remodeling is similar to that happening in DCM. Focal and widespread interstitial fibrosis is present as well. Fiber disarray, disorientation of connexins, increased fibrosis and reduced excitability—all favor conduction delay and form an electrically unstable myocardial substrate supporting the occurrence of arrhythmias.

Arrhythmogenic right ventricular cardiomyopathy

Arrhythmogenic right ventricular cardiomyopathy (ARVC) is an inherited disorder, which involves predominantly the right ventricle. Arrhythmias in patients with ARVC include idiopathic ventricular fibrillation, ventricular extrasystoles, supraventricular tachycardia and ventricular tachycardia of right ventricular origin. The histopathology of ARVC is characterized by progressive replacement of right ventricular myocardium by fatty and fibrous tissue. Affected myocardium reveals sparse myocytes interspersed among adipocytes and fibrous tissue. Remodeling of connexin43 has been observed in Naxos disease, a plakoglobin mutation causing ARVC [30]. This form of ARVC shows a high incidence of arrhythmias and sudden cardiac death probably related to reentrant arrhythmias caused by impaired conduction. Myocardial fibrosis is related to late potentials and seems to play a major role in arrhythmias.

Summary

The healthy heart is electrophysiologically not homogeneous but characterized by spatial differences in ion channel expression. Although differences between RV and LV are present, most striking are the transmural and basico-apical gradients in potassium and sodium channel expression. These intrinsic differences might be important in case of remodeling due to pathology. Pathology of the heart is accompanied by both structural and electrical remodeling. Increased interstitial collagen deposition, replacement fibrosis and reactive fibrosis are the hallmarks of most cardiac disease processes, but are usually escorted by reduced connexin and ion channel expression. This usually leads to reduced conduction velocity and changes in action potential duration—parameters that together with the increased collagen content will make the heart vulnerable for arrhythmias. In addition, remodeling may increase the already existing differences in ion and gap junction channel expression and may add to the vulnerability to arrhythmias.

References

1 Imanishi S, Surawicz B. Automatic activity in depolarized guinea pig ventricular myocardium. Characteristics and mechanisms. Circ Res 1976;39:751–9.

2 Katzung BG, Morgenstern JA. Effects of extracellular potassium on ventricular automaticity and evidence for a pacemaker current in mammalian ventricular myocardium. Circ Res 1977;40:105–11.

3 Friedman PL, Stewart JR, Fenoglio JJ Jr, Wit AL. Survival of subendocardial Purkinje fibers after extensive myocardial infarction in dogs. Circ Res 1973;33:597–611.

4 de Bakker JM, Hauer RN, Bakker PF, Becker AE, Janse MJ, Robles de Medina EO. Abnormal automaticity as mechanism of atrial tachycardia in the human heart – electrophysiologic and histologic correlation: a case report. J Cardiovasc Electrophysiol 1994;5:335–44.

5 Cranefield PF, Aronson RS. *Cardiac arrhythmias: the role of triggered activity and other mechanisms.* Mount Kisco: New York Futura; 1988.

6 Sicouri S, Antzelevitch C. Afterdepolarizations and triggered activity develop in a select population of cells (M cells) in canine ventricular myocardium: the effects of acetylstrophanthidin and Bay K 8644. Pacing Clin Electrophysiol 1991;14:1714–20.

7 Liu J, Laurita KR. The mechanism of pause-induced torsade de pointes in long QT syndrome. J Cardiovasc Electrophysiol 2005;16:9817.

8 Qin D, Zhang ZH, Caref EB, Boutjdir M, Jain P, el-Sherif N. Cellular and ionic basis of arrhythmias in postinfarction remodeled ventricular myocardium. Circ Res 1996;79:461–73.

9 Fozzard HA. Afterdepolarizations and triggered activity. Basic Res Cardiol 1992;87 Suppl 2:105–13.

10 Valdivia CR, Chu WW, Pu J, et al. Increased late sodium current in myocytes from a canine heart failure model and from failing human heart. J Mol Cell Cardiol 2005;38:475–83.

11 Bigger JT Jr. Implications of the Cardiac Arrhythmia Suppression Trial for antiarrhythmic drug treatment. Am J Cardiol 1990;65:3D–10D.

12 Icardo JM, Colvee E. Collagenous skeleton of the human mitral papillary muscle. Anat Rec 1998;252:509–18.

13 Kostin S, Rieger M, Dammer S, et al. Gap junction remodeling and altered connexin43 expression in the failing human heart. Mol Cell Biochem 2003;242:135–44.

14 Liu DW, Gintant GA, Antzelevitch C. Ionic bases for electrophysiological distinctions among epicardial, midmyocardial, and endocardial myocytes from the free wall of the canine left ventricle. Circ Res 199;72:671–87.

15 Szentadrassy N, Banyasz T, Biro T, et al. Apico-basal inhomogeneity in distribution of ion channels in canine and human ventricular myocardium. Cardiovasc Res 2005;65:851–60.

16 London B, Baker LC, Petkova-Kirova P, Nerbonne JM, Choi BR, Salama G. Dispersion of repolarization and refractoriness are determinants of arrhythmia phenotype in transgenic mice with long QT. J Physiol 2007;578:115–29.

17 Roden DM. Early after-depolarizations and torsade de pointes: implications for the control of cardiac arrhythmias by prolonging repolarization. Eur Heart J 1993;Suppl H:56–61.

18 Viswanathan PC, Rudy Y. Cellular arrhythmogenic effects of congenital and acquired long-QT syndrome in the heterogeneous myocardium. Circulation 2000;101:1192–8.

19 I Li GR, Lau CP, Leung TK, Nattel S. Ionic current abnormalities associated with prolonged action potentials in cardiomyocytes from diseased human right ventricles. Heart Rhythm 2004;1:460–8.

20 Hund TJ, Rudy Y. Rate dependence and regulation of action potential and calcium transient in a canine cardiac ventricular cell model1. Circulation 2004;110:3168–74.

21 Pogwizd SM. Increased Na(+)-Ca(2+) exchanger in the failing heart. Circ Res 2000;87:641–3.

22 Akar FG, Spragg DD, Tunin RS, Kass DA, Tomaselli GF. Mechanisms underlying conduction slowing and arrhythmogenesis in nonischemic dilated cardiomyopathy. Circ Res 2004;95:717–25.

23 van Rijen HV, Eckardt D, Degen J, et al. Slow conduction and enhanced anisotropy increase the propensity for ventricular tachyarrhythmias in adult mice with induced deletion of connexin43. Circulation 2004;109:1048–55.

24 van Veen TA, Stein M, Royer A, et al. Impaired impulse propagation in Scn5a-knockout mice: combined contribution of excitability, connexin expression, and tissue architecture in relation to aging. Circulation 2005;112:1927–35.

25 Kawara T, Derksen R, de Groot JR, et al. Activation delay after premature stimulation in chronically diseased human myocardium relates to the architecture of interstitial fibrosis. Circulation 2001;104:3069–75.

26 Maltsev VA, Sabbah HN, Undrovinas AI. Late sodium current is a novel target for amiodarone: studies in failing human myocardium. J Mol Cell Cardiol 2001;33:923–32.

27 Kitamura H, Ohnishi Y, Yoshida A, et al. Heterogeneous loss of connexin43 protein in nonischemic dilated cardiomyopathy with ventricular tachycardia. J Cardiovasc Electrophysiol 2002;13:865–70.

28 Pogwizd SM, McKenzie JP, Cain ME. Mechanisms underlying spontaneous and induced ventricular arrhythmias in patients with idiopathic dilated cardiomyopathy. Circulation 1998;98:2404–14.

29 Varnava AM, Elliott PM, Sharma S, McKenna WJ, Davies MJ. Hypertrophic cardiomyopathy: the interrelation of disarray, fibrosis, and small vessel disease. Heart 2000;84:476–82.

30 Kaplan SR, Gard JJ, Protonotarios N, et al. Remodeling of myocyte gap junctions in arrhythmogenic right ventricular cardiomyopathy due to a deletion in plakoglobin (Naxos disease). Heart Rhythm 2004;1:3–11.

CHAPTER 3

Time-dependent gender differences in the clinical course of patients with the congenital long-QT syndrome

Ilan Goldenberg, Arthur J. Moss, & Wojciech Zareba

Mutations in cardiac ion channels have been identified as the basis of the congenital long-QT syndrome (LQTS). Interest in this genetic disorder has increased in recent years because of the association of LQTS with the high risk for sudden cardiac death (SCD) in a relatively young and otherwise healthy population with no structural heart disease. The growing data regarding identification of the gene defects in this disorder have contributed to current knowledge of the basic mechanisms of cardiac arrhythmias and the genotype–phenotype expression of inherited cardiac disorders.

The International LQTS Registry was established in 1979 with the objective of providing a better understanding and management of LQTS [1]. In recent years, studies on the registry have provided important information regarding genotype–phenotype relationship and risk factors for cardiac events in LQTS patients [2–10]. Importantly, data from the registry have shown that the clinical course of LQTS patients is not uniform due to variable penetrance, and is influenced by interactions among gender age, gender, genotype, environmental factors, therapy, and possibly other modifier genes [2]. These findings have demonstrated that improved risk stratification in this genetic disorder can be

obtained if the clinical course of affected patients is evaluated within prespecified age groups, and by assessing age–gender interactions in the risk.

In this report we provide a summary of current knowledge from previous and ongoing registry analyses regarding age–gender differences in the clinical course of LQTS patients. We also discuss possible mechanisms that underlie these differences, and the therapeutic implications of the variable phenotypic expression in affected patients.

Methods

The International LQTS Registry
Data regarding the clinical course of male and female LQTS patients were obtained from studies that were carried out among patients enrolled in the International LQTS Registry and from ongoing registry analyses. Enrolled subjects from proband-identified families were diagnosed with LQTS by prolonged corrected QT interval (QTc) criteria for age and gender as previously reported [2]. For each enrolled patient, data on personal and family history, cardiac events, and therapy were systematically recorded at each visit or medical contact. Clinical data were recorded on prospectively designed forms and included patient and family history and demographic, electrocardiographic, therapeutic, and cardiac event information. The LQTS genotype was determined using standard mutational analytic

Ventricular Arrhythmias and Sudden Cardiac Death, 1st edition.
Edited by P.J. Wang, A. Al-Ahmad, H. Hsia, and P.C. Zei
© 2008 Blackwell Publishing, ISBN: 978-1-4051-6114-5.

techniques involving five established genetic laboratories associated with the International LQTS Registry.

All patients or their guardians provided informed consent agreeing to inclusion in the registry and subsequent clinical studies. The protocol was approved by the University of Rochester Medical Center Institutional Review Board.

End points in LQTS studies

Early LQTS studies traditionally assessed the combined end point of a first cardiac event (comprising syncope, aborted cardiac arrest [ACA]), or LQTS-related SCD. In these studies the predominant component in the combined end point was syncope due to sample size limitations.

Recent data from the International LQTS Registry have facilitated a comprehensive analysis of risk factors for life-threatening cardiac events (ACA or SCD) that are clinically more important in affected patients. For the end point of life-threatening cardiac events, a history of syncope is considered as a time-dependent risk factor rather than as a component of a combined cardiac events end point.

Gender differences in the risk for both end points will be considered separately in the current report.

Statistical analyses

The Kaplan–Meier life-table method was used to assess the time to first occurrence of an end point and the cumulative event rates by gender and age groups. The results were compared using the log-rank statistic.

Multivariate Cox proportional hazards regression modeling was used to assess the independent contribution of gender and age–gender interactions to development of the end points during follow-up. The occurrence of syncope in an affected individual and the effect of β-blocker therapy were evaluated in a time-dependent manner in the multivariate models.

Results

We assessed the clinical course of 3779 LQTS patients enrolled in the registry, of whom 2319 patients (60%) were female. The cumulative probability of a first cardiac event from age 1 through 75 years and the corresponding probability of a first life-threatening cardiac event, by gender, are shown in Figures 3.1A and B, respectively. Data from previous and ongoing registry analyses regarding gender differences in the risk of the two end points, by age groups, are shown in Tables 3.1A–C.

The results of these analyses consistently demonstrate that during childhood, male patients display a higher event rate than females, whereas after this time period, risk reversal occurs, and females maintain a higher risk than males during adulthood. Notably, when the combined end point of any cardiac event is considered, gender risk reversal is shown to occur during adolescence (Figure 3.1A), whereas when the more severe end point of ACA or SCD is evaluated, the change in the male–female risk occurs later, usually during the third decade of life (Figure 3.1B).

Time-dependent differences in gender-related risk in LQTS patients, within age groups, and among patients with the Jervell and Lange–Nielsen syndrome (JLNS), are considered separately below.

Clinical course of preadolescent male and female LQTS patients

In a study of 479 probands (70% females) and 1041 affected family members (QTc >440 ms, 58% females) from the registry, Locati et al. [5] showed that the cumulative probability of a first cardiac event of any type from birth through age 14 years was significantly higher in males than in females, among both probands (74% versus 51%, $P < 0.0001$) and affected family members (20% versus 16%, $P < 0.01$). A similar pattern was also present in 181 family members with unexplained sudden death, in whom the death rate before age 15 years was twice as high in males as in females (57% versus 29%, $P < 0.0001$). In multivariate analysis, male gender was independently associated with a significant 85% and 72% increase in the risk of cardiac events before age 15 years among probands and affected family members, respectively (Table 3.1A).

Zareba et al. [6] studied 533 registry patients who were genetically tested and found to be carriers of the LQT1 ($n = 243$), LQT2 ($n = 209$), and LQT3 ($n = 81$) genotypes. During childhood, the rate of cardiac events was significantly higher in

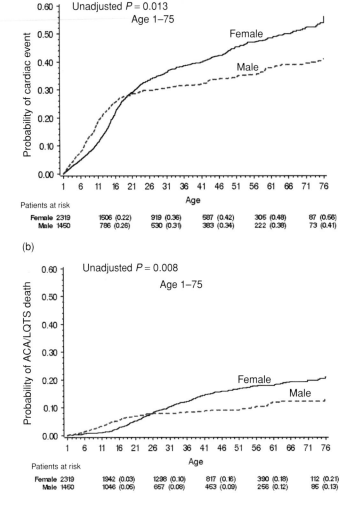

(a)

(b)

Figure 3.1 Kaplan–Meier estimates of (A) a first cardiac event (syncope, aborted cardiac arrest or sudden cardiac death); and (B) a first life-threatening cardiac event (aborted cardiac arrest or sudden cardiac death) from age 1 through 75 years by gender in 3779 LQTS patients from the International LQTS Registry.

LQT1 males than in LQT1 females (56% versus 44%), corresponding to a 71% increase in the risk of a first cardiac event during childhood in males (Table 3.1A), whereas there was no significant gender-related difference in the risk of cardiac events among LQT2 and LQT3 carriers during the same time period.

In a recent analysis of the International LQTS Registry we assessed the end point of ACA or SCD in 3015 LQTS children (1893 males and 1122 females) from proband-identified families who were diagnosed by QTc criteria. In this study population, the cumulative probability of a first life-threatening cardiac event from age 1 through 12 years was 5% in males as compared to only 1%

among females ($P < 0.001$). Accordingly, the multivariate analysis showed that male gender was associated with a threefold increase in the risk of ACA or SCD during childhood, and with more than a fourfold increase in the risk of this end point in a subgroup of 803 genotype positive LQTS children (Table 3.1A).

Ongoing genotype-specific registry analyses further demonstrate that gender differences in the risk during childhood can be identified among LQT1 genotype carriers (Figure 3.2A), whereas among LQT2 genotype carriers the rate of life-threatening cardiac events is relatively low during childhood, and does not exhibit a significant difference between males and females (Figure 3.2B).

Table 3.1 Data from the International LQTS Registry regarding gender-related risk of cardiac events by age groups

A. Preadolescence period

Population	N	Age range, (yr)	End point	Male:female adjusted HR[†] (95% CI)	Data source
Probands	479	0–14	Any cardiac event	1.85 (1.59–2.70)	Locati et al. [5]
Affected family members	1041	0–14	Any cardiac event	1.72 (1.23–2.39)	Locati et al. [5]
LQT1	247	0–15	Any cardiac event	1.72 (1.19–2.33)	Zareba et al. [6]
LQT2	209	0–15	Any cardiac event	1.37 (0.80–2.33)	Zareba et al. [6]
LQT3	81	0–15	Any cardiac event	0.54 (0.14–2.13)	Zareba et al. [6]
Registry pts diagnosed by QTc criteria or genetic testing	3015	1–12	ACA or SCD	3.03 (1.80–5.12)	Current Registry analyses
Registry pts diagnosed by genetic testing*	805	1–12	ACA or SCD	4.31 (1.14–20.50)	Current Registry analyses
Registry pts diagnosed by QTc criteria or genetic testing	2772	10–12	ACA or SCD	4.0 (1.8–9.2)	Hobbs et al. [8]
Registry pts diagnosed by QTc criteria or genetic testing	2772	10–12	SCD	11.6 (1.4–94.2)	Hobbs et al. [8]

B. Adolescence through age 40 years

Population	N	Age range, (yr)	End point	Male:female adjusted HR[†] (95% CI)	Data source
Probands	479	15–40	Any cardiac event	0.53 (0.27–1.06)	Locati et al. [5]
Affected family members	1041	15–40	Any cardiac event	0.31 (0.17–0.56)	Locati et al. [5]
LQT1	247	16–40	Any cardiac event	0.30 (0.12–0.71)	Zareba et al. [6]
LQT2	209	16–40	Any cardiac event	0.27 (0.09–0.73)	Zareba et al. [6]
LQT3	81	16–40	Any cardiac event	1.11 (0.35–3.45)	Zareba et al. [6]
Registry pts diagnosed by QTc criteria or genetic testing	2772	13–20	SCD	1.6 (0.2–0.8)	Hobbs et al. [8]
Registry pts diagnosed by genetic testing	812	18–40	Any cardiac event	3.05 (2.13–4.38)	Sauer et al. [9]
Registry pts diagnosed by genetic testing	812	18–40	ACA or SCD	2.77 (1.66–4.62)	Sauer et al. [9]

C. After the fourth decade of life

Population	N	Age range, (yr)	End point	Male:female adjusted HR[†] (95% CI)	Data source
Registry pts diagnosed by QTc criteria	540	41–75	Any cardiac event	0.54 (0.28–0.87)	Current Registry analyses
Registry pts with QTc ≥ 470 ms	860	41–60	All-cause mortality	0.97 (0.52–1.81)	Current Registry analyses
Registry pts with QTc ≥ 470 ms	314	61–75	All-cause mortality	0.69 (0.37–1.26)	Current Registry analyses

Note: *Subgroup of the 3015 patients in the previous row.

[†]Findings adjusted for QTc duration, time-dependent β-blocker therapy; for the end point of ACA or SCD findings were also adjusted for a history of time-dependent syncope.

ACA, aborted cardiac arrest; LQT1, 2, and 3, long-QT syndrome types 1, 2 and 3, respectively; SCD, sudden cardiac death.

Clinical course of male and female LQTS patients from adolescence through age 40 years

In the registry analysis of 479 probands and 1041 affected family members carried out by Locati et al.

[5], a gender risk-reversal was shown to occur after age 14 years when the end point of a first cardiac event of any type was assessed. Thus, in the age range of 15–40 years, females had an 87% increase in the risk of cardiac events as compared to males among

(a)

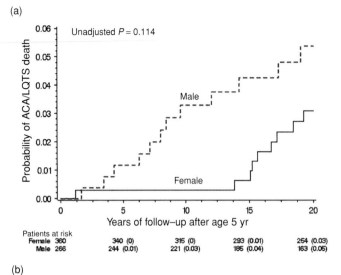

Patients at risk

Female 360	340 (0)	315 (0)	293 (0.01)	254 (0.03)
Male 266	244 (0.01)	221 (0.03)	185 (0.04)	163 (0.05)

(b)

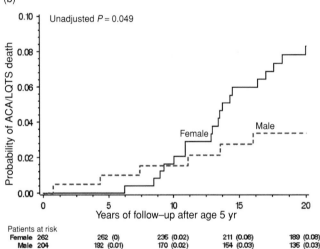

Patients at risk

Female 262	252 (0)	235 (0.02)	211 (0.06)	189 (0.08)
Male 204	192 (0.01)	170 (0.02)	154 (0.03)	135 (0.03)

Figure 3.2 Kaplan–Meier estimates of aborted cardiac arrest or sudden cardiac death from age 5 through 25 years in (A) LQT1; and (B) LQT2 patients from the International LQTS Registry.

probands, and a 3.3-fold increase in the risk among affected family members (Table 3.1B). Consistently, Zareba et al. [6] showed that in the age range of 16–40 years the risk of cardiac events of any type was more than threefold higher among both LQT1 and LQT2 females as compared to the respective males (Table 3.1B), whereas among LQT3 genotype carriers no significant gender difference in the risk was detected.

As noted above, when the end point of ACA or SCD is considered, gender-risk reversal occurs at a later stage than the age shown for the less severe cardiac event end point that includes also syncope

(Figure 3.1). In a recent study of 2772 registry patients that were followed between the ages of 10 and 20 years, Hobbs et al. [8] showed that in the age range of 10–12 years males had a fourfold increase in the risk of ACA or SCD and an 11-fold increase in the risk of SCD compared to females (Table 3.1A), whereas in the age range of 12–20 years no significant gender difference in the risk of life-threatening of cardiac events was shown (Table 3.1B). Subsequently, Sauer et al. [9], in an analysis of 812 mutation-confirmed LQTS patients from the registry who were followed-up between the ages of 18 and 40 years, showed that during adulthood females have nearly a threefold increase in the risk of ACA or SCD as compared to males (Table 3.1B). In this study, the cumulative probability of ACA or SCD at age 40 years was 11% among females as compared to only 2% among males ($P < 0.001$) [9]. The two latter studies further demonstrate that gender risk-reversal occurs at a later age when the end point of life-threatening cardiac events is considered.

Current genotype-specific analyses show that a higher rate of life-threatening cardiac events after adolescence can be identified in females that are carriers of both the LQT1 and LQT2 genotypes (Figures 3.2A and B, respectively).

Clinical course of male and female LQTS patients after the fourth decade of life

Published studies on the clinical course of LQTS patients are limited to the first four decades of life due to lack of appropriate follow-up information in the older age group. The International LQTS Registry has recently expanded the duration of follow-up in enrolled subjects, and current updated data now facilitate a comprehensive analysis of the clinical course of affected patients beyond the age of 40 years.

We assessed the end point of a first cardiac event of any type after age 40 years in 540 LQTS patients. In this analysis, the cumulative probability of LQTS-related cardiac events at age 75 years was 32% in females as compared to 18% in males ($P = 0.005$), corresponding to an 85% increase in the adjusted risk of cardiac event in females compared to males (Table 3.1C). Since in the older age group the competing risks cardiovascular comorbidities are higher among males, and may counterbalance the higher risk of LQTS-related cardiac events in females, we also assessed the end point of all-cause mortality in affected subjects after age 40 years. In an analysis of 860 LQTS patients, the cumulative probability of all-cause mortality from age 41 years through 75 years was 27% among females as compared to 32% in males ($P = 0.37$). Consistently, the risk associated with female gender was not significant when the end point of all-cause mortality was assessed in age ranges of 41–60 years and of 61–75 years (Table 3.1C). Thus, it appears that LQTS continues to confer a high risk of arrhythmic events among females even after the fourth decade of life that counterbalances the higher risk of acquired cardiovascular morbidity and mortality of males in this age group. These age-specific risk interactions lead to a neutral effect of gender on the end point of all-cause mortality in the older age group.

Clinical course of male and female patients affected by the Jervell and Lange–Nielsen syndrome

Jervell and Lange–Nielsen syndrome is the autosomal recessive form of LQTS, and is associated with a more severe clinical course than the more common autosomal dominant form. The clinical course of 44 JLNS patients was recently assessed in a study from the US portion of the International LQTS Registry [11]. Males affected by JLNS who were ≤16 years were found to have a 4.4-fold increase in the risk of cardiac events of any type as compared to females in the same age category (HR = 4.43 [95% CI 2.01–9.80]; $P < 0.001$). Similarly, a 9.5-fold increase in the risk of life-threatening cardiac events was shown among <20-year-old JLNS males as compared to females in the same age category (HR = 9.95 [95% CI 1.14–78.70]; $P = 0.04$). After these respective time periods, only a relatively small number of events occur in JLNS patients, and no significant gender-related difference in the risk of both endpoints was observed. Accordingly, the cumulative probability of cardiac events in JLNS patients at age 20 years was 93% in males and 79% in females, with relatively few events thereafter (Figure 3.3).

Discussion

Accumulating data from the International LQTS Registry consistently demonstrate that the phenotype expression of LQTS displays major time-dependent gender differences in the risk of non-fatal and life-threatening cardiac events. These findings have important pathophysiologic and therapeutic implications in the understanding and risk-management of affected patients.

Possible mechanisms underlying differences in the clinical course of male and female LQTS patients

Currently, the mechanisms behind the age-dependent differences in gender-related risk are unknown. Data from recent studies suggest possible

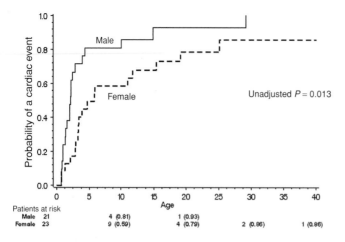

Figure 3.3 Kaplan–Meier estimates of a first cardiac event by gender in 44 patients with the Jervell and Lange–Nielsen syndrome from the US portion of the International LQTS Registry.

interactions among genetic, hormonal, and environmental factors.

Ventricular tachyarrhythmias have been shown to occur more frequently during physical effort in patients carrying the common LQT1 genotype who harbor mutations that impair the I_{Ks} current. It has been shown that 79% of the lethal arrhythmic episodes in LQT1 patients are associated with exercise and faster heart rates [7]. This may be due to the fact that the repolarizing current I_{Ks} activates during increased heart rate, and is essential for QT interval adaptation during tachycardia. Thus, impaired adaptive QT shortening with decreasing RR intervals during tachycardia in LQT1 patients can lead to life-threatening ventricular arrhythmias during physical activities [1]).

Environmental factors may predispose boys to more intensive physical activity during childhood than girls, possibly leading to a higher risk of life-threatening cardiac events that are associated with fast heart rates in males who carry the LQT1 genotype during this time period. Consistently, our data show that the highest rate of life-threatening cardiac events during childhood occurs in males who carry the LQT1 genotype (Figure 3.2). With the onset of adolescence, hormonal factors may affect the clinical course of LQTS males and females. Androgens were shown to blunt QT interval prolongation to quinidine [1]), and thus may be associated with QT shortening in males after childhood. In contrast, estrogens were demonstrated to modify the expression of potassium channels, and may have a dose-dependent blocking effect on IKs [17]. Female LQTS patients with mutations impairing potassium channel activity may therefore be specifically sensitive to estrogen activity. Consistently, registry data demonstrate that after childhood, both LQT1 and LQT2 females have a higher risk of LQTS-related life-threatening cardiac events than the respective males (Figure 3.2). Furthermore, adult female patients may be exposed to conditions such as menses and pregnancy, in which hormonal changes favor QT prolongation and vulnerability to arrhythmias [18]. The possible relationship between female hormones and arrhythmic risk is also supported by a recent study on the registry that showed a significant increase in the risk of cardiac events in the 9-month postpartum period, mainly among females who were identified as LQT2 genotype carriers [10].

Female predominance in population studies of the long-QT syndrome

Age–gender differences in clinical manifestations may contribute to the unexplained sex imbalance among patients referred to the LQTS Registry. Previous studies have shown that among enrolled registry patients there is a higher frequency of females (approximately 60%) than males [2,3,5,8,9]. Locati et al. [5] have demonstrated that while the referral of patients to the registry during childhood appears to be similar by gender, probands and affected family members that are referred to the LQTS Registry during adulthood are virtually all females [5].

Furthermore, females predominate in registry analyses even when a more stringent cutoff (i.e., QTc >470 ms) is applied [5]. The age–gender imbalance may reflect the fact that among males the risk of fatal-LQTS-related events is confined mostly to the first two decades of life, whereas among females most first cardiac events occur after this time period. This survival bias can also possibly explain the findings in a recent study by Imboden et al. [19] that assessed allele transmission in 484 LQT1 and 269 LQT2 families. The study showed that LQTS alleles were transmitted more often to females than to males. Notably, this analysis was conducted in families with fully genotyped offspring (e.g., all members of families in which a member had a fatal event before being genotyped were excluded from the study). Thus, the female predominance in this report may also reflect the fact that males have a significantly higher risk of fatal events from early childhood before being genotyped, thereby excluding this higher-risk population from the genetic analysis.

Clinical and therapeutic implications

The long-QT syndrome represents a cardiac genetic disorder with substantial phenotypic variability. Therefore, time-dependent risk factors need to be continually assessed in affected patients in order to provide an appropriate therapeutic management strategy for the primary prevention of life-threatening ventricular arrhythmias. Importantly, risk stratification in LQTS should incorporate age- and gender-specific factors.

β-blocker therapy was shown to be associated with a significant survival benefit in high-risk LQTS patients [8,9]. Other, more invasive therapeutic modalities, including left cervical sympathetic denervation (LCSD) and implantation of an implantable cardioverter-defibrillator (ICD), have been shown to be effective in patients who remain symptomatic despite β-blocker therapy [20,21]. Our data suggest that these LQTS therapies should be considered in male patients during childhood due a high risk for life-threatening cardiac events in affected males prior to adolescence, while after the onset of adolescence, asymptomatic males without additional risk factors may be carefully observed, and initiation of preventive therapy should

be strongly considered in females who maintain a high risk for cardiac events throughout adulthood.

Conclusions and future directions

LQTS studies have provided novel and important insight into the fundamental nature of the electrical activity of the human heart and to the relationship between disturbances in ion flow and cardiac disease. Further exploration of the mechanisms that underlie time-dependent gender differences in the phenotypic expression of LQTS patients will provide a better understanding of the interactions among environmental, hormonal, and possible modifier genes, with the age and gender specific expression of this genetic disorder. These may lead to improved criteria for risk stratifications, and possible gender-specific therapeutic strategies in affected patients.

References

1 Moss AJ, Schwartz PJ. Circulation. 25th anniversary of the International Long-QT Syndrome Registry: an ongoing quest to uncover the secrets of long-QT syndrome. Circulation 2005;111:1199–201.

2 Moss AJ, Schwartz PJ, Crampton RS, et al. The long QT syndrome. Prospective longitudinal study of 328 families. Circulation 1991;84:1136–44.

3 Zareba W, Moss AJ, Schwartz PJ, et al. Influence of genotype on the clinical course of the long-QT syndrome. International Long-QT Syndrome Registry Research Group. N Engl J Med 1998;339:960–5.

4 Priori SG, Schwartz PJ, Napolitano C, et al. Risk stratification in the long-QT syndrome. N Engl J Med 2003;348:1866–74.

5 Locati EH, Zareba W, Moss AJ, et al. Age- and sex-related differences in clinical manifestations in patients with congenital long-QT syndrome: findings from the International LQTS Registry. Circulation 1998;97:2237–44.

6 Zareba W, Moss AJ, Locati EH, et al. Modulating effects of age and gender on the clinical course of long QT syndrome by genotype. J Am Coll Cardiol 2003;42:103–9.

7 Schwartz PJ, Priori SG, Spazzolini C, et al. Genotype-phenotype correlation in the long-QT syndrome: gene-specific triggers for life-threatening arrhythmias. Circulation 2001;10389–95.

8 Hobbs JB, Peterson DR, Moss AJ, et al. Risk of aborted cardiac arrest or sudden cardiac death during adolescence in the long-QT syndrome. JAMA 2006;296:1249–54.

9 Sauer AJ, Moss AJ, McNitt S, et al. Long QT syndrome in adults. J Am Coll Cardiol 2007;49:329–37.

10 Seth R, Moss AJ, McNitt S, et al. Long QT syndrome and pregnancy. J Am Col Cardiol 2007;49:1092–8.

11 Goldenberg I, Moss AJ, Zareba W, et al. Clinical course and risk stratification of patients affected with the Jervell and Lange-Nielsen syndrome. J Cardiovasc Electrophysiol 200617:1161–8.

12 Swan H, Viitasalo M, Piippo K, Laitinen P, Kontula K, Toivonen L. Sinus node function and ventricular repolarization during exercise stress test in long QT syndrome patients with KvLQT1 and HERG potassium channel defects. J Am Coll Cardiol 1999;34:823–9.

13 Bidoggia H, Maciel JP, Capalozza N, et al. Sex differences on the electrocardiographic pattern of cardiac repolarization: possible role of testosterone. Am Heart J 2000;140:678–83.

14 Drici MD, Burklow TR, Haridasse V, Glazer RI, Woosley RL. Sex hormones prolong the QT interval and downregulate potassium channel expression in the rabbit heart. Circulation 1996;94:1471–4.

15 Liu XK, Katchman A, Drici MD, et al. Gender difference in the cycle length-dependent QT and potassium currents in rabbits. J Pharmacol Exp Ther 1998;285:672–9.

16 Boyle MB, MacLusky NJ, Naftolin F, Kaczmarek LK. Hormonal regulation of K+-channel messenger RNA in rat myometrium during oestrus cycle and in pregnancy. Nature 1987;330:373–5.

17 Boyle M, MacLusky N, Naftolin F, Kaczmarek L. Hormonal regulation of K+ channel messenger RNA in rat myometrium during oestrus cycle and in pregnancy. Nature 1987;330:373–5.

18 Kadish AH. The effect of gender on cardiac electrophysiology and arrhythmias. In: Zipes DP, Jalife J, eds. *Cardiac Electrophysiology: From Cell to Bedside*, 2nd ed. Philadelphia, PA: WB Saunders; 1995:1268–75.

19 Imboden M, Swan H, Denjoy I, et al. Female Predominance and Transmission Distortion in the Long-QT Syndrome. N Engl J Med 2006;355:2744–51.

20 Schwartz PJ, Priori SG, Cerrone M, et al. Left cardiac sympathetic denervation in the management of high-risk patients affected by the long-QT syndrome. Circulation 2004;109:1826–33.

21 Zareba W, Moss AJ, Daubert JP, Hall WJ, Robinson JL, Andrews M. Implantable cardioverter defibrillator in high-risk long QT syndrome patients. J Cardiovasc Electrophysiol 2003;14:337–41.

CHAPTER 4

Genetics of ventricular arrhythmias

Zian H. Tseng, & Jeffrey Olgin

Summary

The last two decades have witnessed significant advances in our understanding of the genetic basis for various forms of inherited cardiac diseases predisposing to ventricular arrhythmias and sudden cardiac death (SCD). Monogenic cardiac diseases are caused by rare mutations in single genes altering the electrical or structural substrate of the ventricular myocardium. These include (1) primary electrical disease, due to mutations affecting ion channels, transporters, and their modifier proteins, and (2) inherited cardiomyopathies, mainly due to mutations affecting the sarcomeric and cell–cell junction proteins. Common genetic variants, single nucleotide polymorphisms (SNPs), at other genetic loci can affect expression and penetrance of these monogenic diseases. Investigation has also begun to examine the genetic basis for polygenic cardiac disease predisposing to ventricular arrhythmias, such as the most common form of SCD—that associated with coronary artery disease (CAD).

Introduction

Cardiac diseases predisposing to ventricular arrhythmias and sudden cardiac death (SCD) can be divided into the monogenic disorders, those caused by a rare single-gene defect, and the polygenic disorders, those in which more common genetic variants at multiple loci contribute to the risk of the disease.

Monogenic disorders are generally caused by rare mutations that result in phenotypes such as congenital long-QT syndrome (LQTS) or Brugada

Ventricular Arrhythmias and Sudden Cardiac Death, 1st edition.
Edited by P.J. Wang, A. Al-Ahmad, H. Hsia, and P.C. Zei
© 2008 Blackwell Publishing, ISBN: 978-1-4051-6114-5.

syndrome. These diseases typically exhibit Mendelian inheritance patterns: autosomal dominant, autosomal recessive, or X-linked. Penetrance and expressivity of these mutations are generally high but can be variable, modified by interaction with genetic variation at other loci as well as environmental factors.

Monogenic diseases predisposing to ventricular arrhythmias are generally classified as either primary electrical diseases, arrhythmogenic diseases in the absence of structural abnormalities, or inherited structural cardiomyopathies. The former are caused by alterations in ion channels, ion exchangers/transporters, and their modifier proteins while the latter are caused by alterations in myocardial structural proteins: cell–cell junction proteins and contractile sarcomeric proteins.

Common diseases such as the most common form of SCD associated with coronary artery disease (CAD), are complex polygenic diseases thought to be caused by the summation of common genetic variants in multiple genes, with the risk further modified by epigenetic influences [1].

Of the nearly half a million SCD occurring in the United States per year [2], approximately 5% are caused by the primary electrical disease, 10–15% by inherited cardiomyopathies, and over 80% by CAD and its sequelae [3].

The majority of mutations causing the disease are due to missense mutations, single-nucleotide point mutations that alter the exonic (protein-coding) sequence of the gene but deletion or insertion mutations can also be responsible for disease. Splice site mutations can also vary the protein product as can intronic (noncoding) mutations. Mutations can result in either gain or loss of function to cause a variety of alterations in protein function, regulation, and expression (Table 4.1). Whereas mutations

Table 4.1 Mutational effects on protein function

Alteration of channel function
    Ion conductance
    Gating
    Binding to subunits
Alteration of channel regulation
    Response to autonomic inputs
Alteration of protein transcription
    Promoter and control element mutations
    Intronic mutations
    Splice site mutations
Alteration of protein trafficking to membrane
Alteration of modifier protein function
Alteration of genetic background
    SNPs at other loci

occur with rare frequency (generally ≪1%), SNPs are more common genetic variants with an allele frequency >1%, occurring in coding or noncoding regions of genes. SNPs in the exonic region of genes are classified as either synonymous (no effect on the amino acid sequence) or nonsynonymous (resulting in an amino acid substitution). Although many SNPs have no effect on protein or cellular function, others may predispose individuals to disease or influence drug response, either alone or in combination.

Primary electrical diseases

The finely coordinated symphony of depolarizing and repolarizing currents across the cell membrane and sarcoplasmic reticulum (SR) in the cardiomyocyte is regulated by ion channels, exchangers, and their modifier proteins to result in the ventricular action potential and ultimately contractile function. Ion channels are composed of an α pore-forming subunit and ancillary β subunits. Gain of function or loss of function mutations in the genes encoding each of the ion channel components cause a characteristic alteration of their respective currents and particular phases of the action potential to result in the electrical substrate for arrhythmias in the absence of structural abnormalities (Figure 4.1).

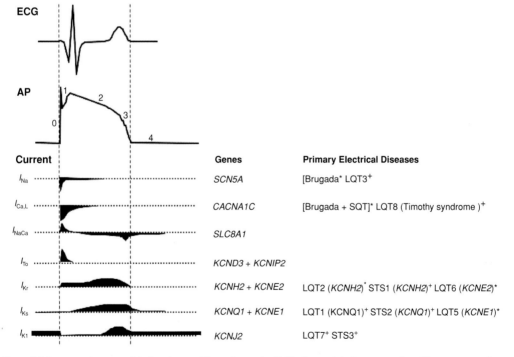

Figure 4.1 Ion currents responsible for phases of the action potential in the ventricular myocardium. Time course and magnitude of currents are depicted schematically. Genes encoding the channels underlying each current are indicated, as are the primary electrical diseases associated with each current. *Loss of function mutation; †Gain of function mutation.

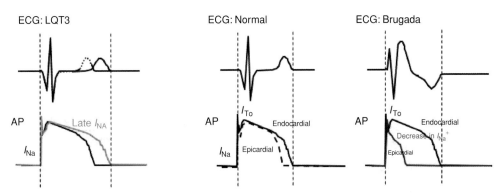

(a) *SCN5A* gain of function mutations

(b) *SCN5A* loss of function mutations

ECG: LQT3

ECG: Normal

ECG: Brugada

Figure 4.2 *SCN5A* mutations cause allelic diseases. (a) Autosomal dominant gain of function mutations cause defective inactivation of the Na$^+$ channel to result in persistent late I_{Na+}, prolongation of action potential plateau, and ECG manifestation of LQT3. (b) Autosomal dominant loss of function mutations cause reduction in I_{Na+} which results in exaggeration of action potential differences between the epicardial and endocardial layers of the right ventricular myocardium and ECG manifestation of Brugada syndrome.

Mutations causing opposite effects on the same gene and current can result in vastly different phenotypes. Gain of function mutations in *SCN5A* result in LQT3, a form of congenital LQTS, while loss of function mutations in the same gene result in Brugada syndrome. Similarly, gain of function mutations in the genes encoding elements of the repolarizing potassium currents result in forms of the short QT syndrome, while loss of function mutations in the same genes result in numerous forms of congenital LQTS. Mutations in modifier proteins ultimately result in increased or decreased current, without affecting the ion channels themselves, to result in disease.

Mutations affecting I_{Na}

The *SCN5A* gene encodes the α subunit of the cardiac sodium channel and has a genomic structure spanning 80 kb, consisting of 28 exons, on chromosome 3p21 [4]. The α subunit combines with up to three β subunits to form the functional sodium channel, which is voltage-gated and regulates the inward sodium current that accounts for phase 0, the rapid upstroke of the action potential. Sodium channels rapidly enter a nonconducting inactivated state during the action potential plateau.

Mutations in *SCN5A* cause allelic diseases (Figure 4.2). Gain of function mutations lead to defective

inactivation of the Na$^+$ channel and a persistent late Na$^+$ current. This causes prolongation of the action potential [5], manifest as a long QT interval on the surface electrocardiogram (ECG) and leads to LQT3 [6]. Loss of function mutations in *SCN5A* result in reduction of myocardial Na$^+$ current, which is associated with Brugada syndrome [7], idiopathic ventricular fibrillation [8], and sudden unexplained nocturnal death syndrome (SUNDS) [9,10]. SUNDS has been recognized in southeast Asia for decades as a disease causing SCD, usually during sleep in young males, and is functionally the same disease as Brugada syndrome [11,12]. A single mutation in *SCN5A* can also cause a combined phenotype of Brugada syndrome and LQT3 [13].

Congenital LQTS is a heterogeneous inherited disease of prolonged myocardial repolarization with a common form transmitted as an autosomal dominant disease (Romano–Ward syndrome) and a rare form transmitted as an autosomal recessive disease associated with congenital deafness (Jervell and Lange-Nielsen syndrome) [14]. Genetic heterogeneity underlies congenital LQTS given that causative mutations in nine genes have thus far have been described. Abnormal dispersion of repolarization in the ventricular myocardium predisposes to early afterdepolarizations and torsade de pointes, causing syncope and SCD [15].

Mutations in *SCN5A* causing LQT3 account for approximately 10% of cases of congenital LQTS [16]. Triggers and clinical features of congenital LQTS vary according to genotype. *SCN5A* mutations are typically associated with bradycardia, and a tendency for syncope or SCD to occur at rest or during sleep [17,18]. Gender can affect the risk for clinical events; male sex was demonstrated to be an independent predictor of cardiac arrest or SCD in congenital LQTS patients with *SCN5A* mutations [19].

Brugada syndrome is associated with a characteristic ECG pattern of right bundle branch block, ST elevation in the right precordial leads, and normal QT intervals, and risk for polymorphic ventricular tachycardia (VT) and ventricular fibrillation (VF) [20,21]. *SCN5A* mutations are inherited in an autosomal dominant pattern, often with incomplete penetrance and male predominance. Thus far, over 60 mutations have been described, including frameshift errors, early stop codons, or splice site mutations that affect the coding region of *SCN5A* [7,22]. Although mechanisms vary, all mutations result in decreased Na$^+$ current. A number of mutations cause failure of the channel to express, impaired pore conductance, or disrupted trafficking to the cell membrane [23–26]. Other mutations cause an alteration in channel kinetics by a shift in voltage and time dependence of gating, slow recovery, or accelerated inactivation [27–29]. Brugada syndrome is also recognized as a genetically heterogeneous disease since only 20% of all cases are linked to *SCN5A* mutations [30]. A recent study [31] demonstrated no abnormalities in location, function, or expression of *SCN5A* protein in some Brugada patients, suggesting the involvement of other proteins in the pathogenesis of this syndrome.

The proposed basis for the ECG abnormalities and arrhythmia susceptibility in Brugada syndrome is an exaggeration of the normal differences in action potential duration (APD) between the right ventricular epicardium and endocardium [32–35]. In normal individuals, unequal transmural distribution of the transient outward current I_{To} results in a more prominent repolarizing current and a shorter APD in the epicardium as compared to the endocardium. A decrease in the Na$^+$ current results in extreme shortening of the epicardial APD due to unopposed I_{To}. The more pronounced transmural

voltage gradient and dispersion of repolarization allow for phase 2 reentry and polymorphic ventricular tachycardia (Figure 4.2b).

The genetic and environmental milieu affects penetrance in individuals with *SCN5A* mutations. An *SCN5A* SNP rescues a missense *SCN5A* mutation carried on a separate chromosome, by allowing trafficking to the cell membrane of mutant channels to restore normal Na$^+$ current, accounting for the fact that not all carriers of the missense mutation exhibit disease [36]. At supraphysiologic temperatures Brugada syndrome may be unmasked, and Brugada patients are at higher risk of arrhythmia during febrile states [37] due to the exaggerated inactivation of mutant channels [27]. Males have more prominent I_{To} current in the right ventricular epicardium as compared to females, which may explain the higher prevalence of Brugada syndrome in males [38]. In different ethnic groups, common *SCN5A* variants occur with variable prevalence and result in phenotypes more subtle than those caused by rare mutations. A common *SCN5A* SNP in African-Americans results in slight acceleration of channel activation, abnormal repolarization, and arrhythmia susceptibility, particularly during conditions such as exposure to QTc-prolonging drugs [39].

Mutations affecting I_K

The rapid and slow components of the delayed rectifier potassium currents, I_{Kr} and I_{Ks}, account for the cardiac action potential plateau. Both of these currents are composed of channels with α pore-forming subunits, encoded by *KCNH2* (I_{Kr}) and *KCNQ1* (I_{Ks}), and modulating β subunit proteins, encoded by *KCNE2* (I_{Kr}) and *KCNE1* (I_{Ks}). The inwardly rectifying potassium current, I_{K1}, stabilizes the resting membrane potential and is responsible for final repolarization of the action potential. *KCNJ2* encodes the α subunit of the channel accounting for I_{K1}.

Mutations with opposite effects in components of these potassium currents cause reverse phenotypes (Table 4.2). Loss of function mutations result in delayed repolarization, QT interval prolongation, and many of the forms of congenital LQTS. Gain of function mutations cause forms of short QT syndrome due to accelerated repolarization and are

Table 4.2 Diseases caused by mutations affecting I_K

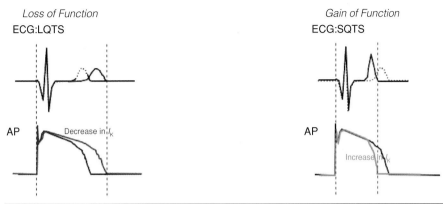

Loss of function	Gene	Locus	Protein	Gain of function
I_{Ks} current				
LQT1 (AD), JLN1 (AR)	*KCNQ1*	11p15.5	α subunit	STS2 (AD)
LQT5 (AD), JLN2 (AR)	*KCNE1*	21q22.1-2	β subunit	
I_{Kr} current				
LQT2 (AD)	*KCNH2*	7q35-36	α subunit	STS1 (AD)
LQT6 (AD)	*KCNE2*	21q22.1	β subunit	
I_{K1} current				
LQT7 (AD)	*KCNJ2*	17q23	Kir2.1 subunit	STS3 (AD)

characterized by a high propensity for ventricular arrhythmias.

Mutations in the genes encoding components of the I_{Ks} channel, *KCNQ1* and *KCNE1*, cause LQT1 and LQT5, respectively. Similarly, LQT2 and LQT6 are caused by mutations in components of I_{Kr} channel encoded by *KCNH2* and *KCNE2*, respectively. These LQTS genotypes result in decreased K^+ currents, but cause the same phenotype of action potential prolongation, decreased repolarization reserve, and susceptibility to early afterdepolarizations and torsade de pointes as do those with gain of function mutations in the Na^+ channel (LQT3) [40]. Many of these mutations are inherited in an autosomal dominant fashion to cause Romano–Ward syndrome, but autosomal recessive mutations in *KCNQ1* and *KCNE1* can cause Jervell and Lange-Nielsen syndrome (JLNS). Loss of function *KCNJ2* mutations account for decreased I_{K1} current and LQT7, Andersen–Tawil syndrome, a multisystem disease with dysmorphic features, ventricular arrhythmias, and periodic paralysis due to expression of *KCNJ2* in cardiac and skeletal muscle [41].

Mutations commonly affect channel function by altering gating kinetics or exerting a dominant-negative effect on subunit assembly, but some *KCNH2* and *KCNJ2* mutations have also been shown to cause abnormal channel trafficking resulting in forms of LQT2 and LQT7, respectively [42,43]. The location of mutations within the coding sequence determines clinical risk of cardiac events. LQTS patients with mutations in the pore regions of *KCNH2* and *KCNQ1* have a higher frequency and earlier incidence of arrhythmic events than patients with nonpore mutations [44,45].

LQTS genotype determines clinical characteristics and response to therapy as well as risk of cardiac events [17]. LQT1 (*KCNQ1*) patients typically experience events during physical activity, such as while swimming, exhibit a broad-based T wave, and respond most effectively to β blocker therapy. LQT2 (*KCNH2*) patients generally develop symptoms following auditory or emotional stimuli and have low amplitude, notched T waves. Gender also has a variable effect on transmission of alleles and risk for cardiac events depending on genotype. *KCNQ1* and *KCNH2* mutations are more likely to be transmitted

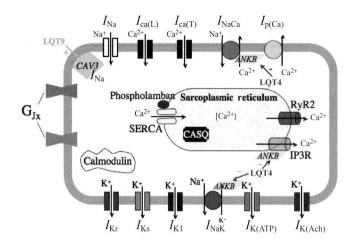

Figure 4.3 Modifier proteins ankyrin B (*ANKB*) and caveolin 3 (*CAV3*) and their relationship to cardiomyocyte ion currents. Associated primary electrical diseases with gain of function (LQT9) and loss of function (LQT4) phenotypes are shown.

to daughters than sons in LQTS families [46]. The incidence of first cardiac arrest or SCD was shown to be higher among female patients than male patients with *KCNH2* mutations [19].

SNPs in K^+ channel genes with more subtle effects underlie between 10–15% of the cases of acquired LQTS [47]. Typically, these variants do not result in prolongation of QT interval until exposure to stressors, such as drugs or hypokalemia. Ethnicity can affect this risk: a *KCNQ1* SNP predisposing to drug-induced LQTS has a high prevalence in the Japanese population [48]. A *KCNE2* SNP common in the US population does not affect the K^+ current but increases the risk of drug-induced LQTS by increasing sensitivity to blockade of K^+ current by sulfa drugs [49].

Short QT syndrome (SQTS) is a disease characterized by familial SCD, short refractory periods with QTc typically between 280 and 300 milliseconds, and easily inducible ventricular arrhythmias [50]. SCD often occurs early in life. Accelerated K^+ channel function caused by autosomal dominant mutations in *KCNH2*, *KCNQ1*, and *KCNJ2* account for the STS1, STS2, and STS3 forms of the disease, respectively [51–53]. A proposed mechanism for the development of ventricular arrhythmias is heterogeneous abbreviation of APD resulting in transmural dispersion of repolarization [54]. In patients with *KCNH2* mutation causing STS1, quinidine restored QTc intervals to normal range and prevented inducibility of ventricular arrhythmias [55].

Mutations affecting modifier proteins

Modifier proteins anchor ion channels to cell membrane elements (Figure 4.3). Loss of function mutations in ankyrin B (*ANKB*), a 220 kDa protein which binds anion exchanger, Na^+/K^+ ATPase, voltage-sensitive Na^+ channels, Na^+/Ca^{2+} exchanger, and inositol-1,4,5-triphosphate receptors, result in disrupted cellular organization of these elements and Ca^{2+} currents, ultimately leading to action potential prolongation and LQT4. Altered Ca^{2+} signaling plays a major role in development of ventricular arrhythmias in LQT4 [56].

Recently, mutations in CAV3, encoding caveolin 3, have been shown to cause LQT9 [57]. Caveolin 3 is the principal protein of caveolae, the plasma vesicles that compartmentalize SCN5A-encoded Na^+ channels. These gain of function mutations cause a twofold to threefold increase in the late Na^+ current and action potential prolongation with a phenotype similar to LQT3.

Mutations affecting $I_{Ca(L)}$

CACNA1C on chromosome 12p13.3 encodes the 24 transmembrane segment, pore-forming α subunit of the L-type voltage-dependent Ca^{2+} channel. Gain of function mutations in *CACNA1C* cause Timothy syndrome (LQT8) by resulting in loss of voltage-dependent channel inactivation and increased Ca^{2+} current, which prolongs APD [58]. Timothy syndrome is a multisystem disorder characterized by markedly prolonged QT intervals and lethal ventricular arrhythmias, autism, cognitive and immune deficiencies, and webbed fingers and toes. Expression of *CACNA1C* has been demonstrated in all tissues involved in Timothy syndrome.

Loss of function mutations in *CACNA1C* have recently been demonstrated to result in a new familial SCD syndrome characterized by Brugada syndrome phenotype with shorter than normal QT intervals [59].

Mutations affecting sarcoplasmic I_{Ca}

The ryanodine receptor, encoded by the 105 exon *RYR2* gene, is responsible for Ca^{2+} release from the SR in response to Ca^{2+} entering the cardiomyocyte during the plateau phase of the action potential. Ryanodine receptor binds to an inhibitory subunit, calstabin 2. During exercise and sympathetic stimulation, ryanodine receptor phosphorylation by protein kinase A partially dissociates calstabin 2 to result in increased intracellular Ca^{2+} release and contractility. Gain of function *RYR2* mutations inherited in an autosomal dominant manner result in catecholaminergic polymorphic ventricular tachycardia (CPVT), a disease characterized by exercise- or stress-induced bidirectional and polymorphic VT and strikingly early age of SCD, with 30–50% mortality by age 35 [60,61].

Mutant *RYR2* channels exhibit reduced binding to calstabin 2, leading to normal sarcoplasmic Ca^{2+} release at rest but augmented Ca^{2+} release during exercise, accounting for the CPVT phenotype [62]. Missense *RYR2* mutations linked to CPVT have also been shown to cause frequent delayed afterdepolarizations and premature ventricular complexes during epinephrine infusion, lending further mechanistic support for the observation of exercise dependence of ventricular arrhythmias [63]. An analysis of *RYR2* mutations causing disease showed that sporadic mutations are associated with a much younger age of SCD than inherited mutations are (8 ± 4 yr versus 20 ± 16 yr), due to the fact that the more severe phenotypes associated with sporadic mutations decrease their chance of inheritance [60].

Autosomal dominant *RYR2* mutations have also been linked in four Italian families to the type 2 form of arrhythmogenic right ventricular dysplasia (ARVD), a disease characterized by progressive fibrofatty replacement of the right ventricular myocardium, monomorphic VT, and SCD [64]. ARVD has a prevalence of approximately 1:5000 and is the most common cause of SCD in competitive athletes in Italy [65]. In addition to *RYR2* mutations, ARVD has also been described in association with TGF-β3 mutations [66], but it is predominantly a disease of desmosomal protein abnormalities, as described later. A murine model of one of the *RYR2* mutations associated with type 2 ARVD, R176Q, exhibited catecholamine-induced VT without structural abnormalities of the myocardium [67]. Moreover, type 2 ARVD is uniquely associated with effort-related VT and early SCD [68], supporting the notion that type 2 ARVD may in fact be an allelic variant of CPVT.

Calsequestrin 2, encoded by the *CASQ2* gene on chromosome 1p13.3-p11, is a glycoprotein that serves as the main Ca^{2+} reservoir within the SR. Mutations in *CASQ2*, inherited in an autosomal recessive fashion, cause a genetic variant of CPVT [69–71]. Investigation thus far suggests that *CASQ2* mutations lead to altered Ca^{2+} handling and delayed afterdepolarizations to facilitate the development of ventricular tachyarrhythmias [69].

Inherited cardiomyopathies

The two major genetic primary structural cardiomyopathies with significant risk for SCD, as classified in the recent American Heart Association scientific statement, are ARVD and hypertrophic cardiomyopathy (HCM) [65]. With some exceptions, ARVD is caused by mutations affecting desmosomal proteins which form an integral component of cell–cell junctions while HCM is caused by mutations affecting sarcomeric proteins of the myocardial contractile apparatus.

Mutations affecting desmosomal proteins

Myocardial desmosomes, along with gap junctions and adherens junctions, comprise the intercalated disc, which provides the structural and mechanical integrity joining cardiomyocytes. Desmosomes connect the plasma membrane with the intermediate filament network and are involved in the structural organization of the intercalated disc [72]. Desmosomes are expressed in tissues that experience mechanical stress, such as myocardium and epidermis.

Table 4.3 Genes encoding desmosomal proteins and associated arrhythmogenic right ventricular dysplasia phenotypes

Gene	Locus	Protein	Phenotypes	Mutations	Inheritance
PKP2	12p11	Plakophilin 2	ARVD	Multiple	AD/AR
DSG2	18q12.1	Desmoglein 2	ARVD	Multiple	AD
DSP	6p24	Desmoplakin	ARVD	N terminus	AD
			ARVD + LV	C terminus	AD
JUP	17q21	Plakoglobin	Naxos	2 bp deletion	AR
DSC2	18q12.1	Desmocollin 2	ARVD	Stop codon	AD

Altered desmosomes are most vulnerable under conditions of excess mechanical stress (e.g., athletic patients) and in the thinnest regions of the right ventricle—the right ventricular outflow tract, the inflow region, and the apex—which demonstrate the most involvement in ARVD (i.e., "triangle of dysplasia"). Disruption and degeneration of cardiomyocytes results in fibrofatty replacement with altered conduction properties to create the substrate for VT and SCD. Desmosomes have recently been found to participate in the Wnt/β-catenin signaling pathway which is involved in cell proliferation and differentiation. Desmosome dysfunction leads to plakoglobin translocation to the nucleus resulting in altered Wnt/β-catenin signaling and may shift cells from cardiomyocyte to adipocyte differentiation [73].

Causal mutations in the five major proteins of the desmosome—plakophilin 2 (*PKP2*), desmoglein 2 (*DSG2*), desmoplakin (*DSP*), plakoglobin (*JUP*), and desmocollin 2 (*DSC2*)—have all been demonstrated in ARVD (Table 4.3). The majority of these mutations are inherited in an autosomal dominant fashion. A notable exception is a rare autosomal recessive mutation in *JUP*, which causes Naxos disease, characterized by ARVD, palmoplantar keratoderma, and woolly hair. *PKP2* mutations are the most common in ARVD patients, accounting for 27–43% of unrelated cases, and up to 70% of familial cases [74,75]. However, no significant difference in the occurrence of ventricular arrhythmias, SCD, or appropriate implantable cardioverter-defibrillator discharges has been found in *PKP2* mutation carriers versus noncarriers [75,76]. In contrast, *DSP* mutations are associated with a high rate of SCD and left ventricular involvement in up to 50% of carriers [77].

The clinical spectrum of ARVD caused by these mutations is highly variable. Mutations have characteristically variable penetrance based on gender (higher in men than women) [78,79] and epigenetic influences, such as exposure to intense physical activity or viral agents [80]. In support of the observation that ARVD patients participating in regular intensive sports have a higher rate of syncope and SCD than sedentary patients [81], heterozygous plakoglobin-deficient mice that underwent daily exercise developed more right ventricular tachycardias and dysfunction than inactive controls [82].

Mutations affecting sarcomeric proteins

Over 400 individual mutations in 10 major sarcomeric myofilament proteins have been described in association with HCM (Table 4.4). HCM is the most prevalent genetic cardiomyopathy (1:500), characterized by unexplained left ventricular hypertrophy (LVH), fibrosis, and myocyte disarray. Myocyte disarray is a direct consequence of mutations in sarcomeric elements [83]. HCM is a phenotypically and genetically heterogeneous disease with manifestations ranging from a symptom-free lifelong course to refractory congestive heart failure, and it is recognized as the most common cause of SCD in individuals under age 35 [84]. Although predominantly a disease of the sarcomere, HCM has also been described as associated with mutations in genes encoding proteins of the closely associated cardiac Z-disc, telethonin (*TCAP*), LIM protein (*CSRP3*), α actinin 2 (*ACTN2*), vinculin/ metavinculin (*VCL*), and LIM domain binding 3 (*LDB3*) [85–87]. Recently, metabolic variants of HCM have been reported, with mutations in two genes

Table 4.4 Genes encoding sarcomeric and nonsarcomeric proteins associated with hypertrophic cardiomyopathy

Gene	Locus	Protein	Inheritance	Frequency
Sarcomeric				
MYH7	14q11.2-12	β-Myosin heavy chain	AD	~35%
TNNT2	1q32	Cardiac troponin T	AD	~20%
MYBPC3	11p11.2	Cardiac myosin-binding protein C	AD	~20%
TPM1	15q22.1	α-Tropomyosin	AD	~5%
TNNI3	19p13.4	Cardiac troponin I	AD	~5%
TTN	2q24.3	Titin	AD	1–5%
MYH6	14q11.2-12	α-Myosin heavy chain	AD	1–5%
MYL2	12q23-24.3	Regulatory myosin light chain	AD	1–5%
MYL3	3p21.2-21.3	Essential myosin light chain	AD	1–5%
ACTC	15q14	α-Cardiac actin	AD	1–5%
Z-Disc				
TCAP	17q12-21.1	Telethonin	AD	Rare
CSRP3	11p15.1	Muscle LIM protein	AD	Rare
ACTN2	1q42-43	α-Actinin 2	AD	Rare
VCL	10q22.1-23	Vinculin/metavinculin	AD	Rare
LDB3	10q22.2-23.3	LIM binding domain 3	AD	Rare
Metabolic				
PRKAG2	7q35-36.36	AMP-activated protein kinase	AD	Rare
LAMP2	Xq24	Lysosome-associated membrane protein 2	X-linked	Rare

associated with glycogen storage disease—*PRKAG2*, encoding protein kinase γ -2, and *LAMP2*, encoding lysosome-associated membrane protein 2 [88,89].

Mutations in sarcomeric proteins causing HCM are inherited in an autosomal dominant fashion. These mutations most commonly encode truncated sarcomeric proteins due to missense, insertion, deletion, or splice site mutations. Mutations in the β myosin heavy chain gene (*MYH7*) are the most common, followed by cardiac myosin-binding protein C (*MYBPC3*), critical to the assembly of the thick filament. Up to 5% of patients harbor multiple mutations [90,91]. Penetrance and phenotypic expression of these mutations are highly variable. One factor is the presence of genetic variation at other loci; SNPs in the renin–angiotensin–aldosterone system can influence the degree of LVH in family members carrying an identical *MYBPC3* mutation [92].

Genotyping of sarcomeric genes has been considered as a means of risk stratification for mortality and SCD in HCM. Initial studies suggested the presence of mutations associated with a benign clinical course and low incidence of SCD [93–98], but later studies did not confirm these observations

[99–101]. The difficulty of such an approach was highlighted by a recent study that genotyped unrelated HCM patients for eight particular "benign" mutations in *MYH7*, *TNNT2*, and *TPM1*. Only 1.7% of the 293 patients were carriers of these mutations, all of who had severe manifestations and most of whom had a family history of SCD. Therefore, out of the context of the families (and cosegregating genetic and environmental milieu) in whom they are described, it is difficult to assign particular risks to individual mutations.

Polygenic cardiac disease predisposing to SCD

CAD and its consequences account for the vast majority of SCDs, which usually occur in the setting of an acute or previous myocardial infarction (MI) and/or resultant left ventricular dysfunction [2,3]. A genetic susceptibility to SCD in the setting of acquired heart disease is supported by several epidemiologic studies, which demonstrate that a family history of SCD, independent of the risk for CAD or MI, is a risk factor for SCD [102–104]. A recent case–control study confirmed the finding that

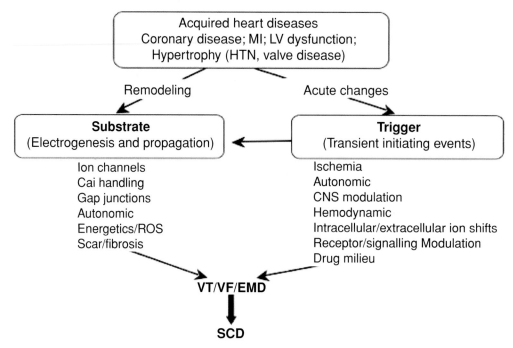

Figure 4.4 Pathophysiology of SCD in the setting of acquired heart disease.

familial SCD is a strong predictor for primary VF in the setting of acute ischemia [102].

Traditional linkage analysis approaches, based on the collection of pedigrees of affected individuals and analysis for linkage of transmission across generations of the phenotype and marker alleles, are ideally suited for investigation of rare mutations causing diseases with high penetrance, such as the monogenic diseases described above. Such an approach has low power to detect causative genetic variants for complex, polygenic diseases such as SCD associated with CAD [105,106], which are likely caused by a combination of multiple common genetic variants (SNPs) with variable penetrance rather than rare single mutations. Therefore, association studies comparing the frequency of SNPs in candidate genes or in the whole genome in affected and nonaffected individuals are the preferred strategy [105]. Independent of genetic variation, environmental influences and triggers also play a significant role in modulating the risk for the common form of SCD [107].

Candidate genes for SCD in the setting of CAD include any of those discussed above, as well as other genes in the pathways (substrate or triggers) involved in the pathophysiology of SCD in the setting of acquired heart disease (Figure 4.4). An SNP in one such candidate gene, the β2 adrenergic receptor, has recently been implicated in the risk for out-of-hospital SCD [108]. Replication of these findings will be critical as false positive findings are common in association studies [109] and study designs evaluating a homogeneous phenotype are essential for the discovery of genetic association. The recent completion of the Human Genome Project and the International HapMap Project, which is a catalog of tag SNPs that identify shared haplotypes throughout the genome, will facilitate future candidate gene and whole genome association studies.

References

1 Risch N, Merikangas K. The future of genetic studies of complex human diseases. Science 1996;273(5281):1516–1517.
2 Zheng ZJ, Croft JB, Giles WH, et al. Sudden cardiac death in the United States, 1989 to 1998. Circulation 2001;104(18):2158–2163.
3 Huikuri HV, Castellanos A, Myerburg RJ. Sudden death due to cardiac arrhythmias. N Engl J Med 2001;345(20):1473–1482.

4 Wang Q, Li Z, Shen J, et al. Genomic organization of the human SCN5A gene encoding the cardiac sodium channel. Genomics 1996;34(1):9–16.

5 Clancy CE, Rudy Y. Linking a genetic defect to its cellular phenotype in a cardiac arrhythmia. Nature 1999;400(6744):566–569.

6 Wang Q, Shen J, Splawski I, et al. SCN5A mutations associated with an inherited cardiac arrhythmia, long QT syndrome. Cell 1995;80(5):805–811.

7 Chen Q, Kirsch GE, Zhang D, et al. Genetic basis and molecular mechanism for idiopathic ventricular fibrillation. Nature 1998;392(6673):293–296.

8 Akai J, Makita N, Sakurada H, et al. A novel SCN5A mutation associated with idiopathic ventricular fibrillation without typical ECG findings of Brugada syndrome. FEBS Lett 2000;479(1–2):29–34.

9 Sangwatanaroj S, Yanatasneejit P, Sunsaneewitayakul B, et al. Linkage analyses and SCN5A mutations screening in five sudden unexplained death syndrome (Lai-tai) families. J Med Assoc Thai 2002;85(Suppl 1):S54–S61.

10 Vatta M, Dumaine R, Varghese G, et al. Genetic and biophysical basis of sudden unexplained nocturnal death syndrome (SUNDS), a disease allelic to Brugada syndrome. Hum Mol Genet 2002;11(3):337–345.

11 Baron RC, Thacker SB, Gorelkin L, et al. Sudden death among Southeast Asian refugees. An unexplained nocturnal phenomenon. JAMA 1983;250(21):2947–2951.

12 Nademanee K, Veerakul G, Nimmannit S, et al. Arrhythmogenic marker for the sudden unexplained death syndrome in Thai men. Circulation 1997;96(8):2595–2600.

13 Bezzina C, Veldkamp MW, van Den Berg MP, et al. A single Na(+) channel mutation causing both long-QT and Brugada syndromes. Circ Res 1999;85(12):1206–1213.

14 Moss AJ, Schwartz PJ, Crampton RS, et al. The long QT syndrome. Prospective longitudinal study of 328 families. Circulation 1991;84(3):1136–1144.

15 Antzelevitch C, Shimizu W. Cellular mechanisms underlying the long QT syndrome. Curr Opin Cardiol 2002;17(1):43–51.

16 George AL Jr. Inherited disorders of voltage-gated sodium channels. J Clin Invest 2005;115(8):1990–1999.

17 Schwartz PJ, Priori SG, Spazzolini C, et al. Genotype-phenotype correlation in the long-QT syndrome: gene-specific triggers for life-threatening arrhythmias. Circulation Jan 2 2001;103(1):89–95.

18 Schwartz PJ, Priori SG, Locati EH, et al. Long QT syndrome patients with mutations of the SCN5A and HERG genes have differential responses to Na$^+$ channel blockade and to increases in heart rate. Implications for gene-specific therapy. Circulation 1995;92(12):3381–3386.

19 Priori SG, Schwartz PJ, Napolitano C, et al. Risk stratification in the long-QT syndrome. N Engl J Med 2003;348(19):1866–1874.

20 Brugada P, Brugada J. Right bundle branch block, persistent ST segment elevation and sudden cardiac death: a distinct clinical and electrocardiographic syndrome. A multicenter report. J Am Coll Cardiol 1992;20(6):1391–1396.

21 Brugada J, Brugada P. Further characterization of the syndrome of right bundle branch block, ST segment elevation, and sudden cardiac death. J Cardiovasc Electrophysiol 1997;8(3):325–331.

22 Schulze-Bahr E, Eckardt L, Breithardt G, et al. Sodium channel gene (SCN5A) mutations in 44 index patients with Brugada syndrome: different incidences in familial and sporadic disease. Hum Mutat 2003;21(6):651–652.

23 Baroudi G, Acharfi S, Larouche C, et al. Expression and intracellular localization of an SCN5A double mutant R1232W/T1620M implicated in Brugada syndrome. Circ Res 2002;90(1):E11–E16.

24 Baroudi G, Napolitano C, Priori SG, et al. Loss of function associated with novel mutations of the SCN5A gene in patients with Brugada syndrome. Can J Cardiol 2004;20(4):425–430.

25 Baroudi G, Pouliot V, Denjoy I, et al. Novel mechanism for Brugada syndrome: defective surface localization of an SCN5A mutant (R1432G). Circ Res 2001;88(12):E78–E83.

26 Valdivia CR, Tester DJ, Rok BA, et al. A trafficking defective, Brugada syndrome-causing SCN5A mutation rescued by drugs. Cardiovasc Res 2004;62(1):53–62.

27 Dumaine R, Towbin JA, Brugada P, et al. Ionic mechanisms responsible for the electrocardiographic phenotype of the Brugada syndrome are temperature dependent. Circ Res 1999;85(9):803–809.

28 Rook MB, Bezzina Alshinawi C, Groenewegen WA, et al. Human SCN5A gene mutations alter cardiac sodium channel kinetics and are associated with the Brugada syndrome. Cardiovasc Res 1999;44(3):507–517.

29 Wang DW, Makita N, Kitabatake A, et al. Enhanced Na(+) channel intermediate inactivation in Brugada syndrome. Circ Res 2000;87(8):E37–E43.

30 Priori SG, Napolitano C, Gasparini M, et al. Natural history of Brugada syndrome: insights for risk stratification and management. Circulation 2002;105(11):1342–1347.

31 Nakano Y, Tashiro S, Kinoshita E, et al. Non-SCN5A related Brugada syndromes: verification of normal splicing and trafficking of SCN5A without exonic mutations. Ann Hum Genet 2007;71(Pt 1):8–17.

32 Antzelevitch C. Ion channels and ventricular arrhythmias: cellular and ionic mechanisms underlying the Brugada syndrome. Curr Opin Cardiol 1999;14(3):274–279.

33 Antzelevitch C, Yan GX, Shimizu W. Transmural dispersion of repolarization and arrhythmogenicity: the Brugada syndrome versus the long QT syndrome. J Electrocardiol 1999;32(Suppl):158–165.

34 Kurita T, Shimizu W, Inagaki M, et al. The electrophysiologic mechanism of ST-segment elevation in Brugada syndrome. J Am Coll Cardiol 2002;40(2):330–334.

35 Yan GX, Antzelevitch C. Cellular basis for the Brugada syndrome and other mechanisms of arrhythmogenesis associated with ST-segment elevation. Circulation 1999;100(15):1660–1666.

36 Poelzing S, Forleo C, Samodell M, et al. SCN5A polymorphism restores trafficking of a Brugada syndrome mutation on a separate gene. Circulation 2006;114(5):368–376.

37 Antzelevitch C, Brugada R. Fever and Brugada syndrome. Pacing Clin Electrophysiol 2002;25(11):1537–1539.

38 Di Diego JM, Cordeiro JM, Goodrow RJ, et al. Ionic and cellular basis for the predominance of the Brugada syndrome phenotype in males. Circulation 2002;106(15): 2004–2011.

39 Splawski I, Timothy KW, Tateyama M, et al. Variant of SCN5A sodium channel implicated in risk of cardiac arrhythmia. Science 2002;297(5585):1333–1336.

40 Keating MT, Sanguinetti MC. Molecular and cellular mechanisms of cardiac arrhythmias. Cell 2001;104(4): 569–580.

41 Plaster NM, Tawil R, Tristani-Firouzi M, et al. Mutations in Kir2.1 cause the developmental and episodic electrical phenotypes of Andersen's syndrome. Cell 2001;105(4):511–519.

42 Bendahhou S, Donaldson MR, Plaster NM, et al. Defective potassium channel Kir2.1 trafficking underlies Andersen-Tawil syndrome. J Biol Chem 2003;278(51):51779–51785.

43 Furutani M, Trudeau MC, Hagiwara N, et al. Novel mechanism associated with an inherited cardiac arrhythmia: defective protein trafficking by the mutant HERG (G601S) potassium channel. Circulation 1999;99(17): 2290–2294.

44 Moss AJ, Zareba W, Kaufman ES, et al. Increased risk of arrhythmic events in long-QT syndrome with mutations in the pore region of the human ether-a-go-go-related gene potassium channel. Circulation 2002;105(7): 794–799.

45 Shimizu W, Horie M, Ohno S, et al. Mutation site-specific differences in arrhythmic risk and sensitivity to sympathetic stimulation in the LQT1 form of congenital long QT syndrome: multicenter study in Japan. J Am Coll Cardiol 2004;44(1):117–125.

46 Imboden M, Swan H, Denjoy I, et al. Female predominance and transmission distortion in the long-QT syndrome. N Engl J Med 2006;355(26):2744–2751.

47 Yang P, Kanki H, Drolet B, et al. Allelic variants in long-QT disease genes in patients with drug-associated torsades de pointes. Circulation 2002;105(16):1943–1948.

48 Kubota T, Horie M, Takano M, et al. Evidence for a single nucleotide polymorphism in the KCNQ1 potassium channel that underlies susceptibility to life-threatening arrhythmias. J Cardiovasc Electrophysiol 2001;12(11):1223–1229.

49 Sesti F, Abbott GW, Wei J, et al. A common polymorphism associated with antibiotic-induced cardiac arrhythmia. Proc Natl Acad Sci U S A 2000;97(19):10613–10618.

50 Gaita F, Giustetto C, Bianchi F, et al. Short QT Syndrome: a familial cause of sudden death. Circulation 2003;108(8):965–970.

51 Bellocq C, van Ginneken AC, Bezzina CR, et al. Mutation in the KCNQ1 gene leading to the short QT-interval syndrome. Circulation 2004;109(20):2394–2397.

52 Brugada R, Hong K, Dumaine R, et al. Sudden death associated with short-QT syndrome linked to mutations in HERG. Circulation 2004;109(1):30–35.

53 Priori SG, Pandit SV, Rivolta I, et al. A novel form of short QT syndrome (SQT3) is caused by a mutation in the KCNJ2 gene. Circ Res 2005;96(7):800–807.

54 Schimpf R, Wolpert C, Gaita F, et al. Short QT syndrome. Cardiovasc Res 2005;67(3):357–366.

55 Borggrefe M, Wolpert C, Antzelevitch C, et al. Short QT syndrome. Genotype-phenotype correlations. J Electrocardiol 2005;38(4 Suppl):75–80.

56 Mohler PJ, Schott JJ, Gramolini AO, et al. Ankyrin-B mutation causes type 4 long-QT cardiac arrhythmia and sudden cardiac death. Nature 2003;421(6923):634–639.

57 Vatta M, Ackerman MJ, Ye B, et al. Mutant caveolin-3 induces persistent late sodium current and is associated with long-QT syndrome. Circulation 2006;114(20):2104–2112.

58 Splawski I, Timothy KW, Sharpe LM, et al. Ca(V)1.2 calcium channel dysfunction causes a multisystem disorder including arrhythmia and autism. Cell 2004;119(1):19–31.

59 Antzelevitch C, Pollevick GD, Cordeiro JM, et al. Loss-of-function mutations in the cardiac calcium channel underlie a new clinical entity characterized by ST-segment elevation, short QT intervals, and sudden cardiac death. Circulation 2007;115(4):442–449.

60 George CH, Jundi H, Thomas NL, et al. Ryanodine receptors and ventricular arrhythmias: emerging trends in mutations, mechanisms and therapies. J Mol Cell Cardiol 2007;42(1):34–50.

61 Priori SG, Napolitano C, Tiso N, et al. Mutations in the cardiac ryanodine receptor gene (hRyR2) underlie catecholaminergic polymorphic ventricular tachycardia. Circulation 2001;103(2):196–200.

62 Wehrens XH, Lehnart SE, Huang F, et al. FKBP12.6 deficiency and defective calcium release channel (ryanodine receptor) function linked to exercise-induced sudden cardiac death. Cell 2003;113(7):829–840.

63 Paavola J, Viitasalo M, Laitinen-Forsblom PJ, et al. Mutant ryanodine receptors in catecholaminergic polymorphic ventricular tachycardia generate delayed afterdepolarizations due to increased propensity to Ca^{2+} waves. Eur Heart J 2007, 28(9):1135–1142.

64 Tiso N, Stephan DA, Nava A, et al. Identification of mutations in the cardiac ryanodine receptor gene in families affected with arrhythmogenic right ventricular cardiomyopathy type 2 (ARVD2). Hum Mol Genet 2001;10(3):189–194.

65 Maron BJ, Towbin JA, Thiene G, et al. Contemporary definitions and classification of the cardiomyopathies: an American Heart Association Scientific Statement from the Council on Clinical Cardiology, Heart Failure and Transplantation Committee; Quality of Care and Outcomes Research and Functional Genomics and Translational Biology Interdisciplinary Working Groups; and Council on Epidemiology and Prevention. Circulation 2006;113(14):1807–1816.

66 Beffagna G, Occhi G, Nava A, et al. Regulatory mutations in transforming growth factor-beta3 gene cause arrhythmogenic right ventricular cardiomyopathy type 1. Cardiovasc Res 2005;65(2):366–373.

67 Kannankeril PJ, Mitchell BM, Goonasekera SA, et al. Mice with the R176Q cardiac ryanodine receptor mutation exhibit catecholamine-induced ventricular tachycardia and cardiomyopathy. Proc Natl Acad Sci USA 2006;103(32):12179–12184.

68 Nava A, Canciani B, Daliento L, et al. Juvenile sudden death and effort ventricular tachycardias in a family with right ventricular cardiomyopathy. Int J Cardiol 1988;21(2):111–126.

69 di Barletta MR, Viatchenko-Karpinski S, Nori A, et al. Clinical phenotype and functional characterization of CASQ2 mutations associated with catecholaminergic polymorphic ventricular tachycardia. Circulation 2006;114(10):1012–1019.

70 Lahat H, Eldar M, Levy-Nissenbaum E, et al. Autosomal recessive catecholamine- or exercise-induced polymorphic ventricular tachycardia: clinical features and assignment of the disease gene to chromosome 1p13-21. Circulation 2001;103(23):2822–2827.

71 Lahat H, Pras E, Olender T, et al. A missense mutation in a highly conserved region of CASQ2 is associated with autosomal recessive catecholamine-induced polymorphic ventricular tachycardia in Bedouin families from Israel. Am J Hum Genet 2001;69(6):1378–1384.

72 Basso C, Czarnowska E, Della Barbera M, et al. Ultrastructural evidence of intercalated disc remodelling in arrhythmogenic right ventricular cardiomyopathy: an electron microscopy investigation on endomyocardial biopsies. Eur Heart J 2006;27(15):1847–1854.

73 Garcia-Gras E, Lombardi R, Giocondo MJ, et al. Suppression of canonical Wnt/beta-catenin signaling by nuclear plakoglobin recapitulates phenotype of arrhythmogenic right ventricular cardiomyopathy. J Clin Invest 2006;116(7):2012–2021.

74 Gerull B, Heuser A, Wichter T, et al. Mutations in the desmosomal protein plakophilin-2 are common in arrhythmogenic right ventricular cardiomyopathy. Nat Genet 2004;36(11):1162–1164.

75 van Tintelen JP, Entius MM, Bhuiyan ZA, et al. Plakophilin-2 mutations are the major determinant of familial arrhythmogenic right ventricular dysplasia/cardiomyopathy. Circulation 2006;113(13):1650–1658.

76 Syrris P, Ward D, Asimaki A, et al. Clinical expression of plakophilin-2 mutations in familial arrhythmogenic right ventricular cardiomyopathy. Circulation 2006;113(3):356–364.

77 Norman M, Simpson M, Mogensen J, et al. Novel mutation in desmoplakin causes arrhythmogenic left ventricular cardiomyopathy. Circulation 2005;112(5):636–642.

78 Hamid MS, Norman M, Quraishi A, et al. Prospective evaluation of relatives for familial arrhythmogenic right ventricular cardiomyopathy/dysplasia reveals a need to broaden diagnostic criteria. J Am Coll Cardiol 2002;40(8):1445–1450.

79 Nava A, Bauce B, Basso C, et al. Clinical profile and long-term follow-up of 37 families with arrhythmogenic right ventricular cardiomyopathy. J Am Coll Cardiol 2000;36(7):2226–2233.

80 Bowles NE, Ni J, Marcus F, et al. The detection of cardiotropic viruses in the myocardium of patients with arrhythmogenic right ventricular dysplasia/ cardiomyopathy. J Am Coll Cardiol 2002;39(5):892–895.

81 Daubert C, Vauthier M, Carre F, et al. Influence of exercise and sport activity on functional symptooms and ventricular arrhythmias in arrhythmogenic right ventricular disease. J Am Coll Cardiol 1994;23:34A.

82 Kirchhof P, Fabritz L, Zwiener M, et al. Age- and training-dependent development of arrhythmogenic right ventricular cardiomyopathy in heterozygous plakoglobin-deficient mice. Circulation 2006;114(17):1799–1806.

83 Varnava AM, Elliott PM, Sharma S, et al. Hypertrophic cardiomyopathy: the interrelation of disarray, fibrosis, and small vessel disease. Heart 2000;84(5):476–482.

84 Maron BJ. Hypertrophic cardiomyopathy: a systematic review. JAMA 2002;287(10):1308–1320.

85 Bos JM, Poley RN, Ny M, et al. Genotype-phenotype relationships involving hypertrophic cardiomyopathy-associated mutations in titin, muscle LIM protein, and telethonin. Mol Genet Metab 2006;88(1):78–85.

86 Geier C, Perrot A, Ozcelik C, et al. Mutations in the human muscle LIM protein gene in families with hypertrophic cardiomyopathy. Circulation 2003;107(10):1390–1395.

87 Hayashi T, Arimura T, Itoh-Satoh M, et al. Tcap gene mutations in hypertrophic cardiomyopathy and dilated cardiomyopathy. J Am Coll Cardiol 2004;44(11):2192–2201.

88 Arad M, Benson DW, Perez-Atayde AR, et al. Constitutively active AMP kinase mutations cause glycogen storage disease mimicking hypertrophic cardiomyopathy. J Clin Invest 2002;109(3):357–362.

89 Arad M, Maron BJ, Gorham JM, et al. Glycogen storage diseases presenting as hypertrophic cardiomyopathy. N Engl J Med 2005;352(4):362–372.

90 Richard P, Charron P, Carrier L, et al. Hypertrophic cardiomyopathy: distribution of disease genes, spectrum of mutations, and implications for a molecular diagnosis strategy. Circulation 2003;107(17):2227–2232.

91 Van Driest SL, Ommen SR, Tajik AJ, et al. Yield of genetic testing in hypertrophic cardiomyopathy. Mayo Clin Proc 2005;80(6):739–744.

92 Ortlepp JR, Vosberg HP, Reith S, et al. Genetic polymorphisms in the renin-angiotensin-aldosterone system associated with expression of left ventricular hypertrophy in hypertrophic cardiomyopathy: a study of five polymorphic genes in a family with a disease causing mutation in the myosin binding protein C gene. Heart 2002;87(3):270–275.

93 Anan R, Shono H, Kisanuki A, et al. Patients with familial hypertrophic cardiomyopathy caused by a Phe110Ile missense mutation in the cardiac troponin T gene have variable cardiac morphologies and a favorable prognosis. Circulation 1998;98(5):391–397.

94 Charron P, Dubourg O, Desnos M, et al. Clinical features and prognostic implications of familial hypertrophic cardiomyopathy related to the cardiac myosin-binding protein C gene. Circulation 1998;97(22):2230–2236.

95 Coviello DA, Maron BJ, Spirito P, et al. Clinical features of hypertrophic cardiomyopathy caused by mutation of a "hot spot" in the alpha-tropomyosin gene. J Am Coll Cardiol 1997;29(3):635–640.

96 Ho CY, Lever HM, DeSanctis R, et al. Homozygous mutation in cardiac troponin T: implications for hypertrophic cardiomyopathy. Circulation 2000;102(16):1950–1955.

97 Niimura H, Bachinski LL, Sangwatanaroj S, et al. Mutations in the gene for cardiac myosin-binding protein C and late-onset familial hypertrophic cardiomyopathy. N Engl J Med 1998;338(18):1248–1257.

98 Watkins H, Rosenzweig A, Hwang DS, et al. Characteristics and prognostic implications of myosin missense mutations in familial hypertrophic cardiomyopathy. N Engl J Med 1992;326(17):1108–1114.

99 Fananapazir L, Epstein ND. Genotype-phenotype correlations in hypertrophic cardiomyopathy. Insights provided by comparisons of kindreds with distinct and identical beta-myosin heavy chain gene mutations. Circulation 1994;89(1):22–32.

100 Havndrup O, Bundgaard H, Andersen PS, et al. The Val606Met mutation in the cardiac beta-myosin heavy chain gene in patients with familial hypertrophic cardiomyopathy is associated with a high risk of sudden death at young age. Am J Cardiol 2001;87(11):1315–1317.

101 Van Driest SL, Ackerman MJ, Ommen SR, et al. Prevalence and severity of "benign" mutations in the beta-myosin heavy chain, cardiac troponin T, and alpha-tropomyosin genes in hypertrophic cardiomyopathy. Circulation 2002;106(24):3085–3090.

102 Dekker LR, Bezzina CR, Henriques JP, et al. Familial sudden death is an important risk factor for primary ventricular fibrillation: a case-control study in acute myocardial infarction patients. Circulation 2006;114(11):1140–1145.

103 Friedlander Y, Siscovick DS, Weinmann S, et al. Family history as a risk factor for primary cardiac arrest. Circulation 1998;97(2):155–160.

104 Jouven X, Desnos M, Guerot C, et al. Predicting sudden death in the population: the Paris prospective study I. Circulation 1999;99(15):1978–1983.

105 Risch NJ. Searching for genetic determinants in the new millennium. Nature 2000;405(6788):847–856.

106 Altmuller J, Palmer LJ, Fischer G, et al. Genomewide scans of complex human diseases: true linkage is hard to find. Am J Hum Genet 2001;69(5):936–950.

107 Zipes DP, Rubart M. Neural modulation of cardiac arrhythmias and sudden cardiac death. Heart Rhythm 2006;3(1):108–113.

108 Sotoodehnia N, Siscovick DS, Vatta M, et al. Beta2-adrenergic receptor genetic variants and risk of sudden cardiac death. Circulation 2006;113(15):1842–1848.

109 Morgan TM, Krumholz HM, Lifton RP, et al. Nonvalidation of reported genetic risk factors for acute coronary syndrome in a large-scale replication study. JAMA 2007;297(14):1551–1561.

CHAPTER 5

Arrhythmogenic right ventricular dysplasia/cardiomyopathy

Rahul Jain, & Hugh Calkins

Introduction

Arrhythmogenic right ventricular dysplasia/ cardiomyopathy (ARVD/C) is a genetic cardiomyopathy characterized by ventricular arrhythmias and structural abnormalities of the right ventricle (RV) [1,2]. Pathologically, ARVD/C is characterized by progressive replacement of right ventricular myocardium with fatty and fibrous tissue [3]. The precise prevalence of ARVD/C is unknown as patients with clinical diagnosis represent only one spectrum of the disease. However, the prevalence of the disease has been estimated to be 1 in 1000 to 1 in 10,000 in the Veneto Region of Italy. Cardiovascular diseases account for 2.1 sudden deaths per 100,000 athletes per year, out of which ARVD/C accounts for 22.4% of deaths in the same region of Italy [4]. Since the first description of the disease in 1977 by Fontaine et al., there have been considerable advancements in our understanding of ARVD/C. The purpose of this chapter is to review the current understanding of ARVD/C and its management. Particular attention has been placed on reviewing new information concerning genetic loci associated with ARVD/C as well as the role of ICD and radiofrequency ablation in the management of patients with ARVD/C.

Clinical presentation and natural history

The clinical characteristics of ARVD/C were first reported by Marcus et al. in 1982 [1]. Patients

Ventricular Arrhythmias and Sudden Cardiac Death, 1st edition.
Edited by P.J. Wang, A. Al-Ahmad, H. Hsia, and P.C. Zei
© 2008 Blackwell Publishing, ISBN: 978-1-4051-6114-5.

with ARVD/C seek clinical attention most commonly for the ventricular arrhythmias. The ventricular arrhythmias, which originate in the diseased right ventricle, may be asymptomatic and detected by routine electrocardiogram (ECG), or they may cause palpitations, syncope, or sudden cardiac death (SCD) [5]. Although ARVD/C is an uncommon cause of SCD, it has been estimated that ARVD/C accounts for approximately 3–10% of SCD in individuals under the age of 65 years. Exercise has been identified as a common precipitant of arrhythmias that occur in ARVD/C [4,6,7].

Diagnosis of ARVD/C

The diagnosis of ARVD/C has been established based on the criteria set by the Task Force of the Working Group of Myocardial and Pericardial Disease of the European Society of Cardiology and of the Scientific Council on Cardiomyopathies of the International Society and Federation of Cardiology [8]. These criteria are presented in Table 5.1. Specific cardiac tests that are recommended in all patients suspected of having ARVD/C include an ECG; a signal-averaged ECG (SAECG), a Holter monitor, and an echocardiogram. Exercise stress testing should also be performed. When appropriate, more detailed analysis of RV size and function can be provided by cardiac MR and/or CT. If the results of the noninvasive tests point toward a diagnosis of ARVD/C, invasive testing including endomyocardial biopsy, right ventricular angiography, and electrophysiology testing are recommended to establish the diagnosis and help provide further information to guide treatment recommendations.

Table 5.1 Diagnostic criteria for ARVD/C

	Major criteria	*Minor criteria*
Structural or functional abnormalities	1. Severe dilation and reduction of RVEF with mild or no LV involvement	1. Mild global RV dilation and/or EF reduction with normal LV
	2. Localized RV aneurysm (akinetic or dyskinetic areas with diastolic bulging)	2. Mild segmental dilation of the RV
	3. Severe segmental dilatation of the RV	3. Regional RV hypokinesis
Tissue characterization	Infiltration of RV by fat with presence of surviving strands of cardiomyocytes	
ECG depolarization/conduction abnormalities	1. Localized QRS complex duration >110 ms in V1, V2, or V3	Late potentials in SAECG
	2. Epsilon wave in V1, V2, or V3	
ECG repolarization abnormalities		Inverted T waves in right precordial leads (V2–3 above age 12 yr in absence of RBBB)
Arrhythmias		1. LBBB VT (sustained or nonsustained) on ECG, Holter or ETT
		2. Frequent PVCs (>1000/24 h on Holter)
Family history	Family history of ARVD confirmed by biopsy or autopsy	1. Family history of premature sudden death (<35 yr) due to suspected ARVD
		2. Family history of clinical diagnosis based on present criteria

Note: The criteria state that an individual must have two major, or one major plus two minor, or four minor criteria from different categories to meet the diagnosis of ARVD/C.

Electrocardiographic evaluation

ECG abnormalities are found in up to 90% of ARVD/C patients. T wave inversion (TWI) in leads V1–V3 is a well-established ECG feature of ARVD/C, and in the absence of a RBBB is considered as a minor diagnostic criterion. The juvenile pattern of TWI (normal variant in children less than 12 yr of age) is present in 1–3% of healthy population that is 19–45 years of age but is present in 87% of patients with ARVD/C. TWI beyond V1 in a patient in the above age group, who have no apparent heart disease but do have ventricular arrhythmias of LBBB morphology, should raise the suspicion of ARVD/C [9,10].

Another typical ECG feature of ARVD/C is the "epsilon wave," which are "post excitation" electrical potentials of small amplitude that occur at the end of the QRS complex and at the beginning of the ST segment. Epsilon waves (Figure 5.1), which are seen in 33% of ARVD/C patients, are considered a major diagnostic criterion for ARVD/C. Slowed electrical conduction in the right ventricle, as a result of ARVD/C may also cause localized widening of QRS complex ($\geq$110 ms) in the right precordial leads, which is seen in 64% of the patients. Prolonged S-wave upstroke in V1 through V3 $\geq$ 55 ms is the most prevalent ECG feature seen in 95% of the patients and correlates with disease severity and induction of ventricular tachycardia on electrophysiological study [10].

Late action potentials on signal-averaged ECG (SAECG) recordings are the counterpart of the epsilon waves and are considered a minor criterion for the diagnosis of ARVD/C. The Task Force on SAECG defines a SAECG as abnormal when two or more of the following are present: (1) the duration of the signal-averaged, high frequency filtered QRS complex (fQRS) $\geq$ 114 ms; (2) the duration of the low-amplitude signal of <40 μV in the terminal portion of the filtered QRS complex (LAS40)

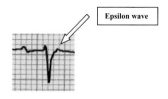

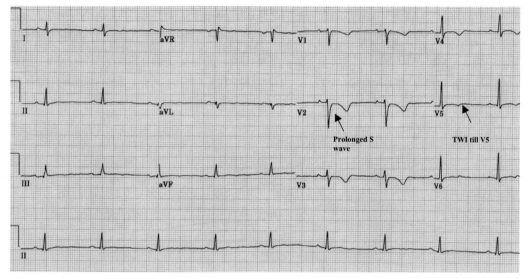

Figure 5.1 A typical ECG in a patient with ARVD/C. The arrow indicates the presence of an "epsilon wave," which represents the "post excitation" small amplitude electrical potential at the end of the QRS complex and at the beginning of the ST segment. Epsilon waves are seen in 33% of ARVD/C patients and are considered a major diagnostic criterion for ARVD/C. There are also T wave inversions that extend in this case to lead V5.

≥ 38 ms; and (3) the root-mean-square voltage of the terminal 40 ms of the filtered QRS complex (RMS40) < 20 µV. The results of several recent studies have shown that probability of an abnormal SAECG, as defined by these criteria, is related to the degree of structural disease [11,12]. The abnormal SAECG has been shown to predict inducibility on electrophysiological testing as well as implantable cardioverter defibrillator (ICD) firing [13].

Imaging of the right ventricle

Right ventricular size and function can be evaluated using a variety of imaging modalities including echocardiography, angiography, CMR, and CT. According to the Task Force criteria, a major criterion for ARVD/ C is defined as the presence of severe dilatation and/or functional loss of the RV. A less severe abnormality of RV size and/or function is considered to be minor criteria for ARVD/C. It may

be appreciated that the Task Force criteria are fairly nonspecific, in that no definition of "severe" versus "less severe" has been agreed on. Although each of the available modalities for evaluation of RV size and function can detect severe structural abnormalities of the RV, the diagnostic accuracy of these tests is less certain when used for evaluation of patients with mild disease. Right ventricular angiography has historically been regarded as the gold standard for the diagnosis of ARVD/C and has been shown to be highly specific (90%). Compared to right ventricular angiography, echocardiography is a noninvasive, widely used technique representing the first-line imaging approach in evaluating patients with suspected ARVD/C or in screening family members [14]. Limitations of echocardiography include the fact that it is subject to obtaining adequate views and that it does not allow for a qualitative evaluation of right ventricular size and function. Newer echo modalities such as three-dimensional echocardiography, strain, and tissue Doppler echocardiography may overcome some of these limitations [15,16]. CMR is an attractive imaging method because it is noninvasive and has the unique ability to characterize tissue, specifically by differentiating fat from muscle [17–19]. CMR also allows for a highly accurate and quantitative evaluation of right ventricular size and function. The newer gadolinium-enhanced MR imaging can localize the fibrosis in the RV myocardium [20,21]. Despite so many advantages, the role of CMR in ARVD/C is limited by the fact that an ICD is generally considered to be a contraindication to performing a CMR. Although we recently defined the extent of interactions between ICDs and CMR, and have shown the feasibility of performing CMR in ICD patients, these results must be considered preliminary. An additional disadvantage is that the results of CMR are highly impacted by the specific protocol with which it is performed, the presence of artifacts caused by ventricular premature beats, and the experience of the physician interpreting these results. It is our experience that CMR is a common cause of "over diagnosis" of ARVD/C [22,23]. Physicians should be careful diagnosing ARVD/C when the only abnormalities that are identified are seen on CMR. In our experience, an abnormality detected with MR imaging will virtually never be the sole abnormality detected in a patient with ARVD/C. It is also important to recognize the fact that the presence of "fat" in the myocardium may be normal and should not be considered diagnostic of ARVD/C. In fact fat, as detected with MR imaging that is not accompanied by wall motion abnormalities, is not one of the criteria for diagnosis of ARVD/C listed by the International Task force.

Myocardial biopsy

Performance of an endomyocardial biopsy is recommended for all patients suspected of having ARVD/C. This technique is most sensitive when performed on the free wall at a site of regional RV dysfunction or thinning. It is important to recognize that ARVD/C can be a patchy disease and that clear evidence for the diagnosis will be obtained in approximately one-third of affected individuals. However, when the biopsy shows fibrosis (24%) and fatty infiltration (26%) along with surviving strands of myocytes, the diagnosis of ARVD/C is

clearly established [3]. An endomyocardial biopsy is also useful in excluding other conditions such as sarcoidosis and myocarditis, which can be confused with ARVD/C [24].

Differential diagnosis

Although it is not difficult to diagnose an overt case of ARVD/C, differentiation of ARVD/C at its early stages from idiopathic ventricular tachycardia (IVT), a usually benign and nonfamilial arrhythmic condition, remains a clinical challenge [25,26]. The major differences in the two conditions are presented in Table 5.2. It is extremely important to determine if a patient has IVT or ARVD/C for two reasons. First, IVT is a benign condition, not associated with a risk of sudden death and therefore is not an indication for placement of an ICD. In contrast, there is a clear association between ARVD/C and SCD. For this reason, many patients with ARVD/C undergo placement of an ICD. Secondly, ARVD/C is hereditary whereas IVT is not. As a result when a diagnosis of ARVD/C is made, screening of all first-degree family members is recommended.

Genetics

ARVD/C is a heritable condition, typically with an autosomal dominant pattern of inheritance and variable penetrance. Most studies have reported a familial pattern of disease in approximately one-third of probands [27]. ARVD/C is primarily a disease of desmosomes. To date, 11 different genetic variants of ARVD/C have been mapped, which have been summarized in Table 5.3. These 11 genomic loci have mutations in plakoglobin (JUP), desmoplakin (DSP), the cardiac ryanodine receptor (RYR2), plakophilin-2 (PKP2), desmoglein-2 (*DSG2*), and desmocollin-2. (*DSC-2*) [28–33].

Desmosomes are complex multiprotein structures of the cell membrane and provide structural and functional integrity to adjacent cells (e.g., epithelial cells and cardiomyocytes). Desmosomal proteins also have a role in cell signaling. At least three groups of molecules contribute to the formation of desmosomes: desmosomal cadherins, armadillo-repeat proteins, and plakins [29]. The plakophilins, which are armadillo-related proteins, contain ten 42-amino-acid armadillo-repeat motifs and are located in the outer dense plaque of

Table 5.2 Differences between idiopathic VT and ARVD/C

Features	Idiopathic VT	ARVD/C
Clinical presentation		
Family history of arrhythmia or sudden cardiac death	No	Frequently yes
Arrhythmias	Morphology/or ventricular arrhythmias LBBB + II, III, AUF, − AVL PVCs, nonsustained VT, or sustained VT at rest or with exercise	May be same, but frequently morphology of ventricular arrhythmias form the basis of RV LBBB − II, III AVF, + AVL
Sudden cardiac death	Rare	1% per year
Electrocardiographic features		
T-wave morphology	T wave upright V2–V5	T wave inverted beyond V1
Parietal block	QRS duration <110 ms in V1, V2, or V3	QRS duration >110 ms
Epsilon wave V1–V3	Absent	Present in 30%
Prolonged S-wave upstroke	Rarely seen	Present in 95%
Signal-averaged ECG	Normal	Usually abnormal
Imaging features		
Echocardiogram	Normal	Increased RV size and/or wall motion abnormalities
RV ventriculogram	Usually normal	Usually abnormal
MRI	Usually normal	Increased signal intensity of RV-free wall; wall motion abnormalities with CINE MRI
Treatment		
Response to therapy	Acute: vagal maneuvers adenosine, β-blockers verapamil	
	Chronic: β-blockers or verapamil ± class one antiarrhythmic drugs	Sotalol Amiodarone ± β blockers
RF ablation	Usually curative	Seldom curative; may modify substrate to permit AA drugs; effective arrhythmias of different morphology tend to occur

desmosomes, linking desmosomal cadherins with desmoplakin and the intermediate filament system. Like other armadillo-repeat proteins, plakophilins are also found in the nucleus, where they may have a role in transcriptional regulation. Plakophilin-2 exists in two alternatively spliced isoforms (2a and 2b), which interact with multiple cell adhesion proteins and is the primary cardiac plakophilin. Gerull et al. [29] reported heterozygous mutations in PKP2, in 32 of 120 unrelated individuals with ARVD/C. Syrris et al. [31] further provided evidence that PKP2 mutation is involved in the pathogenesis of ARVD/C. Lack of plakophilin-2 or incorporation of mutant plakophilin-2 into cardiac desmosomes impairs cell–cell contact, consequently disrupting adjacent cardiomyocytes, particularly in response to mechanical stress or stretch. This provides a potential explanation for the high prevalence of the disorder in athletes, the frequent occurrence of ventricular tachyarrhythmias and sudden death during exercise and the predominant involvement of the right ventricle. Intercellular disruption would occur first in areas of high stress and stretch: the right ventricular outflow tract, apex, and inferobasal (subtricuspid) area, which are pathological predilection areas in ARVD/C (forming the "triangle of dysplasia") [29]. We recently reported a study validating the frequency of PKP2 mutations in large series of ARVD/C patients and examined the frequency of phenotypic characteristics associated

Table 5.3 Gene defects associated with ARVD/C

Genetic variant	Inheritance	Chromosome	Gene	Comment
ARVD1	AD	14q23-q24	TGFB$_3$	Characterized by progressive degeneration of RV myocardium Causes cytokine stimulating fibrosis and modulates cell adhesion
ARVD2	AD	1q41.2-q43	Cardiac ryanodine receptor	Identification of four different mutations in different families. Associated with catecholaminergic polymorphic VT. Whether ARVD2 and CPMT are different diseases due to different mutations of the RYR2 gene still remains unsettled
ARVD3	AD	14q12-q22	—	—
ARVD4	AD	2q32.1-q32.3	—	Associated with localized LV involvement with left bundle branch block in some affected members
ARVD5	AD	3p21.3,3p23	—	Seen in ARVD/C cases in Newfoundland. LAMR1 (Laminin receptor 1) gene is the possible implicated gene
ARVD6	AD	10p14-p12	—	Early onset, high penetrance
ARVD7	AD	10q22.3	—	Associated with myofibrillar myopathy. Mutation in ZASP (Z-band alternatively spliced PDZ motif- containing protein) gene in patients with myofibrillar myopathy
ARVD8 (Naxos)	AD/AR	6p24	Desmoplakin	Associated with palmoplantar keratoderma and woolly hair (Naxos disease)
ARVD9	AR	12p11	Plakophilin 2	Patients with PKP2 mutations present with arrhythmia earlier than do patients with ARVD/C who do not have the mutation
ARVD10	AD	18q12.1-q12.2	Desmoglein 2	Component of desmosome
ARVD11	AD	18q12.2	Desmocollin 2	Component of desmosome. Mutation resulted in frameshifts and premature truncation of the desmocollin-2 protein

Note: AD, autosomal dominant; AR, autosomal recessive.

with PKP2 mutations [32]. The current study highlights the fact that the presence of a PKP2 mutation in ARVD/C correlates with the earlier onset of symptoms and arrhythmias, and that the patients with PKP2 mutation experience ICD interventions irrespective of the classic risk factors determining ICD intervention in ARVD/C patients.

Identification of a gene abnormality in a family member does not provide definitive information regarding risk. The presence of an abnormal gene does not indicate the phenotypic expression, which can vary. For example, family members with plakophilin 2 have been identified who are in middle age or are the parents of an affected proband. These family members have the gene abnormality but no evidence of the disease. At the present time we feel that genetic analysis may be of clinical value in identifying those offspring that need to be followed most intensively for the development of ARVD/C. For example, assuming a PKP2 mutation is identified in a proband with ARVD/C, it would be of potential clinical value to screen the offspring for this mutation. While absence of this mutation does not totally exclude the risk of development of ARVD/C, our experience suggests that it is much less likely to develop. In contrast, if the offspring does carry the PKP2 mutation, more intensive screening for identification of early ARVD/C (i.e., biannual non-invasive testing after puberty) and/or restriction of athletic activity may be warranted.

Pathophysiologic basis of ARVD

Mutations in six genes, including four encoding desmosomal proteins (Junctional plakoglobin (JUP), Desmoplakin (DSP), Plakophilin 2, and Desmoglein have been identified in patients with ARVD/C. The *in vitro* and *in vivo* analyses done of the mutated proteins by Yang et al. [34] supported the fact that ARVD/C is a disease of the desmosomes and elucidated the possible pathogenesis. They did mutation analysis of 66 probands and identified four variants in DSP: V30M, Q90R, W233X, and R2834H. To establish a cause and effect relationship between those DSP missense mutations and ARVD/C, they performed *in vitro* and *in vivo* analyses of the mutated proteins. Unlike wild-type (WT) DSP, the N-terminal mutants (V30M and Q90R) failed to localize to the cell membrane in desmosome-forming cell line and failed to bind to and coimmunoprecipitate JUP. Multiple attempts to generate N-terminal DSP (V30 and Q90R) cardiac-specific transgenes failed: analysis of embryos revealed evidence of profound ventricular dilation, which likely resulted in embryonic lethality. They were able to develop transgenic (Tg) mice with cardiac-restricted overexpression of the C-terminal mutant (R2834H) or WT DSP. Whereas mice overexpressing WT DSP had no detectable histologic, morphologic, or functional cardiac changes, the R234H-Tg mice had increased cardiomyocyte apoptosis, cardiac fibrosis, and lipid accumulation, along with ventricular enlargement and cardiac dysfunction in both ventricles. These mice also displayed interruption of DSP–desmin interaction at intercalated discs (IDs) and marked ultrastructural changes of IDs. This data suggested DSP expression in cardiomyocyte is crucial for maintaining cardiac tissue integrity, and DSP abnormalities

result in ARVD/C by cardiomyocyte death, changes in lipid metabolism, and defects in cardiac development.

Kirchhof et al. [35] recently published a study demonstrating the age- and training-dependent development of ARVD/C in heterozygous plakoglobin-deficient mice. Ten-month old heterozygous plakoglobin-deficient mice (plakoglobin$^{+/-}$) had increased right ventricular volume, reduced right ventricular function, and spontaneous ventricular ectopy (all $P < 0.05$). Left ventricular size and function were not altered. Isolated perfused plakoglobin$^{+/-}$ hearts had spontaneous ventricular tachycardia of right ventricular origin and prolonged right ventricular conduction times compared to wild-type hearts. Endurance training accelerated the development of right ventricular dysfunction and arrhythmias in plakoglobin$^{+/-}$ mice. Histology and electron microscopy did not identify right ventricular abnormalities in affected animals. This study demonstrates that reduced expression of the junctional protein is sufficient for the development of an ARVD/C-like phenotype.

Management

In patients who have ARVD/C the risk of sudden death is higher than the normal population [36–38]. Once the patient is diagnosed as a case of ARVD/C the most important management decision is whether to implant an ICD. We will also discuss the role of antiarrhythmic therapy and catheter ablation.

ICD implantation

A decision to implant an ICD is critically important because these are young patients with few or no symptoms who are expected to live many years with a device that is not complication free. Furthermore, ICDs require replacement every 5 years and the probability of lead failure increases with time since this is a progressive disease. In addition, magnetic resonance imaging, which is valuable in the evaluation and follow up of patients with ARVD/C, is presently contraindicated after ICD implantation.

We recently reported the predictors of appropriate implantable defibrillator therapies in patients with ARVD/C [39]. The patient population

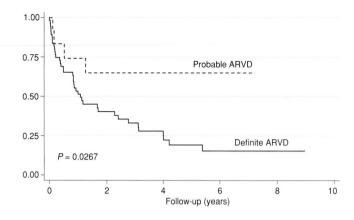

Figure 5.2 Kaplan–Meier event-free analysis (appropriate ICD intervention) according to Task Force diagnosis (definite versus probable ARVD).

consisted of 67 patients, of whom 55 had definite ARVD/C and 12 probable ARVD/C—all of whom received ICD. Thirty-five patients were males and the mean age at time of ICD placement was 36 ± 14 years (range 2–78 yr). Over a mean follow-up of 4.4 ± 2.9 years, 44 (66%) of the patients had an appropriate therapy for treatment of a sustained ventricular arrhythmia. The mean time to ICD therapy was 1.1 ± 1.4 years and the mean number of appropriate ICD intervention during follow-up was 11.6 ± 14.6 (range 1–69). Thirty-eight patients (57%) received therapy for sustained VT ≤ 240 bpm and 14 patients (21%) received therapy for life-threatening arrhythmias (VT/VF > 240 bpm). Sixteen patients (24%) received inappropriate therapy.

Based on the study results, we can conclude that the incidence of appropriate therapy was greater for patients with definite ARVD/C compared to probable ARVD/C ($P = 0.027$) (Figure 5.2) and for patients with positive electrophysiologic study ($P = 0.002$). Patients who underwent ICD placement for secondary prevention had a higher rate of appropriate ICD therapies (Figure 5.3), and there was no difference in the occurrence of life-threatening arrhythmia (VT/VF > 240 bpm) between the primary and secondary groups ($P = 0.29$). Multivariate analysis of the data identified prior sustained VT/VF (secondary prevention) as an independent predictor of receiving an appropriate ICD intervention. ($P = 0.15$) in the study.

We reported another important study that validated the frequency of PKP2 mutations in large series of ARVD/C patients and examined the frequency of phenotypic characteristics associated with PKP2 mutations [32]. DNA from 58 ARVD/C patients was sequenced to determine the presence of mutations in PKP2. Clinical features of ARVD/C were compared between two groups of patients:

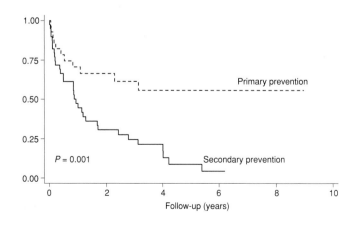

Figure 5.3 Kaplan–Meier event-free analysis (appropriate ICD intervention) according to the indication for device implantation (primary versus secondary prevention).

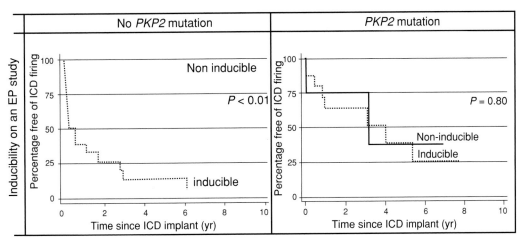

Figure 5.4 Kaplan–Meier analysis demonstrating cumulative rates of appropriate ICD intervention stratified by presence of PKP2 mutation and inducibility on EP study. EP indicates electrophysiology.

those with a PKP2 mutation and those with no detectable PKP2 mutation. Thirteen different PKP2 mutations were identified in 25 (43%) patients. Six of these mutations had not been reported previously; four occurred in multiple, apparently unrelated, families. The mean age at presentation was lower among those with a PKP2 mutation (28 ± 11 yr) than in those without (36 ± 16 yr) ($P < 0.05$). The age at both median cumulative symptom–free survival (32 versus 42 yr) and median cumulative arrhythmia–free survival (34 versus 46 yr) was lower among patients with a PKP2 mutation than among those without a PKP2 mutation ($P < 0.05$). Inducibility of ventricular arrhythmias on an electrophysiological study, diffuse nature of right ventricular disease, and presence of prior spontaneous ventricular tachycardia were identified as predictors of implanted cardioverter/defibrillator (ICD) intervention only among patients without a PKP2 mutation ($P < 0.05$) (Figure 5.4). The current study highlights the fact that the presence of a PKP2 mutation in ARVD/C correlates with earlier onset of symptoms and arrhythmias, and those patients with a PKP2 mutation experience ICD interventions irrespective of the classic risk factors determining ICD intervention in ARVD/C patients. This is an important study as it highlights the potential role of genetic analysis in management decisions. Although the precise indications for ICD implantation in patients with ARVD/C are not well defined,

we recommend ICD implantation for all patients who meet the strict Task Force criteria for ARVD/C.

Radiofrequency ablation

We recently reported the outcome of radiofrequency catheter ablation of ventricular tachycardia (VT) in ARVD/C patients enrolled in the Hopkins ARVD data base [40]. Particular focus was placed on defining the single-procedure efficacy over long-term follow up. These procedures were performed at centers throughout the United States. The study population comprised of 24 patients (age 36 ± 9 yr, 11 male) who underwent one or more RFA procedures for treatment of VT. Patients were followed for 32 ± 36 months (range 1 day–12 yr). Recurrence was defined as the documentation of VT subsequent to the procedure.

A total of 48 RFA procedures were performed using 3D electroanatomic ($n = 10$) or conventional ($n = 38$) mapping. In these procedures, 22 (46%), 15 (31%), and 11 (23%) resulted in elimination of all inducible VTs, clinical VT but not all, and none of the inducible VTs, respectively. Forty (85%) procedures were followed by recurrence. The cumulative VT recurrence-free survival was 75%, 50%, and 25% after 1.5, 5, and 14 months, respectively (Figure 5.5). The cumulative survival did not differ by procedural success, mapping technique or repetition of procedures. The cumulative incidence of VT after the repeat procedures did not differ

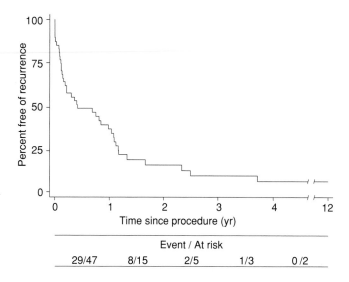

Figure 5.5 Survival analysis showing the overall cumulative VT recurrence-free survival in the entire study population. Table below the graph presents the number of events during each interval indicated on the X-axis, and the number of patients at risk at the beginning of that interval.

significantly from that after the first procedure (Figure 5.6).

Our study calls into question the value of catheter ablation in the management of patients with ARVD/C. In this regard, it is important to recognize the fact that even in the absence of catheter ablation, that VT storms are not uncommon and that they commonly respond to β-blocker or antiarrhythmic therapy. Given the high rate of recurrence during follow-up, an apparently successful ablation procedure should not be considered an appropriate reason to avoid ICD implantation in a patient with ARVD/C. We recommend that catheter ablation of VT in patients with ARVD/C should only be considered to be a palliative procedure to reduce the frequency of VT episodes, particularly after failure of one or more antiarrhythmic drugs.

Medical therapy

Symptomatic ventricular arrhythmias are treated initially with β-blocker therapy [41,42]. If this is inadequate to control patient symptoms or to

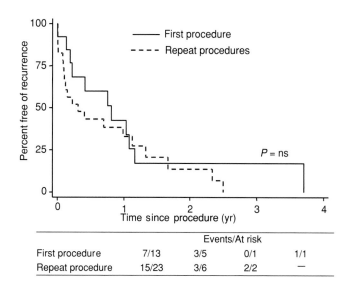

Figure 5.6 Survival analysis showing the comparison in the cumulative VT recurrence-free survival between patients undergoing first and subsequent catheter ablation procedures. Table below the graph presents the number of events during each interval indicated on the X-axis, and the number of patients at risk at the beginning of that interval.

prevent recurrence of VT, membrane-active antiarrhythmic agents such as sotalol and if necessary amiodarone are considered [43]. Further research is needed to determine if other commonly used treatments for heart failure such as angiotensin-converting enzyme inhibitors are of value for treatment of patients with ARVD/C.

Surgical treatment

Simple ventriculotomy at the site of earliest epicardial activation, total or partial disconnection of RV free wall from rest of heart has been performed in some European centers with good short-term success rates [44,45]. Since the RV may continue to enlarge after the surgery, there remains concern about progressive right heart failure. Cardiac transplantation is considered in patients with progressive heart failure and intractable recurrent ventricular arrhythmias [46]. We examined the need for cardiac transplantation in our series of 66 living patients with ARVD/C; only two underwent cardiac transplantation for incessant VT [27].

Avoidance of competitive athletics

There are several other standard recommendations, which are made for treatment of patients with this condition. First, it is recommended that all patients with ARVD/C avoid competitive athletics. Activities such as golf or walking are encouraged whereas activities such as marathon running or weight lifting should be strongly discouraged as they may hasten the progression of the disease [47].

Unanswered questions

A large number of questions remain unanswered regarding the diagnosis, treatment, and pathophysiology of ARVD/C. The natural history of the disease has yet to be defined well. Regarding treatment, further research is needed to better define which patients suspected of having ARVD/C benefit from placement of an ICD. Further work is also needed to better understand the genetic basis of ARVD/C. At the present time a mutation can be identified in approximately 50% of ARVD/C patients. In addition, the identification of the specific genetic defects may ultimately have specific therapeutic implications for gene therapy.

References

1 Marcus FI, Fontaine GH, Guiraudon G, et al. Right ventricular dysplasia: a report of 24 adult cases. Circulation 1982;65:384–398.

2 Marcus FI, Fontaine G. Arrhythmogenic right ventricular dysplasia/cardiomyopathy: a review. Pacing Clin Electrophysiol 1995;18:1298–1314.

3 Chimenti C, Pieroni M, Maseri A, Frustaci A. Histologic findings in patients with clinical and instrumental diagnosis of sporadic arrhythmogenic right ventricular dysplasia. J Am Coll Cardiol 2004;43:2305–2313.

4 Corrado D, Basso C, Rizzoli G, Schiavon M, Thiene G. Does sports activity enhance the risk of sudden death in adolescents and young adults? J Am Coll Cardiol 2003;42:1959–1963.

5 Corrado D, Basso C, Thiene G, et al. Spectrum of clinico-pathologic manifestations of arrhythmogenic right ventricular cardiomyopathy/dysplasia: a multicenter study. J Am Coll Cardiol 1997;30:1512–1520.

6 Hulot JS, Jouven X, Empana JP, Frank R, Fontaine G. Natural history and risk stratification of arrhythmogenic right ventricular dysplasia/cardiomyopathy. Circulation 2004;110:1879–1884.

7 Tabib A, Loire R, Chalabreysse L, et al. Circumstances of death and gross and microscopic observations in a series of 200 cases of sudden death associated with arrhythmogenic right ventricular cardiomyopathy and/or dysplasia. Circulation 2003;108:3000–3005.

8 McKenna WJ, Thiene G, Nava A, et al. Diagnosis of arrhythmogenic right ventricular dysplasia/ cardiomyopathy. Task Force of the Working Group Myocardial and Pericardial Disease of the European Society of Cardiology and of the Scientific Council on Cardiomyopathies of the International Society and Federation of Cardiology. Br Heart J 1994;71:215–218.

9 Marcus FI. Prevalence of T-wave inversion beyond V (1) in young normal individuals and usefulness for the diagnosis of arrhythmogenic right ventricular cardiomyopathy/dysplasia. Am J Cardiol 2005;95:1070–1071.

10 Nasir K, Bomma C, Tandri H, et al. Electrocardiographic features of arrhythmogenic right ventricular dysplasia/cardiomyopathy according to disease severity: a need to broaden diagnostic criteria. Circulation 2004;110:1527–1534.

11 Nasir K, Rutberg J, Tandri H, Berger R, Tomaselli G, Calkins H. Utility of SAECG in arrhythmogenic right ventricle dysplasia. Ann Noninvasive Electrocardiol 2003;8:112–120.

12 Nasir K, Bomma C, Khan FA, et al. Utility of a combined signal-averaged electrocardiogram and QT dispersion algorithm in identifying arrhythmogenic right ventricular dysplasia in patients with tachycardia of right ventricular origin. Am J Cardiol 2003;92:105–109.

13 Nasir K, Tandri H, Rutberg J, et al. Filtered QRS duration on signal-averaged electrocardiography predicts inducibility of ventricular tachycardia in arrhythmogenic right ventricle dysplasia. Pacing Clin Electrophysiol 2003;26:1955–1960.

14 Yoerger DM, Marcus F, Sherrill D, et al. Echocardiographic findings in patients meeting task force criteria for arrhythmogenic right ventricular dysplasia: new insights from the multidisciplinary study of right ventricular dysplasia. J Am Coll Cardiol 2005;45:860–865.

15 Donal E, Raud-Raynier P. Transthoracic tissue Doppler study of right ventricular regional function in a patient with an arrhythmogenic right ventricular cardiomyopathy. Heart 2004;90:980.

16 Lopez-Fernandez T, Garcia-Fernandez MA, Perez David E, Moreno Yanguela M. Usefulness of contrast echocardiography in arrhythmogenic right ventricular dysplasia. J Am Soc Echocardiogr 2004;17:391–393.

17 Tandri H, Calkins H, Nasir K, et al. Magnetic resonance imaging findings in patients meeting task force criteria for arrhythmogenic right ventricular dysplasia. J Cardiovasc Electrophysiol 2003;14:476–482.

18 Tandri H, Friedrich MG, Calkins H, Bluemke DA. MRI of arrhythmogenic right ventricular cardiomyopathy/dysplasia. J Cardiovasc Magn Reson 2004;6:557–563.

19 Bluemke DA, Krupinski EA, Ovitt T, et al. MR Imaging of arrhythmogenic right ventricular cardiomyopathy: morphologic findings and interobserver reliability. Cardiology 2003;99:153–162.

20 Tandri H, Saranathan M, Rodriguez ER, et al. Noninvasive detection of myocardial fibrosis in arrhythmogenic right ventricular cardiomyopathy using delayed-enhancement magnetic resonance imaging. J Am Coll Cardiol 2005;45:98–103.

21 Tandri H, Bomma C, Calkins H, Bluemke DA. Magnetic resonance and computed tomography imaging of arrhythmogenic right ventricular dysplasia. J Magn Reson Imaging 2004;19:848–858.

22 Tandri H, Calkins H, Marcus FI. Controversial role of magnetic resonance imaging in the diagnosis of arrhythmogenic right ventricular dysplasia. Am J Cardiol 2003;92:649.

23 Bomma C, Rutberg J, Tandri H, et al. Misdiagnosis of arrhythmogenic right ventricular dysplasia/ cardiomyopathy. J Cardiovasc Electrophysiol 2004;15:300–306.

24 Shiraishi J, Tatsumi T, Shimoo K, et al. Cardiac sarcoidosis mimicking right ventricular dysplasia. Circ J 2003;67:169–171.

25 O'Donnell D, Cox D, Bourke J, Mitchell L, Furniss S. Clinical and electrophysiological differences between patients with arrhythmogenic right ventricular dysplasia and right ventricular outflow tract tachycardia. Eur Heart J 2003;24:801–810.

26 Tandri H, Bluemke DA, Ferrari VA, et al. Findings on magnetic resonance imaging of idiopathic right ventricular outflow tachycardia. Am J Cardiol 2004;94:1441–1445.

27 Dalal D, Nasir K, Bomma C, et al. Arrhythmogenic right ventricular dysplasia: a United States experience. Circulation 2005;112:3823–3832.

28 Ahmad F. The molecular genetics of arrhythmogenic right ventricular dysplasia-cardiomyopathy. Clin Invest Med 2003;26:167–178.

29 Gerull B, Heuser A, Wichter T, et al. Mutations in the desmosomal protein plakophilin-2 are common in arrhythmogenic right ventricular cardiomyopathy. Nat Genet 2004;36:1162–1164.

30 Heuser A, Plovie RE, Ellinor TP, et al. Mutant desmocollin-2 causes arrhythmogenic right ventriclular cardiomyopathy. Am J Hum Genet 2006;79:1081–1088.

31 Syrris P, Ward D, Asimaki A, et al. Clinical expression of Plakophilin-2 mutations in familial arrhythmogenic right ventricular dysplasia. Circulation 2006;113;356–364.

32 Dalal D, Lorraine H, Calkins H, et al. Clinical features of arrhythmogenic right ventricular dysplaisa/cardiomyopathy associated with mutations in Plakophilin-2. Circulation 2006;113:1641–1649.

33 Pilichou K, Nava A, Basso C, et al. Mutations in Demoglein-2 gene are associated with arrhythmogenic right ventricular cardiomyopathy. Circulation 2006;113;1171–1179.

34 Zhao Y, Neil EB, Hugh C, et al. Desmosomal dysfunction due to mutations in Desmoplakin causes arrhythmogenic right ventricular dysplasia/cardiomyopathy. Circ Res 2006;99;646–655.

35 Kirchhof P, Fabritz L, Wichter T, et al. Age and training-dependent development of arrhythmogenic right ventricular cardiomyopathy in heterozygous Plakoglobin-deficient mice. Circulation 2006;114;1799–1806.

36 Corrado D, Basso C, Thiene G, et al. Does sports activity enhance the risk of sudden death in young people? Eur Heart J 1999;20:444.

37 Marcus Fl, Fontaine GH, Gallagher FR, et al. Long term follow up in patients with arrhythmogenic right ventricular disease. Eur Heart J 1989;10(Suppl D):68–73.

38 Blomstöm-Lundqvist C, Sabel CG, Oisson SB, et al. A long term follow up of 15 patients with arrhythmogenic right ventricular dysplasia. Br Heart J 1987;58:477–488.

39 Piccini JP, Dalal D, Calkins H, et al. Predictors of inappropriate implantable defibrillator therapies in patients with arrhythmogenic right ventricular dysplasia. Heart Rhythm 2005;2:1188–1194.

40 Dalal D, Jain R, Marine EJ, et al. Long term efficacy of catheter ablation of ventricular tachycardia in patients with arrhythmogenic right ventricular dysplasia/carcardiomyopathy. J Am Coll Cardiol 2007 (in press).

41 Wichter T, Borggrefe M, Haverkamp W, Chen X, Breithardt G. Efficacy of antiarrhythmic drugs in patients with arrhythmogenic right ventricular disease. Results in patients with inducible and noninducible ventricular tachycardia. Circulation 1992;86:29–37.

42 Hiroi Y, Fujiu K, Komatsu S, et al. Carvedilol therapy improved left ventricular function in a patient with arrhythmogenic right ventricular cardiomyopathy. Jpn Heart J 2004;45:169–177.

43 Tonet J, Frank R, Fontaine G, Grosgogeat Y. Efficacy and safety of low doses of beta-blocker agents combined with amiodarone in refractory ventricular tachycardia. Pacing Clin Electrophysiol 1988;11:1984–1989.

44 Misaki T, Watanabe G, Iwa T, et al. Surgical treatment of arrhythmogenic right ventricular dysplasia: long-term outcome. Ann Thorac Surg 1994;58:1380–1385.

45 Morita K, Takeuchi M, Oe K, et al. Perioperative management of Fontan operation for two patients with arrhythmogenic right ventricular dysplasia. J Anesth 2002;16:169–172.

46 Lacroix D, Lions C, Klug D, Prat A. Arrhythmogenic right ventricular dysplasia: catheter ablation, MRI, and heart transplantation. J Cardiovasc Electrophysiol 2005;16:235–236.

47 Furlanello F, Bertoldi A, Dallago M, et al. Cardiac arrest and sudden death in competitive athletes with arrhythmogenic right ventricular dysplasia. Pacing Clin Electrophysiol 1998;21:331–335.

CHAPTER 6

Risk stratification and the implantable defibrillator for the prevention of sudden death in hypertrophic cardiomyopathy

Barry J. Maron

Sudden and unexpected death has been recognized as the most devastating consequence of hypertrophic cardiomyopathy (HCM) since the initial description of this disease almost 50 years ago [1]. Over this period of time, considerable investigative interest has been generated with regard to risk stratification, definition of the mechanisms responsible for sudden death, and treatment strategies to prevent these unexpected catastrophes [2–24]. This review focuses on observations linking ventricular tachyarrhythmias with sudden death in HCM and the current role of preventive interventions such as the implantable cardioverter-defibrillator (ICD).

Historical context

Since Teare's original pathologic report of this disease [1], recognition that a small yet important subgroup of young patients with HCM are at increased risk of sudden cardiac death has for many years generated considerable interest in the role of arrhythmias and the process of risk stratification [2–5,8–14,20–23]; it is also stimulating a continuing debate regarding the most appropriate measures for effective prevention of these unpredictable events [13,24]. Indeed, over the years, many authors have emphasized that sudden death in HCM occurs

Ventricular Arrhythmias and Sudden Cardiac Death, 1st edition. Edited by P.J. Wang, A. Al-Ahmad, H. Hsia, and P.C. Zei © 2008 Blackwell Publishing, ISBN: 978-1-4051-6114-5.

disproportionately in young and asymptomatic patients [1–26].

Pharmacologic treatment

Historically, the management of high-risk HCM patients had been confined to prophylactic pharmacologic treatment with β-blockers, verapamil, and antiarrhythmic agents (such as procainamide and quinidine) and subsequently with amiodarone [2–5,15,20]. However, in HCM there are virtually no data supporting the efficacy of prophylactic drug treatment for sudden death [2–5,15,20]. For example, there are no controlled studies in the literature addressing the effects of β-blockers or verapamil on sudden death. Type IA antiarrhythmic agents have been largely abandoned as prophylactic treatment for HCM patients with isolated or infrequent runs of nonsustained ventricular tachycardia on ambulatory (Holter) ECG, due to the potential proarrhythmic effects of these drugs [5,8,16].

Following that sole study (retrospective and nonrandomized with historical controls) which over 20 years ago reported protective effects of amiodarone against sudden death in HCM with nonsustained ventricular tachycardia [15], no further data regarding the long-term protective efficacy of this drug have been published. Also, the not-infrequent adverse side effects associated with the chronic administration of amiodarone severely limits the application of this drug to sudden-death prevention in

35 yr – Brother SD
(age 39)

(a)

36 yr – ICD

5 yr 40 yr – Generator
replaced

(b)

41 yr – Appropriate
Shock #1

9 yr

(c)

50 yr – Appropriate
Shock # 2

52 yr – Present

(d)

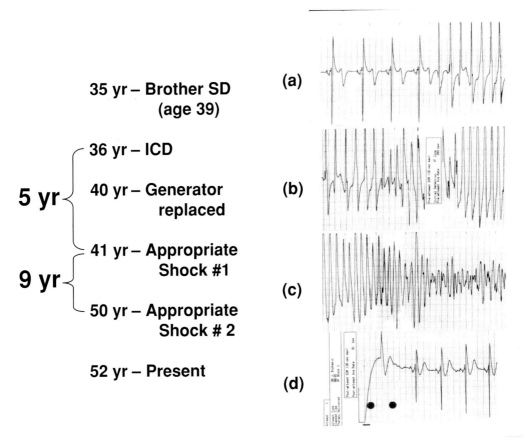

Figure 6.1 Primary prevention of sudden cardiac death in HCM. Stored ventricular electrogram from an asymptomatic 35-year-old man who received an ICD prophylactically for a family history of HCM-related sudden death and marked ventricular septal hypertrophy (i.e., wall thickness 31 mm). Intracardiac electrogram was triggered almost 5 years after the defibrillator implant (at 1:20 a.m., in sleep). Continuous recording at 25 mm/s, shown in four contiguous panels with the tracing recorded left to right in each segment. (a) Begins with 4 beats of sinus rhythm and, thereafter, ventricular tachycardia begins abruptly (at 200 beats/min); (b) Device senses ventricular tachycardia and charges; (c) Ventricular tachycardia deteriorates into ventricular fibrillation; (d) Defibrillator discharges appropriately (20-J shock) during ventricular fibrillation and restores sinus rhythm. From Maron BJ et al. [13], reproduced with permission of the Massachusetts Medical Society.

young patients with HCM who harbor extended periods of risk [7,13,20]. Therefore, due to the proven efficacy of ICD [13] the lack of pharmacologic efficacy [27] as well as unpredictable patient compliance with drugs over the many years of potential risk, pharmacologic prevention of sudden death has largely been abandoned in HCM [27].

Ventricular tachyarrhythmias and mechanisms of sudden death

Although supraventricular arrhythmias (particularly atrial fibrillation) are of great clinical importance for a substantial proportion of HCM patients by virtue of an association with heart failure, acute hemodynamic decompensation, and the risk for embolic stroke [7,19,20,28,29], ventricular arrhythmias have been most devastating due to a clear linkage with risk for sudden unexpected death [2,3,5,10,11,13,18,23,30–33] (Figures 6.1 and 6.2).

Ventricular tachyarrhythmias, as recorded by ambulatory Holter ECG, are particularly common in HCM including premature ventricular depolarizations and complex forms such as couplets and nonsustained ventricular tachycardia (VT) [8,10,11,30,34] (Figure 6.3). Short bursts of

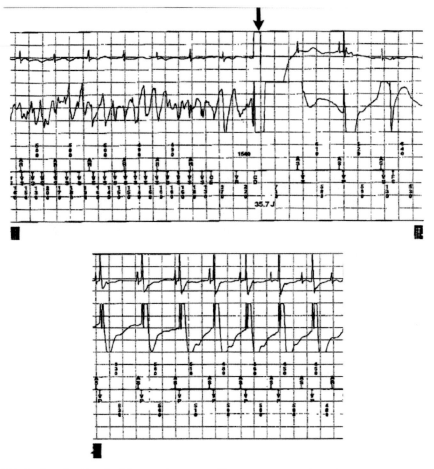

Figure 6.2 Mechanism of sudden death in HCM demonstrated by continuous recording of a stored intracardiac ventricular electrogram from a 28-year-old asymptomatic patient with extreme LV hypertrophy (ventricular septal thickness, 36 mm) who received an implantable cardioverter-defibrillator for primary prevention of sudden death. Spontaneous onset of ventricular fibrillation is automatically sensed and terminated by a defibrillation shock (arrow), immediately restoring sinus rhythm.

nonsustained VT (usually 3–6 beats) were initially identified in the 1980s as a marker for sudden death in two studies from tertiary HCM centers [10,11].

More recently, arrhythmia sequences in HCM have been documented with stored electrocardiographic recordings in patients with ICDs experiencing appropriate device interventions [13,32,35,36] (Figures 6.1 and 6.2). These observations offer a unique window to understanding the mechanisms responsible for sudden death in HCM. For example, a multicenter ICD study in high-risk HCM patients showed that VT or ventricular fibrillation (VF) triggered appropriate device activations [13], supporting the long-standing hypothesis that primary ventricular tachyarrhythmias are most commonly responsible for unexpected catastrophes in this disease [2–5,17,18,32]. Sinus tachycardia is often the initiating rhythm, suggesting that high sympathetic drive may be proarrhythmic when a susceptible substrate is present. However, it has not been possible to conclusively exclude bradycardia-mediated events because of the back-up pacing capability operative in many of the devices; indeed, other more diverse arrhythmia mechanisms may ultimately explain appropriate device interventions in HCM [19,32,33].

Ventricular tachyarrhythmias probably emanate from an electrically unstable myocardial substrate with distorted electrophysiologic propagation and

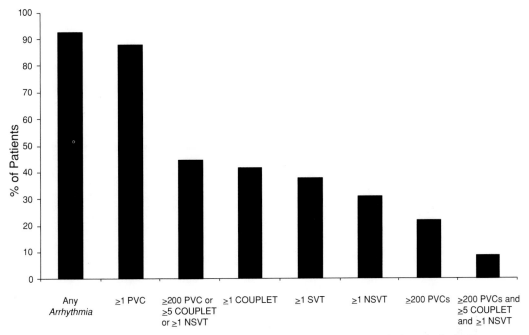

Figure 6.3 Prevalence of ventricular and supraventricular tachyarrhythmias on 24-hour ambulatory (Holter) ECG recording in HCM. NSVT, nonsustained ventricular tachycardia; PVC, premature ventricular contraction; SVT, supraventricular tachycardia. From Adabag et al. [34], reproduced with permission of American College of Cardiology.

repolarization created by disorganized cellular architecture and/or areas of replacement scarring. This fibrosis emanates from the repair process following silent bursts of myocardial ischemia that lead to myocyte necrosis (probably due to structurally abnormal, narrowed intramural arterioles) [1–5,17,20,37–41] (Figure 6.4). This arrhythmogenic myocardial substrate may be vulnerable to a variety of incompletely defined triggers, either intrinsic to the HCM disease process, or extrinsically as environmental factors such as intense physical exertion [42,43]. Undoubtedly, substantial individual patient susceptibility plays an important role in determining which individual HCM patients experience clinical events.

Risk stratification

Sudden cardiac death is a well-recognized and devastating complication of HCM, but occurs in only a minority of patients [1–24,30,32–34,42,43]. Therefore, a major clinical challenge has been the identification of that high-risk subset among all patients within the broad HCM disease spectrum. Certainly,

a measure of uncertainty and lack of precision persist regarding the stratification of sudden death risk for individual HCM patients, and no single test is capable of reliably stratifying all patients eligible for primary prevention within the HCM patient population.

Nevertheless, at present, based on the available evidence it is reasonable to conclude that the highest levels of risk are associated with one or more of the following noninvasive clinical markers (Figure 6.5) [2,3,5,8–14,21–23,30]: (1) prior cardiac arrest due to VF or sustained (and spontaneous) episodes of VT; (2) family history of premature HCM-related death, particularly if sudden, occurring in close relatives and multiple; (3) unexplained syncope, particularly in the young (and except for remote events); (4) bursts of nonsustained VT on serial ambulatory (Holter) ECGs, particularly if multiple, repetitive, or prolonged; (5) extreme phenotypic disease expression with massive left ventricular (LV) hypertrophy (maximum wall thickness ≥30 mm), particularly in the young; and (6) hypotensive (or attenuated) blood pressure response to exercise. Of note, however, in customary clinical practice it is

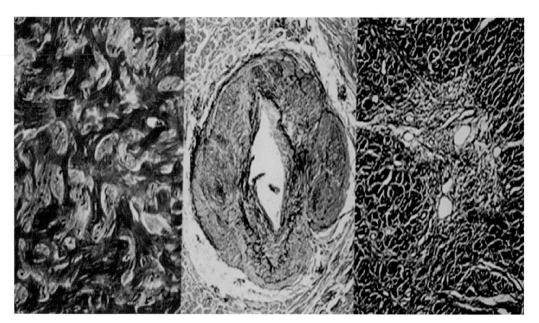

Figure 6.4 Arrhythmogenic substrate in HCM. Left: Disorganized cellular architecture. Center: Abnormal intramural coronary artery responsible for silent myocardial ischemia. Right: Myocardial scar, the repair process following ischemia and cell death (consequence of small muscle disease shown in center panel).

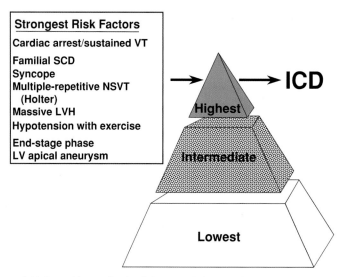

Figure 6.5 Assessment of risk for sudden cardiac death in the HCM population. At present, treatment with ICDs for prevention of sudden death is focused on the small subset of patients perceived to be at the highest risk. Secondary prevention patients are those with prior cardiac arrest or sustained VT. Primary prevention candidates are those with risk factors, i.e., family history of HCM–sudden death, unexplained syncope, multiple/repetitive/prolonged nonsustained ventricular tachycardia (NSVT) on ambulatory Holter ECG, hypotensive blood pressure response to exercise, and massive LVH. Patients in other selected high-risk patient subgroups, such as those with LV apical aneurysm (and apical scarring) or the end stage with systolic dysfunction are also candidates for a primary prevention ICD. ICD, implantable cardioverter defibrillator; LVH, left ventricular hypertrophy; SCD, sudden cardiac death; VT, ventricular tachycardia.

rare for a HCM patient to be judged at high risk based solely or largely on an abnormal blood pressure response to exercise.

Evidence is insufficient to conclude that LV outflow tract obstruction, [44–48] occurrence of atrial fibrillation [28], or myocardial ischemia [49,50] generally constitute primary independent risk factors for sudden death in HCM patients. However, the possibility that these mechanisms play a role in determining events in individual selected patients cannot be completely excluded. For example, two studies have reported a relationship between LV outflow obstruction at rest and risk for sudden death, although the particularly low positive predictive value for this marker argues against using obstruction as a sole indication for a primary prevention ICD [48].

Despite early enthusiasm, it is now apparent that defining the precise mutation in a given HCM patient cannot predict future events nor provide reliable prognostic information, i.e., with 11 genes and >400 mutations known to cause HCM the extreme intergenetic and intragenetic heterogeneity makes it virtually impossible to discern favorable from unfavorable genetic substrates [51,52]. While rapid commercial genetic testing is now available (http://www.hpcgg.org//LMM/tests.html), the principal role for gene identification is to achieve a definitive HCM diagnosis in family members or in individuals with an equivocal phenotype.

The role of electrophysiologic testing (with programmed ventricular stimulation) in defining the substrate for VF and sudden death risk in individual HCM patients [20], has been largely abandoned [2,3,5,20]. Acknowledged limitations to this technique include both the infrequency with which monomorphic VT is inducible in HCM (only 10% of patients) and the likelihood that the provoked ventricular arrhythmias are highly dependent on the precise laboratory protocol employed. For example, aggressive electrophysiologic testing utilizing three premature ventricular extra-stimuli may trigger sustained polymorphic VT/VF in a substantial proportion of patients, a result that has largely been regarded as a nonspecific response in patients with ischemic heart disease [5]. Since most high-risk HCM patients who are eligible for primary prevention can now be identified by noninvasive clinical markers [2,20,23,35,36], routine use of invasive laboratory-based testing to replicate arrhythmias now appears to have little practical value in clinical practice for predicting outcome in HCM. The vulnerable electrophysiologic substrate for reentrant arrhythmias in HCM has also been investigated by an extra-stimulus-based method assessing paced electrogram fractionation, which reflects asynchronous delayed activation and the disrupted myocardial architecture in this disease [53].

Prevention of sudden death with ICD

Since its introduction in clinical medicine by Michel Mirowski [54] nearly 30 years ago, ICD has achieved widespread acceptance as a preventive treatment for sudden death, by virtue of indisputable evidence of its efficacy in terminating life-threatening ventricular tachyarrhythmias and prolonging life, principally in high-risk patients with ischemic heart disease [55–58]. The superiority of ICD to antiarrhythmic drug treatment has been documented in several prospective, randomized trials, for both primary and secondary prevention [55–58]. ICD represents one of the major advances in cardiovascular medicine in the last 100 years [54] and for the past 25 years it has been used extensively to prevent sudden death, saving and prolonging lives of thousands of largely older patients with advanced acquired heart disease and failure [55–58].

However, the cardiovascular community has been slow to translate this powerful therapeutic strategy to the genetic heart diseases, which nevertheless are responsible for most of the sudden deaths in both young and middle-aged patients [1–7,59]. Indeed, it was not until the year 2000 that data reported from a large group of patients with HCM promoted the efficacy of the ICD for this disease [13]. Importantly, that publication triggered a considerable rise in the number of implants in the HCM patient population [31,35,36]. Indeed, despite the widespread and dramatic increase in ICD utilization in patients with coronary artery disease over more than two decades, until recently there has been relatively little application of the ICD, to less common genetic cardiovascular diseases also associated with sudden death risk in the young such as ion channelopathies (long-QT and Brugada syndromes), and arrhythmogenic right ventricular cardiomyopathy [60–63].

Specifically, there is at present a somewhat understandable reluctance on the part of pediatric cardiologists to implant prophylactic ICDs in children considering the necessary long-term commitment to device maintenance and the perhaps greater likelihood of lead or other ICD-related complications occurring over many years. However, while adolescence can represent a psychologically difficult age to be encumbered by an ICD, it should also be emphasized that this is also the period of life with the greatest predilection for sudden death in HCM [7]. Therefore, without aggressive preventive strategies utilizing ICDs, the specter of sudden death in youthful people due to HCM will continue.

When contemporary criteria judge the level of risk for sudden death to be unacceptably high and deserving of intervention, the ICD has proven to be the most effective and reliable treatment option available, harboring the potential for absolute protection and altering the natural history of this disease in some patients [13,20,31,33,35,36,54,64]. Efficacy of ICD for aborting potentially life-threatening arrhythmias has been assessed in HCM patients judged to be at high risk for sudden death, in both retrospective and prospective studies [13,31–33,35,36,64,65]. The largest of these cohorts comprised 506 HCM patients, all of whom had ICDs implanted for sudden death prevention, and were followed for an average period of about $3^1/_2$ years (up to 16) [36] (Figure 6.6). Appropriate device interventions (either defibrillation shocks or antitachycardia pacing), triggered by VT/VF, occurred in 20% of patients with an overall annual discharge rate of 5%. Appropriate intervention rate was 11%/year for secondary and 4%/year for primary prevention. Of note, almost 30% of the young patients implanted ≤20 years of age had appropriate ICD interventions at 18 ± 4 years of age (including 35% of those implanted ≤15 years old). Therefore, ICD proved effective in HCM despite the substantially increased cardiac mass characteristic of this disease (Figures 6.1 and 6.2) and the not infrequent occurrence of left ventricular outflow tract obstruction [14,44,66,67]. Furthermore, about 60% of those patients who received appropriate defibrillator therapy had experienced multiple such interventions.

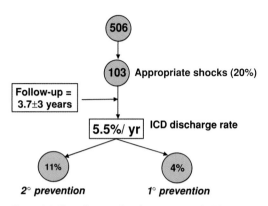

Figure 6.6 Flow diagram showing outcome of 506 high-risk HCM patients with implantable defibrillators for primary prevention (≥1 risk factors) or secondary prevention following ventricular fibrillation or sustained ventricular tachycardia.

There is general consensus and virtually no controversy that secondary sudden death prevention (i.e., with ICD) is strongly warranted in those patients with fortuitous resuscitation from prior cardiac arrest (with documented VF) or sustained and spontaneously occurring VT [13,20,33,68,69].

While the presence of multiple clinical risk factors conveys greater comfort in judging increased risk, it is also apparent that a single risk factor may be sufficient evidence to justify a recommendation for a prophylactic ICD for prevention of sudden death. Preliminary data from a large multicenter international registry showed no difference in the likelihood of an appropriate shock with ICDs implanted for 1, 2, or ≥3 risk markers [36]. Therefore many investigators, particularly in the US, favor strong consideration for a prophylactic ICD even in the presence of only one major risk factor and that one-risk-factor patients cannot be ignored in the important considerations for primary prevention [20,35]. Other (largely European) investigators are generally more conservative and restrictive in requiring two or more risk factors before raising consideration for prophylactic device implantation [22–24].

While a single risk factor may be sufficient to consider and offer the option of a prophylactic ICD to HCM patients, there are numerous clinical circumstances for which ambiguities and gray areas arise with respect to the presence, strength or number of risk factors. One such specific clinical situation is the elderly patient with a single risk factor who may not be candidates for primary prevention, given that HCM-related sudden death is uncommon in this age group [7] and survival to advanced age without complications itself generally means lower risk status in this disease [2,20,46,70]. Ultimately, many of the complex clinical scenarios regarding prophylactic ICD decisions in one-risk-factor patients may require a measure of physician judgment in the context of the individual clinical profile. Patient autonomy in combination with full physician disclosure [71–73] allows an informed HCM patient to contribute significantly to resolving such uncertainties which often arise in clinical situations We also recognize that physician and patient attitudes toward ICDs (and access to such devices within various healthcare systems) can vary considerably among countries and cultures, and thereby impact importantly on clinical decision-making and the threshold for device implant in HCM [69].

By extrapolating the reported primary prevention discharge rate, it can be estimated that within 10 years about 40% of the defibrillators prophylactically implanted in young patients will intervene to abort an important ventricular tachyarrhythmia. Indeed, the annual discharge rate achieved in this subset of patients represents a figure reminiscent of that previously reported for sudden death in the selected high-risk HCM patient cohorts evaluated at tertiary referral centers [2,3,20,25]. It should be emphasized that using prophylactic ICD in cases of sudden death as practiced in HCM, represents a novel and particularly pure form of primary prevention, given that it is based solely on the assessment of noninvasive risk factors in asymptomatic (or only mildly symptomatic) patients and that the ICD is used typically in the absence of major cardiovascular events or evidence of spontaneous sustained arrhythmias. Nevertheless, there was only a 4:1 ratio of devices implanted to lives saved in the multicenter ICD in HCM study, a favorable excess compared to that in primary prevention trials in coronary artery disease following myocardial infarction in which that ratio may be >10:1 [56]. ICD therapy in HCM has also been shown to be cost-effective (and even cost-saving) due to additional years of productive life in young high-risk patients [74].

At the time of appropriate defibrillator interventions, more than half of the patients were taking amiodarone or other antiarrhythmic drugs [13,36]. This observation, even though ancillary to the main end-points of the trial, substantiates the superiority of ICD over pharmacologic strategies for preventing sudden death as well as disputing previous claims that amiodarone provides absolute protection against sudden death in HCM patients [15].

Crucial to understanding the role of ICD within the broad HCM disease spectrum is an appreciation of certain demographic distinctions from ICD therapy in ischemic heart disease. The latter patients are of relatively advanced age at the time of implant (average, about 65 years), often with severe and progressive heart failure as a consequence of prior myocardial infarction and LV dysfunction. In sharp contrast, ICDs in HCM often involve young asymptomatic patients with an extended period of risk for sudden death and potentially many decades of productive life ahead [13,20,46,70]. Indeed, in the multicenter ICD-HCM registry [13,36] mean age at implant (and also age at first appropriate device intervention) was only 40 years. Furthermore, almost 25% of the patients were <30 years old when they received an ICD, usually for primary prevention.

Therefore, although annual appropriate intervention rates for HCM are lower than those reported in coronary artery disease [55–58], they are nevertheless significant since that experience must be placed in the context of a much younger patient population usually free of significant heart failure and noncardiac disease. Protected by ICD, these patients could survive many decades with little or no symptoms, even achieving normal or near-normal life expectancy if not encumbered by other major HCM-related or other disease complications. Therefore, ICD therapy can be regarded as potentially altering the natural history of HCM for many patients.

Of particular note, the time interval between implant and first appropriate ICD intervention may be quite variable, with particularly long delays of up to 10 years not uncommon for the initial life-saving intervention (Figure 6.7) [13,35,36]. This observation underlines the unpredictable timing of sudden death in HCM in which ICD may remain dormant for substantial periods of time before it is ultimately required to intervene appropriately.

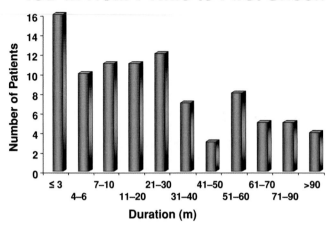

ICD in HCM : Time to First Shock

Figure 6.7 Time elapsed from implantation of the cardioverter-defibrillator (ICD) to first appropriate shock.

Conversely, some appropriate shocks occur early after implant, and not uncommonly within the first 12 months [75]. The mechanisms underlying such early interventions are unresolved and remain controversial [76].

Indeed, the decision to prophylactically implant an ICD in an HCM patient is often fortuitously based on the precise time at which risk stratification is undertaken and high-risk status identified. Once potential risk is recognized, it is difficult and probably imprudent to temporize or delay the potentially preventive treatment [75]. Indeed, a patient identified as high-risk at age 20 (and implanted with a device prophylactically) will still be young and at increased risk for an event at age 35, even if ICD has not been triggered appropriately during that 15-year period. Consequently, once the decision to implant an ICD in a high-risk HCM patient is made, it is likely to represent a life-long preventive measure.

end-stage heart failure or embolic stroke [29,77]. The single notable exception in our substantial multicenter experience was a 21-year-old college student with extreme LV hypertrophy and syncope (and normal systolic function) who died suddenly when his mechanically defective ICD (known only to the manufacturer) failed due to massive electrical overstress while delivering a defibrillation shock [71–73].

Finally, even with the life-saving potential of the ICD in HCM, it is also important to recognize the potential complications of ICD therapy that may impact on implant decisions, including inappropriate and spurious device discharges [13,36] fractured or disrupted leads, and the small risk for infection. In the ICD in HCM registry experience, such complications occurred in about 25% of patients. These possibilities must always be weighed against the ultimate potential benefit of ICD for each individual high-risk patient, i.e., preservation of life.

Conclusions

The central message of this discussion is indisputable, i.e., that ICDs are highly effective and life-saving in HCM and deserve an important role in the management of this complex disease, even in the presence of only one primary prevention risk factor. Indeed, ICDs restored sinus rhythm in virtually every HCM patient with a typical phenotypic expression and in the absence of progressive

References

1 Teare D. Asymmetrical hypertrophy of the heart in young patients. Br Heart J 1958;20:1–8.
2 Maron BJ. Hypertrophic cardiomyopathy: a systematic review. JAMA 2002;287:1308–1320.
3 Maron BJ. Hypertrophic cardiomyopathy. Lancet 1997;350:127–133.
4 Wigle ED, Rakowski H, Kimball BP, et al. Hypertrophic cardiomyopathy. Clinical spectrum and treatment. Circulation 1995;92:1680–1692.

5 Spirito P, Seidman CE, McKenna WJ, Maron BJ. The management of hypertrophic cardiomyopathy. N Engl J Med 1997;336:775–785.

6 Maron BJ, Roberts WC, Epstein SE. Sudden death in hypertrophic cardiomyopathy: profile of 78 patients. Circulation 1982;65:1388–1394.

7 Maron BJ, Olivotto I, Spirito P, et al. Epidemiology of hypertrophic cardiomyopathy-related death: revisited in a large non-referral based patient population. Circulation 2000;102:858–864.

8 Spirito P, Rapezzi C, Autore C, et al. Prognosis of asymptomatic patients with hypertrophic cardiomyopathy and nonsustained ventricular tachycardia. Circulation 1994;90:2743–2747.

9 Olivotto I, Maron BJ, Montereggi A, et al. Prognostic value of systemic blood pressure response during exercise in a community-based patient population with hypertrophic cardiomyopathy. J Am Coll Cardiol 1999;33:2044–2051.

10 Maron BJ, Savage DD, Wolfson JK, et al. Prognostic significance of 24-hour ambulatory electrocardiographic monitoring in patients with hypertrophic cardiomyopathy: a prospective study. Am J Cardiol 1981;48:252–257.

11 McKenna WJ, Camm AJ. Sudden death in hypertrophic cardiomyopathy: assessment of patients at high risk. Circulation 1989;80:1489–1492.

12 Maron BJ, Cecchi F, McKenna WJ. Risk factors and stratification for sudden cardiac death in patients with hypertrophic cardiomyopathy. Br Heart J 1994;72(Suppl):S-13–S-18.

13 Maron BJ, Shen W-K, Link MS, et al. Efficacy of implantable cardioverter-defibrillators for the prevention of sudden death in patients with hypertrophic cardiomyopathy. N Engl J Med 2000;342:365–373.

14 Spirito P, Bellone P, Harris KM, et al. Magnitude of left ventricular hypertrophy predicts the risk of sudden death in hypertrophic cardiomyopathy. N Engl J Med 2000;324:1778–1785.

15 McKenna WJ, Oakley CM, Krikler DM, et al. Improved survival with amiodarone in patients with hypertrophic cardiomyopathy and ventricular tachycardia. Br Heart J 1985;53:412–416.

16 Cecchi F, Olivotto I, Montereggi A, et al. Prognostic value of non-sustained ventricular tachycardia and the potential role of amiodarone treatment in hypertrophic cardiomyopathy: assessment in an unselected non-referral based patient population. Heart 1998;79:331–336.

17 Maron BJ, Bonow RO, Cannon RO, et al. Hypertrophic cardiomyopathy: interrelation of clinical manifestations, pathophysiology, and therapy (Parts I and II). N Engl J Med 1987;316:780–789 and 844–852.

18 Nicod P, Polikar R, Peterson KL. Hypertrophic cardiomyopathy and sudden death. N Engl J Med 1988;318:1255–1256.

19 Stafford WJ, Trohman RG, Bilsker M, et al. Cardiac arrest in an adolescent with atrial fibrillation and hypertrophic cardiomyopathy. J Am Coll Cardiol 1986;7:701–704.

20 Maron BJ, McKenna WJ, Danielson GK, et al. American College of Cardiology/European Society of Cardiology Clinical Expert Consensus Document on Hypertrophic Cardiomyopathy. A report of the American College of Cardiology Task Force on Clinical Expert Consensus Documents and the European Society of Cardiology Committee for Practice Guidelines Committee to Develop an Expert Consensus Document on Hypertrophic Cardiomyopathy. J Am Coll Cardiol 2003;42:1687–1713.

21 Sadoul N, Prasad L, Elliott PM, et al. Prospective diagnostic assessment of blood pressure response during exercise in patients with hypertrophic cardiomyopathy. Circulation 1997;96:2987–2991.

22 Elliott PM, Gimeno JR, Mahon NG, et al. Relation between severity of left-ventricular hypertrophy and prognosis in patients with hypertrophic cardiomyopathy. Lancet 2001;357:420–424.

23 Elliott PM, Poloniecki J, Dickie S, et al. Sudden death in hypertrophic cardiomyopathy: identification of high risk patients. J Am Coll Cardiol 2000;36:2212–2218.

24 Watkins H. Sudden death in hypertrophic cardiomyopathy (editorial). N Engl J Med 2000;342:422–424.

25 Maron BJ, Spirito P. Impact of patient selection biases on the perception of hypertrophic cardiomyopathy and its natural history. Am J Cardiol 1993;72:970–972.

26 Spirito P, Chiarella F, Carratino L, et al. Clinical course and prognosis of hypertrophic cardiomyopathy in an outpatient population. N Engl J Med 1989;320:749–755.

27 Melacini P, Maron BJ, Bobbo F, et al. Evidence that pharmacologic strategies lack efficacy for the prevention of sudden death in hypertrophic cardiomyopathy. Heart, in press.

28 Olivotto I, Cecchi F, Casey SA, et al. Impact of atrial fibrillation on the clinical course of hypertrophic cardiomyopathy. Circulation 2001;104:2517–2524.

29 Maron BJ, Olivotto I, Bellone P, et al. Clinical profile of stroke in 900 patients with hypertrophic cardiomyopathy. J Am Coll Cardiol 2002;39:301–307.

30 Monserrat L, Elliott PM, Gimeno JR, Sharma S, Penas-Lado M, McKenna WJ. Non-sustained ventricular tachycardia in hypertrophic cardiomyopathy: an independent marker of sudden death risk in young patients. J Am Coll Cardiol 2003;42:873–879.

31 Jayatilleke I, Doolan A, Ingles J, et al. Long-term follow-up of implantable cardioverter defibrillator therapy for hypertrophic cardiomyopathy. Am J Cardiol 2004;93:1192–1194.

32 Cha Y-M, Gersh BJ, Maron BJ, et al. Electrophysiologic manifestations of ventricular tachyarrhythmias provoking appropriate defibrillator interventions in high risk patients with hypertrophic cardiomyopathy. J Cardiovasc Electro, in press.

33 Elliott PM, Sharma S, Varnava A, et al. Survival after cardiac arrest in patients with hypertrophic cardiomyopathy. J Am Coll Cardiol 1999;33:1596–1601.

34 Adabag AS, Casey SA, Kuskowski MA, Zenovich AG, Maron BJ. Spectrum and prognostic significance of arrhythmias on ambulatory Holter electrocardiogram in hypertrophic cardiomyopathy. J Am Coll Cardiol 2005;45:697–704.

35 Maron BJ, Estes NAM III, Maron MS, Almquist AK, Link MS, Udelson J. Primary prevention of sudden death as a novel treatment strategy in hypertrophic cardiomyopathy. Circulation 2003;107:2872–2875.

36 Maron BJ, Spirito P, Shen W-K, et al. Implantable cardioverter-defibrillators and prevention of sudden cardiac death in hypertrophic cardiomyopathy. JAMA 2007;298:405–412.

37 Maron BJ, Roberts WC. Quantitative analysis of cardiac muscle cell disorganization in the ventricular septum of patients with hypertrophic cardiomyopathy. *Circulation* 1979;59:689–706.

38 Maron BJ, Wolfson JK, Epstein SE, et al. Intramural ("small vessel") coronary artery disease in hypertrophic cardiomyopathy. J Am Coll Cardiol 1986;8:545–557.

39 Tanaka M, Fujiwara H, Onodera T, et al. Quantitative analysis of myocardial fibrosis in normal, hypertensive hearts, and hypertrophic cardiomyopathy. Br Heart J 1986;55:575–581.

40 Tanaka M, Fujiwara H, Onodera T, et al. Quantitative analysis of narrowing of intramyocardial small arteries in normal hearts, hypertensive hearts, and hearts with hypertrophic cardiomyopathy. Circulation 1987;75:1130–1139.

41 Cannon RO, Rosing DR, Maron BJ, et al. Myocardial ischemia in hypertrophic cardiomyopathy: contribution of inadequate vasodilator reserve and elevated left ventricular filling pressures. Circulation 1985;71:234–243.

42 Maron BJ, Shirani J, Poliac LC, et al. Sudden death in young competitive athletes: clinical, demographic and pathological profiles. JAMA 1996;276:199–204.

43 Maron BJ. Sudden death in young athletes. N Engl J Med 2003;349:1064–1075.

44 Maron MS, Olivotto I, Betocchi S, et al. Effect of left ventricular outflow tract obstruction on clinical outcome in hypertrophic cardiomyopathy. N Engl J Med 2003;348:295–303.

45 Maki S, Ikeda H, Muro A, et al. Predictors of sudden cardiac death in hypertrophic cardiomyopathy. Am J Cardiol 1998;82:774–778.

46 Maron BJ, Casey SA, Poliac LC, et al. Clinical consequences of hypertrophic cardiomyopathy in an unselected regional United States cohort. JAMA 1999;281:650–655.

47 Elliott PM, Gimeno JR, Tome MT, et al. Left ventricular outflow tract obstruction and sudden death risk in patients with hypertrophic cardiomyopathy. Eur Heart J 2006;27:1933–1941.

48 Maron BJ, Olivotto I, Maron MS. The dilemma of left ventricular outflow tract obstruction and sudden death in hypertrophic cardiomyopathy: do patients with gradients really deserve prophylactic defibrillators? Eur Heart J 2006;27:1895–1897.

49 Yetman AT, McCrindle BW, MacDonald C, Freedom RM, Gow R. Myocardial bridging in children with hypertrophic cardiomyopathy – a risk factor for sudden death. N Engl J Med 1998;339:1201–1209.

50 Cecchi F, Olivotto I, Gistri R, et al. Coronary microvascular dysfunction and prognosis in hypertrophic cardiomyopathy. N Engl J Med 2003;349:1027–1035.

51 Ackerman MJ, Van Driest SL, Ommen SR, et al. Prevalence and age dependence of malignant mutations in the beta-myosin heavy chain and troponin T genes in hypertrophic cardiomyopathy: a comprehensive outpatient perspective. J Am Coll Cardiol 2002;39:2042–248.

52 Van Driest SL, Ackerman MJ, Ommen SR, et al. Prevalence and severity of "benign" mutations in the beta-myosin heavy chain, cardiac troponin T, and alpha-tropomyosin genes in hypertrophic cardiomyopathy. Circulation 2002;106:3085–3090.

53 Saumarez RC, Chojnowska L, Derksen R, et al. Sudden death in noncoronary heart disease is associated with delayed paced ventricular activation. Circulation 2003;42:889–894.

54 Mirowski M, Reid PR, Mower MM, et al. Termination of malignant ventricular arrhythmias with an implanted automatic defibrillator in human beings. N Engl J Med 1980;303:322–324.

55 The Antiarrhythmics Versus Implantable Defibrillators (AVID) Investigators. A comparison of anitarrhythmic-drug therapy with implantable defibrillators in patients resuscitated from near-fatal ventricular arrhythmias. *N Engl J Med* 1997;337:1576–1583.

56 Moss AJ, Zareba W, Hall WJ, et al. Prophylactic implantation of a defibrillator in patients with myocardial infarction and reduced ejection fraction. N Engl J Med 2002;346:877–883.

57 Buxton AE, Lee KL, Fisher JD, et al. A randomized study of the prevention of sudden death in patients with coronary artery disease. N Engl J Med 1999;341:1882–1890.

58 Bardy GH, Lee KL, Mark DB, et al. Amiodarone or an implantable cardioverter- defibrillator for congestive heart failure. N Engl J Med 2005;352:225–237.

59 Maron BJ, Chaitman B, Ackerman MJ, et al. American Heart Association Scientific Statement: recommendations for Physical Activity and Recreational Sports Participation for Young Patients with Genetic Cardiovascular Diseases. Circulation 2004;109:2807–2816.

60 Corrado D, Leoni L, Link MS, et al. Implantable cardioverter-defibrillator therapy for prevention of sudden death in patients with arrhythmogenic right ventricular cardiomyopathy/dysplasia. Circulation 2003;108:3084–3091.

61 Roguin A, Bomma CS, Nasir K, et al. Implantable cardioverter-defibrillators in patients with arrhythmogenic right ventricular dysplasia/cardiomyopathy. J Am Coll Cardiol 2004;43: 1843–1852.

62 Zareba W, Moss AJ, Daubert JP, Hall WJ, Robinson JL, Andrews M. Implantable cardioverter defibrillator in high-risk long QT syndrome patients. J Cardiovasc Electrophysiol 2003;14:337–341.

63 Sacher F, Probst V, Iesaka Y, et al. Outcome after implantation of a cardioverter- defibrillator in patients

with Brugada syndrome. A multicenter study. Circulation 2006;114:2317–2324.

64 Primo J, Geelen P, Brugada J, et al. Hypertrophic cardiomyopathy: role of the implantable cardioverter-defibrillator. J Am Coll Cardiol 1998;31:1081–1085.

65 Marín F, Gimeno JR, Payá E, et al. Implantable cardioverter-defibrillator in hypertrophic cardiomyopathy. Experience of three centers. Rev Esp Cardiol 2006; 59:537–544.

66 Klues HG, Schiffers A, Maron BJ. Phenotypic spectrum and patterns of left ventricular hypertrophy in hypertrophic cardiomyopathy: morphologic observations and significance as assessed by two-dimensional echocardiography in 600 patients. J Am Coll Cardiol 1995;26:1699–1708.

67 Maron BJ, Gross BW, Stark SI. Extreme left ventricular hypertrophy. Circulation 1995;92:2748.

68 Gregoratos G, Abrams J, Epstein AE, et al. ACC/AHA/NASPE 2002 Guideline Update for Implantation of Cardiac Pacemakers and Antiarrhythmia Devices: summary article: a report of the American College of Cardiology/American Heart Association Task Force on Practice Guidelines. Circulation 2002;106:2145–2161.

69 Camm AJ, Nisam S. The utilization of the implantable defibrillator – a European enigma. Eur Heart J 2000;21:1998–2004.

70 Maron BJ, Casey SA, Hauser RG, Aeppli DM. Clinical course of hypertrophic cardiomyopathy with survival to advanced ages. J Am Coll Cardiol 2003;42:882–888.

71 Hauser RG, Maron BJ. Lessons from the failure and recall of an implantable cardioverter defibrillator. Circulation 2005;112:2040–2042.

72 Steinbrook R. The controversy over Guidant's implantable defibrillators. N Engl J Med 2005;253:221–224.

73 Maron BJ, Hauser RG. Past and future perspectives on the failure of pharmaceutical and medical device industries to protect the public health interests. Am J Cardiol, 2007;100:147–151.

74 Goldenberg I, Moss AJ, Maron BJ, Dick AW, Zareba W. Cost effectiveness of implanted defibrillators in young people with inherited cardiac arrhythmias. Ann Noninvas Electrocardiol 2005;10(Suppl. 4):67–83.

75 Almquist AK, Hanna CA, Haas TS, Maron BJ. Significance of appropriate defibrillator shock 3 hours and 20 minutes following implantation in hypertrophic cardiomyopathy. J Cardiovasc Electrophys, in press.

76 Germano JJ, Reynolds M, Essebag V, Josephson ME. Frequency and causes of implantable cardioverter-defibrillator therapies: is device therapy proarrhythmic? Am J Cardiol 2006;97:1255–1261.

77 Harris KM, Spirito P, Maron MS, et al. Prevalence, clinical profile and significance of left ventricular remodeling in the end-stage phase of hypertrophic cardiomyopathy. Circulation 2006;114:216–225.

CHAPTER 7

Mapping and ablation of ventricular tachycardia after myocardial infarction

William G. Stevenson, & Usha Tedrow

Introduction

Implantable cardioverter defibrillators (ICDs) are the first line therapy for patients with ventricular tachycardia (VT) after myocardial infarction. Of patients who receive an ICD after a spontaneous episode of sustained VT, 40–60% will experience recurrent episodes [1]. Electrical storm, commonly defined as three separate episodes of sustained VT within 24 hours, occurs in up to 20% of patients, some with incessant VT [2–5]. Approximately 20% of patients with an ICD implanted for primary prevention of sudden death will experience one or more episodes of spontaneous VT within 3–5 years after ICD implantation [6–8]. ICD shocks can be painful and traumatic, and some patients consequently require therapy to reduce or prevent even infrequent episodes [7,9]. In addition, spontaneous VT episodes are associated with an increased mortality risk even when the arrhythmia is effectively treated by an ICD [6,8]. Antiarrhythmic drug therapy with amiodarone or sotalol can reduce VT episodes but have potential side effects and the efficacy is poor [6]. Catheter ablation is useful for reducing VT episodes and can be life-saving when VT is incessant [4,10,11].

In ischemic cardiomyopathy, the majority of recurrent VTs are monomorphic, related to reentry through regions of ventricular scar. Monomorphic

VTs involving the Purkinje system and recurrent polymorphic VTs that are not caused by acute myocardial ischemia are also susceptible to catheter ablation [12]. Several factors make catheter ablation of VT more difficult than ablation of supraventricular arrhythmias. Multiple morphologies of VT are commonly present. The infarct region containing the arrhythmogenic area is often large. The induced VTs can be "unmappable" or "unstable" due to hemodynamic intolerance. Additionally, shifting VT morphology can occur during attempted mapping, and the clinical VT may not be reliably induced in the laboratory. Further, reaching the critical portions of the reentry circuit can be difficult since the arrhythmogenic area, while most commonly located in the subendocardium, can occasionally be epicardial or intramural in location. Advances in understanding of the pathophysiology and in mapping and ablation technology have facilitated catheter ablation for these arrhythmias.

Sustained monomorphic VT late after myocardial infarction

The substrate

Reentry involving regions of infarct scars is the most common cause of sustained monomorphic VT in this patient population. Infarct scars are comprised of variable regions of dense fibrosis that create conduction block. Surviving myocyte bundles with interstitial fibrosis and diminished coupling produces circuitous slow conduction paths through the scar that promote reentry [13]. Many of these circuits

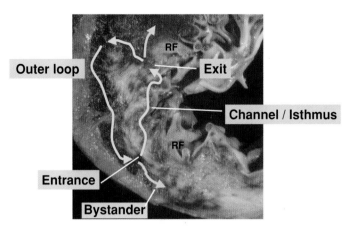

Figure 7.1 Depicted is a cross-section through an infarct scar from a patient with uncontrollable VT and failed ablation. A theoretical reentry circuit path is indicated by yellow arrows. Areas of white fibrosis create the conduction block. A long potential isthmus exists with an exit at the superior margin of the infarct region. After emerging from the exit the circulating wavefront propagates through tissue along the border of the infarct (outer loop). Bystander regions that are not in the circuit are also noted. Two areas with discoloration and hemorrhage are RF ablation lesions from the failed ablation attempt.

can be modeled as having an isthmus or channel consisting of a small mass of tissue, whose depolarization is not detected on the surface ECG [14]. The QRS complex is inscribed when the reentrant excitation wavefront emerges from an exit along the border of the scar and spreads across the ventricles (Figure 7.1). Areas of conduction block that define the isthmus may be fixed, bordering on a valve annulus (most often mitral or aortic), or area of dense myocardial fibrosis. Critical areas of slow conduction may also be related either to collision of wavefronts or to functional conduction block [15,16]. Reentry circuit configurations and locations vary from patient to patient. Large macroreentry circuits spanning several centimeters are common [17].

Repeated programmed stimulation typically induces multiple morphologies of monomorphic VT, with most studies reporting a mean of three different VTs inducible (Table 7.1). Multiple morphologies of VT can be due to different circuits in disparate areas of the infarct, different exits from the same circuit, or changes in activation remote from the circuit due to alteration in functional regions of block. Ablation at one region often abolishes more than one VT [15,18,19].

QRS morphology

The QRS morphology of VT is an indication of the likely location of the circuit exit. VTs with a left bundle branch block-like configuration in lead V1, with a dominant s-wave, usually have an exit in interventricular septum or the right ventricle (RV). This QRS configuration is also the most common morphology of bundle branch reentry VT [20]. Dominant R waves in V1 usually indicate a left ventricular (LV) exit. An inferiorly directed frontal plane axis indicates that the exit is on the anterior wall. A superiorly directed frontal plane exit suggests an inferior wall exit location. A rightward frontal plane axis suggests a lateral or posterior exit, while dominant r-waves in lead I suggest a septal exit. The mid-precordial leads—V3 and V4—provide an indication of exit location between the mitral annulus and apex. Apical exits produce dominant S waves in these leads; basal exits generate dominant R waves. VTs that originate in the subepicardium generally produce a longer QRS duration and slower QRS upstrokes in the precordial leads compared to those with an endocardial exit [21].

Substrate mapping

Identification of the likely arrhythmogenic substrate during a stable sinus or paced rhythm is commonly referred to as substrate mapping. This method often allows identification of likely exits and channels without mapping during VT, facilitating ablation in patients with multiple and unstable VTs [22–25].

Table 7.1 RF ablation for VT after MI since 2000

Author	N	Age (yr)	LVEF	Amiodarone therapy	VTs/Pt	VT CL	Unstable VTs targeted (% pts)	Mapping: S = substrate VT = during VT	Ablation lesion Set	RF method
Cesario et al. *[22]	20	64	0.28	100%	N/A	N/A	89% of VTs	S, VT	Line	4 & 8 mm
Bogun et al. [35]	48	66	0.27	79%	1.8	491	0	S, VT	Focal	Std
Segal et al. [37]	40	65	0.36	83%	3.5	401	N/A	VT – balloon	Focal, line	Std
Deneke et al. [48]	25	62	0.37	100%	2.4	440	100%	S	Lines	8 mm
Arenal et al. [33]	26	68	0.31	N/A	N/A	374	N/A	S, VT	Focal RF	Std
Della Bella et al. [18]	137	67	0.31–0.36	99%	2–3	338–385	53%	S; VT – balloon	Focal	Std
Kottkamp et al. [27]	28	64	0.29	50%	2.3	392	39%	S, VT	Line	Ext Irrig
Reddy et al. [25]	11	66	0.31	64%	3.7	340	100%	S	Line	Ext Irrig
Arenal et al. [28]	24	66	0.3	N/A	N/A	367	69%	S, VT	Focal, line	Std
Kautzner et al. [49]	28	63	0.28	71%	2.9	399	50%	S,VT	Focal	Std
O'Donnell et al. [47]	112	64	<0.35 in 42%	N/A	2.4	N/A	30%	VT	Line	4 & 8 mm, Irrig
de Chillou et al. [17]	21	66	0.34	N/A	1 or 2	432	0	VT	Focal	Std
Soejima et al. [15]	14	65	0.29	N/A	N/A	N/A	N/A	S, VT	Line	Irrig
van der Burg et al. [46]	89	66	0.29	N/A	N/A	345	N/A	S,VT	Focal	Std
Soejima et al. [24]	40	66	0.29	68%	3.6	391	83%	S, VT	Line	4 & 8 mm, Irrig
Sra et al. [55]	19	70	0.27	89%	2.4	336	82% of targeted VTs	S, VT	Line, focal	Std
Strickberger et al. [39]	13	71	0.33	60%	N/A	441–314	54%	VT – balloon	Focal, line	Std
Calkins et al. [51]	146	62	0.31	40%	3	N/A	0	VT	Focal	Closed Irrig

*60% of patients with CAD.

Focal, focal set of RF lesions placed; Irrig, irrigated RF; N/A, not available; S, substrate mapping; Std, standard solid RF electrode of 4– 5 mm length; VT, mapping during VT.
(Modified with permission from Ref [12].)

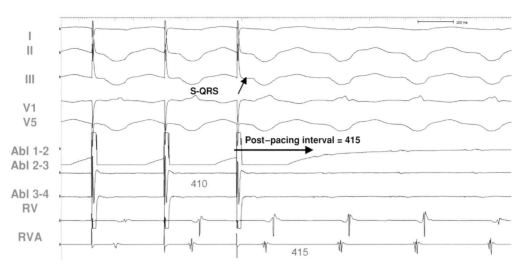

Figure 7.2 Entrainment from the exit site shown in Figure 7.2 is shown. From the top are surface ECG leads, bipolar recordings from the distal, mid, and proximal pairs of the mapping and ablation catheter (Abl 1-2, 2-3, and 3-4, respectively), and the right ventricle (RV and RVA). VT with a cycle length of 415 milliseconds is present. Pacing at a cycle length of 410 milliseconds entrains tachycardia with concealed fusion. The post-pacing interval approximates the tachycardia cycle length indicating that the site is in the circuit. The S-QRS is relatively short, consistent with an exit site. (Modified with permission from Ref. [12].)

Areas of myocyte loss and replacement with fibrosis due to infarction are characterized by low-amplitude bipolar electrograms (typically <1.55 mV). Plots of peak-to-peak electrogram amplitude displayed in three-dimensional electroanatomic reconstructions are referred to as voltage maps (Figure 7.2) [23,25]. The low-voltage region contains the reentry circuit, but is usually extensive, often exceeding 20 cm in circumference, such that ablation of the entire region may not be feasible or attractive [24]. Additional markers of the circuit exit or isthmus are sought for ablation.

Exit regions can be located during sinus rhythm by pace mapping along the scar border (Figure 7.2). Pacing in the exit region replicates the QRS morphology of VT [26,27]. The interval between the stimulus and QRS onset is typically short consistent with its location in the infarct border.

Several markers of potential isthmuses or critical channels within low-voltage regions have been identified. Delayed activation of a channel during sinus or paced rhythm can create isolated potentials that occur after the end of the QRS, even late in diastole in some cases [28–32]. Pacing in a channel produces a QRS that emerges after a delay due to slow conduction through the channel (Figures 7.3 and 7.4). When the stimulated wavefront propagates through the channel to a reentry circuit exit region, the paced QRS morphology resembles VT, strongly suggesting that the pacing site is in a reentry circuit isthmus [26,31]. If the wavefront leaves the scar by another path, the paced QRS morphology may differ from VT, or resemble a different VT.

Potential channels can also be exposed by assessing the relative electrogram amplitudes through the low-voltage region [33,34]. In some patients potential channels appear as paths of relatively higher voltage delineated by lower voltage region. This can be appreciated by obtaining a high-density map of the low-voltage region and then gradually reducing the upper maximal range for the color scale.

Areas of dense fibrosis causing conduction block that defines some isthmuses, designated as electrically unexcitable scar (EUS), can be identified from a high pacing threshold (>10 mA at 2 ms pulse width with unipolar pacing) [15]. Marking these EUS areas (gray area on the voltage map in Figure 7.2) creates a visual map of potential channels in some patients. The detection of these regions likely depends on the size of the "virtual electrode" produced by the pacing stimulus, relative to the size of the region of fibrosis beneath the electrode. Narrow bands of fibrosis likely escape detection with this method. EUS cannot be reliably detected

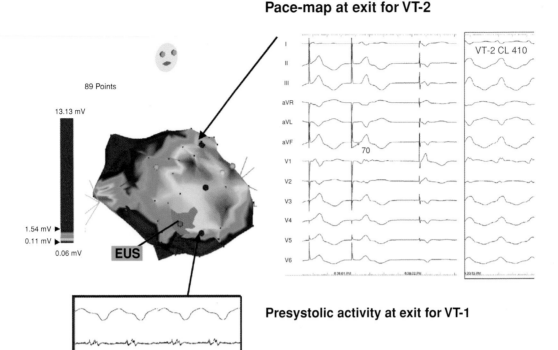

Figure 7.3 A voltage map from a patient with an anterior wall infarction is shown. Colors indicate peak-to-peak bipolar voltage, with purple >1.5 mV consistent with normal, and red, the lowest amplitude region. This patient had two morphologies of VT. VT-1 had a superiorly directed frontal plane axis due to an exit at the inferior septal margin of the scar adjacent to an area of electrically unexcitable scar (EUS). During VT presystolic electrical activity was recorded at this site (bottom panel). VT-2 had an inferiorly directed frontal plane axis due to an exit at the superior margin of the scar. The pace-map at this site during sinus rhythm produced a QRS that matched VT with a stimulus – QRS interval of 70 milliseconds consistent with slow conduction in the region (right panels). (Modified with permission from Ref. [12].)

based on electrogram amplitude alone. Pacing captures at a substantial number of very low amplitude sites where the electrogram amplitude is less than 0.25 mV. In contrast some EUS sites have electrogram amplitude >0.5 mV, that are likely due to far-field potentials generated by depolarization of a substantial mass of ventricular tissue that is remote from the pacing site (Figure 7.5). Inadequate electrode myocardial contact is also a potential source of error with this method.

The electrogram characteristics and pace-mapping findings provide complementary information during substrate mapping. We typically acquire data from both nearly simultaneously as the voltage map is created. At each low-voltage site, pace mapping at 10 mA is briefly performed and then analyzed as the catheter is moved to the next site.

Many recent ablation series include patients with multiple and unstable VTs targeted by one or a combination of these substrate mapping methods (Table 7.1) [15,23,27,28,33]. When VT is stable, substrate mapping can be used to identify regions for further evaluation during VT (see below), minimizing the time spent in VT. Even for unstable VTs brief entrainment is often possible, to confirm the location of a reentry circuit, potentially allowing ablation with a smaller number of RF lesions than when ablation is guided only by substrate mapping [24].

Mapping during VT

When VT is stable for mapping the exit or isthmus can be targeted for ablation during VT [17,24,35,36]. During VT the circuit exit and

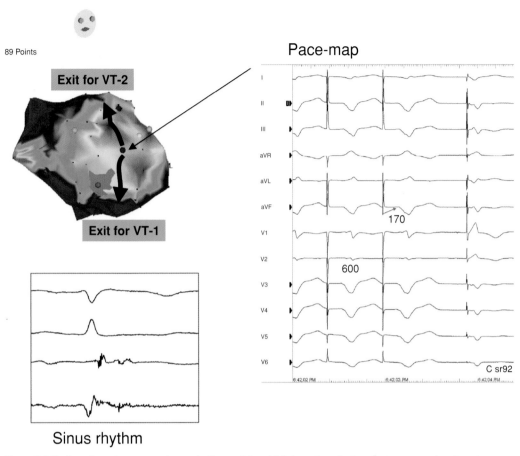

Figure 7.4 Findings from the same patient as in Figures 7.2 and 7.3 show sinus rhythm electrogram and pacing at an isthmus site within the scar. The sinus rhythm electrogram shows a late potential, indicating depolarization of tissue after the end of the QRS consistent with slow conduction. Pacing at this site during sinus rhythm produces a long S-QRS of 170 milliseconds consistent with slow conduction. The QRS morphology matches that of VT-1 consistent with pacing in an isthmus proximal to the exit region for that VT. All times are in ms. (Modified with permission from Ref. [12].)

isthmus have presystolic (prior to the QRS onset) and diastolic activation (Figures 7.3 and 7.5). Entrainment mapping (see below) can be used to distinguish these from abnormal bystander areas. Radiofrequency ablation during VT often terminates the arrhythmia.

Both multielectrode and noncontact mapping systems allow acquisition of electrograms from multiple sites simultaneously allowing an assessment of activation over a broad area even during a single beat of tachycardia. Detection of low-amplitude signals in isthmuses is limited, however, and often these are not seen unless electrodes of the array are fortuitously in close proximity to the isthmus. The larger amplitude signals that occur in

the border of the scar are more easily detected with these systems. Thus the exit region along the border of the infarct is often identifiable as the region of earliest endocardial activation [37–39].

Due to heterogeneity of ventricular scars with multiple potential conduction paths and channels, electrogram timing alone is not a reliable guide for targeting a specific reentry circuit isthmus [40]. Confirmation that a site is involved in the reentry circuit can be obtained by entrainment mapping (Figures 7.3 and 7.5) [24,35,40,41]. At pacing sites in the reentry circuit, stimuli that capture during VT can reset the circuit. The conduction time required for the stimulated wavefront to complete one revolution through the circuit is equal to the

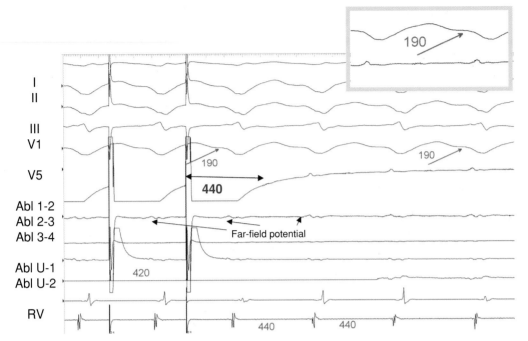

Figure 7.5 Recordings from the isthmus site shown in Figure 7.4 during VT-1. The top right panel shows an enlargement of the electrograms revealing two low-amplitude potentials, one inscribed during the QRS and a second during diastole. Pacing at the site entrains VT with concealed fusion, with S-QRS interval of 190 milliseconds consistent with a location in the central portion of the isthmus. Pacing indicates that the electrogram inscribed during the QRS is a far-field potential due to depolarization of tissue remote from the pacing site. The post-pacing interval measured to the low amplitude diastolic potential approximates the VT cycle length. All measures are in ms. (Modified with permission from Ref. [12].)

tachycardia cycle length, and thus the postpacing interval (PPI) following the pacing train approximates the tachycardia cycle length. Entrainment may occur at pacing sites removed from the circuit, but the PPI increases as a function of the conduction time between the site and the reentry circuit. If the site is an isthmus in the circuit, entrainment occurs without changing the QRS morphology (entrainment with concealed fusion) because the stimulated wavefronts follow the path of the reentry circuit and propagate through its exit. In this case, the S-QRS interval indicates the conduction time from the pacing site to the reentry circuit exit and matches the electrogram to QRS interval during VT.

Other features that indicate that a site is in the reentry circuit include reproducible VT termination by catheter-induced mechanical pressure, termination by ablation during VT, and termination by a pacing stimulus that does not produce a response that propagates away from the pacing site, such that no QRS complex follows the pacing stimulus

[35,42,43]. It is not necessary to define the entire circuit if an isthmus can be identified for ablation.

Purkinje system and VT after myocardial infarction

Approximately 7% of patients with VT after myocardial infarction have bundle branch reentry as the cause of one of their VTs, although scar-related reentry is often also present [20]. Bundle branch reentry VT is more common when the HV interval is prolonged in sinus rhythm. The QRS complex in tachycardia most commonly shows a left bundle branch block pattern, or a pattern resembling the QRS morphology in sinus rhythm. A right bundle potential and/or His bundle electrogram preceding and linked to the QRS helps establish the diagnosis. Ablation of the right bundle branch typically eliminates this VT. Occasionally, interfascicular reentry requires ablation of left bundle fascicles. Rarely, automaticity in the Purkinje system is the cause of VT, and is often induced with sympathetic stimulation. [20]. The Purkinje system can also be involved as a portion of a scar-related reentry circuit that can be targeted for ablation [44,45].

Acute procedural endpoints

Patients in the reported series have generally had recurrent episodes of VT despite antiarrhythmic drug therapy (Table 7.1). In the electrophysiology laboratory an average of three different monomorphic VTs are usually induced (Table 7.1). Those that have been observed to occur spontaneously are often referred to as "clinical VTs"; the others are often designated "nonclinical," implying that they are unlikely to occur spontaneously. This distinction is often problematic. Some "nonclinical" VTs subsequently occur spontaneously [18,37,46]. The ECG morphology of spontaneous VT is often not known in patients where an ICD promptly terminates VT.

Abolishing incessant VT and inducible "clinical" VT is generally considered the minimum end point for acute success of ablation [35,41]. The ablation strategy usually targets the isthmus or exit region. Some centers attempt to abolish all inducible VTs, or all inducible mappable VTs, aiming to reduce recurrences [18,24,47,48]. When multiple and unstable VTs are present, several different strategies for placing ablation lesions have been reported (Table 7.1). These include ablation lines through exit regions, ablation through all identified isthmuses, ablation through isthmuses or exits extending to the border of the scar, and ablation of all diastolic potential sites. For unstable VTs approached by substrate mapping, multiple RF applications are usually employed. These different acute ablation strategies and endpoints have not been directly compared.

At the end of the ablation procedure at least one VT is no longer inducible in 73–100% of patients and no monomorphic VT of any type can be induced in 38–95% of patients (Table 7.1). Remaining inducible VTs are often faster and require more aggressive stimulation for initiation than the initial VTs [18,24,48,49].

When the targeted VT remains inducible after ablation the recurrence risk exceeds 60% [46,47]. Absence of inducible VT has been shown to be associated with a lower yet significant incidence of recurrence ranging from less than 3% to 27% in single-center reports [15,18,24,46–48]. Inducible,

"nonclinical" VTs are associated with increased risk of recurrence in some studies [48,50]. Healing of initial ablation lesions and reduction of antiarrhythmic medications likely contribute to recurrences; and some patients benefit from a repeat procedure. In a multicenter trial in 146 patients, acute results did not predict outcomes; VT recurred in 44% of patients who had no inducible VT and 46% of those who had inducible VT [51].

Acute failure of endocardial ablation often appears to be due to anatomic constraints. Epicardial or intramural reentry circuits that either are difficult to locate or cannot be adequately damaged are the greatest challenge. The availability of large electrodes and saline-irrigated ablation catheters likely improves the ability to create deeper RF lesions compared to 4 or 5 mm solid electrodes [43].

Epicardial circuits are likely present in 10–30% of patients, more often in inferior wall as opposed to anterior wall infarctions [10,22,52,53]. These circuits can often be located and ablated using the method for percutaneous access to the percutaneous space described by Sosa and colleagues (Chapter 14) [52]. If pericardial scarring from prior cardiac surgery precludes this approach, a surgical subxiphoid pericardial window has been used to allow epicardial catheter ablation [54].

Major complications are reported in 5–10% of patients (Table 7.1) including cardiac tamponade, shock, stroke (0–2.7%), aortic valve injuries, vascular injuries, and A-V block due to ablation of septal VTs. Procedure mortality, 2.7% in one multicenter trial, is often caused by failure to control VT rather than complications of the procedure [51].

Long-term outcomes

In most series, previously ineffective antiarrhythmic drugs, often amiodarone, have been continued during follow-up (Table 7.2). VT recurs in 19–50% of patients, although the frequency is reduced in the majority (Figures 7.6 [23,24,51,55] and 7.7 [24]). Multiple morphologies of VT and unstable VTs are associated with a higher recurrence risk [18,24].

During follow-up after ablation, the annual mortality ranges from 5% to more than 20%, with death from progressive heart failure being the most common cause [50,51,56]. This substantial mortality is consistent with the severity of heart disease, depressed ventricular function, and the

Table 7.2 Ablation outcomes

Author	Proc. time (h)	At least one VT ablated	All inducible VTs abolished	Proc. mortality	Proc. complications	Follow-up (mo)	Antiarrhythmic drug in Follow-up	No VT in F/U	Death in F/U
Cesario et al. *[22]	8	N/A	N/A	0	10% tamponade, vascular	12	100%	75%	10%
Bogun et al. [35]	N/A	86% of VTs	N/A	0	N/A	16	≥ 79%	88% free of targeted VT	
Segal et al. [37]	6	N/A	73%	0	28% (shock, stroke, TIA, tamponade vascular; hemothorax, A-V block)	36	100%	50%	32%
Deneke et al. [48]	3.4	92%	70%	0	0	10	100%	84%	
Arenal et al. [33]	N/A	96%	69%	0	0	17	N/A	73%	15%
Della Bella et al. [18]	N/A	77%	57%	0	N/A	36	99%	51%	9%
Kottkamp et al. [27]	2	86%	79%	0	3.5% TIA	15	>50%	64%	7%
Reddy et al. [25]	7	82%	64%	0	9% tamponade	13	≥ 64%	81%	0
Arenal et al. [28]	4	95%	67%	0	0	9	N/A	78%	17%
Kautzner et al. [49]	4	86%	57%	0	3.5% TIA	11	N/A	79%	7%
O'Donnell et al. [47]	N/A	N/A	38%	0	2% tamponade	72	58%	78%	
de Chillou et al. [17]	4	95%	57%	0	N/A	16	N/A	81%	10%
Soejima et al. [15]	N/A	86%	71%	0	0	6	93%	71%	0
van der Burg et al. [46]	N/A	79%	N/A	2%	9% stroke, incess VT, tamponade, A-V block	34	approx 55%	73%	14%
Soejima et al. [24]	7	83%	55%	0	10% all minor vascular access	10	63%	63%	22%
Sra et al. [55]	1.4	79%	N/A	0	5% tamponade	7	47%	66%	0%
Strickberger et al. [39]	N/A	77%	N/A	8%	23% tamponade, stroke	1	N/A	71%	N/A
Calkins et al. [51]	5	>75%	41%	3%	8% stroke, tamponade, A-V block, Aortic valve injury	8	66%	54%	18%

F/U, follow-up: incess, incessant; N/A, not available; Proc, procedure; TIA, transient ischemic attack.

(Modified with permission from Reference [12].)

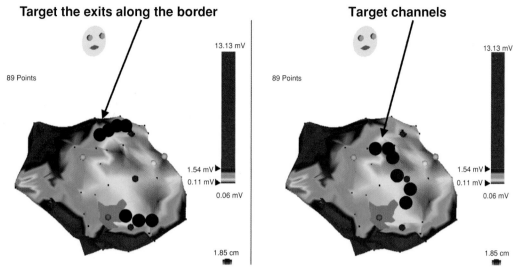

Figure 7.6 Voltage maps from the same patient as in Figures 7.2–7.5 illustrating potential ablation strategies for targeting the multiple VTs. Potential ablation lesions are indicated by dark red circles. Ablation targeting the exit region is shown on the left. Ablation targeting the channel is shown on the right. (Modified with permission from Ref. [12].)

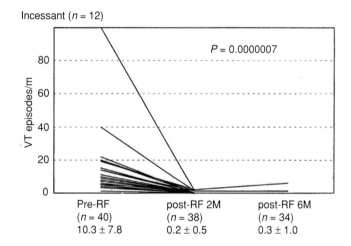

Figure 7.7 Impact of ablation on frequency of recurrent VT in 40 patients referred for catheter ablation. From Ref. [24].

observation that spontaneous VT is a marker for mortality and heart failure despite presence of an ICD [8]. Older age and greater LV size and dysfunction are associated with worse mortality [50,56]. The potential for ablation to adversely affect LV function is cause for concern, although assessment of LV ejection fraction after ablation has not shown deterioration [23,57]. Confining ablation lesions to regions of low-amplitude scar and attention to appropriate medical therapy for LV dysfunction are prudent means to minimize this concern.

Summary

Catheter ablation has an important role for reducing episodes of VT in patients with scar-related LV dysfunction and implantable defibrillators. Substrate mapping approaches have facilitated ablation even in the presence of multiple and hemodynamically unstable VTs formerly considered "unmappable." Efficacy remains less than that for ablation of many supraventricular arrhythmias. Failure of VT ablation often seems to be due to anatomic difficulties, such as unreachable deep intramural reentry circuits in areas of thick myocardium. Further technologic developments are needed and will require careful assessment of risks and efficacy.

References

1 Klein RC, Raitt MH, Wilkoff BL, et al. Analysis of implantable cardioverter defibrillator therapy in the antiarrhythmics versus implantable defibrillators (AVID) trial. J Cardiovasc Electrophysiol 2003;14: 940–948.

2 Schreieck J, Zrenner B, Deisenhofer I, et al. Rescue ablation of electrical storm in patients with ischemic cardiomyopathy: a potential-guided ablation approach by modifying substrate of intractable, unmappable ventricular tachycardias. Heart Rhythm 2005;2:10–14.

3 Exner DV, Pinski SL, Wyse DG, et al. Electrical storm presages nonsudden death: the antiarrhythmics versus implantable defibrillators (AVID) trial. Circulation 2001;103:2066–2071.

4 Bansch D, Oyang F, Antz M, et al. Successful catheter ablation of electrical storm after myocardial infarction. Circulation 2003;108:3011–3016.

5 Silva RM, Mont L, Nava S, et al. Radiofrequency catheter ablation for arrhythmic storm in patients with an implantable cardioverter defibrillator. Pacing Clin Electrophysiol 2004;27:971–975.

6 Connolly SJ, Dorian P, Roberts RS, et al. Comparison of beta-blockers, amiodarone plus beta-blockers, or sotalol for prevention of shocks from implantable cardioverter defibrillators: the OPTIC Study: a randomized trial. JAMA 2006;295:165–171.

7 Schron EB, Exner DV, Yao Q, et al. Quality of life in the antiarrhythmics versus implantable defibrillators trial: impact of therapy and influence of adverse symptoms and defibrillator shocks. Circulation 2002;105: 589–594.

8 Moss AJ, Greenberg H, Case RB, et al. Long-term clinical course of patients after termination of ventricular tachyarrhythmia by an implanted defibrillator. Circulation 2004;110:3760–3765.

9 Irvine J, Dorian P, Baker B, et al. Quality of life in the Canadian Implantable Defibrillator Study (CIDS). Am Heart J 2002;144:282–289.

10 Brugada J, Berruezo A, Cuesta A, et al. Nonsurgical transthoracic epicardial radiofrequency ablation: an alternative in incessant ventricular tachycardia. J Am Coll Cardiol 2003;41:2036–2043.

11 Zipes DP, Camm AJ, Borggrefe M, et al. ACC/AHA/ESC 2006 guidelines for management of patients with ventricular arrhythmias and the prevention of sudden cardiac death: a report of the American College of Cardiology/ American Heart Association Task Force and the European Society of Cardiology Committee for Practice Guidelines (Writing Committee to Develop Guidelines for Management of Patients With Ventricular Arrhythmias and the

Prevention of Sudden Cardiac Death). J Am Coll Cardiol 2006;48:e247–e346.

12 Stevenson WG, Soejima K. Catheter ablation for ventricular tachycardia. Circulation 2007; 115:2750–2760.

13 de Bakker JM, van Capelle FJ, Janse MJ, et al. Slow conduction in the infarcted human heart. 'Zigzag' course of activation. Circulation 1993;88:915–926.

14 Stevenson WG, Khan H, Sager P, et al. Identification of reentry circuit sites during catheter mapping and radiofrequency ablation of ventricular tachycardia late after myocardial infarction. Circulation 1993;88:1647–1670.

15 Soejima K, Stevenson WG, Maisel WH, et al. Electrically unexcitable scar mapping based on pacing threshold for identification of the reentry circuit isthmus: feasibility for guiding ventricular tachycardia ablation. Circulation 2002;106:1678–1683.

16 Wilber DJ, Kopp DE, Glascock DN, et al. Catheter ablation of the mitral isthmus for ventricular tachycardia associated with inferior infarction. Circulation 1995;92:3481– 3489.

17 de Chillou C, Lacroix D, Klug D, et al. Isthmus characteristics of reentrant ventricular tachycardia after myocardial infarction. Circulation 2002;105:726–731.

18 Della Bella P, Riva S, Fassini G, et al. Incidence and significance of pleomorphism in patients with postmyocardial infarction ventricular tachycardia. Acute and long-term outcome of radiofrequency catheter ablation. Eur Heart J 2004;25:1127–1138.

19 Bogun F, Li YG, Groenefeld G, et al. Prevalence of a shared isthmus in postinfarction patients with pleiomorphic, hemodynamically tolerated ventricular tachycardias. J Cardiovasc Electrophysiol 2002;13:237–241.

20 Lopera G, Stevenson WG, Soejima K, et al. Identification and ablation of three types of ventricular tachycardia involving the His-Purkinje system in patients with heart disease. J Cardiovasc Electrophysiol 2004;15:52–58.

21 Berruezo A, Mont L, Nava S, et al. Electrocardiographic recognition of the epicardial origin of ventricular tachycardias. Circulation 2004;109:1842–1847.

22 Cesario DA, Vaseghi M, Boyle NG, et al. Value of high-density endocardial and epicardial mapping for catheter ablation of hemodynamically unstable ventricular tachycardia. Heart Rhythm 2006;3:1–10.

23 Marchlinski FE, Callans DJ, Gottlieb CD, et al. Linear ablation lesions for control of unmappable ventricular tachycardia in patients with ischemic and nonischemic cardiomyopathy. Circulation 2000;101:1288–1296.

24 Soejima K, Suzuki M, Maisel WH, et al. Catheter ablation in patients with multiple and unstable ventricular tachycardias after myocardial infarction: short ablation lines guided by reentry circuit isthmuses and sinus rhythm mapping. Circulation 2001;104:664–669.

25 Reddy VY, Neuzil P, Taborsky M, et al. Short-term results of substrate mapping and radiofrequency ablation of ischemic ventricular tachycardia using a saline-irrigated catheter. J Am Coll Cardiol 2003;41:2228–2236.

26 Brunckhorst CB, Delacretaz E, Soejima K, et al. Identification of the ventricular tachycardia isthmus after infarction by pace mapping. Circulation 2004;110:652–659.

27 Kottkamp H, Wetzel U, Schirdewahn P, et al. Catheter ablation of ventricular tachycardia in remote myocardial infarction: substrate description guiding placement of individual linear lesions targeting noninducibility. J Cardiovasc Electrophysiol 2003;14:675–681.

28 Arenal A, Glez-Torrecilla E, Ortiz M, et al. Ablation of electrograms with an isolated, delayed component as treatment of unmappable monomorphic ventricular tachycardias in patients with structural heart disease. J Am Coll Cardiol 2003;41:81–92.

29 Harada T, Stevenson WG, Kocovic DZ, et al. Catheter ablation of ventricular tachycardia after myocardial infarction: relation of endocardial sinus rhythm late potentials to the reentry circuit. J Am Coll Cardiol 1997;30:1015–1023.

30 Brunckhorst CB, Stevenson WG, Jackman WM, et al. Ventricular mapping during atrial and ventricular pacing. Relationship of multipotential electrograms to ventricular tachycardia reentry circuits after myocardial infarction. Eur Heart J 2002;23:1131–1138.

31 Bogun F, Good E, Reich S, et al. Isolated potentials during sinus rhythm and pace-mapping within scars as guides for ablation of post-infarction ventricular tachycardia. J Am Coll Cardiol 2006;47:2013–2019.

32 Bogun F, Bender B, Li YG, et al. Analysis during sinus rhythm of critical sites in reentry circuits of postinfarction ventricular tachycardia. J Interv Card Electrophysiol 2002;7:95–103.

33 Arenal A, del Castillo S, Gonzalez-Torrecilla E, et al. Tachycardia-related channel in the scar tissue in patients with sustained monomorphic ventricular tachycardias: influence of the voltage scar definition. Circulation 2004;110:2568–2574.

34 Hsia HH, Lin D, Sauer WH, et al. Anatomic characterization of endocardial substrate for hemodynamically stable reentrant ventricular tachycardia: identification of endocardial conducting channels. Heart Rhythm 2006;3:503–512.

35 Bogun F, Kim HM, Han J, et al. Comparison of mapping criteria for hemodynamically tolerated, postinfarction ventricular tachycardia. Heart Rhythm 2006;3:20–26.

36 Verma A, Marrouche NF, Schweikert RA, et al. Relationship between successful ablation sites and the scar border zone defined by substrate mapping for ventricular tachycardia post-myocardial infarction. J Cardiovasc Electrophysiol 2005;16:465–471.

37 Segal OR, Chow AW, Markides V, et al. Long-term results after ablation of infarct-related ventricular tachycardia. Heart Rhythm 2005;2:474–482.

38 Della Bella P, Pappalardo A, Riva S, et al. Non-contact mapping to guide catheter ablation of untolerated ventricular tachycardia. Eur Heart J 2002;23:742–752.

39 Strickberger SA, Knight BP, Michaud GF, et al. Mapping and ablation of ventricular tachycardia guided by virtual electrograms using a noncontact, computerized mapping system. J Am Coll Cardiol 2000;35:414–421.

40 Delacretaz E, Stevenson WG. Catheter ablation of ventricular tachycardia in patients with coronary heart disease: Part I: Mapping. Pacing Clin Electrophysiol 2001;24:1261–1277.

41 El-Shalakany A, Hadjis T, Papageorgiou P, et al. Entrainment/mapping criteria for the prediction of termination of ventricular tachycardia by single radiofrequency lesion in patients with coronary artery disease. Circulation 1999;99:2283–2289.

42 Bogun F, Good E, Han J, et al. Mechanical interruption of postinfarction ventricular tachycardia as a guide for catheter ablation. Heart Rhythm 2005;2:687–691.

43 Soejima K, Delacretaz E, Suzuki M, et al. Saline-cooled versus standard radiofrequency catheter ablation for infarct-related ventricular tachycardias. Circulation 2001;103:1858–1862.

44 Hayashi M, Kobayashi Y, Iwasaki YK, et al. Novel mechanism of postinfarction ventricular tachycardia originating in surviving left posterior Purkinje fibers. Heart Rhythm 2006;3:908–918.

45 Bogun F, Good E, Reich S, et al. Role of Purkinje fibers in post-infarction ventricular tachycardia. J Am Coll Cardiol 2006;48:2500–2507.

46 van der Burg AE, de Groot NM, van Erven L, et al. Long-term follow-up after radiofrequency catheter ablation of ventricular tachycardia: a successful approach? J Cardiovasc Electrophysiol 2002;13:417–423.

47 O'Donnell D, Bourke JP, Furniss SS. Standardized stimulation protocol to predict the long-term success of radiofrequency ablation of postinfarction ventricular tachycardia. Pacing Clin Electrophysiol 2003;26:348–351.

48 Deneke T, Grewe PH, Lawo T, et al. Substrate-modification using electroanatomical mapping in sinus rhythm to treat ventricular tachycardia in patients with ischemic cardiomyopathy. Z Kardiol 2005;94:453–460.

49 Kautzner J, Cihak R, Peichl P, et al. Catheter ablation of ventricular tachycardia following myocardial infarction using three-dimensional electroanatomical mapping. Pacing Clin Electrophysiol 2003;26:342–347.

50 Della Bella P, De Ponti R, Uriarte JA, et al. Catheter ablation and antiarrhythmic drugs for haemodynamically tolerated post-infarction ventricular tachycardia; long-term outcome in relation to acute electrophysiological findings. Eur Heart J 2002;23:414–424.

51 Calkins H, Epstein A, Packer D, et al. Catheter ablation of ventricular tachycardia in patients with structural heart disease using cooled radiofrequency energy: results of a prospective multicenter study. Cooled RF Multi Center Investigators Group. J Am Coll Cardiol 2000;35:1905–1914.

52 Sosa E, Scanavacca M, d'Avila A, et al. Nonsurgical transthoracic epicardial catheter ablation to treat recurrent ventricular tachycardia occurring late after myocardial infarction. J Am Coll Cardiol 2000;35:1442–1449.

53 Svenson RH, Littmann L, Gallagher JJ, et al. Termination of ventricular tachycardia with epicardial laser photocoagulation: a clinical comparison with patients undergoing successful endocardial photocoagulation alone [see comments]. J Am Coll Cardiol 1990;15:163–170.

54 Soejima K, Couper G, Cooper JM, et al. Subxiphoid surgical approach for epicardial catheter-based mapping and ablation in patients with prior cardiac surgery or difficult pericardial access. Circulation 2004;110:1197–1201.

55 Sra J, Bhatia A, Dhala A, et al. Electroanatomically guided catheter ablation of ventricular tachycardias causing multiple defibrillator shocks. Pacing Clin Electrophysiol 2001;24:1645–1652.

56 Nabar A, Rodriguez LM, Batra RK, et al. Echocardiographic predictors of survival in patients undergoing radiofrequency ablation of postinfarct clinical ventricular tachycardia. J Cardiovasc Electrophysiol 2002;13:S118–S121.

57 Khan HH, Maisel WH, Ho C, et al. Effect of radiofrequency catheter ablation of ventricular tachycardia on left ventricular function in patients with prior myocardial infarction. J Interv Card Electrophysiol 2002;7:243–247.

CHAPTER 8

Mapping and ablation of ventricular tachycardia in nonischemic cardiomyopathy

Henry H. Hsia, & Pirooz S. Mofrad

Introduction

Nonischemic cardiomyopathy constitutes a heterogeneous group of disorders in which the predominant feature is myocardial systolic dysfunction in the absence of significant coronary artery disease. It is often associated with cardiac chamber dilatation with the clinical syndrome of heart failure. The etiology of nonischemic dilated cardiomyopathy is diverse (Table 8.1). Although the cause of nonischemic cardiomyopathy is often not definable, it is likely that this condition represents a final common pathway resulting from myocardial damage produced by a variety of toxic, metabolic, infectious, or hemodynamic insults [1,2]. Ventricular arrhythmias, both sustained monomorphic ventricular tachycardia and nonsustained ventricular arrhythmias, are prevalent (60–87%) in patients with idiopathic cardiomyopathy [3,4].

Autopsy study in patients with idiopathic dilated cardiomyopathy demonstrated a high incidence of mural endocardial plaque (69–85%) and myocardial fibrosis (57%) with a relative paucity of dense scar (14%) [5]. The ventricular myocardium in idiopathic cardiomyopathy is characterized by multiple patchy areas of interstitial and replacement fibrosis and myofiber disarray with variable degrees of myocyte hypertrophy [5,6]. Histological and electrophysiologic correlations have been studied in

transplanted hearts from patients with idiopathic nonischemic cardiomyopathy. Generalized, nonspecific diffuse presence of reactive fibrosis, with heterogeneous patterns of activations and conduction disturbances were observed at both epicardial and endocardial layers. The degree of conduction abnormalities/nonuniform anisotropy seemed to correlate with the amount of fibrosis/myofiber disarray as well as generations of reentrant wavefronts [2,7–10].

The mechanisms of monomorphic VT in nonischemic cardiomyopathy include: (1) myocardial reentry, (2) reentrant arrhythmias utilizing the cardiac conduction system, such as bundle branch reentry or interfascicular reentry, and (3) focal automaticity [11,12].

Mapping and ablation of focal ventricular arrhythmia

Focal ectopic automaticity or triggered activity arising from subepicardial or subendocardial sites presents mostly as nonsustained arrhythmias in 10–25% of the VTs in patients with nonischemic cardiomyopathy [10,13]. It may originate from the distal Purkinje system; in that case a Purkinje-like potential may be recorded with a short potential to QRS interval (Figure 8.1). Mapping and ablation can be approached using, either activation mapping for the earliest activation or using pace mapping. Similar focal VTs involving the distal His–Purkinje system have been reported in patients with ischemic heart disease [14,15].

Ventricular Arrhythmias and Sudden Cardiac Death, 1st edition. Edited by P.J. Wang, A. Al-Ahmad, H. Hsia, and P.C. Zei © 2008 Blackwell Publishing, ISBN: 978-1-4051-6114-5.

Table 8.1 Etiologies of nonischemic cardiomyopathy

Idiopathic	46.5%
Myocarditis	12%
HIV	4.9%
Peripartum cardiomyopathy	4.9%
Chronic alcohol use	3.4%
Drug-induced	3.1%
Connective tissue disease	2.2%
Amyloidosis	2.1%
Hypertension	2.1%
Familial	1.8%
Valvular	1.5%
Congenital	1%

Ventricular tachycardia related to the His–Purkinje system

Reentrant VTs utilizing the cardiac conduction system such as bundle branch reentry has been reported in 11–30% of the VTs in nonischemic cardiomyopathy [11,16–18]. The prerequisite for bundle branch reentry is conduction delay in the His–Purkinje system, with an averaged HV interval of 80 milliseconds (range 60–110 ms) [19]. The most common electrocardiographic abnormality in patients with bundle branch reentrant VT is a non-specific intraventricular conduction defect (IVCD) of the left bundle branch block (LBBB) pattern [16,18]. Although dilated nonischemic cardiomyopathy is the most common clinical setting for bundle branch reentrant VT, this arrhythmia can occur in cardiomyopathy of any etiology. Bundle branch reentrant VT often coexist with other myocardial reentrant arrhythmias in patients with structural heart disease [16,18].

The electrophysiologic mechanism of macroreentrant bundle branch reentry (BBR) VT consists of anterograde conduction down the right bundle, retrograde conduction up the left bundle, and slow trans-septal intramyocardial conduction. Bundle branch reentry involving circus movement

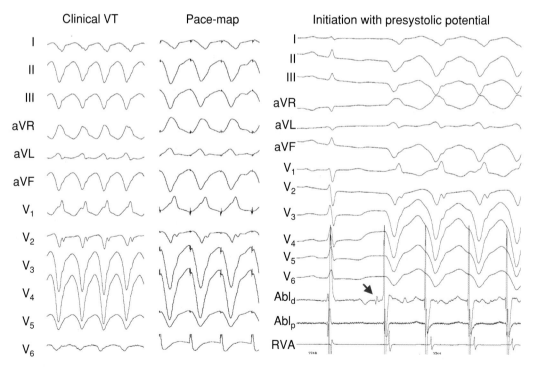

Figure 8.1 Focal ectopic automaticity triggered from subepicardial or subendocardial sites represents 10–25% of the VTs in nonischemic cardiomyopathy. Focal arrhythmia in this setting may arise from damaged Purkinje fibers and a Purkinje-like potential may be recorded with a short potential to QRS interval. Mapping and ablation can be approached using either activation mapping for earliest activation or pace mapping.

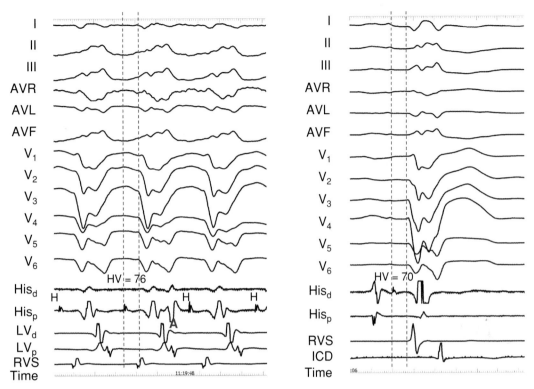

Figure 8.2 Bundle branch reentry (BBR) ventricular tachycardia. The QRS morphology during VT often bears similarity to the sinus rhythm. The baseline HV interval was prolonged at 70 milliseconds. During BBR VT, VA dissociation was noted and a one-to-one HV relationship was observed with further prolongation of the HV interval to 76 milliseconds.

in the opposite direction or interfascicular reentry in the left ventricular (LV) fascicular system has also been observed [16,18,20]. The QRS morphology during BBR VT often bears similarity to the sinus rhythm QRS (Figure 8.2), has a typical LBBB (more common) or RBBB appearance, depending on whether the anterograde ventricular activation is via the right or left bundle branches, respectively [14,16].

The diagnosis of bundle branch reentry is based on careful detailed electrogram recordings, including recordings from the bundle branches and the His, both during the initiation and sustained reentry. During a typical LBBB BBR VT, the onset of the QRS is often preceded by the right-bundle potential or the His deflection, with an HV interval typically equal to or longer than that found during sinus rhythm (Figure 8.3). Cycle length oscillations of the V–V intervals are preceded by similar changes in the H–H intervals. Entrainment of the bundle

branch circus movement reentry can be achieved by pacing and capturing either the right bundle branch or the left fascicle (Figure 8.4). Catheter ablation of the right or left bundle branches interrupts the circuit and provides an effective treatment of this arrhythmia [14,17]. However, a comprehensive electrophysiologic evaluation is essential in patients with cardiomyopathy since ventricular tachycardias related to the His–Purkinje system often coexist with other myocardial reentry arrhythmias.

Myocardial reentrant ventricular tachycardia

The predominant mechanism (62–89%) of ventricular tachycardia in nonischemic cardiomyopathy is myocardial scar-based reentry [11,12,21]. Early catheter mapping studies demonstrated less frequent abnormal fractionated and/or late electrogram recordings in patients with nonischemic

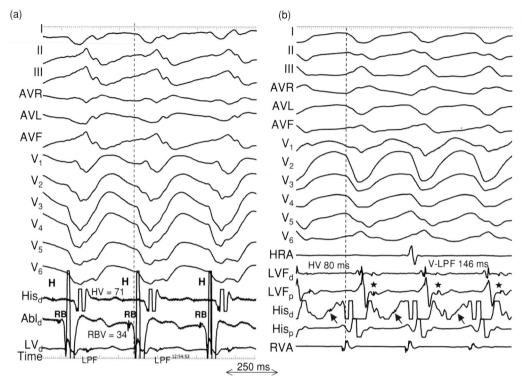

(a)   (b)

Figure 8.3 Bundle branch reentry ventricular tachycardia with an LBBB QRS morphology. Panel (a) During LBBB VT, His deflections (HV interval of 71 ms) precedes right bundle activation (RBB–V interval of 34 ms), followed by onset of the QRS. The left posterior fascicle (LPF) potentials followed right ventricular activations suggesting retrograde penetration up the LPF during a counterclockwise reentry BBR VT. Panel (b) Similar observation in a different patient with nonischemic cardiomyopathy. Presystolic His activation (marked by small arrows) with a HV interval of 80 milliseconds. This is followed by slow trans-septal propagation and late retrograde left posterior fascicular activation (marked by stars) with a V–LPF interval of 146 milliseconds.

cardiomyopathy compared to those with coronary artery disease (Table 8.2). Furthermore, the extent of electrogram abnormality seems to correlate with the type of arrhythmia presentation in this population. Namely, abnormal endocardial electrograms were more prevalent in the population with sustained VT, compared to those with no inducible arrhythmia, nonsustained VT, or cardiac arrest (Table 8.3) [22,23].

High-density electroanatomical mapping provided a unique description of the size and location of the endocardial voltage abnormalities that were not previously attainable with conventional mapping technologies. The endocardial electrophysiologic substrate for monomorphic ventricular tachycardia in the setting of nonischemic cardiomyopathy is characterized by modest distribution of abnormal low-voltage electrogram recordings. The extent of endocardial abnormalities is highly variable and rarely involves more than 25% of the LV endocardial surface. Importantly, the predominant distribution of the endocardial electrogram abnormality

Table 8.2 Influence of underlying heart disease on endocardial electrogram characteristics

	CAD	Cardiomyopathy
Patients (*n*)	132	26
Normal sites (%)	50 ± 24	84 ± 16**
Abnormal sites (%)	43 ± 21	15 ± 18**
Fractionated sites (%)	7 ± 11	1 ± 3*
Late sites (%)	12 ± 14	2 ± 5**

Note: ** $P < 0.001$, * $P < 0.005$.

CAD, coronary artery disease. Adapted from Cassidy et al., Circulation, 1986, with permission.

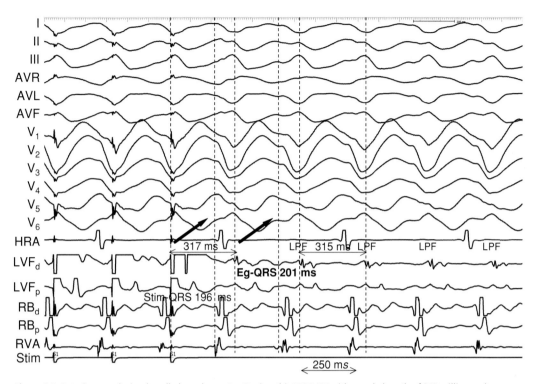

Figure 8.4 Entrainment during bundle branch reentry. During this LBBB VT with a cycle length of 315 milliseconds, entrainment of the tachycardia was achieved at the left posterior fascicle with concealed fusion, with a postpacing interval (PPI) of 201 milliseconds. Markedly prolonged stimuli–QRS (Stim–QRS = 196 ms) and electrogram–QRS intervals (Eg–QRS = 201 ms) were noted, suggesting capturing from sites far away from the exit (with early right ventricular apical activation) of this counterclockwise reentry tachycardia.

is located at the ventricular base, frequently involving the perivalvular regions (Figure 8.5). Ventricular tachycardias in these patients were carefully mapped and they typically (88%) originate from the basal region of the left ventricle, corresponding to the locations of the anatomic endocardial substrate (Figure 8.6) [11,12,24]. The predilection of basal location of scar has been observed by contrast-enhanced cardiac MRI [25]. Compared to patients with coronary artery disease, the overall extent of the abnormal endocardial low-voltage areas is significantly smaller in size in patients with nonischemic cardiomyopathy (approximately one-third) [20,26] (Figure 8.7).

Table 8.3 Influence of clinical arrhythmias on endocardial electrogram characteristics in patients with cardiomyopathy

	No VT	NSVT	CA	VT
Normal sites (%)	87 ± 7	90 ± 10	91 ± 11	$60 \pm 25^*$
Abnormal sites (%)	13 ± 7	10 ± 10	9 ± 11	$37 \pm 27^*$
Fractionated sites (%)	0 ± 0	0 ± 0	0 ± 0	3 ± 7
Late sites (%)	4 ± 6	5 ± 8	0 ± 0	0 ± 0

Note: $P < 0.05$ VT versus No VT, NSVT, and CA.
NSVT, nonsustained ventricular tachycardia; CA, cardiac arrest.
Adapted from Cassidy et al., Circulation, 1986, with permission.

Endocardial versus epicardial electrogram characteristics

The relationship between inducible arrhythmias and the extent of abnormal endocardial and/or epicardial substrate in patients with nonischemic cardiomyopathy was initially evaluated during surgical epicardial defibrillator patch placement [20,27].

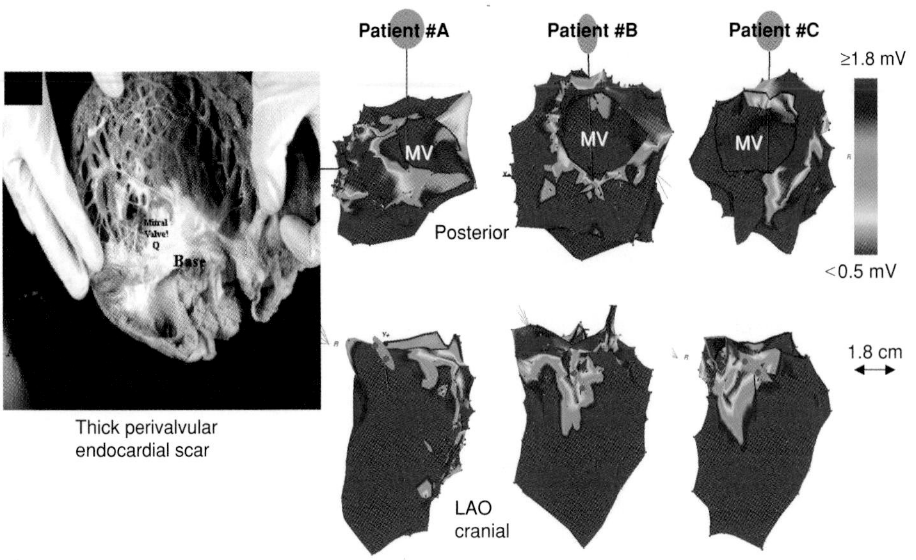

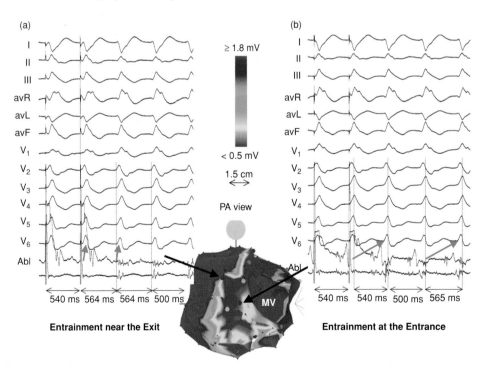

Figure 8.5 Endocardial 3D electroanatomic mapping in patients with nonischemic cardiomyopathy presenting with monomorphic VT. Purple areas represent normal endocardium (amplitude $\geq$1.8 mV) with dense scar depicted as red (amplitude <0.5 mV). The border zone (amplitude 0.5–1.8 mV) is defined as areas with the color gradient between red and purple. The voltage maps typically demonstrate a modest-sized low-voltage endocardial electrogram abnormalities or scar, located near the ventricular base in the perivalvular region. On the left is a pathologic specimen that demonstrates perivalvular scarring at the ventricular base and corresponds to the observed low-voltage areas on the voltage maps.

Figure 8.6 Comparison of endocardial voltage abnormalities between patients with nonischemic cardiomyopathy (a) and coronary artery disease (b) with prior myocardial infarctions. The color gradient of the voltage maps has been previously described. Compared to patients with coronary artery disease, the overall extent of the abnormal endocardial scar areas is significantly smaller in size in patients with nonischemic cardiomyopathy (approximately one-third), and is primarily located near the basal left ventricle.

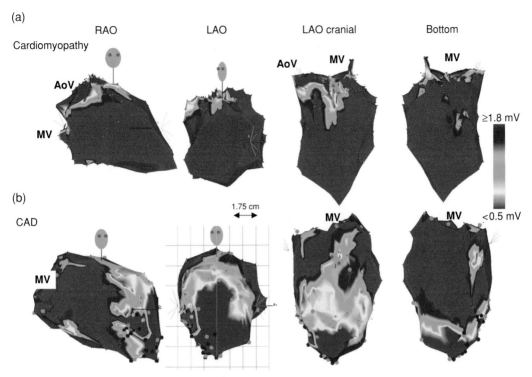

Figure 8.7 Electroanatomic voltage map coupled with entrainment mapping for localization of ventricular tachycardia circuit. The color gradient corresponds to the left ventricular endocardial bipolar electrogram amplitude as described in Figure 8.5. Entrainment with minimal surface fusion was observed near the exit site with a short stimulus–QRS interval (Panel a). The entrance site was identified with perfect entrainment and concealed fusion and a long stimulus–QRS interval that matched the electrogram–QRS interval (Panel b). The VT circuit was located near the left ventricular base, corresponding to the locations of the abnormal endocardial substrate at the perivalvular region defined by the voltage map.

The relationship of arrhythmia inducibility to the extent of electrogram abnormalities was demonstrated. Forty-seven percent of epicardial electrograms were considered abnormal in patients with inducible sustained monomorphic VT, compared to 6% in patients who were noninducible or with only inducible polymorphic arrhythmia or ventricular fibrillation. A similar relationship of VT inducibility with the presence of abnormal endocardial electrograms was also observed. In patients with inducible sustained monomorphic VT, 38% of endocardial electrograms were abnormal, while in patients with no inducible VT, only 18% of endocardial electrograms were abnormal. The extent of abnormal endocardial compared to epicardial electrograms was similar and represented approximately 40–50% of the recordings in patients with inducible sustained monomorphic VT, compared to only 10–20% in those without inducible monomorphic VT.

The electroanatomic substrate for sustained monomorphic VT appears to be associated with more extensive myocardial fibrosis, electrogram abnormalities and nonuniform anisotropy, involving both the endocardium and epicardium, compared to those without sustained reentry. The relatively equal distributions of electrogram abnormalities suggest some VT circuits may be located in the mid-myocardial or epicardial layers, whereas other tachycardia may originate from the subendocardium. Importantly, although the overall distribution of electrogram abnormalities was equal for the group as a whole, the results were patient specific. Abnormal epicardial substrate predominated in some patients while endocardial abnormalities were more common in others (Figure 8.8). With

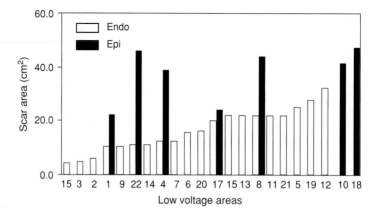

Figure 8.8 Abnormal low voltage (<1.5 mV) areas in selected patients with nonischemic cardiomyopathy, who had both epicardial and endocardial mapping. The area of scar **(y axis)** was larger on the epicardial surface than on the endocardial surfaces. Endocardial **(white bars)** and epicardial **(black bars)** scars in patients with myocardial re-entry. (Adopted from Soejima K, JACC 2004;43(10):1834) (permission pending).

programmed electrical stimulation, inducibility of monomorphic VT in patients with nonischemic cardiomyopathy is usually lower than in those with ischemic heart disease [28]. Furthermore, the response of these patients to ventricular stimulation is variable with poor prediction of clinical outcomes and prognosis.

High-density epicardial and endocardial substrate mapping provided further understanding of the relationship of recurrent monomorphic VT to low-voltage areas [12,26,29]. Most (63%) endocardial scars were again identified adjacent to a valve annulus. Scar can be deep in the endocardium, and can be greater in extent on the epicardium than on the endocardium in nonischemic cardiomyopathy (Table 8.4). Evidence of slow conduction and VT circuit isthmus may be identified in large areas of epicardial scar (Figure 8.9).

The success of endocardial ablation was lower than that which we have observed for postinfarct VT [12,29]. Reentry circuits deep to the endocardium and in the epicardium appear to be a likely explanation. Epicardial mapping led to successful ablation in a significant portion of patients who failed prior endocardial procedures. The use of either a combined [26] or a staged [12] endocardial–epicardial mapping/ablation approach is likely to improve success.

Noninvasive imaging

The recent advancement in noninvasive imaging such as cardiac magnetic resonance (MR) has provided new insight into the anatomical substrate in patients with nonischemic cardiomyopathy. Late gadolinium enhancement on cardiac MR scan has been used to evaluate the differences between the nonischemic and ischemic subgroups in patients with LV dysfunction and heart failure [30]. None of the control subjects with normal ventricular function had abnormal enhancement on MR, while all patients with coronary artery disease had enhancement, which was subendocardial or transmural, consistent with the typical locations of infarcted scars. However, in patients with nonischemic cardiomyopathy, no evidence of late gadolinium enhancement was observed in over half (59%) of the population. Patchy or longitudinal striae of mid-wall enhancement patterns were seen in one-third (28%) of the patients that were clearly different from the distribution associated with coronary artery disease. The mid-wall myocardial enhancement in

Table 8.4 Substrate in sustained monomorphic ventricular tachycardia: Endocardial versus Epicardial sites

Total area of scar	Epicardial	Endocardial
Nonischemic cardiomyopathy		
Area of abnormal Egm (cm²)	37.5 ± 10.4	16.5 ± 8.1
Ischemic cardiomyopathy		
Area of abnormal Egm (cm²)	15 ± 1.5	42.2 ± 1.1

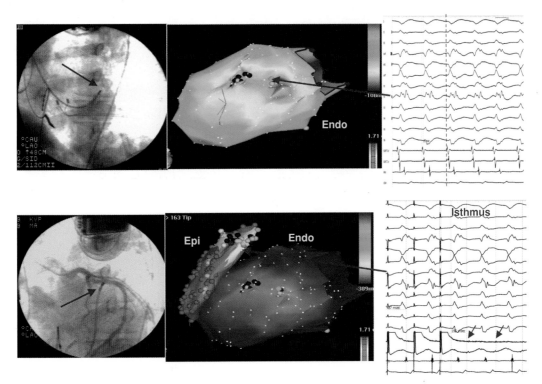

Figure 8.9 Endocardial and epicardial mapping in a patient with sustained ventricular tachycardia. Upper panel shows an endocardial electroanatomic activation map with the corresponding fluoroscopic image in left anterior oblique (LAO) projection. Red color represents early activation with late activation areas depicted in blue. The electroanatomic map demonstrated a diffuse area of early activation on the endocardial surface during VT. This suggests the site-of-origin was distant from the endocardium. The activation sequence showed minimally early presystolic recordings. The lower panel shows an epicardial electroanatomic activation map superimposed over the endocardial location map (in blue). The gray area represents dense scar in the epicardial surface. Low-amplitude presystolic electrograms were recorded (small arrow) over the epicardial surface and the VT isthmus was identified by perfect entrainment with concealed fusion and a long stimulus–QRS that equaled electrogram–QRS interval. The corresponding fluoroscopic image showed an epicardial catheter positioned in the high lateral basal area near the Circumflex artery.

patients with nonischemic cardiomyopathy is similar to the fibrosis found at autopsy [5]. The remaining patients (13%) had patterns of subendocardial or transmural enhancement that was indistinguishable from that of ischemic heart disease.

A similar incidence (35%) of mid-wall MR enhancement consistent with fibrosis was also observed by Assomull et al. [31]. In this prospective study, patients with mid-wall myocardial fibrosis had a significantly worse outcome of all-cause death or cardiac hospitalization during a mean duration of follow-up of 658 ± 355 days. In addition, despite the relatively low number of events, patients with fibrosis had a significantly greater incidence of sudden cardiac death and sustained ventricular tachycardia (Figure 8.10).

The substrate for inducible sustained monomorphic VT, as determined by contrast-enhanced cardiac MRI, has also been described in patients with nonischemic cardiomyopathy [25]. The presence of scar was most common in the basal and septal walls, but their location was not predictive of inducible ventricular tachycardia at electrophysiological study. Patients who were inducible for monomorphic VT had a greater myocardial scar volume with a predominance of mid-wall scar distribution, involving the 26–75% of wall thickness. Catheter mapping studies of patients

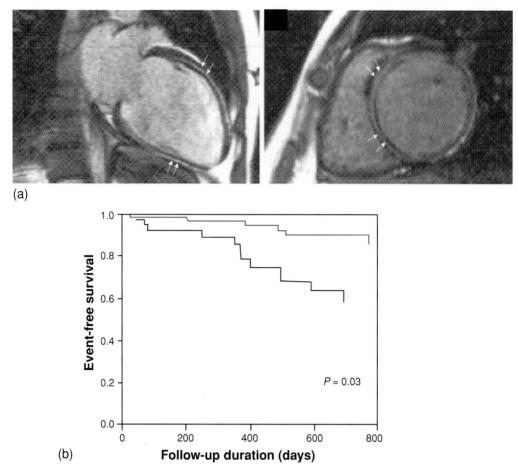

Figure 8.10 Late gadolinium enhancement (LGE) patterns in dilated cardiomyopathy. Marked mid-wall enhancement (small white arrows) is shown in vertical long axis and short axis (a). Kaplan–Meier survival estimates for sudden cardiac death or sustained ventricular tachycardia, adjusted for baseline differences in left ventricular ejection fraction (b). In nonischemic cardiomyopathy, the presence of mid-wall fibrosis determined by contrast-enhanced cardiac MR is a predictor of poor clinical and arrhythmic outcomes, which is independent of ventricular remodeling.

with nonischemic cardiomyopathy point to reentry around scar deep in the myocardium, near the ventricular base and in the perivalvular region, as the underlying mechanism for ventricular tachycardia.

In patients with nonischemic cardiomyopathy, the presence and morphology of myocardial scar, as determined by contrast-enhanced MRI, appear to be an independent risk factor in predicting clinical and arrhythmic outcome, as well as inducibility of monomorphic VT. Similar findings have been observed in patients with ischemic heart disease, in whom the cardiac MRI is a better identifier of substrates for inducible monomorphic VT than ejection fraction [32].

In summary, contrast-enhanced cardiac MR has a potential role in the risk stratification of patients with nonischemic cardiomyopathy. Furthermore, detection and localization of the abnormal myocardial scar by MR has the potential to abbreviate voltage/substrate mapping in the electrophysiology laboratory, and may be utilized for defining an ablation strategy for ventricular tachycardia [33].

Conclusions

The mechanism of monomorphic ventricular tachycardia in patients with nonischemic cardiomyopathy is predominantly myocardial-based reentry associated with scar; however, bundle-branch

Table 8.5 Outcomes* of catheter ablation of myocardial reentrant VT in nonischemic cardiomyopathy

	Number of patients	Follow-up (mo)	Ablation Approach	No recurrence	Infrequent VT (< 1/3 mo)
Soejima et al. (2004)	22	12	Endo ±Epi (7)	12 (54%)	N/A
Marchlinski et al. (2000)	8	10	Endo	3 (38%)	1 (12%)
Hsia et al. (2003)	19	22	Endo	5 (26%)	8 (42%)

Note: *With or without antiarrhythmic drugs.
Soejima, JACC 2004;43:1834; Hsia, Circ 2003;108:704; Marchlinski, Circ 2000;101:1288.

reentry and nonreentrant focal VT must also be considered.

The pathophysiologic substrate in patients with nonischemic cardiomyopathy and scar-based reentry clearly differs from that of coronary artery disease. In patients with sustained monomorphic VT, a greater degree of myocardial fibrosis is present compared to those with only nonsustained arrhythmia. Compared to patients with monomorphic VT and coronary artery disease, only modest (~1/3) endocardial scar is present with a predominant scars distribution adjacent to valve annuli, deep in the endocardium, and can be greater in extent on the epicardium than on the endocardium. Such variable distributions of epicardial and endocardial electrogram abnormalities with significant patient-to-patient variability suggest that the location for reentrant VT may be epicardial, endocardial, or extend transmurally. Approximately one-third of the patients with nonischemic cardiomyopathy may require epicardial ablation. Recognition of this unique anatomic distribution of the electrophysiologic substrate has important implications for designing strategies for VT mapping and ablation in this setting. Aggressive attempts to target all morphologies of VT with detailed endocardial and epicardial mapping and pacing protocols will be required. Recordings made from noncontact mapping during VT may also provide insight into the relationship of the VT circuit and the electroanatomic substrate. With the development of exciting new thoracoscopic or intrapericardial approaches, epicardial mapping and radiofrequency is likely to improve success.

Noninvasive imaging, such as contrast-enhanced cardiac MR imaging, may provide diagnostic information regarding the extent of electroanatomical substrate and possible locations of VT circuit. In addition, the presence of mid-wall fibrosis is an independent predictor of arrhythmic and clinical outcome, and may be useful in risk stratification in determining the need for device therapy.

Future directions

Catheter ablation in patients with nonischemic cardiomyopathy remains a challenge, especially in those with myocardial reentrant VT (Table 8.5). The substrate associated with monomorphic VT in the setting of nonischemic cardiomyopathy needs to be further defined. Future investigations will focus on improving our understanding of the heterogeneous pathophysiologic processes of this disease. In patients undergoing cardiac transplantation, characterization of the anatomy as it relates to clinical history of spontaneous or inducible sustained monomorphic VT needs to be completed. Future noninvasive imaging technologies that provide rapid, detailed description of the electroanatomical substrate is essential and can abbreviate our mapping effort, as well as provide the capacity for serial assessment of temporal changes and progressions of the disease process and risk stratification. Lastly, effective access to epicardial or mid-myocardial layers, coupled with novel energy delivery, such as cryo-, laser-, or focused ultrasound, will result in successful ablative interventions.

References

1 Kasper E, Agema W, Hutchins G, Deckers J, Hare J, Baugham K. The causes of dilated cardiomyopathy: a clinicopathologic review of 673 consecutive patients. J Am Coll Cardiol 1994;23:586–590.

2 de Leeuw N, Ruiter D, Balk A, Melchers W, Galama J. Histopathologic findings in explanted heart tissue from patients with end-stage idiopathic dilated cardiomyopathy. Transpl Int 2001;1:299–306.

3 Meinertz T, Hofmann T, Kasper W, et al. Significance of ventricular arrhythmias in idiopathic dilated cardiomyopathy. Am J Cardiol 1984;53:902–907.

4 Huang S, Messer J, Denes P. Significance of ventricular tachycardia in idiopathic dilated cardiomyopathy: observation in 35 patients. Am J Cardiol 1982;51:507–512.

5 Roberts W, Siegel R, McManus B. Idiopathic dilated cardiomyopathy: analysis of 152 necropsy patients. Am J Cardiol 1987;60:1340–1355.

6 Unverferth D, Magorien R, Moeschberger M, Baker P, Fetters J, Leier C. Factors influencing the one-year mortality of dilated cardiomyopathy. Am J Cardiol 1984;54:147–152.

7 Anderson K, Walker R, Urie P, et al. Myocardial electrical propagation in patients with idiopathic dilated cardiomyopathy. J Clin Invest 1993;92:122–140.

8 Wu T, Ong J, Hwang C, et al. Characteristics of wave fronts during ventricular fibrillation in human hearts with dilated cardiomyopathy: role of increased fibrosis in the generation of reentry. J Am Coll Cardiol 1998;32:187–96.

9 de Bakker J, van Capelle F, Janse M, et al. Fractionated electrograms in dilated cardiomyopathy: origin and relation to abnormal conduction. J Am Coll Cardiol 1996;27:1071–1078.

10 Pogwizd S. Nonreentrant mechanisms underlying spontaneous ventricular arrhythmias in a model of nonischemic heart failure in rabbits. Circulation 1995;92:1034–1048.

11 Delacretaz E, Stevenson W, Ellison K, Maisel W, Friedman P. Mapping and radiofrequency catheter ablation of the three types of sustained monomorphic ventricular tachycardia in nonischemic heart disease. J Cardiovasc Electrophysiol 2000;11:11–17.

12 Soejima K, Stevenson W, Sapp J, Selwyn A, Couper G, Epstein L. Endocardial and epicardial radiofrequency ablation of ventricular tachycardia associated with dilated cardiomyopathy: the importance of low-voltage scars. J Am Coll Cardiol 2004;43:1834–1842.

13 Pogwizd S, McKenzie J, Cain M. Mechanisms underlying spontaneous and induced ventricular arrhythmias in patients with idiopathic dilated cardiomyopathy. Circulation 1998;98:2404–2414.

14 Lopera G, Stevenson W, Soejima K, et al. Identification and ablation of three types of ventricular tachycardia involving the His-Purkinje system in patients with heart disease. J Cardiovasc Electrophysiol 2004;15:52–58.

15 Bogun F, Good E, Reich S, et al. Role of Purkinje fibers in post-infarction ventricular tachycardia. J Am Coll Cardiol 2006;48:2500–2507.

16 Akhtar M. Clincial spectrum of ventricular tachycardia. Circulation 1990;82:1561–1573.

17 Tchou P, Jazayeri M, Denker S, Dongas J, Caceres J, Akhtar M. Transcatheter electrical ablation of right bundle branch. A method of treating macroreentrant ventricular tachycardia attributed to bundle branch reentry. Circulation 1988;78:246–257.

18 Caceres J, Jazayeri M, McKinnie J, et al. Sustained bundle branch reentry as a mechanism of clinical tachycardia. Circulation 1989;79:256–270.

19 Blanck Z, Dhala A, Deshpande S, Sra J, Jazayeri M, Akhtar M. Bundle branch reentrant ventricular tachycardia:

cumulative experience in 48 patients [see comments]. J Cardiovasc Electrophysiol 1993;4:253–262.

20 Hsia H, Marchlinski F. Characterization of the electroanatomical substrate for monomorphic ventricular tachycardia in patients with nonischemic cardiomyopathy. PACE 2002;25:1114–1127.

21 Hsia H, Callans D, Marchlinski F. Characterization of endocardial electrophysiological substrate in patients with nonischemic cardiomyopathy and monomorphic ventricular tachycardia. Circulation 2003;108:704–710.

22 Cassidy D, Vassallo J, Buxton A, Doherty J, Marchlinski F, Josephson M. The value of catheter mapping during sinus rhythm to localize site of origin of ventricular tachycardia. Circulation 1984;69:1003–1010.

23 Cassidy D, Vassallo J, Miller J, et al. Endocardial catheter mapping in patients in sinus rhythm: relationship to underlying heart disease and ventricular arrhythmias. Circulation 1986;73:645–652.

24 Hsia H, Callans D, Marchlinski F. Characterization of the electrophysiologic substrate in patients with nonischemic cardiomyopathy and monomorphic ventricular tachycardia. Circulation 2003;108:704–710.

25 Nazarian S, Bluemke D, Lardo A, et al. Magnetic resonance assessment of the substrate for inducible ventricular tachycardia in nonischemic cardiomyopathy. Circulation 2005;112:2821–2825.

26 Cesario D, Vaseghi M, Boyle N, et al. Value of high-density endocardial and epicardial mapping for catheter ablation of hemodynamically unstable ventricular tachycardia. Heart Rhythm 2006;3:1–10.

27 Perlman R, Miller J, Kindwall K, Buxton A, Josephson M, Marchlinski F. Abnormal epicardial and endocardial electrograms in patients with idiopathic dilated cardiomyopathy: relationship to arrhythmias. Circulation 1990;82:I-708.

28 Hsia H, Marchlinski F. Electrophysiology studies in patients with dilated cardiomyopathies. Card Electrophysiol Rev 2002;6:472–481.

29 Marchlinski F, Callans D, Gottlieb C, Zado E. Linear ablation lesions for control of unmappable ventricular tachycardia in patients with ischemic and nonischemic cardiomyopathy. Circulation 2000;101:1288–1296.

30 McCrohon J, Moon J, Prasad S, et al. Differentiation of heart failure related to dilated cardiomyopathy and coronary artery disease using gadolinium-enhanced cardiovascular magnetic resonance. Circulation 2003;108:54–59.

31 Assomull R, Prasad S, Lyne J, et al. Cardiovascular magnetic resonance, fibrosis, and prognosis in dilated cardiomyopathy. J Am Coll Cardiol 2006;48:1977–1985.

32 Bello D, Fieno D, Kim R, et al. Infarct morphology identifies patients with substrate for sustained ventricular tachycardia. J Am Coll Cardiol 2005;45:1104–1108.

33 Bello D, Kipper S, Valderrábano M, Shivkumar K. Catheter ablation of ventricular tachycardia guided by contrast-enhanced cardiac computed tomography. Heart Rhythm 2004;4:490–492.

CHAPTER 9

Mapping to define scars and isthmuses: a new paradigm for guiding ventricular tachycardia ablation

Kyoko Soejima

Myocardial infarction, cardiomyopathies, and repaired congenital heart disease are very different entities. Yet a common theme has emerged when considering sustained monomorphic VT in these patients: the vast majority is caused by reentry associated with areas of ventricular scar. These scars provide slow conduction and areas of conduction block that facilitate reentry. Areas of slow conduction are caused by fibrotic tissue between myocardial fibers causing zigzag conduction [1]. Dense fibrosis contributes to conduction block that defines the reentry circuit borders. In most of the reentry circuits, these features lead to formation of critical isthmuses that are desirable targets for ablation [2].

Conventional mapping techniques

The traditional ablation methods to identify the reentry circuit are as follows: (1) activation sequence mapping, (2) pace mapping during sinus rhythm to identify the exit site for the VT, and (3) entrainment mapping during VT. The type of mapping technique depends on the types of VT, whether VT is stable or unstable.

Activation sequence mapping

For activation sequence mapping, the VT has to be stable hemodynamically, with the patient remaining

Ventricular Arrhythmias and Sudden Cardiac Death, 1st edition. Edited by P.J. Wang, A. Al-Ahmad, H. Hsia, and P.C. Zei © 2008 Blackwell Publishing, ISBN: 978-1-4051-6114-5.

in the same VT during mapping. Even when activation mapping is possible, entrainment mapping is often necessary to determine which potential of a multicomponent electrogram is the local electrogram, rather than a far-field signal, and to correctly identify abnormal bystander regions [3]. After obtaining the activation sequence map to define the circuit, one can decide where to place RF lesions to transect the reentry circuit.

Pace mapping

Pace mapping is useful when the VT is unstable and cannot be mapped during VT. Pacing near the exit of the reentry circuit often produces a QRS similar to that of the VT, although the area over which pacing matches VT can be relatively large. Also, the QRS during pace mapping may look very different from that of the VT even when the site is in the reentry circuit, as the wavefront is able to propagate away from the circuit over a different path than it follows during VT.

In addition to the exit site identification, pace mapping provides evidence of slow conduction, evident as a long stimulus to the QRS onset (S-QRS). Stevenson et al. [4] reported that the S-QRS interval was more than 40 milliseconds at 70% of isthmus sites. Brunckhorst et al. [5] evaluated pace mapping at isthmus sites, including exits and more proximal sites in the isthmus. Sites where pace mapping produced the same QRS with different S-QRS intervals were identified to attempt to trace the course of the

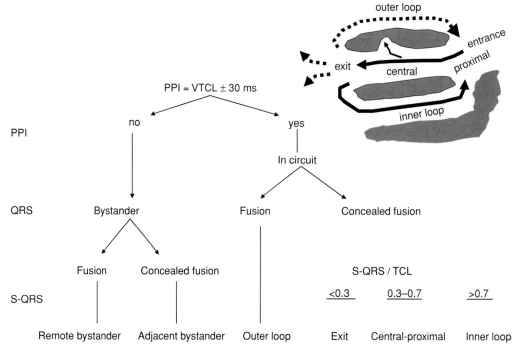

Figure 9.1 Diagram showing the identification of the isthmus by entrainment mapping (see details in Ref. [6]).

isthmus. All sites with an S-QRS >40 milliseconds were located in the low-voltage area, identified by the electroanatomical mapping system. A total of 13 isthmuses in 13 scars were identified. The shortest S-QRS interval in each isthmus averaged 51 ± 18 (range 23–84) milliseconds. The longest S-QRS was 94 ± 33 (49–141) milliseconds. The QRS morphology during pace mapping at the longest S-QRS isthmus sites matched VT only in 27% patients, suggesting that the pace-map QRS is less likely to resemble that of VT at more proximal sites in the isthmus. However, the pace mapping matched VT at 85% of the identified isthmus sites.

Entrainment mapping

Entrainment is continuous resetting of the circuit by a series of stimuli. Pacing during the VT at a slightly faster rate accelerates all QRS complexes and electrograms to the pacing rate. The QRS morphology during entrainment can be compared to VT QRS morphology, then the postpacing interval can be measured to compare with the VT cycle length. Finally, by comparing the S-QRS interval to the VT

cycle length, the location in relation to the reentry circuit exit can be decided [6]. A diagram is shown in Figure 9.1.

Identification of the isthmus with substrate mapping

It is not uncommon for VT to be unstable for mapping. It may be hemodynamically unstable, or change morphology either spontaneously or during catheter manipulation or pacing. Some VTs are not reliably inducible during the electrophysiological study. Using only fluoroscopic guidance, repeated assessment of the catheter ablation procedure was challenging, time-consuming, and difficult to rely on. One approach to this problem is to characterize the arrhythmia substrate during a hemodynamically stable rhythm, which may be sinus, paced, or a stable VT. This assessment has been called substrate mapping. The recent development of nonfluoroscopic electroanatomical mapping systems has greatly facilitated this approach. These systems reconstruct the three-dimensional anatomical information and display electrical information, such as voltage and activation sequence. Importantly, sites of interest, such as those with a "perfect pace match" or "isthmus" can be tagged for precise return to the site later. Plots of electrogram amplitude, known as voltage maps, are particularly useful for patients with scar-related arrhythmias. Marchlinski et al. [7], have shown that more than 95% of normal bipolar ventricular electrograms have an amplitude exceeding 1.5 mV. Using this value to define the maximum of the display range, all of the normal voltage area is shown as one color (purple in Figure 9.2, with permission), and abnormal low-voltage areas that contain scar are delineated.

Brunckhorst et al. [13] evaluated whether the direction of activation produced by sinus rhythm compared to ventricular pacing influences the voltage maps employed to detect areas of scar. The correlation of bipolar electrogram amplitude during one rhythm with that during the other was excellent ($r = 0.77$, $P < 0.0001$); so either rhythm seems acceptable for voltage maps.

Finding an isthmus can be crucial for successful ablation. The identification of an isthmus is associated with better acute success rate, shorter ablation line, and a tendency to fewer arrhythmia recurrences [8]. The width of these reentry circuit isthmuses, when carefully defined in patients with mappable VTs, is typically in the range of 1.5 cm with a length of 3 cm [9]. Therefore usually linear ablation is preferred over a single RF lesion to transect the reentry circuit isthmus. However, strict mapping criteria to identify single sites for successful RF site were evaluated by El-Shalakany et al. [10]. They reported that ablation at a single site is likely to be successful if the following combination of features is present: (1) entrainment with concealed fusion, (2) postpacing interval difference from the VT cycle length (CL) ≤ 10 milliseconds, and (3) presystolic potential ($<70\%$ of VTCL) with Eg-QRS and S-QRS difference ≤ 10 milliseconds. At the sites which meet all these three criteria, termination of VT occurred in 10 seconds in 75% VTs, and termination within 32 seconds in 95% VTs. Nineteen of the 20 targeted VTs were terminated with an RF application at a single site. The positive predictive value of these strict mapping criteria to predict

VT termination with single RF was 100%, whereas the negative predictive value was 96%. The sensitivity was 94%, and specificity was 100%.

Sinus rhythm electrogram with delayed isolated component [11]

Areas of slow conduction and block can give rise to delayed activation during sinus rhythm. It has been hypothesized that identification of electrograms displaying an isolated, delayed component (IDC), characterized by double or multiple components separated by very low amplitude signals or isoelectric intervals, could better identify the VT-related slow conduction areas than low-amplitude electrograms. Substrate mapping for these potentials is performed during sinus rhythm or RV pacing. These electrograms were characterized by double or multiple components separated by ≥ 50 milliseconds. By tagging the sites with IDC, an area was identified with cluster of tags. To define the limits of the area demonstrating IDC, once an IDC was identified, multiple sites were explored around it to obtain a distance of ≤ 1 cm between the mapped sites. It was more frequent to identify the area with delayed isolated potential during RV pacing, probably due to the activation direction. After the maps were complete, pace mapping was used to relate a particular IDC area to clinical VT. Pace mapping started at sites of the latest IDC. When the QRS morphology of the clinical VT was not reproduced, VT morphology was analyzed and a site from the limits of the IDC area was selected for pacing. Then the VT was induced with the catheter positioned in this area. The diagram is shown in Figure 9.3. In their series of 24 patients, one area of IDC was recorded in 20 patients, and two or more areas were recorded in four patients. These areas were detected more often during RVA pacing (23 patients) that during SR (14 patients) ($P < 0.01$). An IDC area related to the clinical VT was identified in each patient (Figure 9.2, with permission). From a total of 28 IDC areas, 24 were related to clinical VTs. Ablation guided by IDC suppressed all but one clinical VT, although inducibility was not tested in all patients. During a follow-up period of 9 ± 4 months, three patients had recurrences of the ablated VT and two had occurrence of a different VT. The merit of this method is that the area of IDC is significantly smaller than

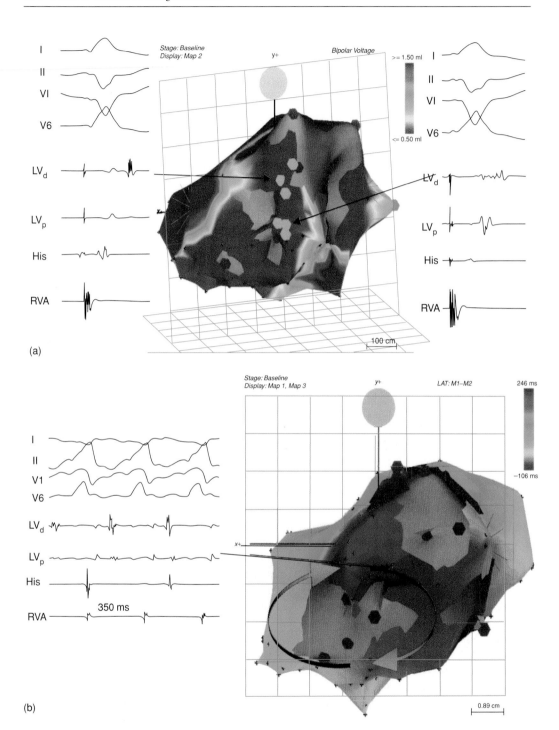

Figure 9.2 (a) Voltage map obtained during RVA pacing. The E-IDCs (seen at the LV distal electrode) were recorded in the space located between the inferior and superior scars. (b) Activation map recorded during VT in the same patient. The color index shows the continuity between the earliest and latest activated areas, suggesting the mechanism of the VT being the reentry. The E-IDC during RVA pacing and mid-diastolic electrogram of VT have the same morphology and are recorded at the same site. LV, left ventricle; RVA, right ventricular apex; d, distal; p, proximal.

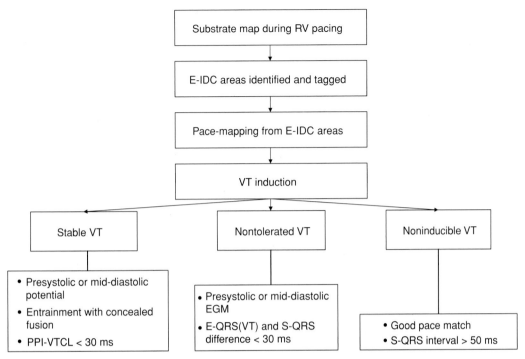

Figure 9.3 Diagram showing the approach to mapping and RF ablation of VT by isolated delayed component area. RV, right ventricle; E-IDC, electrogram displaying isolated, delayed component; VT, ventricular tachycardia; PPI, postpacing interval; CL, cycle length; S-QRS, stimulus to the QRS interval; E-QRS, electrogram to the QRS interval.

the low-voltage area <0.5 mV, therefore it permits focusing further mapping techniques and ablation on the defined area (3.5 ± 2.6 versus 22 ± 11 cm^2, $P < 0.01$).

Similar findings were reported by Bogun et al. [12]. In ischemic VT patients, substrate mapping was performed during sinus rhythm and pace mapping was performed at sites with abnormal electrograms or isolated potentials. Isolated potentials were recorded in all 19 patients, and were more frequent at sites with good or perfect pace maps than at sites with abnormal electrograms ($P <$ 0.0001). Pace maps at 65% of sites with isolated potentials were either perfect or good, compared to 5% of sites with abnormal/fragmented electrograms ($P < 0.0001$). At sites with isolated potentials the S-QRS was longer (108 ± 43 versus 81 ± 54 ms, $P < 0.0001$). With a cutoff isoelectric interval of ≥20 milliseconds for the definition of isolated potentials, the sensitivity and specificity for identifying the isthmus area were 54% and 90%, respectively.

Electrically unexcitable scar [8]
(see Figure 9.4)

We hypothesized that areas of fibrosis that form conduction block could be identified based on pacing threshold, such that delineating electrically unexcitable scar (EUS) within low-voltage infarct regions would locate reentry circuit isthmuses by defining their borders. EUS was defined as a pacing threshold >10 mA/2 milliseconds. In 14 consecutive patients, mapping and ablation of VT were performed using an electroanatomic mapping system. During sinus rhythm, unipolar pacing was performed at sites with bipolar electrogram amplitude <1.5 mV, and EUS regions were marked on the maps. Following the voltage map, VT was reinduced and entrainment mapping used to confirm the isthmus. Then a series of ablation lesions were made to transect the isthmuses (Figure 9.5). Reentry circuit isthmuses were identified by entrainment mapping or pace mapping, and ablation was performed. EUS was identified in the infarct in all 14 patients (11.8 ± 13.9 cm^2) in comparison with the low-voltage area (41.1 ±

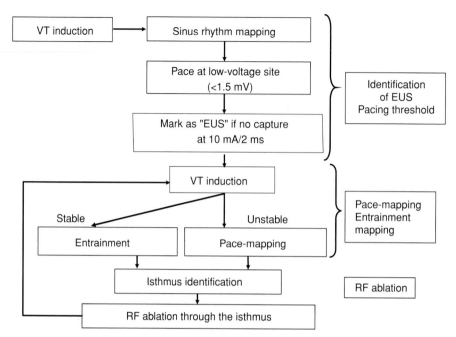

Figure 9.4 Diagram showing the approach to mapping and RF ablation of VT by the identification of electrically unexcitable scar (EUS).

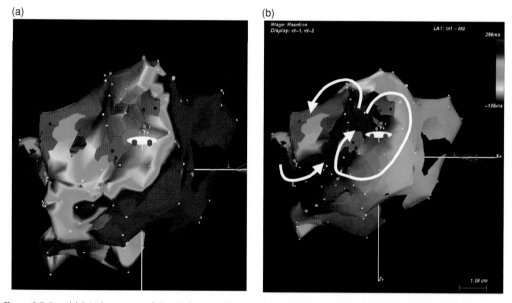

Figure 9.5 Panel (a): Voltage map of the RV from a patient with previous RV and LV infarctions. Lowest-amplitude areas are shown as red, progressing to greater-amplitude areas indicated by yellow, green, blue, and purple. Purple areas have an electrogram amplitude >1.5 mV. There is an extensive low-voltage area close to the RV outflow tract. Two EUS (gray areas) are located in the RV outflow. Panel (b): Activation map of VT with earliest activation shown as red, followed by yellow, green, blue, and purple, showing a complete reentry loop with an isthmus between the two areas of EUS.

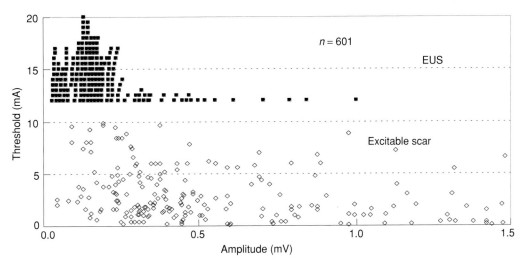

Figure 9.6 The bipolar electrogram amplitude (x axis) versus unipolar pacing threshold (y axis). See text. ◇ Sites with threshold ≤10 mA; • Sites with threshold >10 mA, specified as having a threshold of 10 mA for the analysis. By the Spearman rank correlation, threshold and electrogram amplitude were found to be highly correlated ($r = 0.64$, $P < 0.0001$).

20.4 cm^2). Average of 2.9 ± 1.0 EUS areas were identified in each patient; and all 20 VT circuit isthmuses were adjacent to EUS. Isthmuses were located in between two areas of EUS (9 isthmuses) or between EUS and a valve annulus (two isthmuses). Interestingly, 11 isthmuses were shared by >1 VT circuit. Although electrogram amplitude correlated with pacing threshold ($r = 0.64$, $P < 0.0001$), many isthmuses had very low-amplitude electrograms, and EUS could not be identified from electrogram amplitude alone (Figure 9.6). RF ablation lines connecting selected EUS regions abolished all inducible VTs in 10 patients (71%). Spontaneous VT was markedly reduced during follow-up (from 142 ± 360 to 0.9 ± 2.0 episodes/mo, $P = 0.002$). This method of identifying EUS provides complementary information to the electrogram amplitude in delineating potential reentry circuit paths, potentially facilitating ablation during sinus rhythm.

Higher voltage in the abnormal low voltage [14]

The reentrant circuit is located in the abnormally low voltage area. Arenal and co-workers [14] hypothesized that defining regional variations of electrogram amplitude might define isthmuses. Left ventricular electroanatomic voltage maps obtained during RV pacing in 26 patients with chronic

myocardial infarction were analyzed to identify conducting channels (CCs) inside the scar tissue. A CC was defined by the presence of a corridor of consecutive electrograms differentiated by higher voltage amplitude than the surrounding area. The effect of different levels of voltage scar definition, from 0.5 to 0.1 mV, was analyzed. Twenty-three potential channels were identified in 20 patients. The majority of CCs were identified when the voltage scar definition was ≤0.2 mV. Electrograms with ≥2 components were recorded more frequently at the inner than at the entrance of CCs (100% versus 75%, $P \leq 0.01$). The activation time of the latest component was longer at the inner than at the entrance of CCs (200 ± 40 versus 164 ± 53 ms, $P \leq 0.001$). Pacing from these CCs gave rise to a long-stimulus QRS interval (110 ± 49 ms). Radiofrequency lesions applied to CCs suppressed the inducibility in 88% of CC-related tachycardias. During a follow-up of 17 ± 11 months, 23% of the patients experienced a VT recurrence. CCs represent areas of slow conduction that can be identified in 75% of patients by analyzing the step-wise reduction of the upper voltage threshold.

Scar border ablation [7]

Prior surgical experience showed that 90% of VTs had their earliest endocardial breakthrough within

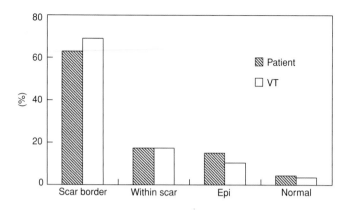

Figure 9.7 Graphs depicting percentage of patients and VT for which a successful ablation site was found in a particular location (X axis).

1–2 cm of the visible/palpable endocardial scar border [15]. Endocardial resection, incision, or cryoablation of these regions of the scar border resulted in low rates of postoperative inducibility and clinical recurrence. Marchlinski et al. [7] reported a method of creating linear RF lesions targeting the border zone identified by the sinus rhythm voltage map. The suggested mechanism of this method was comparable to that of surgical subendocardial resection. Subendocardial linear lesions extend from dense scar to normal endocardium. Linear lesions guided by pace mapping may interrupt potential for reentry, much like subendocardial resection. Oza and Wilber [16] also reported excellent results targeting exit regions at the scar border. In 32/35 VTs (91%), an exit site was identified within 1.5 cm of the scar border. Also, the important finding from their study was that the orientation of the circuit central isthmus was either perpendicular or tangential to the scar border, suggesting that lesions placed parallel to the scar border should be effective. In circuits adjacent to the mitral annulus, the isthmus is usually oriented parallel to the annulus, and ablation lesions do not need to extend to the margin of the scar.

Are all isthmuses located at the scar border?

Verma et al. [17] evaluated the relationship between successful ablation sites of hemodynamically stable VTs associated with ischemic heart disease as determined by traditional mapping techniques during VT with the scar border zone mapped in sinus rhythm in 46 patients. In 39/46 patients an

endocardial location of the critical isthmus was clearly demonstrated (77/86 VTs, 90%). In the seven remaining patients (10% VTs) epicardial mapping was performed after ablation at the earliest endocardial site was unsuccessful, and the site failed to demonstrate either critical isthmus characteristics or very early activation. Successful ablation sites were localized to the endocardial scar border zone in 29/46 patients (59/86 VTs, 68%) as shown in Figure 9.7. In 7/46 patients (15%) representing 9/86 VTs (11%), the successful ablation site was on the epicardium. In the remaining two patients (3/86 VTs, 3.5%) the successful ablation site was outside of both the endocardial scar and border zone within normal myocardium. Therefore, central and exit regions of isthmuses were not always found at the scar border zone as assessed by three-dimensional substrate maps. Therefore, the ablation method to target the endocardial scar border zone will likely address the majority of VTs post-MI, but not all of them.

Substrate map versus VT activation map with electroanatomical mapping system

Substrate mapping during sinus rhythm or pacing is frequently used to identify the substrate for VT by differentiating scar tissue, anatomical, and functional barriers and areas of slow conduction. In patients with stable VT, the activation can be performed to identify the reentrant circuit. Volkmer [18] compared substrate versus activation mapping in 47 patients with prior myocardial infarct.

Twenty-two patients were mapped during stable VT and 25 patients during pacing or sinus rhythm due to the mechanical block ($n = 6$) or unstable VT ($n = 19$). In the VT activation map group, entrainment mapping was performed at sites with diastolic potentials to confirm the isthmus. In the substrate map group, pace mapping was performed and sites with S-QRS >50 milliseconds were tagged as "potential targets." Ablation catheter was placed at a potential target site and VT was induced and entrainment mapping was performed. As soon as diastolic activity was recorded, RF was applied. If the VT continued, RF application was stopped and VT was terminated by overdrive pacing or DC cardioversion, and mapping was continued. In VT map group, the acute success rate was 77%, but reablation with irrigated catheter during the same hospitalization increased the success rate to 91%. The mean length of all linear lesions was 50 ± 35 mm (20–158 mm) and the mean number of RF application was 17 ± 9 (5–31). In substrate mapping group, acute success rate was 81%, and reablation using irrigation catheter increased the success rate to 86%. A median of two lines was found from the mean length of all lines, 64 ± 36 (25–141) mm. There was no statistical difference between these two groups, except a higher median number of applications in the substrate mapping group.

Stimulus strength considerations for substrate mapping and ablation

We have routinely used pacing to confirm that an RF lesion has been produced. Failure to capture at 10 mA/2 milliseconds stimulus strength is an indication of unexcitable tissue or RF lesions [8]. This assessment is based on the idea that the pacing stimulus creates a "virtual electrode" in the tissue that describes the area of tissue that is directly depolarized by the stimulus. An excitation wavefront is launched from the margins of this virtual electrode. The size of the virtual electrode is unclear, and likely varies with electrode tissue orientation and a number of other factors. To assess the change in size of the virtual electrode we assessed the effect of pacing stimulus strength on conduction time during pacing in normal ventricles. We assumed that as stimulus strength increased, the margin of the larger

virtual electrode would move closer to the recording site, such that the time from stimulus to activation at the recording site would decrease. Catheters at the RV apex and His bundle position (RV base) were used as reference catheters, their locations were tagged on the three-dimensional electroanatomical map, and the distance from the pacing site to each reference site was measured. Pacing was performed from the mapping catheter, which had a 4-mm-tip electrode and 1-mm interelectrode spacing, positioned between the RV base and RV apex recording sites. Unipolar pacing was performed using the tip electrode as the cathode and an indifferent electrode in the inferior vena cava as the anode. Pacing at a fixed cycle length of 600 milliseconds was performed at stimulus strengths of threshold, 5, 10, 15, and 20 mA with pulse width of 2 milliseconds. Activation time at the RV base and apex were measured from the stimulus onset to the first peak of the bipolar electrogram. The mean conduction velocities from the pacing site to the RV apex and RV base were calculated as the distance/conduction time. The minimum virtual electrode was assumed to occur during pacing at threshold. The increase in radius of myocardium captured along the radian toward each recording site for each increase in stimulus strength was calculated from the difference in conduction time compared to that measured at threshold, multiplied by the conduction velocity at the threshold (Figure 9.8). We found that increasing the stimulus strength from the threshold to 10 mA increased the apparent radius of the virtual electrode by 6 mm.

Kadish et al. [19] have shown increasing current strength alters the QRS morphology produced by pace mapping with most marked changes at 10 mA and with bipolar as compared to unipolar pacing. Their findings are consistent with our study. That the size of the virtual electrode can be manipulated by altering stimulus strength suggests that pacing can be used to assess creation of ablation lesions. Numerous factors affect the size of the ablation lesion, such as the contact between the ablation electrode and the cardiac tissue, magnitude and duration of power delivery, the characteristics of the ablation electrode, the orientation of the electrode in reference to the tissue, energy delivery protocol, and the tissue heat dissipation characteristics. The size of ablation lesions has been reported as around

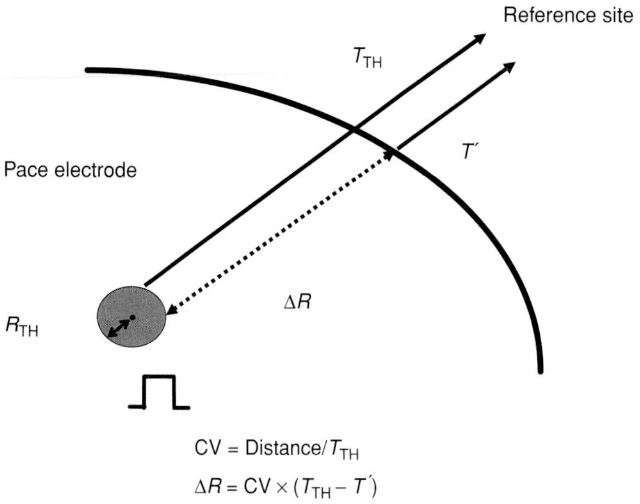

Figure 9.8 Calculation of the radius of the virtual electrode is shown. The gray area represents the area captured during pacing at threshold (virtual electrode). The conduction time to the reference site during pacing at threshold is T_{TH}, and that with the greater strength stimulus is T. The conduction velocity (CV) is calculated as: (distance between pacing and the reference sites)/T_{TH}. The tissue captured with higher stimulus strength (virtual electrode) is indicated by the arc. The increase in the radius of the virtual electrode (ΔR) is calculated as the CV X conduction time difference ($T_{TH} - T$). T, conduction time; CV, conduction velocity; ΔR, increase in the radius of the virtual electrode.

3–5 mm in radius [20],which maybe compatible with the virtual electrode size with 10 mA/2 milliseconds based on our study.

VTs in nonischemic cardiomyopathy

Ventricular tachycardia associated with ischemic heart disease has been reported to have epicardial location of reentry circuit in 15% in inferior myocardial infarction [21]. However, in nonischemic cardiomyopathy, it is more frequent to have epicardial origin of the VT. Hsia et al. [22] reported the left ventricular endocardial low-voltage area distribution near the ventricular base in the perivalvular region. The majority of the VTs (50/57 VTs) originated from the perivalvular scar area in all 19 patients. As a result, 39 out of 57 VTs were targeted for ablation. Three VTs were not targeted due to the epicardial origin. Fourteen of 19 patients had no VT inducible at the end of procedure. Our series of 28 patients, although most of the scars were located in perivalvular area (63%), only 23% patients did have successful ablation from the endocardium [23]. In seven patients out of 10 patients who were failed in ablation underwent epicardial mapping and ablation. All patients had extensive epicardial scar, and six patients had identified isthmus of VT and successfully ablated. Therefore, if mapping from the endocardium does not reveal any low-voltage area, which may be attributable to reentrant circuit, epicardial mapping should be performed during the session or another session.

Summary

Paradigm for ventricular tachycardia ablation has shifted from mapping during VT, to the substrate mapping during the stable rhythm, such as sinus rhythm or pacing. The substrate mapping identifies scars of two types: voltage and EUS. The channels can be identified from their borders or from the conducting tissue in them. Three-dimensional mapping has facilitated this method.

References

1 de Bakker JM, van Capelle FJ, Janse MJ, et al. Slow conduction in the infarcted human heart. 'Zigzag' course of activation. Circulation 1993;88(3):915–926.

2 Stevenson WG, Friedman PL, Sager PT, et al. Exploring postinfarction reentrant ventricular tachycardia with entrainment mapping. J Am Coll Cardiol 1997;29(6):1180–1189.

3 Tung S, Soejima K, Maisel WH, et al. Recognition of far-field electrograms during entrainment mapping of ventricular tachycardia. J Am Coll Cardiol 2003;42(1):110–115.

4 Stevenson WG, Sager PT, Natterson PD, et al. Relation of pace mapping QRS configuration and conduction delay to ventricular tachycardia reentry circuits in human infarct scars. J Am Coll Cardiol 1995;26(2):481–488.

5 Brunckhorst CB, Delacretaz E, Soejima K, et al. Identification of the ventricular tachycardia isthmus after infarction by pace mapping. Circulation 2004;110(6):652–659.

6 Stevenson WG, Khan H, Sager P, et al. Identification of reentry circuit sites during catheter mapping and radiofrequency ablation of ventricular tachycardia late after myocardial infarction. Circulation 1993;88(4 Pt 1):1647–1670.

7 Marchlinski FE, Callans DJ, Gottlieb CD, et al. Linear ablation lesions for control of unmappable ventricular tachycardia in patients with ischemic and nonischemic cardiomyopathy. Circulation 2000;101(11):1288–1296.

8 Soejima K, Stevenson WG, Maisel WH, et al. Electrically unexcitable scar mapping based on pacing threshold for identification of the reentry circuit isthmus: feasibility for guiding ventricular tachycardia ablation. Circulation 2002;106(13):1678–1683.

9 de Chillou C, Lacroix D, Klug D, et al. Isthmus characteristics of reentrant ventricular tachycardia after myocardial infarction. Circulation 2002;105(6):726–731.

10 El-Shalakany A, Hadjis T, Papageorgiou P, et al. Entrainment/mapping criteria for the prediction of termination of ventricular tachycardia by single radiofrequency lesion in patients with coronary artery disease. Circulation 1999;99(17):2283–2289.

11 Arenal A, Glez-Torrecilla E, Ortiz M, et al. Ablation of electrograms with an isolated, delayed component as treatment of unmappable monomorphic ventricular tachycardias in patients with structural heart disease. J Am Coll Cardiol 2003;41(1):81–92.

12 Bogun F, Good E, Reich S, et al. Isolated potentials during sinus rhythm and pace-mapping within scars as guides for ablation of post-infarction ventricular tachycardia. J Am Coll Cardiol 2006;47(10):2013–2019.

13 Brunckhorst CB, Delacretaz E, Soejima K, et al. Impact of changing activation sequence on bipolar electrogram amplitude for voltage mapping of left ventricular infarcts causing ventricular tachycardia. J Interv Card Electrophysiol 2005;12(2):137–141.

14 Arenal A, del Castillo S, Gonzalez-Torrecilla E, et al. Tachycardia-related channel in the scar tissue in patients with sustained monomorphic ventricular tachycardias: influence of the voltage scar definition. Circulation 2004;110(17):2568–2574.

15 Horowitz LN, Josephson ME, Harken AH. Epicardial and endocardial activation during sustained ventricular tachycardia in man. Circulation 1980;61(6):1227–1238.

16 Oza S, Wilber DJ. Substrate-based endocardial ablation of postinfarction of ventricular tachycardia. Heart Rhythm 2006;3(5):607–609.

17 Verma A, Marrouche NF, Schweikert RA, et al. Relationship between successful ablation sites and the scar border zone defined by substrate mapping for ventricular tachycardia post-myocardial infarction. J Cardiovasc Electrophysiol 2005;16(5):465–471.

18 Volkmer M, Ouyang F, Deger F, et al. Substrate mapping vs. tachycardia mapping using CARTO in patients with coronary artery disease and ventricular tachycardia: impact on outcome of catheter ablation. Europace 2006;8(11):968–976.

19 Kadish AH, Schmaltz S, Morady F. A comparison of QRS complexes resulting from unipolar and bipolar pacing: implications for pace-mapping. Pacing Clin Electrophysiol 1991;14(5 Pt 1):823–832.

20 Simmers TA, Wittkampf FH, Hauer RN, et al. In vivo ventricular lesion growth in radiofrequency catheter ablation. Pacing Clin Electrophysiol 1994;17(3 Pt 2):523–531.

21 Svenson RH, Littmann L, Gallagher JJ, et al. Termination of ventricular tachycardia with epicardial laser photocoagulation: a clinical comparison with patients undergoing successful endocardial photocoagulation alone. J Am Coll Cardiol 1990;15(1):163–170.

22 Hsia HH, Callans DJ, Marchlinski FE. Characterization of endocardial electrophysiological substrate in patients with nonischemic cardiomyopathy and monomorphic ventricular tachycardia. Circulation 2003;108(6):704–710.

23 Soejima K, Stevenson WG, Sapp JL, et al. Endocardial and epicardial radiofrequency ablation of ventricular tachycardia associated with dilated cardiomyopathy: the importance of low-voltage scars. J Am Coll Cardiol 2004;43(10):1834–1842.

CHAPTER 10

Ablation of idiopathic ventricular tachycardias

Nitish Badhwar, & Melvin M. Scheinman

Introduction

Most causes of ventricular tachycardia (VT) are caused by an underlying structural heart disease (mainly ischemia or cardiomyopathy). A small subgroup of patients with VT develop this arrhythmia in structurally normal hearts and are designated as idiopathic. Idiopathic VT accounts for 10–20% of VT cases evaluated by electrophysiology centers [1,2]. It is important to recognize these patients as they frequently respond to nonpharmacologic ablative techniques. Idiopathic VT can be broadly classified as polymorphic VT and monomorphic VT (Table 10.1). In this chapter we focus on the clinical, electrocardiographic (ECG), and electrophysiologic findings for patients with monomorphic idiopathic VT with emphasis on ablative therapy.

Outflow tract ventricular tachycardia (OT-VT)

This form of idiopathic VT arises from the outflow tract of the right or the left ventricle. Based on its origin it can be classified as:

1 VT that arises from the right ventricular outflow tract (RVOT VT).
2 VT that arises from the left ventricular outflow tract (LVOT VT).
3 VT that arises from the aortic cusps (cusp VT).
RVOT VT is more common in females and is usually seen in the third to fifth decade of life while LVOT

Ventricular Arrhythmias and Sudden Cardiac Death, 1st edition.
Edited by P.J. Wang, A. Al-Ahmad, H. Hsia, and P.C. Zei
© 2008 Blackwell Publishing, ISBN: 978-1-4051-6114-5.

VT is equally distributed between males and females [3]. Symptoms include palpitations, dizziness, atypical chest pain and syncope. There are two predominant clinical forms of this syndrome: (i) non-sustained repetitive monomorphic VT (RMVT) alternating with periods of sinus rhythm or (ii) paroxysmal exercise-induced sustained VT. [4] There is overlap between these two clinical presentations. Frequently these patients have isolated PVCs that match the tachycardia morphology. An episode consists of rapid succession of short bursts of tachycardia lasting for minutes.

RVOT VT

This form of VT is associated with a characteristic ECG morphology of LBBB with inferior axis suggesting origin from the right ventricle outflow tract. Jadonath et al. [5] evaluated the utility of 12-lead ECG in localizing the site of origin of RVOT VT in 11 patients undergoing catheter ablation. They used pace-mapping techniques and divided the RVOT into nine quadrants. A QS pattern in lead avR and monophasic R waves in leads II, III, avF, and V_6 were noted in each patient at all pacing sites. The anterior sites showed a dominant Q wave or a qR complex in lead I and QS complex in avL. Pacing at the posterior sites produced a dominant R wave in lead I, QS, or R wave in avL and an early precordial transition ($R/S \geq 1$ by V_3). Coggins et al. [6] showed that septal RVOT VT was associated with negative QRS complex in avL while RVOT VT arising from the lateral wall produced a positive QRS complex in avL. Dixit et al. [7] used pace-mapping techniques to differentiate between RVOT VT arising from the free wall versus septal wall (Figure 10.1). They showed that free-wall RVOT VT was associated with wider and

Table 10.1 Idiopathic ventricular tachycardia

Monomorphic ventricular tachycardia	Polymorphic ventricular tachycardia
• Outflow tract VT: RVOT-VT, LVOT-VT, aortic cusp VT	• Long-QT syndrome
• Fascicular VT: LAF-VT, LPF-VT, septal VT	• Brugada syndrome
• Adrenergic monomorphic VT	• Short coupled torsades
• Annular VT: Mitral annular, tricuspid annular	• Short-QT syndrome
	• Catecholaminergic polymorphic VT
	• Idiopathic VF

LAF, left anterior fascicular; LPF, left posterior fascicular; LVOT, left ventricular outflow tract; RVOT, right ventricular outflow tract; VF, ventricular fibrillation; VT, ventricular tachycardia.

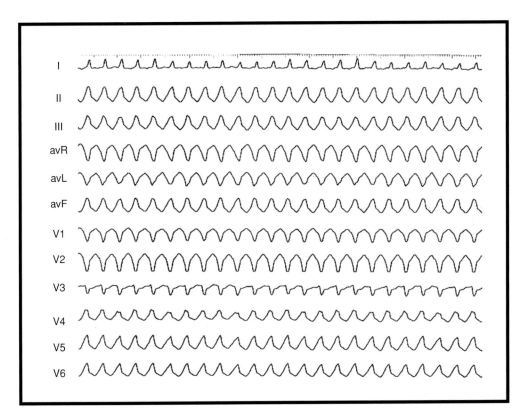

Figure 10.1 Twelve-lead ECG showing pace-maps from anterior, intermediate, and posterior sites (labeled 3, 2, and 1, respectively) in the free wall (right) and septum of the RVOT. All of them have LBBB inferior axis morphology. Lead I is positive in the posterior sites and negative in the anterior sites. The free-wall sites show broader, shorter, and notched R waves in the inferior leads and a later transition in precordial leads. PV, pulmonary valve. (Reprinted from J Cardiovasc Electrophysiol, Volume 14, Dixit et al., Electrocardiographic patterns of superior right ventricular outflow tract tachycardias: distinguishing septal and free-wall sites of origin, Pages 1–7, Copyright (2003).)

Table 10.2 Electrocardiographic findings in outflow tract VT

RVOT VT	LVOT/aortic cusp VT
• QS in avR	• Early precordial transition (V_2–V_3)
• Monophasic R wave in II, III, avF, V_6	• Taller and broader R wave or RBBB in V_1–V_2
• Septal sites have negative QRS in avL	• Septal LVOT has dominant Q in V_1, qrs II/qrs III > 1
• Free-wall sites have wider notched QRS in inferior leads and later precordial transition (V_4)	• Aortomitral LVOT has qR in V_1, qrs II/qrs III < 1
• Lead I shows Q wave in anterior sites and dominant R wave in posterior sites	• Cusp VT—notch in V_5, lack of S in V_5–V_6, taller R in inferior leads
• Phase analysis as measured from the earliest QRS onset to:	• Lead I—rS in left cusp VT, notched R in noncoronary cusp VT
a. Earliest QRS onset is V_2	• Phase analysis (Cusp VT) as measured from the earliest QRS onset to:
b. Initial peak/nadir in III ≤ 120 ms	d. Earliest QRS onset not in V_2
c. Initial peak/nadir in V_2 ≤ 78 ms	e. Initial peak/nadir in III ≥ 120 ms
	f. Initial peak/nadir in V_2 ≥ 78 ms

LVOT, left ventricular outflow tract; RVOT, right ventricular outflow tract.

notched QRS complexes in the inferior leads and the precordial R wave transition was late (R/S ≥ 1 by V_4). Recently, OT-VTs arising from near the His-bundle region have been described [8,9]. The characteristic ECG abnormalities for VT arising from this site include an R/RSR′ pattern in avL, taller R wave in I, small R waves in inferior leads, taller R waves in V_5, V_6, and QS pattern in V_1 (Figure 10.2).

VT arising from the pulmonary artery (PA VT)

Idiopathic VT arising from the pulmonary artery has also been described [10,11]. The origin of VT from the PA is thought to be from remnants of embryonic muscle sleeves that have been noted in amphibian and mammalian outflow tract [12]. This is supported by the presence of a sharp potential at these sites that preceded the onset of ventricular activation during VT [10]. Sekiguchi et al. [11] noted the following ECG characteristics during VT that favor PA VT as compared to RVOT VT: (i) Larger R-wave amplitude in inferior leads; (ii) The ratio of the Q-wave amplitude in avL/avR was larger in the PA group; (iii) Significantly larger R/S amplitude in lead V_2 in patients with PA VT than in those with RVOT VT.

LVOT VT

VT arising from the LVOT shares characteristics similar to the RVOT VT because of a common embryonic origin. This form of VT can be differentiated from the RVOT VT by differences in QRS morphology. LVOT VT is suggested by LBBB morphology with inferior axis with small R waves in V_1 and early precordial transition (R/S ≥ 1 by V_2 or V_3) or RBBB morphology with inferior axis [13–16] and presence of S wave in V_6 [17,18]. LVOT VT arising from the septal para-Hisian region has an ECG pattern of QS or Qr in V_1 with early precordial transition and ratio of QRS in leads II/III > 1 while LVOT VT arising from the aortomitral continuity has a characteristic qR pattern in V_1 with a ratio of QRS in leads II/III ≤ 1 [19] (Table 2).

Cusp VT

Case reports of idiopathic VT with LBBB morphology and inferior axis that failed ablation in the RVOT but were successfully ablated in the left coronary cusp [20, 21] were described in 1999. Kanagaratnam et al. [22] reported the ECG characteristics of 12 patients with outflow tract VT that required ablation in the aortic sinus of Valsalva. All patients had LBBB inferior axis morphology with taller monophasic R waves in inferior leads and an early precordial R wave transition by V_2 or V_3. VT arising from the left cusp had an rS pattern in lead I, and VT arising from the noncoronary cusp had a notched R wave in lead I. Ouyang et al. [23] evaluated the ECG differences between eight patients with RVOT VT and seven patients with VT

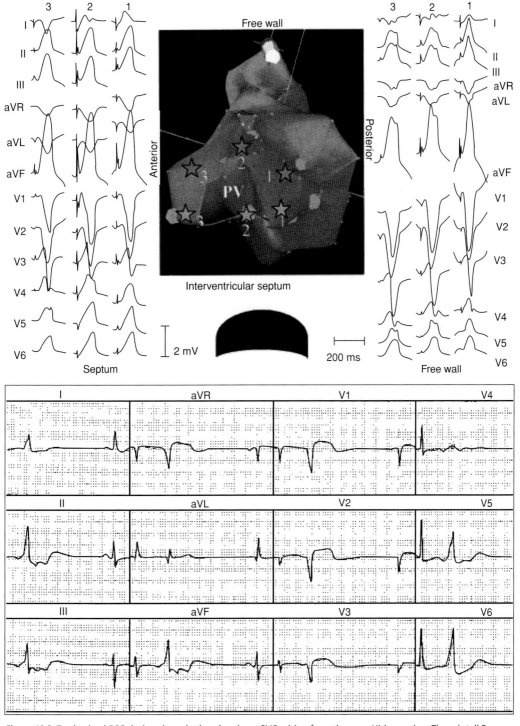

Figure 10.2 Twelve-lead ECG during sinus rhythm showing a PVC arising from the para-Hisian region. There is tall R wave in lead I, QS in V_1, R in lead II > R in lead III, taller R waves in V_5 and V_6, and a characteristic rSR' in lead avL. Local intracardiac signal at this site preceded the QRS onset by 25 milliseconds.

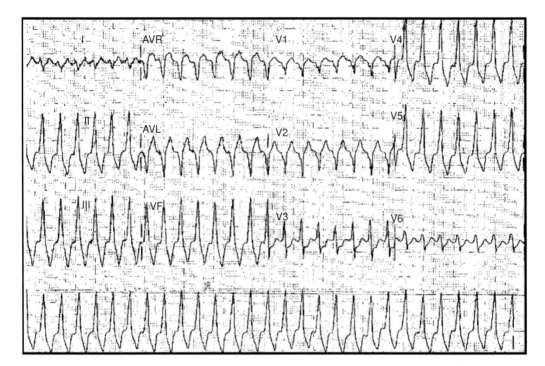

Figure 10.3 Twelve-lead ECG of VT arising from the left coronary cusp. Lead V_1 satisfies the Kindwall criteria for VT based on a notch in the S wave and the duration from the onset of the QRS complex to the nadir of the S wave more than 60 milliseconds. This LBBB inferior axis VT has a transition in V_3 that would be consistent with septal RVOT VT as well as cusp VT. However, the tall R waves in the inferior leads along with a phase analysis showing a longer duration form the earliest QRS onset to peak in III and nadir in V_2 is consistent with cusp VT. The rS complex in lead I favors origin from the left coronary cusp. (Reprinted from Curr Probl Cardiol Volume 32, Badhwar et al., Idiopathic ventricular tachycardia: diagnosis and management, Pages 7–43, Copyright (2007).)

arising from the aortic sinus cusp (five from left sinus and two from right sinus). They found that a broader R wave duration and a taller R/S wave amplitude in V_1 and V_2 favored VT arising from the aortic cusp. Yang et al. [24] used phase differences in the 12-lead ECG to differentiate between RVOT VT (32 patients) and aortic cusp VT (15 patients). They showed that RVOT VT was associated with earliest ventricular activation in V_2 and a shorter time from onset of ECG to peak/nadir in lead III and V_2. Figure 10.3 shows the 12-lead ECG from a patient with VT arising from the left coronary cusp.

Epicardial LV VT originating remote from the sinus of Valsalva

Outflow tract VT occasionally arises from the epicardial surface of the heart that requires ablation in the great cardiac vein or via pericardial approach [8,25–27]. Ito et al. [8] showed that the Q wave ratio of avL to avR > 1.4 or an S wave amplitude in V_1 > 1.2 mV was useful in differentiating between epicardial VT from aortic cusp VT. Daniels et al. [27] showed that 9% of the patients with idiopathic VT referred to their institution had an epicardial focus. They found that a delayed precordial maximum deflection index ≥55 (calculated by measuring the time from the QRS onset to the earliest maximum deflection (nadir or peak) in precordial leads and dividing it by the total QRS duration) differentiates this form of idiopathic epicardial VT from other forms of outflow tract VT.

Management

The majority of the patients with outflow tract VT has a benign course with a very low risk of sudden death [28–30]. It can be associated with tachycardia-induced cardiomyopathy that improves after successful treatment [31,32]. It is important to differentiate this form of VT from VT associated with arrhythmogenic right ventricular cardiomyopathy (ARVC) that is also associated with LBBB morphology. ARVC is associated with a worse prognosis and is responsible for sudden death, especially in young adults less than 35 years old [33,34].

Acute termination of RVOT VT can be achieved with adenosine, carotid sinus massage, verapamil, and lidocaine. Beta-blockers are especially effective for those with exercise-induced outflow tract VT and a synergistic action is noted with calcium channel blockers. Antiarrhythmic agents such as procainamide, flecainide, amiodarone, and sotalol are also effective in these patients. There was a trend toward greater efficacy with sotalol in a study of 23 patients with RVOT VT [35]. Nicorandil, a potassium channel opener, has been reported to terminate and suppress adenosine-sensitive VT [36].

Catheter ablation

Catheter ablation using radiofrequency energy to cure patients with outflow tract VT is associated with a high success rate due to the focal origin of this form of VT. The 12-lead ECG is a useful initial guide to localize the site of origin of the tachycardia. Intracardiac mapping to select the optimal site for ablation includes activation mapping (earliest local intracardiac electrogram that precedes the onset of surface QRS during VT) and pace-mapping (pacing the ventricle from a selected site in sinus rhythm to match the 12-lead morphology of the spontaneous or induced VT). The use of three-dimensional (3D) electroanatomical mapping systems (Figure 10.4) reduces fluoroscopic exposure and improves the efficacy of catheter ablation [37,38]. Application of radiofrequency energy to the successful site usually leads to acceleration of tachycardia followed by termination [39]; catheter ablation during sinus rhythm may lead to induction of PVCs or non-sustained tachycardia with QRS morphology similar to that seen during spontaneous VT [40]. The success rate of catheter ablation for right ventricular outflow tract VT reported from various series is greater than 90% [41,42] with a recurrence rate of 5% (mainly in the first year). The predictors of

recurrence included poor 12-lead ECG pace match, later activation at target site, multiple morphologies of VT, and delta-wave-like beginning of the QRS [43, 44]. Serious complications include induction of RBBB (2%), cardiac perforation, and tamponade (1%); there has been one death reported secondary to complications from RVOT perforation [6]. Ablation for LVOT VT has been associated with occlusion of a coronary artery [45]. Failure of endocardial radiofrequency ablation can be due to epicardial location of the VT focus. Epicardial ablation can be achieved by a subxiphoid technique of pericardial puncture as described by Sosa et al. [46] or by ablating within the great cardiac vein. Coronary angiograms are performed prior to epicardial ablation and ablation in the aortic sinus to avoid ablation close to the coronary arteries that can lead to arterial damage and thrombus formation. Intracardiac echocardiography has also been used to provide real-time visualization of the relationship between the ablation site and the coronary arteries during ablation in the aortic sinus [47].

Idiopathic left ventricular tachycardia (ILVT) or fascicular VT

This form of VT arises from the fascicles in the left ventricle. Based on the QRS morphology and the site of origin, it can be classified as follows [48]:
1. Left posterior fascicular VT (LPF VT)
2. Left anterior fascicular VT (LAF VT)
3. Left upper septal VT (septal VT)

This form of idiopathic VT was first described by Zipes et al. [49] in 1979 with the following characteristic triad: (i) induction with atrial pacing, (ii) RBBB morphology with left axis deviation, and (iii) occurrence in patients without structural heart disease. In 1981, Belhassen et al. [50] showed that this form of VT could be terminated by verapamil, the fourth identifying feature. In 1988 Ohe et al. [51] described another form of this VT with RBBB and right axis deviation. Shimoike et al. [52] and Nogami [48] described a form of idiopathic VT with narrow QRS that required ablation in the upper LV septum.

ILVT is typically seen in patients between the ages of 15 and 40 years with an earlier presentation

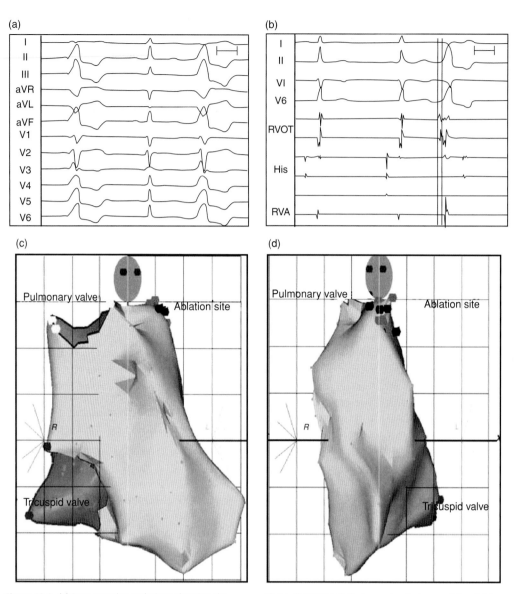

Figure 10.4 (a) Pace-mapping technique showing the 12-lead ECG during pacing from the anteroseptal RVOT region on the left-hand side that matches the 12-lead during VT on the right-hand side with a sinus beat in between. (b) Intracardiac electrogram recording from the RVOT region, His bundle region and right ventricular apex (RVA) during sinus rhythm and during PVC (last beat). The signal from the RVOT precedes the surface QRS by 51 milliseconds and it shows a split potential.

Three-dimensional electroanatomical map of the right ventricle using the Carto mapping system showing the successful ablation site. (c) RAO projection showing anterior location. (d) LAO projection showing the septal location of the ablation site. (Reprinted from Curr Probl Cardiol Volume 32, Badhwar et al., Idiopathic ventricular tachycardia: diagnosis and management, Pages 7–43, Copyright (2007).)

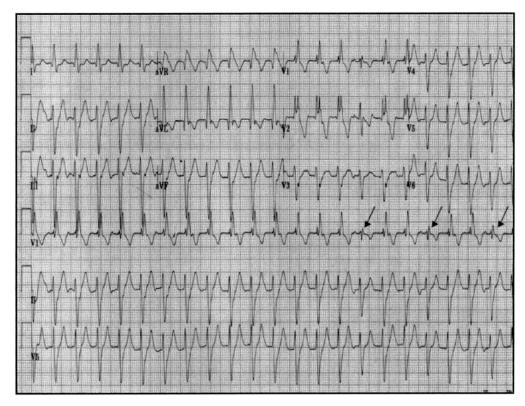

Figure 10.5 Twelve-lead ECG of VT arising from the left posterior fascicle (ILVT) with a RBBB superior axis morphology. The duration of the QRS complex and the RS interval are narrower than that noted in VT associated with structural heart disease. However, the presence of AV dissociation and fusion beats (arrows) is diagnostic of VT. (Reprinted from Curr Probl Cardiol Volume 32, Badhwar et al., Idiopathic ventricular tachycardia: diagnosis and management, Pages 7–43, Copyright (2007).)

in females [3,53–58]. Most of the affected patients are males (60–70%). The symptoms include palpitations, fatigue, dyspnea, dizziness, and presyncope. Syncope and sudden death are very rare [53]. Most of the episodes occur at rest; however, this form of VT can be triggered by exercise and emotional stress [58,59]. Incessant tachycardia leading to tachycardia-induced cardiomyopathy has also been described [56].

ECG recognition

The baseline 12-lead ECG is normal in most patients or it may show transient T wave inversions related to T wave memory shortly after a tachycardia episode terminates. The 12-lead ECG of left posterior fascicular VT (LPF VT) shows RBBB with left axis deviation suggesting an exit site from the inferoposterior ventricular septum (Figure 10.5). Nogami et al. [60]

reported six patients with left anterior fascicular VT (LAF VT) that showed a RBBB with right axis deviation with the earliest ventricular activation in the anterolateral wall of the LV in all patients. Three patients had a distal type of LAF VT with QS or rS morphology in leads I, V_5, and V_6 and the other three had proximal type of LAF VT with RS or Rs morphology in the same leads. Figure 10.6 shows an example of distal LAF VT that was successfully ablated at our center. The QRS duration in fascicular VT varies from 140 to 150 milliseconds and the duration from the beginning of the QRS onset to the nadir of the S-wave (RS interval) in the precordial leads is 60–80 milliseconds unlike VT associated with structural heart disease that is usually associated with longer duration of QRS and RS intervals. This makes it difficult to differentiate fascicular VT from supraventricular tachycardia with aberrancy

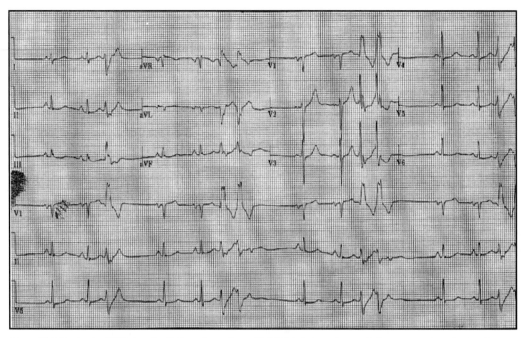

Figure 10.6 Twelve-lead ECG showing PVCs and couplets with RBBB inferior axis morphology suggestive of origin from the left anterior fascicle. The QRS complex in leads I, V_5, and V_6 show an rS morphology that is consistent with an exit site in the distal part of the left anterior fascicle where this VT was successfully ablated. (Reprinted from Curr Probl Cardiol Volume 32, Badhwar et al., Idiopathic ventricular tachycardia: diagnosis and management, Pages 7–43, Copyright (2007).)

using the criteria based on QRS morphology and RS interval [61–63].

Management

The long-term prognosis of patients with fascicular VT without structural heart disease is very good. Patients with mild symptoms without medical therapy did not show progression of their arrhythmias in a study of 37 patients with verapamil-sensitive VT during an average follow-up of 5.8 years [57]. However, those with incessant tachycardia can develop a cardiomyopathy [56]. Acute termination of VT can be achieved with intravenous verapamil (adenosine and Valsalva maneuvers are ineffective). Patients with moderate symptoms can be treated with oral verapamil (120–480 mg/day).

Catheter ablation

Radiofrequency catheter ablation is an appropriate management strategy for patients with severe symptoms or those intolerant or resistant to antiarrhythmic therapy. Initial ablation strategies using pace-mapping are not very effective as a perfect pace-map can be obtained by pacing the Purkinje network that is not critical to the reentrant circuit. Nakagawa et al. [59] and Wen et al. [64] showed that successful ablation could be performed by targeting the earliest high-frequency Purkinje potential (and not the earliest ventricular activation) during VT and this could be recorded far from the exit site that shows the perfect pace-map. Tsuchiya et al. [65] targeted a site recording both a late diastolic potential and a presystolic potential and showed tachycardia termination with catheter pressure at these sites. It is noteworthy that Nakagawa's ablation site was at the apical inferior septal region while Tsuchiya's successful site was in the basal septal region close to the main trunk of the left bundle branch. Nogami et al. [66] used an octapolar catheter to record double potentials during VT from the mid-septal region and successfully terminated VT during catheter ablation at these sites. Ouyang et al. [67] used a 3D electroanatomical mapping system to record sites with retrograde Purkinje (retro PP) potential during sinus rhythm (sharp low-amplitude potentials that followed a Purkinje

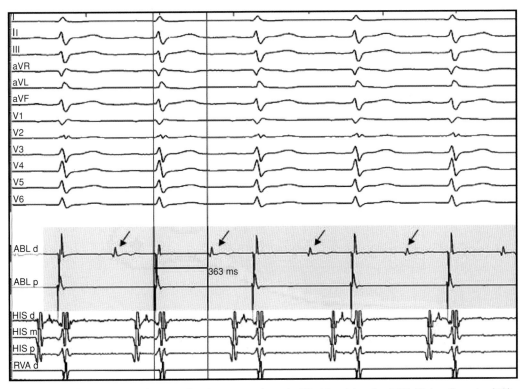

Figure 10.7 Twelve-lead ECG and intracardiac electrograms from the LV mid-septal region (ABL), His bundle region (HIS), and right ventricular apex (RVA) during sinus rhythm in a patient with idiopathic left ventricular fascicular VT (ILVT). Retrograde Purkinje potentials (arrows) are noted after the local ventricular signal in the ABL catheter that correlated with early diastolic potential during VT. Catheter ablation at this site terminated VT. (Reprinted from Curr Probl Cardiol Volume 32, Badhwar et al., Idiopathic ventricular tachycardia: diagnosis and management, Pages 7–43, Copyright (2007).)

potential and local ventricular electrogram) in patients with ILVT. They showed that the site recording the earliest retro PP during sinus rhythm correlated with early diastolic potential during VT and catheter ablation at this site lead to noninducibility of tachycardia. Figure 10.7 shows retro PP recorded on intracardiac signals during sinus rhythm in a patient with idiopathic LPF VT. Chen et al. [68] used a noncontact mapping system to create a successful linear ablation line perpendicular to the wave front propagation direction of the left posterior fascicle in sinus rhythm in patients with nonsustained or noninducible VT. Ma et al. [69] have used development of a left posterior fascicular block pattern on the surface ECG as an end point for successful ablation in patients with noninducible ILVT. Long-term success after catheter ablation is more than 92% with rare complications that include mitral regurgitation due to catheter entrapment in the chordae

of the mitral valve leaflet and aortic regurgitation due to damage to the aortic valve using a retrograde aortic approach [6,58,59,64,70–72].

Mitral annular VT (MAVT)

There have been case reports of adenosine-sensitive monomorphic VT that was successfully ablated at the anterobasal LV [73–75]. Tada et al. [76] were the first group to describe the prevalence and ECG characteristics of MAVT. Their definition was based on the ratio of atrial to ventricular electrograms <1 and the amplitude of the atrial and ventricular electrograms >0.08 and 0.5 mV, respectively, at the successful ablation site.

Tada et al. reported that MAVT was noted in 5% of all the cases of idiopathic VT while Kumagai et al. [77] showed that MAVT accounts for 49% of idiopathic repetitive monomorphic VT arising

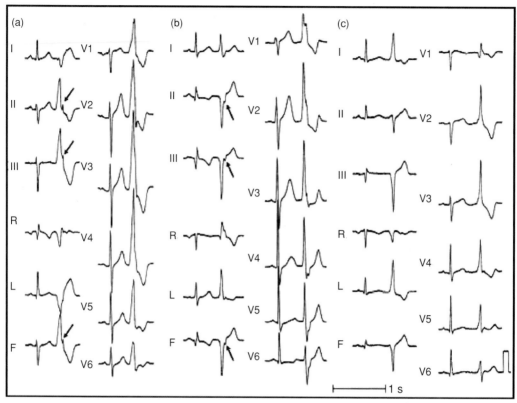

Figure 10.8 Representative 12-lead ECG of premature ventricular contractions originating from the anterolateral (a), posterior (b), and posteroseptal (c) portions of the mitral annulus. Arrows indicate "notching" of the late phase of the QRS complex in the inferior leads. (Reprinted from J Am Coll Cardiol, Volume 45, Tada et al., Idiopathic ventricular arrhythmia arising from the mitral annulus: a distinct subgroup of idiopathic ventricular arrhythmias, Pages 877–886, Copyright (2005).)

from the left ventricle (others sites included coronary cusps and inferoseptal region). Patients presented with palpitations and were noted to have repetitive monomorphic VT or frequent monomorphic PVCs. Tachycardia was noted spontaneously or initiated with isoproterenol. Tada et al. showed initiation with programmed stimulation from the RV in some patients [76]; it was found to be ineffective in the series by Kumagai et al. [77]. Termination was noted with adenosine (10–40 mg) and intravenous verapamil in some patients. VT entrainment was not observed in any of the sustained episodes.

ECG recognition

Tada et al. [76] showed that the surface ECG in all patients with MAVT had a RBBB pattern (transition in V_1 or V_2), S-wave in V_6, and monophasic R or Rs in leads V_2–V_6. They further classified MAVT into three categories depending on the site of origin:

1. Anterolateral (AL) MAVT (58%)
2. Posterior (Pos) MAVT (11%)
3. Posteroseptal (PS) MAVT (31%)

In AL-MAVT, the polarity of the QRS complex in leads I and avL was negative and positive in the inferior leads; Pos-MAVT and PS-MAVT showed a negative polarity in the inferior leads and positive in leads I and avL. AL-MAVT and Pos-MAVT showed a longer QRS duration and "notching" in the late phase of the R wave/Q wave in the inferior leads, suggesting an origin from the free wall. This feature was not observed in PS-MAVT. Pos-MAVT showed a dominant R in V_1 while PS-MAVT had a negative QRS component in V_1 (qR, qr, rs, rS, or QS). The Q-wave amplitude ratio of lead III to lead II was greater in PS-MAVT than in Pos-MAVT. Figure 10.8 shows

Posterolateral portion of the tricuspid annulus

Anterior portion of the tricuspid annulus

Anteroseptal portion of the tricuspid annulus

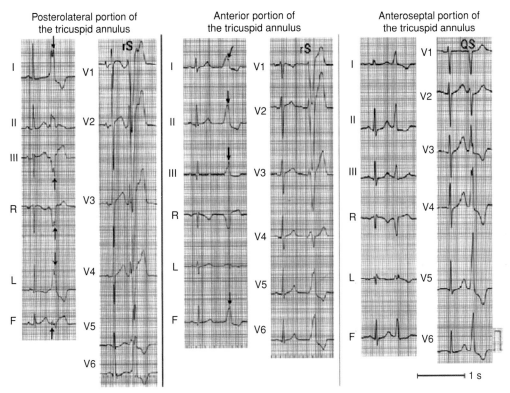

Figure 10.9 Representative 12-lead ECG of premature ventricular contractions originating from the posterolateral (a), anterior (b), and anteroseptal (c) portions of the tricuspid annulus. Arrows indicate the second peak of the "notched" QRS complex in the limb leads. (Reprinted from Heart Rhythm, Volume 4, Tada et al., Idiopathic ventricular arrhythmias originating from the tricuspid annulus: prevalence, electrocardiographic characteristics, and results of radiofrequency catheter ablation, Pages 7–16, Copyright (2007).)

the representative ECG from all three subtypes of MAVT. Kumagai et al. [77] illustrated the δ-wave like beginning on the QRS complex during VT and showed a similarity between the MAVT and left-sided WPW with highly preexcited δ waves in terms of QRS morphology.

Catheter ablation

Electrophysiology mapping was performed using activation mapping and pace-mapping to localize the site of origin of the VT. All successful sites had an adequate atrial and ventricular electrogram satisfying the criteria for mitral annular origin and a potential was noted before the local ventricular electrogram in most of the patients. Pace-mapping was useful in patients with nonsustained tachycardia. Acute success was obtained in all the patients in both the series; however, there was a recurrence rate of 8% in one series [77].

Tricuspid annular VT

Recently, VT arising from the tricuspid annulus has been described. This form of VT was noted in 8% of the patients presenting with idiopathic VT [78]. This was preferentially seen to originate from the septal region (74%) than the free wall (26%). Most of the septal VT was seen to arise from the anteroseptal region (72%). The septal VT had an early transition in precordial leads (V_3), narrower QRS complexes, Qs in lead V_1 with absence of "notching" in the inferior leads while the free-wall VT was associated with late precordial transition ($>V_3$), wider QRS complexes, absence of Q wave in lead V_1, and "notching" in the inferior leads (the timing of the second peak of the "notched" QRS complex in the inferior leads corresponded precisely with the left ventricular free-wall activation). Figure 10.9 shows ECG characteristics of PVCs originating from different sites on the tricuspid annulus. The success rate for catheter ablation of the free-wall VT was 90% as compared to 57% in the septal group due to the presence of junctional rhythm and the likelihood of impairing AV nodal conduction with RFCA.

Summary

There has been an explosion of our understanding of the multiple forms of ventricular tachycardia occurring in patients without structural heart disease. These arrhythmias are known to account for approximately 10–20% of VTs evaluated at large referral centers. Recognition of this type of tachycardia has important practical value. First, since they occur on younger patients with normal hearts, they must be distinguished from supraventricular tachycardia with aberration since the treatment will often be very different. Depending on tachycardia mechanism the arrhythmia may respond to β-blockers, Ca^{2+} channel blockers, or to vagal maneuvers. In addition, these arrhythmias are susceptible to cure by catheter ablation.

References

1 Brooks R, Burgess JH. Idiopathic ventricular tachycardia. A review. Medicine (Baltimore) 1988;67(5):271–294.

2 Okumura K, Tsuchiya T. Idiopathic left ventricular tachycardia: clinical features, mechanisms and management. Card Electrophysiol Rev 2002;6(1–2):61–67.

3 Nakagawa M, Takahashi N, Nobe S, et al. Gender differences in various types of idiopathic ventricular tachycardia. J Cardiovasc Electrophysiol 2002;13(7):633–638.

4 Altemose GT, Buxton AE. Idiopathic ventricular tachycardia. Annu Rev Med 1999;50:159–177.

5 Jadonath RL, Schwartzman DS, Preminger MW, Gottlieb CD, Marchlinski FE. Utility of the 12-lead electrocardiogram in localizing the origin of right ventricular outflow tract tachycardia. Am Heart J 1995;130(5):1107–1113.

6 Coggins DL, Lee RJ, Sweeney J, et al. Radiofrequency catheter ablation as a cure for idiopathic tachycardia of both left and right ventricular origin. J Am Coll Cardiol 1994;23(6):1333–1341.

7 Dixit S, Gerstenfeld EP, Callans DJ, Marchlinski FE. Electrocardiographic patterns of superior right ventricular outflow tract tachycardias: distinguishing septal and free-wall sites of origin. J Cardiovasc Electrophysiol 2003;14(1):1–7.

8 Ito S, Tada H, Naito S, et al. Development and validation of an ECG algorithm for identifying the optimal ablation site for idiopathic ventricular outflow tract tachycardia. J Cardiovasc Electrophysiol 2003;14(12):1280–1286.

9 Yamauchi Y, Aonuma K, Takahashi A, et al. Electrocardiographic characteristics of repetitive monomorphic right ventricular tachycardia originating near the His-bundle. J Cardiovasc Electrophysiol 2005;16(10):1041–1048.

10 Timmermans C, Rodriguez LM, Crijns HJ, Moorman AF, Wellens HJ. Idiopathic left bundle-branch block-shaped ventricular tachycardia may originate above the pulmonary valve. Circulation 2003;108(16):1960–1967.

11 Sekiguchi Y, Aonuma K, Takahashi A, et al. Electrocardiographic and electrophysiologic characteristics of ventricular tachycardia originating within the pulmonary artery. J Am Coll Cardiol 2005;45(6):887–895.

12 Moorman AF, Christoffels VM. Cardiac chamber formation: development, genes, and evolution. Physiol Rev 2003;83(4):1223–1267.

13 Callans DJ, Menz V, Schwartzman D, Gottlieb CD, Marchlinski FE. Repetitive monomorphic tachycardia from the left ventricular outflow tract: electrocardiographic patterns consistent with a left ventricular site of origin. J Am Coll Cardiol 1997;29(5):1023–1027.

14 Kamakura S, Shimizu W, Matsuo K, et al. Localization of optimal ablation site of idiopathic ventricular tachycardia from right and left ventricular outflow tract by body surface ECG. Circulation 1998;98(15):1525–1533.

15 Krebs ME, Krause PC, Engelstein ED, Zipes DP, Miles WM. Ventricular tachycardias mimicking those arising from the right ventricular outflow tract. J Cardiovasc Electrophysiol 2000;11(1):45–51.

16 Lamberti F, Calo L, Pandozi C, et al. Radiofrequency catheter ablation of idiopathic left ventricular outflow tract tachycardia: utility of intracardiac echocardiography. J Cardiovasc Electrophysiol 2001;12(5):529–535.

17 Hachiya H, Aonuma K, Yamauchi Y, et al. Electrocardiographic characteristics of left ventricular outflow tract tachycardia. Pacing Clin Electrophysiol 2000;23 (11 Pt 2):1930–1934.

18 Tada H, Nogami A, Naito S, et al. Left ventricular epicardial outflow tract tachycardia: a new distinct subgroup of outflow tract tachycardia. Jpn Circ J 2001;65(8):723–730.

19 Dixit S, Gerstenfeld EP, Lin D, et al. Identification of distinct electrocardiographic patterns from the basal left ventricle: distinguishing medial and lateral sites of origin in patients with idiopathic ventricular tachycardia. Heart Rhythm 2005;2(5):485–491.

20 Shimoike E, Ohnishi Y, Ueda N, Maruyama T, Kaji Y. Radiofrequency catheter ablation of left ventricular outflow tract tachycardia from the coronary cusp: A new approach to the tachycardia focus. J Cardiovasc Electrophysiol 1999;10(7):1005–1009.

21 Sadanaga T, Saeki K, Yoshimoto T, Funatsu Y, Miyazaki T. Repetitive monomorphic ventricular tachycardia of left coronary cusp origin. Pacing Clin Electrophysiol 1999;22(10):1553–1556.

22 Kanagaratnam L, Tomassoni G, Schweikert R, et al. Ventricular tachycardias arising from the aortic sinus of valsalva: an under-recognized variant of left outflow tract ventricular tachycardia. J Am Coll Cardiol 2001;37(5):1408–1414.

23 Ouyang F, Fotuhi P, Ho SY, et al. Repetitive monomorphic ventricular tachycardia originating from the aortic sinus cusp: electrocardiographic characterization for guiding catheter ablation. J Am Coll Cardiol 2002;39(3):500–508.

24 Yang Y, Saenz LC, Varosy PD, et al. Analyses of phase differences from surface electrocardiogram recordings to distinguish the origin of outflow tract tachycardia (abstract). Heart Rhythm 2005;2(5 Suppl. 1):S80.

25 Tanner H, Hindricks G, Schirdewahn P, et al. Outflow tract tachycardia with R/S transition in lead V3: six different anatomic approaches for successful ablation. J Am Coll Cardiol 2005;45(3):418–423.

26 Meininger GR, Berger RD. Idiopathic ventricular tachycardia originating in the great cardiac vein. Heart Rhythm 2006;3(4):464–466.

27 Daniels DV, Lu YY, Morton JB, et al. Idiopathic epicardial left ventricular tachycardia originating remote from the sinus of Valsalva: electrophysiological characteristics, catheter ablation, and identification from the 12-lead electrocardiogram. Circulation 2006;113(13):1659–1666.

28 Buxton AE, Waxman HL, Marchlinski FE, Simson MB, Cassidy D, Josephson ME. Right ventricular tachycardia: clinical and electrophysiologic characteristics. Circulation 1983;68(5):917–927.

29 Lemery R, Brugada P, Bella PD, Dugernier T, van den Dool A, Wellens HJ. Nonischemic ventricular tachycardia. Clinical course and long-term follow-up in patients without clinically overt heart disease. Circulation 1989;79(5):990–999.

30 Rowland TW, Schweiger MJ. Repetitive paroxysmal ventricular tachycardia and sudden death in a child. Am J Cardiol 1984;53(11):1729.

31 Yarlagadda RK, Iwai S, Stein KM, et al. Reversal of cardiomyopathy in patients with repetitive monomorphic ventricular ectopy originating from the right ventricular outflow tract. Circulation 2005;112(8):1092–1097.

32 Chugh SS, Shen WK, Luria DM, Smith HC. First evidence of premature ventricular complex-induced cardiomyopathy: a potentially reversible cause of heart failure. J Cardiovasc Electrophysiol 2000;11(3):328–329.

33 Thiene G, Nava A, Corrado D, Rossi L, Pennelli N. Right ventricular cardiomyopathy and sudden death in young people. N Engl J Med 1988;318(3):129–133.

34 Marcus FI, Fontaine GH, Guiraudon G, et al. Right ventricular dysplasia: a report of 24 adult cases. Circulation 1982;65(2):384–398.

35 Gill JS, Mehta D, Ward DE, Camm AJ. Efficacy of flecainide, sotalol, and verapamil in the treatment of right ventricular tachycardia in patients without overt cardiac abnormality. Br Heart J 1992;68(4):392–397.

36 Kobayashi Y, Miyata A, Tanno K, Kikushima S, Baba T, Katagiri T. Effects of nicorandil, a potassium channel opener, on idiopathic ventricular tachycardia. J Am Coll Cardiol 1998;32(5):1377–1383.

37 Gepstein L, Hayam G, Ben-Haim SA. A novel method for nonfluoroscopic catheter-based electroanatomical mapping of the heart. In vitro and in vivo accuracy results. Circulation 1997 18;95(6):1611–1622.

38 Fung JW, Chan HC, Chan JY, Chan WW, Kum LC, Sanderson JE. Ablation of nonsustained or hemodynamically unstable ventricular arrhythmia originating from the right ventricular outflow tract guided by noncontact mapping. Pacing Clin Electrophysiol 2003;26(8):1699–1705.

39 Wilber DJ, Baerman J, Olshansky B, Kall J, Kopp D. Adenosine-sensitive ventricular tachycardia. Clinical characteristics and response to catheter ablation. Circulation 1993;87(1):126–134.

40 Chinushi M, Aizawa Y, Ohhira K, et al. Repetitive ventricular responses induced by radiofrequency ablation for idiopathic ventricular tachycardia originating from the outflow tract of the right ventricle. Pacing Clin Electrophysiol 1998;21(4 Pt 1):669–678.

41 Scheinman MM, Huang S. The 1998 NASPE prospective catheter ablation registry. Pacing Clin Electrophysiol 2000;23(6):1020–1028.

42 Joshi S, Wilber DJ. Ablation of idiopathic right ventricular outflow tract tachycardia: current perspectives. J Cardiovasc Electrophysiol 2005;16(Suppl. 1):S52–S58.

43 Wen MS, Taniguchi Y, Yeh SJ, Wang CC, Lin FC, Wu D. Determinants of tachycardia recurrences after radiofrequency ablation of idiopathic ventricular tachycardia. Am J Cardiol 1998 15;81(4):500–503.

44 Rodriguez LM, Smeets JL, Timmermans C, Wellens HJ. Predictors for successful ablation of right- and left-sided idiopathic ventricular tachycardia. Am J Cardiol 1997;79(3):309–314.

45 Friedman PL, Stevenson WG, Bittl JA, et al. Left main coronary artery occlusion during radiofrequency catheter ablation of idiopathic outflow tract ventricular tachycardia (abstract). Pacing Clin Electrophysiol 1997;20 (Part II):1184.

46 Sosa E, Scanavacca M, D'Avila A, et al. Endocardial and epicardial ablation guided by nonsurgical transthoracic epicardial mapping to treat recurrent ventricular tachycardia. J Cardiovasc Electrophysiol 1998;9(3):229–239.

47 Cole CR, Marrouche NF, Natale A. Evaluation and management of ventricular outflow tract tachycardias. Card Electrophysiol Rev 2002;6(4):442–447.

48 Nogami A. Idiopathic left ventricular tachycardia: assessment and treatment. Card Electrophysiol Rev 2002;6(4):448–457.

49 Zipes DP, Foster PR, Troup PJ, Pedersen DH. Atrial induction of ventricular tachycardia: reentry versus triggered automaticity. Am J Cardiol 1979;44(1):1–8.

50 Belhassen B, Rotmensch HH, Laniado S. Response of recurrent sustained ventricular tachycardia to verapamil. Br Heart J 1981;46(6):679–682.

51 Ohe T, Shimomura K, Aihara N, et al. Idiopathic sustained left ventricular tachycardia: clinical and electrophysiologic characteristics. Circulation 1988;77(3):560–568.

52 Shimoike E, Ueda N, Maruyama T, Kaji Y. Radiofrequency catheter ablation of upper septal idiopathic left ventricular tachycardia exhibiting left bundle branch block morphology. J Cardiovasc Electrophysiol 2000;11(2):203–207.

53 German LD, Packer DL, Bardy GH, Gallagher JJ. Ventricular tachycardia induced by atrial stimulation in patients without symptomatic cardiac disease. Am J Cardiol 1983;52(10):1202–1207.

54 Lin FC, Finley CD, Rahimtoola SH, Wu D. Idiopathic paroxysmal ventricular tachycardia with a QRS pattern of right bundle branch block and left axis deviation: a unique clinical entity with specific properties. Am J Cardiol 1983;52(1):95–100.

55 Klein GJ, Millman PJ, Yee R. Recurrent ventricular tachycardia responsive to verapamil. Pacing Clin Electrophysiol 1984;7(6 Pt 1):938–948.

56 Ward DE, Nathan AW, Camm AJ. Fascicular tachycardia sensitive to calcium antagonists. Eur Heart J 1984;5(11):896–905.

57 Ohe T, Aihara N, Kamakura S, Kurita T, Shimizu W, Shimomura K. Long-term outcome of verapamil-sensitive sustained left ventricular tachycardia in patients without structural heart disease. J Am Coll Cardiol 1995;25(1):54–58.

58 Kottkamp H, Chen X, Hindricks G, et al. Idiopathic left ventricular tachycardia: new insights into electrophysiological characteristics and radiofrequency catheter ablation. Pacing Clin Electrophysiol 1995;18(6):1285–1297.

59 Nakagawa H, Beckman KJ, McClelland JH, et al. Radiofrequency catheter ablation of idiopathic left ventricular tachycardia guided by a Purkinje potential. Circulation 1993;88(6):2607–2617.

60 Nogami A, Naito S, Tada H, et al. Verapamil-sensitive left anterior fascicular ventricular tachycardia: results of radiofrequency ablation in six patients. J Cardiovasc Electrophysiol 1998;9(12):1269–1278.

61 Akhtar M, Shenasa M, Jazayeri M, Caceres J, Tchou PJ. Wide QRS complex tachycardia. Reappraisal of a common clinical problem. Ann Intern Med 1988;109(11):905–912.

62 Wellens HJ, Bar FW, Lie KI. The value of the electrocardiogram in the differential diagnosis of a tachycardia with a widened QRS complex. Am J Med 1978;64(1):27–33.

63 Brugada P, Brugada J, Mont L, Smeets J, Andries EW. A new approach to the differential diagnosis of a regular tachycardia with a wide QRS complex. Circulation 1991;83(5):1649–1659.

64 Wen MS, Yeh SJ, Wang CC, Lin FC, Wu D. Successful radiofrequency ablation of idiopathic left ventricular tachycardia at a site away from the tachycardia exit. J Am Coll Cardiol 1997;30(4):1024–1031.

65 Tsuchiya T, Okumura K, Honda T, et al. Significance of late diastolic potential preceding Purkinje potential in verapamil-sensitive idiopathic left ventricular tachycardia. Circulation 1999;99(18):2408–2413.

66 Nogami A, Naito S, Tada H, et al. Demonstration of diastolic and presystolic Purkinje potentials as critical potentials in a macroreentry circuit of verapamil-sensitive idiopathic left ventricular tachycardia. J Am Coll Cardiol 2000;36(3):811–823.

67 Ouyang F, Cappato R, Ernst S, et al. Electroanatomic substrate of idiopathic left ventricular tachycardia: unidirectional block and macroreentry within the Purkinje network. Circulation 2002;105(4):462–469.

68 Chen M, Yang B, Zou J, et al. Non-contact mapping and linear ablation of the left posterior fascicle during sinus rhythm in the treatment of idiopathic left ventricular tachycardia. Europace 2005;7(2):138–144.

69 Ma FS, Ma J, Tang K, et al. Left posterior fascicular block: a new endpoint of ablation for verapamil-sensitive idiopathic ventricular tachycardia. Chin Med J (Engl) 2006;119(5):367–372.

70 Thakur RK, Klein GJ, Sivaram CA, et al. Anatomic substrate for idiopathic left ventricular tachycardia. Circulation 1996;93(3):497–501.

71 Lin FC, Wen MS, Wang CC, Yeh SJ, Wu D. Left ventricular fibromuscular band is not a specific substrate for idiopathic left ventricular tachycardia. Circulation 1996;93(3):525–528.

72 Page RL, Shenasa H, Evans JJ, Sorrentino RA, Wharton JM, Prystowsky EN. Radiofrequency catheter ablation of idiopathic recurrent ventricular tachycardia with right bundle branch block, left axis morphology. Pacing Clin Electrophysiol 1993;16(2):327–336.

73 Yeh SJ, Wen MS, Wang CC, Lin FC, Wu D. Adenosine-sensitive ventricular tachycardia from the anterobasal left ventricle. J Am Coll Cardiol 1997;30(5):1339–1345.

74 Nagasawa H, Fujiki A, Usui M, Mizumaki K, Hayashi H, Inoue H. Successful radiofrequency catheter ablation of incessant ventricular tachycardia with a delta wave-like beginning of the QRS complex. Jpn Heart J 1999;40(5):671–675.

75 Kondo K, Watanabe I, Kojima T, et al. Radiofrequency catheter ablation of ventricular tachycardia from the anterobasal left ventricle. Jpn Heart J 2000;41(2):215–225.

76 Tada H, Ito S, Naito S, et al. Idiopathic ventricular arrhythmia arising from the mitral annulus: a distinct subgroup of idiopathic ventricular arrhythmias. J Am Coll Cardiol 2005;45(6):877–886.

77 Kumagai K, Yamauchi Y, Takahashi A, et al. Idiopathic left ventricular tachycardia originating from the mitral annulus. J Cardiovasc Electrophysiol 2005;16(10):1029–1036.

78 Tada H, Tadokoro K, Ito S, et al. Idiopathic ventricular arrhythmias originating from the tricuspid annulus: prevalence, electrocardiographic characteristics, and results of radiofrequency catheter ablation. Heart Rhythm 2007;4(1):7–16.

CHAPTER 11

Ablation of ventricular fibrillation

Karen P. Phillips, J. David Burkhardt, Robert A. Schweikert, Walid I. Saliba, & Andrea Natale

Introduction

Ventricular fibrillation (VF) is the most common arrhythmia underlying sudden cardiac death. While implantable cardiac defibrillators have become the mainstay of therapy for the established arrhythmia in at-risk patients, recent advances in our understanding of the mechanisms of initiation of VF have allowed the development of novel approaches to catheter ablation of this lethal arrhythmia.

Mechanisms of initiation of ventricular fibrillation

Current knowledge supports that fibrillation can be initiated with stimulation of the ventricles during the vulnerable phase of systole or repolarization. This has been demonstrated to result either from application of electric shock, multisite stimulation protocols, or successive stimulation from a single electrode [1]. Observations and modeling of the spontaneous initiation of VF have confirmed the importance of a reentrant mechanism in the generation of multiple wavelets or rotors that characterize the turbulent cardiac electrical activity in VF [1]. Experimental studies support a critical dynamic interaction between tissue excitability, gradients of refractoriness, and the impact of anatomical and functional obstacles as a prerequisite for this reentry [1].

Studies in pacing-stimulation-induced VF in patients with left ventricular systolic dysfunction and previous myocardial infarction have demonstrated

interval-dependent development of functional lines of block and regions of slow conduction that were associated with fibrillatory initiation [2]. Surprising consistency of the location of VF initiation was noted despite varying rates of stimulation and pacing site [2]. There is preliminary evidence to support that substrate modification of the scar border zone during ablation for ventricular tachycardia can also modify susceptibility to VF [3].

Interest in the sources of initiation of VF has also focused on the role of the Purkinje system. There is little doubt from *in vitro* studies that the Purkinje system has a peculiar capacity to generate and maintain arrhythmias by way of triggered activity, automaticity, and reentrant mechanisms. The unique propagation properties of the Purkinje muscle system, in addition to its complex anatomical distribution and high degree of heterogeneity of action potential duration under varying conditions, provide credible conditions for the initiation and maintenance of VF. Three-dimensional computerized modeling of the interaction between the Purkinje fiber system and ventricular myocardium following a focal trigger at a Purkinje–muscle junction, has enabled accurate simulation of the initiation of reentry during polymorphic ventricular tachycardia (PMVT) [4]. Reentry in this model was initially dependent on the coexistence of Purkinje system and myocardium, but in later stages stabilized as intramyocardial reentry independent of the presence of the Purkinje fibers. The mode of initiation of VF has been suggested to be similar [4].

The observation that Purkinje tissue cells have a greater resistance to ischemia and, experimentally, have been shown to survive within necrotic or scarred muscle areas [5] has also focused interest on their possible role in generating ventricular

Ventricular Arrhythmias and Sudden Cardiac Death, 1st edition. Edited by P.J. Wang, A. Al-Ahmad, H. Hsia, and P.C. Zei © 2008 Blackwell Publishing, ISBN: 978-1-4051-6114-5.

arrhythmias in structural heart disease. Surviving Purkinje fibers have been demonstrated to exhibit a range of arrhythmogenic properties including heightened automaticity, triggered activity, and prolongation of action potential duration [6]. Several groups have now shown that targeting Purkinje tissue along the scar border zone in patients with a prior myocardial infarction [7–10] or at triggering foci within the distal Purkinje arborization in other types of structural heart disease [11,12] can successfully modify the inducibility and recurrence of PMVT and VF in a subset of patients.

VF ablation in structurally normal hearts

As the causes and mechanisms of "idiopathic ventricular fibrillation" are gradually elucidated, a variety of clinical syndromes are now recognized as associated with VF in structurally normal hearts. By definition, structural myopathic disease and coronary ischemia have been rigorously excluded from these patient subgroups. The frequent observation of focal triggers initiating malignant ventricular arrhythmias across these various syndromes lends a commonality to approaches to ablation.

Idiopathic VF originating from the right ventricular outflow tract

Clinical characteristics

There are reports of a malignant entity of idiopathic right ventricular outflow tract ventricular tachycardia (RVOT VT) associated with polymorphic VT or VF [13–19]. The majority of these cases are reported in patients of Asian origin. In the largest series to date from Japan the mean age of patients at presentation was 39 ± 10 years with no predilection for gender noted [13]. A family history of sudden cardiac death is almost uniformly absent. Frequent monomorphic ventricular ectopy has been observed on ECG monitoring typical of RVOT myocardial origin (left bundle branch block pattern, inferior axis, with broad QRS 130–180 ms). The coupling interval of ectopic beats initiating polymorphic VT or VF is intermediate, ranging from 320 to 400 milliseconds and may be identical to coupling intervals of other single PVCs [13]. Coexistence of monomorphic VT with episodes of PMVT or VF is also reported [13]. The onset of malignant ventricular arrhythmias typically occurs at rest or night time and is most commonly heralded symptomatically by presyncope or syncope, although a minority of patients reported only palpitations [13].

Electrophysiological characteristics and catheter ablation

Activation mapping and pace mapping have been successfully used to identify a discrete focus in the RVOT that is amenable to ablation in an approach similar to the benign form of idiopathic RVOT VT [13–19]. Similarly, spontaneous ectopy is reportedly facilitated by the use of isoproterenol, epinephrine, methoxamine, and programmed ventricular stimulation [13]. In the largest series to date from Japan, multiple energy applications delivered over an estimated area of 2–4 cm diameter were reportedly required in 11 of 16 patients following changes in morphology of the target PVC at the onset of initial radiofrequency delivery [13]. Procedural success was achieved in 13 of 16 patients, with persistent inducibility of VF or nonsustained PMVT in the remainder.

Follow-up

In the Japanese series a mean follow-up time of 54 ± 39 months saw no recurrences of syncope, VF or cardiac arrest in the 16 patients who underwent catheter ablation (Table 11.1).

Idiopathic VF originating from Purkinje tissue

Clinical characteristics

A range of unifying characteristics attests to the existence of a subgroup of patients whose triggers for VF originate from Purkinje or Purkinje-like tissue [14,20,21]. The morphology of ventricular ectopy is appreciably narrower (QRS duration 80–150 ms) and may be right bundle branch block pattern or left bundle branch block pattern reflecting an origin from either the left or right ventricular Purkinje system. A tendency toward polymorphic PVCs rather than a monomorphic appearance has also been reported. The coupling interval of the PVC initiating PMVT or VF is characteristically short (240–270 ms) and pause-dependency onset has not been observed. Variability has been noted in the frequency of spontaneous ventricular ectopy with

Table 11.1 Characteristics of RVOT VF cases reported in the literature

Reference	Sex (M/F)	Age (yr)	QRS duration of PVC (ms)	PVC daily count (n)	PVC coupling interval (ms)	Local V-QRS (ms)	Ablation site RVOT	RF applications (n)	Follow-up (mo)
Ashida et al., 1997 [16]	1F	18	N/A	11,800	340	20	Septal	40	36
Kusano et al. 2000 [17]	1F	65	N/A	N/A	410	N/A (pace map)	Mid free wall	N/A	18
Takatsuki et al., 2001 [18]	1M	62	N/A	37,000	320–330	30	Posteroseptal	4	20
Haïssaguerre et al., 2002 [14]	1M/3F	27 ± 8	145 ± 12	N/A	355 ± 30	32 ± 15	RVOT	8 ± 3	75 ± 23
Yu et al., 2006 [19]	1F	42	N/A	Frequent	N/A	N/A (pace map)	RVOT	N/A	15
Noda et al., 2004 [13]	7M/9F	39 ± 10	148 ± 8	17,554 ± 11,338	409 ± 62	17 ± 11	Septal 13/free wall 3	9 ± 4	54 ± 39
Viskin et al., 2005 [15]	3F	55 ± 9	N/A	N/A	350 ± 20	30	Midseptal 1	N/A	5

PVC, premature ventricular contraction; Local V-QRS, local ventricular electrogram to QRS onset at ablation site; RF, radiofrequency.

small numbers of patients reported to have very frequent PVCs between intercurrent ventricular arrhythmias. More commonly, however, PVCs were only identified in temporal association with ventricular arrhythmia storm [14].

In the largest series to date reported by Haissaguerre's group [14], the mean age of patients at presentation was 43 ± 14 years with equal prevalence in males and females. Arrhythmia onset occurred during nonexertional daily activities or, more rarely, during sleep and the most common symptom reported was syncope. A family history of sudden cardiac death was elicited in a minority of patients.

Modulating factors associated with electrical storm are also reported in some patients [23] and share similarities with those described in ion channelopathies such as Brugada syndrome and long-QT syndrome, including fever, electrolyte disturbances, and drug exposure.

Considerable clinical overlap is observed between reported cases of idiopathic Purkinje VF [14,17–19] and the previously described short-coupled variant Torsade de Pointes [21]. A frequent coexistence of PMVT and VF is described in both patient series [14,21]. Varying, divergent responses to a range of provocative pharmacological maneuvers amongst subsets of patients in these series suggest the possibility that different etiologies might be responsible for similar outward manifestations of arrhythmia. An almost uniform observation in cases of Purkinje VF or short-coupled variant Torsade de Pointes, however, is the reported ability of intravenous verapamil to acutely suppress ventricular ectopy and arrhythmias [14,20,21,24]. In our experience, however, administration of very large doses may be required, often limited by the development of A-V nodal conduction block. The effectiveness of chronic oral verapamil therapy in preventing recurrence of the arrhythmia has also been disappointing [14,21,24]. An underlying abnormality of calcium transport associated with triggered activity and delayed after depolarizations has been proposed as an explanation by several authors [14,22,24] and would be consistent with the findings of a short-coupled PVC in the presence of an otherwise normal appearance to the surface electrocardiogram. Additionally, Leenhardt's group [24] found evidence for an autonomic nervous system abnormality in the series of 14 patients with short-coupled variant Torsade de Pointes, specifically depressed heart

rate variability suggestive of low parasympathetic drive.

The intriguing combination of features of onset of arrhythmia at rest or during nonexertional activity and intercurrent nature of triggering ectopy suggests the possibility that a complex interplay of modulating environmental, metabolic, and autonomic factors contributes to unmask a primary abnormality of the Purkinje muscle system.

Electrophysiological characteristics

Activation mapping has been utilized to localize the earliest electrogram relative to the onset of ventricular ectopy or PMVT [14,21]. At these sites sharp potentials were observed to precede the earliest local ventricular electrogram by 15–120 milliseconds during ectopy [14]. The same potential was also identified to precede or fuse with the local ventricular electrogram during sinus rhythm in the majority of patients suggesting true Purkinje system origin. In one case report the potential was reported to have a variable relationship to or follow the ventricular electrogram during sinus rhythm and was proposed to originate from Purkinje-like tissue located in the inferolateral border of the right ventricular wall [21]. The Purkinje sources have been mapped to the right ventricle anterior wall and from a wide region over the lower half of the left ventricular septum. The Purkinje potential was noted to precede local ventricular activation during ectopy to a greater degree in the left than the right ventricle (46 ± 29 versus 19 ± 10 ms) [14]. Multiple Purkinje deflections were observed at the earliest site in several patients. Purkinje–ventricular myocardial conduction block has been observed as the mechanism of termination of episodes of PMVT in several patients [14,22].

Isoproterenol infusion and programmed ventricular stimulation have not been consistently reported useful in the facilitation of spontaneous ectopy during electrophysiological study [14,21,22]. Leenhardt et al. [24] reported a variable response to intravenous atropine and calcium gluconate for an increase in the frequency of spontaneous PVCs and the repetitive form of arrhythmia.

Catheter ablation

Successful approaches to catheter ablation have included both activation and pace-mapping techniques. Haissaguerre's group [14,20] reported the successful targeting of Purkinje tissue at the earliest recorded Purkinje potential, which preceded local ventricular muscle activation during premature beats. Pace mapping in association with identification of a presystolic Purkinje potential was utilized in a single case report by Nogami's group and purported to target the distal Purkinje network to achieve Purkinje system–ventricular muscle disconnection [22]. In several patients without spontaneous arrhythmia during the procedure, pace mapping of previously documented 12-lead ECG morphology PVCs was utilized and local Purkinje potentials targeted for successful ablation [14]. Several observations from groups, however, highlight the potential pitfalls of pace-mapping techniques. Multiple morphology PVCs have been found to result from a single trigger in the Purkinje network, but with different exit points to ventricular muscle as evidence of changing propagation in the distal Purkinje arborization [14,22]. The variable ability to capture Purkinje tissue versus local ventricular muscle [22] also impacts the potential for accurate localization of the trigger source.

Successful sites of energy application were associated with a transient exacerbation of arrhythmia followed by complete disappearance of spontaneous ventricular ectopy [14,21]. Local abolition of the targeted Purkinje sharp potentials was observed in addition to a delay in occurrence of the local ventricular electrogram or a slight prolongation of the QRS duration [14].

Follow-up

Successful ablation appears to be associated with a complete abolition of PVCs or short-coupled PVCs on extended monitoring or device diagnostic logs [14,21,22]. The clinical course of this patient group is, however, only reported out to a mean of 24 ± 28 months [14]. Late recurrence of premature beats of the same preablation morphology is reported in two patients from a series of 23 and was associated with recurrent ventricular arrhythmia (Table 11.2) [14].

VF associated with long-QT and Brugada syndromes

Clinical and electrophysiological characteristics

Strikingly similar findings of RVOT myocardial triggers and PVCs of Purkinje origin initiating PMVT or

VF have been identified in small subsets of patients with long-QT syndrome and Brugada syndrome [25,26]. Patients presented with multiple episodes of PMVT or VF or ventricular electrical storm and on monitoring were found to have a triggering role of ventricular premature beats in the onset of arrhythmia.

In four patients with long-QT syndrome, PVCs had a longer coupling interval of 503 ± 29 milliseconds with a monomorphic typical RVOT or right bundle branch block superior axis morphology in two patients [25]. A polymorphic, sometimes bidirectional appearance of PVCs with a positive morphology in V1, was seen in two patients, associated with intermediate coupling intervals of 280–420 milliseconds. Purkinje potentials were identified at successful sites of ablation in the latter three patients.

In three patients with Brugada syndrome monomorphic PVCs were identified in all—two with a typical RVOT morphology and intermediate coupling intervals of 340 ± 20 and 408 ± 15 milliseconds, and one patient with a left bundle branch block superior axis with a short coupling interval of 278 ± 29 milliseconds [25]. The latter case was associated with Purkinje potentials at electrophysiological study. An additional case report of successful ablation for electrical storm in Brugada syndrome also noted triggering monomorphic PVCs of typical RVOT morphology with QRS duration of 180 milliseconds and a long coupling interval [26].

Further supportive evidence for a focal origin of arrhythmogenesis in Brugada syndrome is provided by a Japanese study [27] which suggested VF was more frequently induced by programmed electrical stimulation at the free wall region of the RVOT, than at other right ventricular or left ventricular sites. Spontaneous PVCs were recorded in only a small percentage of the largely asymptomatic study population and were associated with a long coupling interval $(423 \pm 62 \text{ ms})$. Pace mapping of PVCs localized the origin to the RVOT in the majority of cases.

Catheter ablation and follow-up

Prolonged application of radiofrequency energy was required to eliminate premature beats in all patients, ranging from 7 to 24 minutes [25].

During a mean follow-up time of 24 ± 20 months in the long QT syndrome patients and 7 ± 6 months

Table 11.2 Characteristics of Purkinje VF and short-coupled variant of Torsade de Pointes cases reported in the literature

Reference	Sex (M/F)	Age (yrs)	Family history of SCD (n)	QRS duration of PVC (ms)	PVC morphology	PVC coupling interval (ms)	Local PP-QRS (ms)	Ablation site	RF applications (n)	Follow-up (mo)
Haissaguerre et al., 2002 [14]	12M/11F	43 ± 14	6	126 ± 18	N/A	280 ± 26	LV 46 ± 29 RV 19 ± 10	RV Purkinje 7/LV Purkinje 9/RV and LV 4	9 ± 5	24 ± 28
Saliba et al., 2002 [21]	1F	41	0	145	LBBB L sup axis	240	60	RV inferolateral	N/A	6
Nogami et al., 2005 [22]	1M	54	0	N/A	RBBB R axis	280	15-60	LV septum	N/A	48
Leenhardt et al., 1994 [24]	7M/7F	35 ± 10	4	N/A	LBBB L axis 9/LBBB R or N axis 2/RBBB 2	245 ± 28	N/A	N/A	N/A	N/A

SCD, sudden cardiac death; PVC, premature ventricular contraction; PP-QRS, Purkinje potential to QRS activation time; RF, radiofrequency.

in the Brugada syndrome group and 6 months in the single Brugada case report [26] no recurrence of VF, syncope or sudden cardiac death occurred (Table 11.3).

VF ablation in structural heart disease

VF electrical storm associated with ischemic cardiomyopathy

Patients with a history of remote myocardial infarction have an increased risk of life-threatening ventricular arrhythmias, and the occurrence of ventricular electrical storm portends a direr prognosis, even in the presence of an implantable cardioverter-defibrillator [30]. While medical and supportive therapy remains the cornerstone of successful management of electrical storm [31] with careful attention to resolution of contributory ischemia, heart failure and other precipitants, small numbers of patients may declare themselves as refractory to these measures. The largest experience to date in ablation of VF electrical storm in patients remote from myocardial infarction is from the Cleveland Clinic group [7]. A collective prospective experience of 29 patients with ischemic cardiomyopathy and prior remote myocardial infarction were observed to have a triggering role of monomorphic PVCs to recurrent episodes of ventricular fibrillation. The PVC had a right bundle branch block pattern in all cases with a mean QRS duration of 178 ± 25 milliseconds. The mean coupling interval of the triggering PVC was short at 195 ± 45 milliseconds. The majority of the cohort ($n = 21$) responded to medical management, however, eight patients proceeded to successful ablation of triggering PVCs at a mean time of 14 ± 20 days following the onset of electrical storm.

Electrophysiological characteristics and catheter ablation

Activation mapping localized the earliest site of activation of the spontaneous PVC to the border zone of the ischemic scar in the left ventricle in five patients. Purkinje-like potentials were found to precede the PVC QRS onset by a mean of 68 ± 20 milliseconds. In the remaining three patients in whom PVCs could not be induced during the procedure, Purkinje-like potentials were mapped along the scar border zone

in sinus rhythm and ablation lesions applied along the length of the border zone with an endpoint of elimination of all detected Purkinje potentials. Successful ablation resulting in the complete elimination of triggering PVCs was achieved in all patients with the acute subsidence of electrical storm.

An additional report from Haissaguerre's group [9] suggests similar findings in two patients successfully ablated for recurrent episodes of PMVT at 150 and 170 days postmyocardial infarction. Triggering PVCs were right bundle branch block morphology with a coupling interval of 400–440 and 500–600 milliseconds. PVCs were mapped to the scar border zone, and in both cases were preceded by Purkinje potentials by 20–116 milliseconds.

Follow-up

Out to 11 months of follow-up in the Cleveland Clinic series, recurrence of a single episode of VF was noted in one patient and the development of a monomorphic VT was reported in another (Figures 11.1 and 11.2).

VF electrical storm associated with post-acute myocardial infarction

The culprit triggering PVCs have also been successfully targeted in small numbers of patients with persistent ventricular electrical storm following acute myocardial infarction [8–10]. Combined substrate and activation mapping in the series from Haissaguerre's group [9] again localized the origin of PVCs to the border-zone of the myocardial infarction. PVCs in all cases were right bundle branch block morphology [8–10], with a QRS duration of 120–160 milliseconds [8], and a coupling interval varying from 270 to 500 milliseconds [8,9].

Electrophysiological characteristics

In all cases at the origin of the PVCs Purkinje potentials were noted to precede the onset of the QRS during the spontaneous PVC (range 20–220 ms) [8–10]. At the same site in two patients, varying conduction times of Purkinje potential to QRS were found to be associated with different clinical PVC morphologies [9]. During initiation of VT or VF, repetitive Purkinje activity was observed to precede each QRS complex [8,9], but thereafter the potential was observed in, at least one case, to follow ventricular activation in random order [8]. Additional

Table 11.3 Clinical conditions associated with VF or PMVT in structurally normal hearts

Clinical entity	Arrhythmia	Primary abnormality	Arrhythmia mechanism	Surface ECG characteristics	PVC morphology	QRS duration of PVC (ms)	PVC coupling interval (ms)
Long-QT syndrome	Torsade de Pointes	Loss of function mutations in KCNQ1, KCNH2, SCN5A genes	Dispersion of repolarization and reentry within M cell layer	Resting or inducible QTc > 450 ms	—	—	Short–long–short sequence 587 ± 65 [28]
Short-QT syndrome	AF/VF	Gain of function mutations in KCNQ1, KCNH2 genes	Dispersion of repolarization ?	Resting or inducible QTc <320 ms	—	—	—
Brugada syndrome	PMVT/VF	Gain of function mutation in SCN5A gene	Dispersion of de/repolarization and Phase 2 reentry	Resting or inducible RBBB, ST elevation V1-3	—	—	—
Catecholaminergic PMVT	PMVT	CASQ2 and RyR2 gene mutations	Sympathetically mediated DADs	Normal	RBBB/LBBB polymorphic	110 ± 20 [29]	330 ± 50 [29]
RVOT VT/VF	MMVT/PMVT/VF	? focal abnormality of RVOT myocardium	cAMP mediated EADs	Normal	LBBB inferior axis, monomorphic	148 ± 8 [13]	320–410 [13–19]
Idiopathic Purkinje VF	PMVT/VF	?	? DADs in Purkinje fibers	Normal	LBBB or RBBB, polymorphic	126 ± 18 [14]	220–320 [14,21,22,24]

PVC, premature ventricular contraction; AF, atrial fibrillation; MMVT, monomorphic ventricular tachycardia; EAD, early afterdepolarization; DAD, delayed afterdepolarization.

(a)   (b)

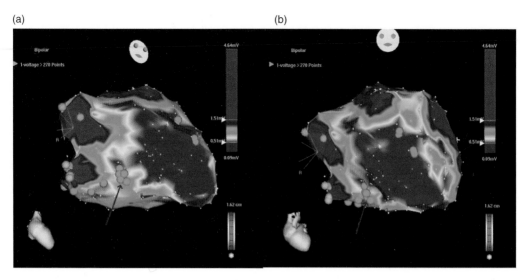

Figure 11.1 Left ventricular endocardial electroanatomic bipolar voltage map in RAO (a) and AP caudal (b) projections of a patient with ischemic cardiomyopathy with monomorphic PVCs observed to trigger VF. Normal voltages (>1.5 mV) are shown in purple and scar (<0.5 mV) is shown in red. The blue tags represent sites of Purkinje potentials. The PVC origin was mapped to the inferoseptal scar border (arrowed), and was preceded by a Purkinje potential as shown in Figure 11.2.

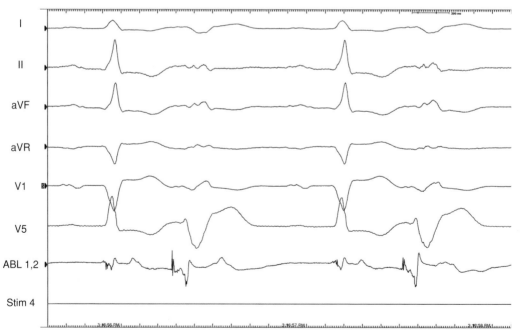

Figure 11.2 Local mapping catheter electrograms at the site of successful ablation of a spontaneous PVC triggering VF. A Purkinje potential precedes the local ventricular electrogram in sinus rhythm and with greater prematurity in the PVC.

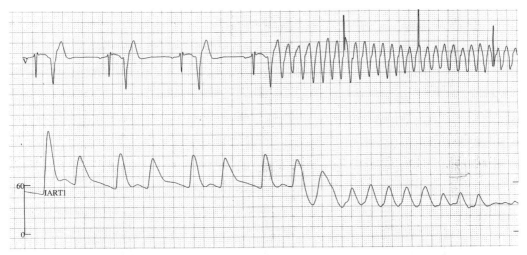

Figure 11.3 Surface ECG and systemic arterial traces capturing the onset of a short-coupled PVC (310 ms) triggering VF in a patient with ventricular electrical storm 15 days following myocardial revascularization. The PVC was localized to the border of an inferoposterior scar (see Figure 11.4) and successfully ablated.

observations of split Purkinje potentials during repetitive runs of PVCs and conduction block between the Purkinje potential and ventricular muscle have also been made in this patient group [9].

Catheter ablation

Multiple radiofrequency applications were required at sites of earliest PVC activation to eliminate PVC occurrence in all patients. Bursts of arrhythmia could be observed during energy delivery before the eventual elimination of ectopy [9]. In one patient without spontaneous PVCs during the procedure, pace-mapping techniques and more extensive ablation targeting all Purkinje potentials in the region was associated with a successful outcome [8].

Follow-up

There was no reported occurrence of ventricular arrhythmia or death over a follow-up time ranging from 5 to 33 months for the seven patients in the combined German [8] and French and Polish [9] experience (Figures 11.3–11.5).

VF electrical storm in other forms of cardiomyopathy

The triggering role of Purkinje tissue-related PVCs to episodes of VF has also been documented in other categories of structural heart disease, including valvular [12] and infiltrative cardiomyopathy

[11]. Successful elimination of Purkinje foci is reported in a young patient following aortic valve surgery for severe aortic regurgitation [12]. Two cases of successful ablation of Purkinje-related PVC triggers are also described in cardiac amyloidosis [11]. Myocardial scar did not appear to be necessarily related to the site of arrhythmogenesis [11]. We ourselves have observed that that monomorphic PVCs triggering VF and PMVT have been noted in several patients of early postoperative corrective mitral and aortic regurgitant valve surgery and in cases of antiarrhythmic drug toxicity, in particular dofetilide. Conservative, supportive management has been associated with resolution of ventricular electrical storm in all cases.

Tips and tricks in the approach to ablation of VF

The decision to proceed with a mapping and ablative procedure for triggers of VF must be weighed against the likelihood that the episode of electrical storm will resolve with medical and supportive management, and the risks that each treatment approach entails. There is undoubtedly a benefit to proceeding with ablation attempts at the time of ventricular electrical storm in order to maximize the ability to map and localize the triggering PVC. It is our experience that antiarrhythmic drug

(a)   (b)

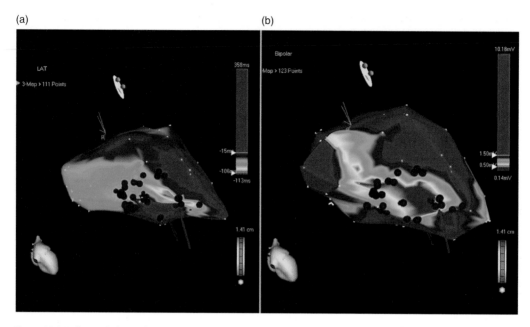

Figure 11.4 Left ventricular endocardial electroanatomic local activation timing map of triggering PVC (a) and bipolar voltage map (b) in RAO caudal projection of the patient with ischemic cardiomyopathy from Figure 11.3. Earliest activation is marked in red and latest activation in purple in map a. Normal voltages (>1.5 mV) are shown in purple and scar (<0.5 mV) is shown in red in map b. The PVC origin was mapped to the inferoposterior scar border (arrowed) and successfully ablated.

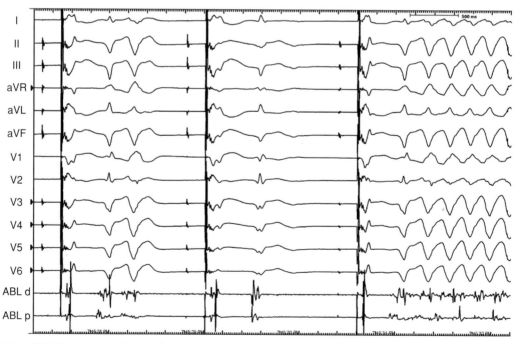

Figure 11.5 Electrograms at the site of successful ablation (see Figure 11.4) of a PVC triggering PMVT in a patient with post-myocardial infarction ventricular electrical storm. A Purkinje potential precedes the local ventricular electrogram by 60 milliseconds in the initiating PVC.

loading, other than β-blockers, should be avoided as it appears to offer limited benefit in a medical management approach [31] and hampers subsequent attempts at mapping and ablation. Procedural sedation should be kept to a minimum to avoid suppression of spontaneous PVCs and arrhythmia activity. In the event of infrequent or absent spontaneous-trigger PVCs during the procedure, a variety of maneuvers should be tried to facilitate their occurrence. Pharmacological agents that are possibly useful for that purpose include infusions or bolus administration of isoproterenol, calcium, and atropine. Programmed stimulation from the atrium or ventricle may also promote arrhythmia including burst pacing and short–long sequences. In the setting of ablation of VF triggers in structurally normal hearts, the spontaneous occurrence of the culprit PVC during mapping is of particular importance given the potential pitfalls of a pace-mapping approach in this group. In the ischemic cardiomyopathy patient, however, substrate and voltage mapping to delineate the scar border zone can be coupled successfully with a pace-mapping approach and targeted ablation of regional Purkinje potentials in the absence of spontaneous PVCs.

Clinical implications

The potential role of Purkinje fibers in ventricular arrhythmogenesis following myocardial infarction has been known for over 30 years [5]. However, the knowledge has lain dormant until the current era of intracardiac mapping. We find ourselves in a unique position with the tools to affect a parallel advancement in our understanding of the mechanisms of ventricular arrhythmias along with the potential to deliver efficacious, targeted therapy.

The concept was once almost inconceivable that focal ablation could be a useful therapy for a chaotic, diffuse arrhythmia such as ventricular fibrillation. However, progress in the field of ablation of atrial fibrillation has helped us to forge a new understanding of the role of triggers, perpetuating factors, and of underlying substrate in complex arrhythmogenesis.

The current follow-up experience for patients who have undergone ablation for triggers of VF in the absence of structural heart disease remains limited. However, as we expand our knowledge on the etiology and mechanisms underlying this condition, there is reason to be hopeful that ablation may represent a potentially curative procedure for such patients. Assessment of the coupling intervals of PVCs appears to be of critical importance to identifying patients with the potentially malignant form of RVOT VT/VF and in patients with intercurrent ectopy in idiopathic Purkinje VF.

In the setting of structural heart disease, catheter ablation must currently play an adjunctive role to optimal medical management and implantable cardioverter-defibrillator therapy in patients with recurrent ventricular fibrillation or ventricular electrical storm. The potential of ablative strategies to modify prognosis following ventricular electrical storm, however, merits closer examination. The future direction of management of ventricular arrhythmias is likely to see the emergence of a greater role of catheter ablation in the proactive prevention and treatment of these life-threatening arrhythmias.

References

1 Jalife J. Ventricular fibrillation: mechanisms of initiation and maintenance. Annu Rev Physiol 2000;62:25–50.
2 Chow AWC, Segal OR, Davies DW, Peters NS. Mechanisms of pacing-induced ventricular fibrillation in the infarcted human heart. Circulation 2004;110:1725–1730.
3 Chow AW, Schilling RJ, Peters NS, Davies DW. Catheter ablation of ventricular tachycardia related to coronary artery disease: the role of noncontact mapping. Curr Cardiol Rep 2000;6:529–536.
4 Berenfeld B, Jalife J. Purkinje-muscle reentry as a mechanism of polymorphic ventricular arrhythmias in a 3-dimensional model of the ventricles. Circ Res 1998;82:1063–1077.
5 Friedman PL, Stewart JR, Fenoglio JJ Jr, Wit AL. Survival of subendocardial Purkinje fibers after extensive myocardial infarction in dogs. Circ Res 1973;33:597–611.
6 Kupersmith J, Li ZY, Maidonado C. Marked action potential prolongation as a source of injury current leading to border zone arrhythmogenesis. Am Heart J 1994;127:1543–1553.
7 Marrouche NF, Verma A, Wazni O, et al. Mode of initiation and ablation of ventricular fibrillation storms in patients with ischemic cardiomyopathy. J Am Coll Cardiol 2004;43:1715–1720.
8 Bansch D, Oyang F, Antz M, et al. Successful catheter ablation of electrical storm after myocardial infarction. Circulation 2003;108:3011–3016.
9 Szumowski L, Sanders P, Walczak F, et al. Mapping and ablation of polymorphic ventricular tachycardia after myocardial infarction. J Am Coll Cardiol 2004;44:1700–1706.

10 Enjoji Y, Mizobuchi M, Shibata K, et al. Catheter ablation for an incessant form of drug-resistant ventricular fibrillation after acute coronary syndrome. PACE 2006;29:102–105.

11 Mlcochova H, Saliba WI, Burkhardt JD, et al. Catheter ablation of ventricular fibrillation storm in patients with infiltrative amyloidosis of the heart. J Cardiovasc Electrophysiol 2006;17:426–430.

12 Li Y-G, Gronefeld G, Israel C, Hohnloser SH. Catheter ablation of frequently recurring ventricular fibrillation in a patient after aortic valve repair. J Cardiovasc Electrophysiol 2004;15:90–93.

13 Noda T, Shimizu W, Taguchi A, et al. Malignant entity of idiopathic ventricular fibrillation and polymorphic ventricular tachycardia initiated by premature extrasystoles originating from the right ventricular outflow tract. J Am Coll Cardiol 2004;46:1288–1294.

14 Haissaguerre M, Shoda M, Jais P, et al. Mapping and ablation of idiopathic ventricular fibrillation. Circulation 2002;106:962–967.

15 Viskin S, Rosso R, Rogowski O, Belhassen B. The "short-coupled" variant of right ventricular outflow ventricular tachycardia: a not-so-benign form of benign ventricular tachycardia? J Cardiovasc Electrophysiol 2005;16:912–916.

16 Ashida K, Kaji Y, Sasaki Y. Abolition of Torsade de Pointes after radiofrequency catheter ablation at the right ventricular outflow tract. Int J Card 1997;59:171–175.

17 Kusano KF, Yamamoto M, Emori T, Morita H, Ohe T. Successful catheter ablation in a patient with polymorphic ventricular tachycardia. J Cardiovasc Electrophysiol 2000;11:682–685.

18 Takatsuki S, Mitamura H, Ogawa S. Catheter ablation of a monofocal premature ventricular complex triggering idiopathic ventricular fibrillation. Heart 2001;86:e3.

19 Yu C-C, Tsai C-T, Lai L-P, Lin J-L. Successful radiofrequency catheter ablation of idiopathic ventricular fibrillation presented as recurrent syncope and diagnosed by an implanted loop recorder. Int J Cardiol 2006;110:112–113.

20 Haissaguerre M, Shah DC, Jais P, et al. Role of Purkinje conducting system in triggering of idiopathic ventricular fibrillation. Lancet 2002;359:677–678.

21 Saliba W, Karim AA, Tchou P, Natale A. Ventricular fibrillation: ablation of a trigger? J Cardiovasc Electrophysiol 2002;13:1296–1299.

22 Nogami A, Sugiyasu A, Kubota S, Kato K. Mapping and ablation of ventricular fibrillation from the Purkinje system. Heart Rhythm 2005;2:646–649.

23 Pasquie JL, Sanders P, Hocini M, et al. Fever as a precipitant of idiopathic ventricular fibrillation in patients with normal hearts. J Cardiovasc Electrophysiol 2004;15:1271–1276.

24 Leenhardt A, Glaser E, Burguera M, Nurnberg M, Maison-Blanche P, Coumel P. Short-coupled variant of Torsade de Pointes: a new electrocardiographic entity in the spectrum of idiopathic ventricular tachyarrhythmias. Circulation 1994;89:206–215.

25 Haissaguerre M, Extramiana F, Hocini M, et al. Mapping and ablation of ventricular fibrillation associated with Long-QT and Brugada syndromes. Circulation 2003;108:925–928.

26 Darmon J-P, Bettouche S, Deswardt P, et al. Radiofrequency ablation of ventricular fibrillation and multiple right and left atrial tachycardia in a patient with Brugada syndrome. J Int Cardiovasc Electrophysiol 2004;11:205–209.

27 Morita H, Fukushima-Kusano K, Nagase S, et al. Site-specific arrhythmogenesis in patients with Brugada syndrome. J Cardiovasc Electrophysiol 2003;14:373–379.

28 Noda T, Shimuzu W, Satomi K, et al. Classification and mechanism of Torsades de Pointes initiation in patients with congenital long QT syndrome. Eur Heart J 2004;25:2149–2154.

29 Sumitomo M, Harada K, Nagashima M, et al. Catecholaminergic polymorphic ventricular tachycardia: electrocardiographic characteristics and optimal therapeutic strategies to prevent sudden death. Heart 2003;89:66–70.

30 Exner DE, Pinski SL, Wyse G, et al. Electrical storm presages nonsudden death: the antiarrhythmics versus implantable defibrillators trial. Circulation 2001;103:2066–2071.

31 Nademanee K, Taylor R, Bailey WE, Rieders DE, Kosar EM. Treating electrical storm: sympathetic blockade versus advanced cardiac life support – guided therapy. Circulation 2000;102:742–747.

CHAPTER 12

Ablation of ventricular tachycardia in congenital heart disease

George F. Van Hare

Ventricular tachycardia remains a difficult management issue in patients who have previously undergone surgical repair of congenital heart defects, and is a cause of sudden cardiac death. This fact is the source of significant disappointment on the part of patients and their families. This is because in most patients, the initial hemodynamic problems posed by such congenital defects have been successfully palliated or repaired by surgery, often years or decades previously. Therefore, the late occurrence of malignant arrhythmias in such successfully repaired patients is distressing. Historically, there has been concern that A-V block may be involved in the etiology of sudden death in a few patients, and atrial flutter with rapid conduction is certainly a potential cause of sudden death of those with extensive atrial surgery [1,2]. However, it is currently felt that ventricular tachycardia is the most important contributor. Clinicians have observed the frequent occurrence of premature ventricular contractions, nonsustained and sustained ventricular tachycardia in patients who have undergone complete repair of tetralogy of Fallot (and related defects such as double outlet right ventricle), and ventricular tachycardia has been implicated in the etiology of sudden death in this patient group. Indeed, it is known that postoperative tetralogy of Fallot is the single-most common condition seen in children between the ages of 1 and 16 years who have experienced sudden death [3], although the risk of sudden death is also elevated in aortic stenosis, coarctation, and transposition of the great vessels [4].

Anatomic and pathological considerations

By far the most information concerning patients with ventricular tachycardia and congenital heart disease pertains to tetralogy of Fallot, as compared to other forms of congenital heart disease. Ventricular arrhythmias occur much more rarely in patients with other lesions [5]. However, for the purposes of management, tetralogy of Fallot can be viewed as a model for other lesions, when patients with other lesions present with ventricular arrhythmias in the setting of ventriculotomy and/or ventricular dysfunction, especially of the anatomic right ventricle.

Controversy exists regarding the role of various risk factors for the occurrence of ventricular tachycardia and sudden death. The exact relationship between ventricular arrhythmias and sudden death is unknown, and the role of electrophysiologic study and other procedures for risk stratification is controversial. Ultimately there is little consensus regarding the appropriate management of postoperative patients with ventricular tachycardia. It is still relatively recently that major advances in understanding the role of antiarrhythmic agents and implantable cardioverter-defibrillators in patients with coronary disease have been made, based on the results of large multicenter trials [6]. One can understand the much greater challenge of answering similar questions in this much smaller patient population. Indeed, Bricker [7] has pointed out that sufficient numbers of operated patients may not be available to perform an adequately powered cohort study to sort out the various likely predictors of sudden death.

Ventricular Arrhythmias and Sudden Cardiac Death, 1st edition. Edited by P.J. Wang, A. Al-Ahmad, H. Hsia, and P.C. Zei. © 2008 Blackwell Publishing, ISBN: 978-1-4051-6114-5.

An extensive review of congenital heart disease anatomy and surgical techniques is beyond the scope of this chapter. However, we may consider the changes in surgical technique that have taken place over the years. Patient age, age at repair, and method of repair clearly interact to increase the risk of arrhythmias. The first complete repair of tetralogy of Fallot was performed in 1954 by Dr W.C. Lillehei, and starting in the 1960s, complete repair became quite common. While infants were corrected from the beginning, the mortality rate was high, and it was more common for patients to undergo repair later, often as late as the second or even third decade of life. Starting in the 1970s, due to improvements both in surgical techniques and postoperative care, many centers chose to perform primary repair in infancy, with good results, and this is the current practice at nearly all programs.

Unoperated patients with tetralogy of Fallot have a ventricular septal defect with some degree, usually severe, of right ventricular outflow tract obstruction, leading to chronic cyanosis. Initial placement of a systemic-to-pulmonary artery shunt as a palliative procedure adds the problem of potential left ventricular volume overload, which may lead to left ventricular dilation and dysfunction. Complete repair of the defect involves patch closure of the ventricular septal defect with relief of right ventricular obstruction. In nearly all patients, this requires resection of a large amount of right ventricular muscle, and early in the experience, this was not done through the tricuspid valve, but required a ventriculotomy. Finally, the pulmonary annulus is usually small, and repair with a simple transannular patch usually leads to chronic pulmonic insufficiency, which may be very severe, especially if it is associated with downstream obstruction due to significant pulmonary arterial narrowing. It seems likely that ventricular arrhythmias are caused by the effect of years of chronic cyanosis and hypertrophy, followed by the placement of a ventriculotomy, with increased right ventricular afterload and preload due to inadequate relief of obstruction and severe pulmonic regurgitation [8–10]. Such factors as wall stress and chronic cyanosis, coupled with the passage of time, may lead to myocardial fibrosis and right ventricular dysfunction, leading to the development of the substrate for reentrant ventricular arrhythmias. This hypothesis is supported by histologic studies of the hearts of patients with tetralogy of Fallot who died suddenly, which have shown such extensive fibrosis [11]. It is also supported by the observation that fractionated electrograms and mid-diastolic potentials may be recorded from the right ventricle at the electrophysiologic study, suggesting the presence of slow conduction [12]. While there is a 5% incidence of coronary artery abnormalities in tetralogy of Fallot, putting the left anterior descending coronary artery or other large branches at risk at the time of complete repair, such potential damage has not been considered to be an important factor in the etiology of ventricular arrhythmias or of sudden death.

Mechanism of ventricular tachycardia

Careful electrophysiologic studies in patients with clinically occurring ventricular tachycardia following surgery for tetralogy of Fallot have supported the concept that the mechanism of tachycardia is macroreentry, which involves the right ventricular outflow tract, either at the site of anterior right ventriculotomy or at the site of a ventricular septal defect patch. Transient entrainment can often be documented, with constant fusion at the paced cycle length and progressive fusion at decreasing cycle lengths, and the evaluation of postpacing intervals strongly suggests that sites in the right ventricular outflow tract are part of a macroreentrant circuit (Figure 12.1).

Anatomically, one may imagine several long circuits that might support macroreentry based on congenital and surgical anatomy, and there have been several circuits reported in postoperative patients with tetralogy of Fallot. While the simplest notion is a circuit that rotates around a right ventricular outflow tract (RVOT) patch, this is only possible if the patch does not extend all the way to the pulmonic annulus, as a transannular patch would. In my opinion, the best delineated proposed circuit was described by Horton et al. [13], who used pacing techniques to document the importance of the right ventricular isthmus between the tricuspid annulus and the right ventricular outflow tract patch. Notably, they did not map the entire circuit in their two patients, and so the rest of the circuit is not identified. Their patients both had

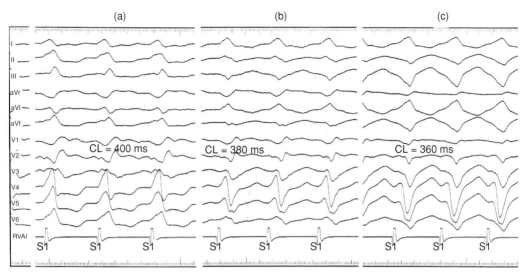

Figure 12.1 Tracings at electrophysiologic study of a 35-year-old man who was status post repair of tetralogy of Fallot at 11 years of age. Ventricular tachycardia was induced by ventricular extrastimulation, with a tachycardia cycle length of 435 milliseconds. Entrainment pacing is performed at (a) 400 milliseconds, (b) 380 milliseconds, and (c) 360 milliseconds. Note that there is progressive fusion at faster paced cycle lengths. CL, cycle length; ms, milliseconds. (From Zipes DP, Jalife J, eds. Cardiac Electrophysiology: From Cell to Bedside. 4th edition. Philadelphia: Saunders, p. 620, 2004, by permission.)

transannular patches, and so there was no possible isthmus between the RVOT patch and pulmonic valve annulus. It seems likely, therefore, that the circuit also involved the interventricular septum. Others, notably Downar et al. [14] have mapped ventricular tachycardia intraoperatively, and have found reentry involving the right ventricular outflow tract in all but only identified sites of earliest ventricular activation rather than the entire circuit. They noted early sites located in the septum, free wall, and parietal band.

Electrocardiographic and electrophysiologic features

By electrocardiogram, despite the fact that most patients with tetralogy of Fallot have macroreentry arising from RVOT, the QRS morphology is often not obviously indicative of this location. As described by Horton et al. [13], the QRS morphology of VT arising from the RVOT mainly depends on the direction of rotation (clockwise versus counterclockwise) around the circuit, which Horton et al. have described as involving the isthmus of tissue in the right ventricle between the tricuspid annulus

and RVOT patch (Figure 12.2). A clockwise rotation gives rise to a negative QRS in lead I and biphasic QRS in V1, whereas a counterclockwise rotation produces an upright QRS in lead I and an entirely negative QRS ("left bundle morphology") in V1.

There are no specific intracardiac electrogram features described in patients with congenital heart disease. Low amplitude and fractionated late potentials have been described, but it is uncertain whether these electrograms are involved in the substrate for VT. Still, Biblo and Carlson [15] used such mid-diastolic potentials to successfully ablate VT in a patient with tetralogy of Fallot in 1993. Stevenson et al. [16] as well as Rostock et al. [17] have emphasized the usefulness of voltage maps for delineating the tachycardia circuit in such patients (see below). Such voltage maps depend on the presence of low-amplitude signals in association with myocardial scarring or patch material as barriers which support macroreentry.

Entrainment pacing may be useful, initially to prove the macroreentrant nature of the tachycardia, prior to mapping of the circuit in the ventricle. Entrainment, of course, depends on the presence of an excitable gap, which might not exist in ventricular

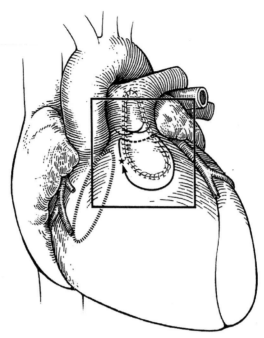

Figure 12.2 Right ventricle and right ventricular outflow tract with transannular patch across outflow tract and pulmonic valve. The location of the tricuspid valve annulus is shown with hatched markings. The proposed macroreentrant circuit (inset) for ventricular tachycardia involves clockwise activation between the patch and tricuspid annulus. The arrow demonstrates a hypothetical pathway for the remainder of the circuit. (From [13], with permission.)

tachycardias that are very rapid. Such rapid tachycardias may not be well tolerated hemodynamically.

Mapping and ablation

As most published evidences support the concept of macroreentry as the mechanism of postoperative ventricular tachycardia, the use of entrainment pacing and mapping techniques is desirable. Several investigators have reported successful procedures using radiofrequency energy [13,18,19]. Stevenson et al. [16] have reported the utility of voltage maps to identify areas of scar in the right ventricle.

While well-tolerated ventricular tachycardia can be mapping in the electrophysiology laboratory, many patients have ventricular dysfunction and/or rapid ventricular tachycardia rates, and will not tolerate this. Several investigators have reported intraoperative mapping and ablation [14,20–22]. In particular, Downar et al. [14] have used intraoperative mapping of the right ventricular outflow tract in the beating heart employing an endocardial electrode balloon and a simultaneous epicardial

electrode sock array. They performed ablation using cryotherapy lesions delivered during normothermic cardiopulmonary bypass with the heart beating, or during anoxic arrest, with success in three patients [14].

Electroanatomic mapping of the arrhythmia circuit may be feasible, when the tachycardia is inducible and is slow enough to be mapped completely. Using the CARTO system (Biosense Webster) or the Nav-X system (St Jude Medical) isochronal and propagation maps may be constructed. As with other arrhythmias, the process of construction of an electroanatomic map may be time consuming and difficult. An additional available modality provided by these systems, the ability to construct three-dimensional voltage maps to better identify the anatomic barriers. For example, Stevenson et al. [16] demonstrated the use of these modalities in the successful mapping and ablation of right ventricular reentrant tachycardia in an adult patient following repair of tetralogy of Fallot. They pointed out the usefulness of tagged ablation sites in constructing a broad line of block between the

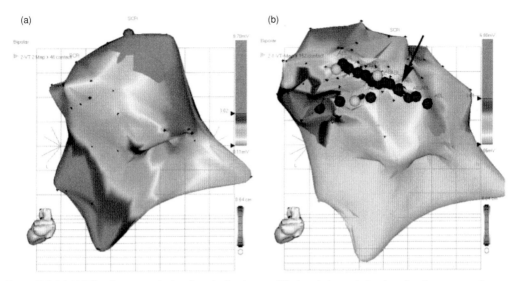

Figure 12.3 (a) CARTO voltage map during sinus rhythm in a modified posterior–anterior view showing an area of low-amplitude signals at the posterior wall of the right ventricular outflow tract confined to the presumed insertion of the homograft. (b) CARTO voltage map during ventricular tachycardia focused on the previously identified area of interest. A Y-shaped ablation line was produced crossing the border zone between the presumed scar region and normal amplitude myocardium. Target sites demonstrating perfect entrainment mapping are depicted by white spots. (From [17], with permission.)

ventriculotomy scar and the tricuspid annulus. Rostock et al. [17] reported a procedure in a 36-year-old patient following surgical repair of tetralogy of Fallot using a homograft conduit, who was mapped using similar methods. They used a combination of entrainment mapping and voltage maps constructed in sinus rhythm, using the CARTO system (Figure 12.3). They defined an area of scar by the recording of intracardiac electrogram amplitudes of less than 0.5 mV, and created a Y-shaped incision blocking conduction of impulses between the RVOT and the homograft.

Appropriate targets for ablation may be determined by relatively simple means, e.g., sites off early ventricular activation that precede surface QRS during tachycardia. Given the macroreentrant nature of these rhythms, however, it makes sense to consider the entire circuit and to focus on sites that are in the circuit by entrainment mapping techniques, and where barriers can be connected by a series of lesions with the effect of bridging the isthmus and creating bidirectional block. These techniques have been well developed in the ablation of typical atrial flutter as well as in the ablation of postsurgical intra-atrial reentrant tachycardia [23]. One of

the best demonstrations of these concepts is the report by Horton et al. [13] in which two patients were found to have ventricular tachycardia involving the isthmus between the RVOT patch and the tricuspid annulus (Figure 12.1). Important contribution made by this case report is the demonstration of a clear method for documenting isthmus block in both clockwise and counterclockwise directions. This capability, of course, allows for the use of a potentially better criterion for ablation success than noninducibility. Horton et al. demonstrated that with the creation of a line of block between the tricuspid annulus and RVOT patch is associated with a characteristic alteration in the paced QRS morphology, as well as a clear change in the order of ventricular activation with pacing from specific sites (Figures 12.4 and 12.5).

As ablation of ventricular tachycardia is, in fact, only rarely attempted in patients with congenital heart disease, each case must be approached in a comprehensive fashion. One starts with a detailed knowledge of the congenital heart anatomy, performing a careful review of the details of the surgical repair that was performed. All imaging studies available should be reviewed, such as echocardiography

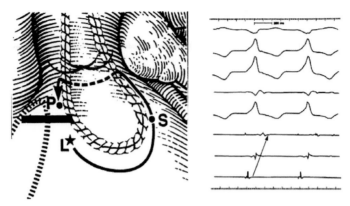

Figure 12.4 Location of the radiofrequency catheter ablation lesion (solid line), extending from the patch to the tricuspid valve annulus. This linear lesion results in bidirectional block and cure of the tachycardia. When pacing from the lateral (L) margin of the patch, there is clockwise block; activation moves counterclockwise around the patch to the septal (S) margin and finally to the pulmonic (P) margin. The surface electrograms (leads I, II, III, V1, and V6) and local electrograms are shown. (From [13], with permission.)

and angiography, as these studies may provide more information concerning the underlying anatomy. If sustained ventricular tachycardia is inducible and is sufficiently well tolerated, then entrainment should be performed in an attempt to make a diagnosis of a macroreentrant tachycardia. Should the tachycardia be stable, entrainment mapping would then be performed, searching for sites where postpacing interval is equivalent to tachycardia cycle length, indicating that such sites are in the macroreentrant circuit. In any case, electroanatomic mapping is an important adjunct, particularly with the use of voltage mapping to identify the scars and other important anatomic details. Lesions may be planned to connect surgical scars and/or anatomic barriers. It is important that a complete line of block is created. One

can also consider documentation of the completed line of block by the use of repeat electroanatomic mapping, or by the recording of double potentials throughout the entire zone.

It is, of course, by no means certain that the successful ablation of a ventricular tachycardia circuit in a patient with congenital heart disease will in any way decrease or eliminate the risk of sudden death, and so many patients will be appropriate candidates of implantation of implantable cardioverter-defibrillators, most prominently those with strong risk factors for sudden death such as severe right ventricular dilation and dysfunction and pulmonic insufficiency.

The potential for irrigated-tip or cooled-tip RF ablation to penetrate the myocardium more deeply

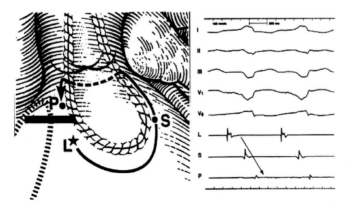

Figure 12.5 Same patient as in Figure 12.4. When pacing from the pulmonic (P) margin on the other side of the lesion, there is counterclockwise block; activation proceeds in a clockwise direction to the septal (S) and the lateral (L) margins. Local electrograms demonstrate this sequence of activation (straight arrows). The bidirectional block is distinct from the normal bidirectional conduction and clockwise ventricular tachycardia seen prior to ablation. (From [13], with permission.)

Table 12.1 Reported ablations in patients with tetralogy of Fallot or other congenital heart disease

Author, year	Method	# procedures	Initial success
Oda et al., 1986 [28]	DC	1	0/1
Burton and Leon, 1993 [29]	RF	2	2/2
Goldner et al., 1994 [30]	RF	1	1/1
Biblo and Carlson, 1994 [15]	RF	1	1/1
Chinushi et al., 1995 [31]	RF	1	1/1
Gonska et al., 1996 [18]	RF	16	15/16
Horton et al., 1997 [13]	RF	2	2/2
Papagiannis et al., 1998 [19]	RF	1	2/2
Stevenson et al., 1998 [16]	RF/CARTO	1	1/1
Saul and Alexander, 1999 [32]	RF	2	2/2
Fukuhara et al., 2000 [33]	RF	1	1/1
Arenal et al., 2003 [34]	RF/CARTO	1	1/1
Rojel et al., 2003 [35]	RF	2	2/2
Morwood et al., 2004 [24]	RF	12	10/12
Rostock et al., 2004 [17]	RF/CARTO	1	1/1
Furushima et al., 2006 [36]	RF	7	4/7
Total reported procedures		45	46/53 (87%)

is clearly a potential advantage when working in the right ventricle, which may well be thick due to the chronic pressure overload and pulmonic insufficiency which often exists in such patients. Furthermore, as Morwood et al. [24] have noted, occasionally the tachycardia circuit involved regions remarkably close to the site where one records the His bundle potential. In such a situation, one might imagine the utility of cryoablation, in which "ice-mapping" lesions are possible, avoiding inadvertent complete A-V block.

Ablation results

Most reports of ablation of ventricular tachycardia in patients with congenital heart disease are single-center reports that involve one or two procedures. A list of ablations reported in patients with tetralogy of Fallot or other congenital heart disease is presented in Table 12.1. This includes one case of 1986, in which DC ablation was attempted, as well as a number of other cases done using RF energy. As can be seen in this table, most procedures are reported as successful. The total success rate, 87%, derived from these reports should be treated with a great deal of suspicion, however. Centers that succeed in ablating this substrate are potentially more

likely to report their results than would be centers who have failed, and this "reporting bias" has the potential to skew the impression of expected results.

Somewhat more useful are reports of multiple cases from a single center, in which a large time-frame is used, and patients are included consecutively. Morwood et al. [24] recently reported the experience at the Children's Hospital in Boston with ablation for ventricular tachycardia in young patients. They reported that of 97 consecutive ablation procedures for VT over 13 years, 20 were in patients with congenital heart disease. In eight of these, mapping and/or ablation was considered not feasible due to tachycardia noninducibility, tachycardia rate, hemodynamic instability, or location close to the His bundle, and ablation was attempted in the other 12, succeeding acutely in 10 (80%). Four of these had recurred at last follow-up (40%).

Another source for data concerning ablations in the pediatric population is the Pediatric Radiofrequency Ablation Registry. Pediatric electrophysiologists at nearly 50 centers have reported their initial results to the Registry since 1991 [25–27]. An analysis of data from both the early and the late registry experience has led to the finding of a total of 74 procedures in patients with congenital heart disease in which ablation of VT was attempted (A. Blaufox, personal communication). Of these, 50/74 (68%) mapped to an anatomic right ventricle, while 24/74 (32%) mapped to a left ventricle. The initial success rate for these ablation attempts was only 47/74 or 64%. In general, the rate of complications of RF ablation for ventricular tachycardia in congenital heart disease patients is similar to those reported for other substrates.

Conclusions

Ablation of ventricular tachycardia is not always feasible, due to the potential for hemodynamic instability during mapping, and most likely will not allow a patient to avoid the implantation of an implantable cardioverter-defibrillator, if significant risk factors are present. For patients in whom the procedure is feasible, current results are encouraging, but the high failure rate of ablation procedures, coupled with the high recurrence risk, need to be remembered. The population of patients at risk for such arrhythmias is growing, however, with recent improvements in surgical techniques leading to increased survival to adulthood of patients with congenital heart disease. Therefore, it is likely that the problem of postoperative ventricular tachycardia is not disappearing; rather it will continue to grow. A great deal of additional work needs to be done to improve on current results.

References

1 Harrison DA, Siu SC, Hussain F, MacLoghlin CJ, Webb GD, Harris L. Sustained atrial arrhythmias in adults late after repair of tetralogy of Fallot. Am J Cardiol 2001;87:584–588.

2 Li W, Somerville J. Atrial flutter in grown-up congenital heart (GUCH) patients. Clinical characteristics of affected population. Int J Cardiol 2000;75:129–137 (discussion 138–139).

3 Garson A Jr, McNamara DG. Sudden death in a pediatric cardiology population, 1958 to 1983: relation to prior arrhythmias. J Am Coll Cardiol 1985;5:134B–137B.

4 Silka MJ, Hardy BG, Menashe VD, Morris CD. A population-based prospective evaluation of risk of sudden cardiac death after operation for common congenital heart defects. J Am Coll Cardiol 1998;32:245–251.

5 Vetter VL, Horowitz LN. Electrophysiologic residua and sequelae of surgery for congenital heart defects. Am J Cardiol 1982;50:588–604.

6 Antiarrhythmics versus Implantable Defibrillators (AVID) Investigators. A comparison of antiarrhythmic-drug therapy with implantable defibrillators in patients resuscitated from near-fatal ventricular arrhythmias. N Engl J Med 1997;337:1576–1583.

7 Bricker JT. Sudden death and tetralogy of Fallot. Risks, markers, and causes. Circulation 1995;92:158–159.

8 Zahka KG, Horneffer PJ, Rowe SA, et al. Long-term valvular function after total repair of tetralogy of Fallot. Relation to ventricular arrhythmias. Circulation 1988;78:III14–III19.

9 Gatzoulis MA, Till JA, Somerville J, Redington AN. Mechanoelectrical interaction in tetralogy of Fallot. QRS prolongation relates to right ventricular size and predicts malignant ventricular arrhythmias and sudden death. Circulation 1995;92:231–237.

10 Gatzoulis MA, Till JA, Redington AN. Depolarization-repolarization inhomogeneity after repair of tetralogy of Fallot. The substrate for malignant ventricular tachycardia? Circulation 1997;95:401–404.

11 Deanfield JE, Ho SY, Anderson RH, McKenna WJ, Allwork SP, Hallidie-Smith KA. Late sudden death after repair of tetralogy of Fallot: a clinicopathologic study. Circulation 1983;67:626–631.

12 Zimmermann M, Friedli B, Adamec R, Oberhansli I. Ventricular late potentials and induced ventricular arrhythmias after surgical repair of tetralogy of Fallot. Am J Cardiol 1991;67:873–878.

13 Horton RP, Canby RC, Kessler DJ, et al. Ablation of ventricular tachycardia associated with tetralogy of Fallot: demonstration of bidirectional block. J Cardiovasc Electrophysiol 1997;8:432–435.

14 Downar E, Harris L, Kimber S, et al. Ventricular tachycardia after surgical repair of tetralogy of Fallot: results of intraoperative mapping studies. J Am Coll Cardiol 1992;20:648–655.

15 Biblo LA, Carlson MD. Transcatheter radiofrequency ablation of ventricular tachycardia following surgical correction of tetralogy of Fallot. Pacing Clin Electrophysiol 1994;17:1556–1560.

16 Stevenson WG, Delacretaz E, Friedman PL, Ellison KE. Identification and ablation of macroreentrant ventricular tachycardia with the CARTO electroanatomical mapping system. Pacing Clin Electrophysiol 1998;21:1448–1456.

17 Rostock T, Willems S, Ventura R, Weiss C, Risius T, Meinertz T. Radiofrequency catheter ablation of a macroreentrant ventricular tachycardia late after surgical repair of tetralogy of Fallot using the electroanatomic mapping (CARTO). Pacing Clin Electrophysiol 2004;27:801–804.

18 Gonska BD, Cao K, Raab J, Eigster G, Kreuzer H. Radiofrequency catheter ablation of right ventricular tachycardia late after repair of congenital heart defects. Circulation 1996;94:1902–1908.

19 Papagiannis J, Kanter RJ, Wharton JM. Radiofrequency catheter ablation of multiple haemodynamically unstable ventricular tachycardias in a patient with surgically repaired tetralogy of Fallot. Cardiol Young 1998;8:379–382.

20 Ressia L, Graffigna A, Salerno-Uriarte JA, Vigano M. The complex origin of ventricular tachycardia after the total correction of tetralogy of Fallot. G Ital Cardiol 1993;23:905–910.

21 Frank G, Schmid C, Baumgart D, Lowes D, Klein H, Kallfelz HC. Surgical therapy of life-threatening tachycardic cardiac arrhythmias in children. Monatsschr Kinderheilkd 1989;137:269–274.

22 Lawrie GM, Pacifico A, Kaushik R. Results of direct surgical ablation of ventricular tachycardia not due to ischemic heart disease. Ann Surg 1989;209:716–727.

23 Kalman JM, VanHare GF, Olgin JE, Saxon LA, Stark SI, Lesh MD. Ablation of 'incisional' reentrant atrial tachycardia complicating surgery for congenital heart disease. Use of entrainment to define a critical isthmus of conduction. Circulation 1996;93:502–512.

24 Morwood JG, Triedman JK, Berul CI, et al. Radiofrequency catheter ablation of ventricular tachycardia in children and young adults with congenital heart disease. Heart Rhythm 2004;1:301–308.

25 Kugler JD, Danford DA, Deal BJ, et al. Radiofrequency catheter ablation for tachyarrhythmias in children and adolescents. The Pediatric Electrophysiology Society. N Engl J Med 1994;330:1481–1487.

26 Van Hare GF, Carmelli D, Smith WM, et al. Prospective assessment after pediatric cardiac ablation: design and implementation of the multicenter study. Pacing Clin Electrophysiol 2002;25:332–341.

27 Van Hare GF, Javitz H, Carmelli D, et al. Prospective assessment after pediatric cardiac ablation: demographics, medical profiles, and initial outcomes. J Cardiovasc Electrophysiol 2004;15:759–770.

28 Oda H, Aizawa Y, Murata M, et al. A successful electrical ablation of recurrent sustained ventricular tachycardia in a postoperative case of tetralogy of Fallot. Jpn Heart J 1986;27:421–428.

29 Burton ME, Leon AR. Radiofrequency catheter ablation of right ventricular outflow tract tachycardia late after complete repair of tetralogy of Fallot using the pace mapping technique. Pacing Clin Electrophysiol 1993;16:2319–2325.

30 Goldner BG, Cooper R, Blau W, Cohen TJ. Radiofrequency catheter ablation as a primary therapy for treatment of ventricular tachycardia in a patient after repair of tetralogy of Fallot. Pacing Clin Electrophysiol 1994;17:1441–1446.

31 Chinushi M, Aizawa Y, Kitazawa H, Kusano Y, Washizuka T, Shibata A. Successful radiofrequency catheter ablation for macroreentrant ventricular tachycardias in a patient with tetralogy of Fallot after corrective surgery. Pacing Clin Electrophysiol 1995;18:1713–1716.

32 Saul JP, Alexander ME. Preventing sudden death after repair of tetralogy of Fallot: complex therapy for complex patients. J Cardiovasc Electrophysiol 1999;10:1271–1287.

33 Fukuhara H, Nakamura Y, Tasato H, Tanihira Y, Baba K, Nakata Y. Successful radiofrequency catheter ablation of left ventricular tachycardia following surgical correction of tetralogy of Fallot. Pacing Clin Electrophysiol 2000;23:1442–1445.

34 Arenal A, Glez-Torrecilla E, Ortiz M, et al. Ablation of electrograms with an isolated, delayed component as treatment of unmappable monomorphic ventricular tachycardias in patients with structural heart disease. J Am Coll Cardiol 2003;41:81–92.

35 Rojel U, Cuesta A, Mont L, Brugada J. Radiofrequency ablation of late ventricular tachycardia in patients with corrected Tetralogy of Fallot. Arch Cardiol Mex 2003;73:275–279.

36 Furushima H, Chinushi M, Sugiura H, et al. Ventricular tachycardia late after repair of congenital heart disease: efficacy of combination therapy with radiofrequency catheter ablation and class III antiarrhythmic agents and long-term outcome. J Electrocardiol 2006;39:219–224.

CHAPTER 13

Role of imaging techniques in catheter ablation of ventricular tachycardia

Mathew D. Hutchinson, & David J. Callans

Introduction

The ablation of ventricular tachycardia has changed fundamentally over the past decade, due in large part to advances in medical and invasive therapies for ischemic heart disease. Catheter ablation is increasingly utilized in a variety of different arrhythmia substrates, often with nonreentrant mechanisms. Even in the setting of reentrant, postinfarct VT, detailed entrainment, and characterization of circuits is often not possible due to: noninducibility at the time of EP study, induction of multiple VT morphologies, or induction of hemodynamically untolerated VT [1]. Thus, successfully targeting modern VT often requires some component of substrate-based ablation [2–4]. Improvements in imaging technology have greatly facilitated this process.

In this chapter, we discuss the utility of specific imaging modalities in catheter ablation of VT. Specifically, we concentrate on the following imaging applications:

- Characterizing arrhythmia substrate
- Guiding lesion formation
- Monitoring for complications

Ventricular Arrhythmias and Sudden Cardiac Death, 1st edition. Edited by P.J. Wang, A. Al-Ahmad, H. Hsia, and P.C. Zei © 2008 Blackwell Publishing, ISBN: 978-1-4051-6114-5.

Characterization of arrhythmia substrate

VT in the setting of left ventricular dysfunction or prior myocardial infarction

Electrocardiogram

The utility of the 12-lead electrocardiogram in identifying the presence and location of previous myocardial infarction is well established [5–8]. Moreover, the site of origin of endocardial, postinfarction VT (or exit site from a reentrant circuit) is readily identified by analysis of the 12-lead electrocardiogram [9]. Algorithms for predicting epicardial sites of origin in idiopathic cardiomyopathy are also available [10–12].

An advantage of the electrocardiogram is its flexibility and reproducibility within a patient, allowing the physician to plan an ablation strategy preoperatively. Assessments can also be made online in the EP lab, allowing the physician to rapidly target the area of interest. Inherent limitations in accurately predicting tachycardia site of origin include: extent and distribution of myocardial scar (e.g., multiple sites of infarction; endocardial and epicardial scar), body habitus, and orientation of the heart with respect to the chest wall.

2D echocardiography

Standard two-dimensional echocardiography provides invaluable information in preparing for VT ablation. It can provide excellent, reproducible assessment of scar burden and location, chronicity

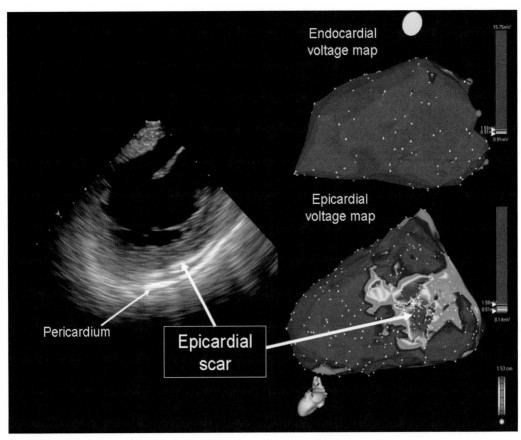

Figure 13.1 Images obtained during ablation of a 48-year-old man with idiopathic cardiomyopathy and repetitive, monomorphic VT. The left panel is an oblique, long-axis view of the lateral wall of the left ventricle obtained with intracardiac echo, which demonstrates a region of hyperintensity involving the epicardial surface of the LV. The corresponding endocardial (top right) voltage map is normal but the epicardial map (bottom right) reveals an area of low voltage that corresponds to the abnormality seen on ICE.

of infarction, and biventricular function [13–15]. It can identify valvular dysfunction and previous valve surgery that necessitate modification of the ablation procedure (e.g., using a trans-septal approach in the setting of a stenotic or prosthetic aortic valve, or an epicardial approach in the setting of prosthetic valves in the aortic and mitral positions). The non-invasive assessment of left atrial and pulmonary arterial pressures, as well as evaluation of biventricular function have important implications in predicting hemodynamic compromise during arrhythmia induction. Technical factors such as inadequate chest wall views and poor tissue resolution limit the utility of standard chest wall echocardiography within the EP lab.

Intracardiac echocardiography

We routinely utilize intracardiac echocardiography (ICE) during complex endocardial or epicardial ablation procedures, both for enhanced characterization of substrate and for monitoring for complications. We have found this extremely useful when performing epicardial ablation with an externally irrigated catheter to assess for fluid accumulation in the pericardial space. We have also frequently noted heterogeneity in the distribution of scar within the myocardium on ICE that was not apparent on a chest wall echo. Early recognition of midmyocardial or epicardial scar allows the physician to move more rapidly either to an irrigated-tip ablation catheter or to an epicardial approach (Figure 13.1).

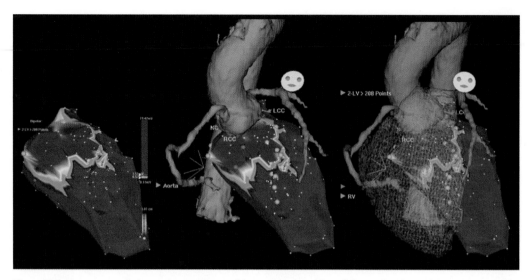

Figure 13.2 Electroanatomical maps from a 50-year-old man with idiopathic cardiomyopathy and repetitive, monomorphic VT. The left panel demonstrates a well-circumscribed LV endocardial scar in front of the aortic valve. In the center panel, the endocardial map has been registered with a previously obtained CT reconstruction of the aortic valve and thoracic aorta using the CARTO Merge™ software. In the right panel, a right ventricular reconstruction has been added. We find this technique extremely valuable in clarifying complex anatomical relationships to facilitate ablation procedures.

Both animal and human studies have demonstrated correlation between regional LV dysfunction as seen on ICE and a reduction in bipolar voltage as measured with electroanatomical mapping [16]. One center also reported intrapericardial ICE views during epicardial ablation, obtaining views complementary to chest wall imaging with higher tissue resolution [17]. In our experience, most operators can rapidly become proficient in obtaining the required views. Limitations of ICE include its cost and requirement of intravascular access. Intrapericardial ICE incurs the risk of pericardial access, and necessitates a double-wire technique if concomitant epicardial ablation is performed.

Electroanatomical mapping

A variety of three-dimensional mapping systems have been developed, all of which permit the assessment of myocardial voltage and local activation time [18–31]. These systems have proven valuable both in defining cardiac anatomy and in providing insight into arrhythmia mechanisms. These mapping systems are flexible and adaptable to either endocardial or epicardial procedures. Such parameters as chamber dimensions and, more recently, surface area of regions of interest can be easily calculated with the CARTO system. In our experience, the ability to collect simultaneous bipolar voltage and local activation time with CARTO provides more flexibility in mapping VT.

We frequently use the CARTO Merge software in our VT cases as it provides valuable anatomical information related to the arrhythmia substrate [32,33]. (Figure 13.2) Accurate registration of the segmented image does require some practice, and the preferred regions vary with the chamber of interest. Fahmy and colleagues [34] have recently demonstrated that tagging posterior pulmonary vein sites with ICE guidance produced less registration error than utilizing anterior sites such as the LAA.

It is well established that the exit sites for VT can be identified from the 12-lead ECG. The anatomy of reentrant circuits has been best characterized historically by the response to entrainment maneuvers [35–40]. Varying bipolar voltage ranges with the CARTO system to elucidate endocardial conduction channels within dense scar is also valuable [41] (Figure 13.3).

Novel applications of noncontact mapping are in development to further investigate the role that channels of apparent preferential conduction play

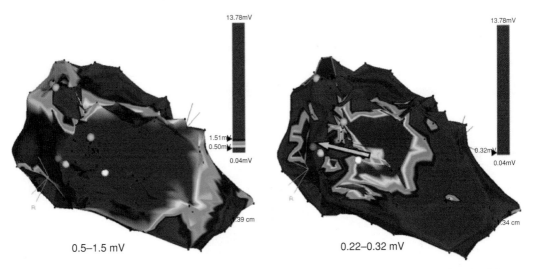

0.5–1.5 mV   0.22–0.32 mV

Figure 13.3 Electroanatomical maps from a patient with recurrent VT in the setting of prior anteroseptal myocardial infarction. By varying the color range from the standard 0.5–1.5 mV to 0.22–0.32 mV, an endocardial channel of relatively preserved voltage is defined. Defining such channels can be useful in substrate-based ablation of ventricular tachycardia. (Courtesy of Henry H. Hsia, MD.)

in the VT circuit. Jacobson and co-workers [42] identified channels that mediate conduction into and out of the infarct substrate using isopotential mapping in a porcine model. These same channels appeared to serve as entrance and exit sites during induced VT. If confirmed in human VT, this observation may allow empiric ablation without the need for VT induction.

Computed tomography

As previously stated, three-dimensional reconstructions of CT images can be useful in procedural planning as well as enhancing the anatomical detail when creating electroanatomical maps. Bello et al. [43] described correlating a preoperative, high-resolution CT with electroanatomical mapping in a patient with unmappable VT. The authors concluded utilizing such preoperative information could facilitate ablation procedures by reducing procedure time and fluoroscopy exposure.

Using previously acquired imaging studies in ablation procedures does incur some limitations. Given dynamic changes in thoracic anatomy (intracardiac, esophageal, etc.), previously acquired images may not fully represent the true anatomical relationships at the time of ablation. Furthermore,

image processing and registration can present significant obstacles to rendering accurate geometries. The development of intraoperative, rotational angiography may provide added fluidity and accuracy to the mapping process. The recent publication by Orlov and colleagues [44] demonstrated comparable image quality between intraoperative rotational angiography and previously acquired CT images for left atrial and esophageal structure, and also noted improved definition of esophageal location when the procedure was combined with intraoperative esophagogram [44]. By modifying the contrast injection procedure to optimize ventricular opacification, rotational angiography may provide an excellent adjunctive imaging modality in VT ablation procedures (Figure 13.4).

VT in the setting of right ventricular cardiomyopathy

Electrocardiogram

The electrocardiographic features of arrhythmogenic right ventricular cardiomyopathy (ARVC) were originally described by Marcus et al. [45] more than 20 years ago and were systematically assessed recently by Nasir and colleagues [46]. Common features of ARVC include: T wave inversions and QRS duration >110 milliseconds in the right precordial

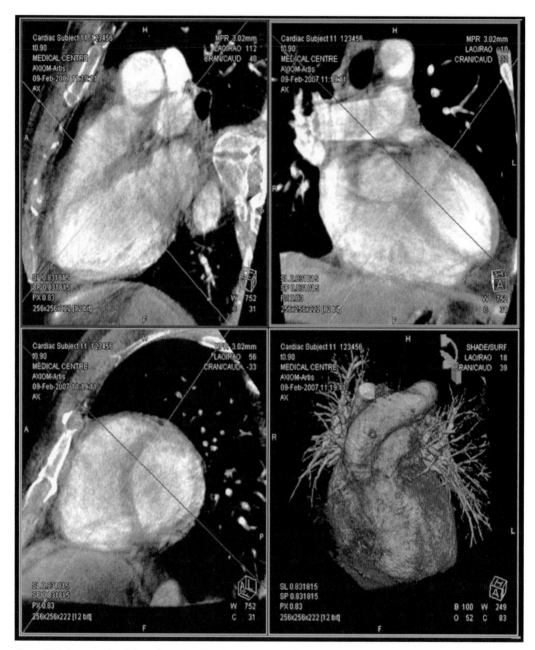

Figure 13.4 An example of three-dimensional cardiac reconstruction (bottom right) obtained with gated rotational angiography. Two-dimensional slices are shown in the RAO cranial (top left), AP cranial (top right), and LAO caudal (bottom left) projections. Courtesy of Amin Al-Ahmad, MD, and Rebecca Fahrig, PhD, Stanford University.

leads, prolonged S wave upstroke (>55 ms) in the absence of RBBB, and epsilon waves. Prolonged S wave upstroke has been found to correlate with inducibility of VT in this cohort.

Electroanatomical mapping

In our experience, patients with RVCM presenting with VT frequently exhibit perivalvular fibrosis [3]. The fibrosis extends for a variable distance apically

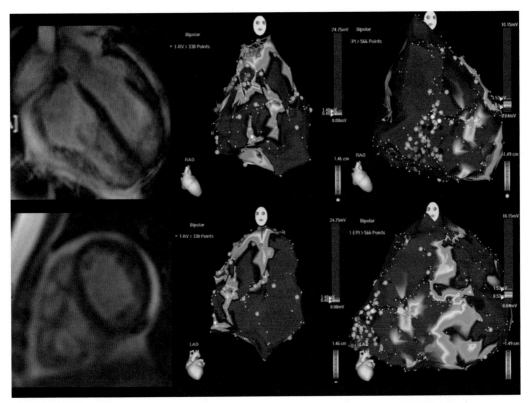

Figure 13.5 Images obtained from a 17-year-old patient with right ventricular cardiomyopathy presenting with recurrent syncope due to ventricular tachycardia. The left upper and lower panels are MR images demonstrating significant RV dilation and hypertrabeculation. There is a perfusion abnormality of the RV free wall and wall motion abnormalities on gated images consistent with the diagnosis of right ventricular cardiomyopathy. The middle upper and lower panels show his endocardial voltage maps in the RAO and LAO projections. There is characteristic low voltage around the tricuspid valve, extending along the RV free wall to the RV outflow tract; the septum is spared. The right upper and lower panels show epicardial voltage maps in the RAO and LAO projections. There is extensive low voltage encompassing the entire surface of the RV with frequent late and fractionated potentials observed (pink dots).

from the tricuspid annulus and superiorly toward the free wall of the outflow tract with relative sparing of the septum. There is also frequently epicardial fibrosis of a variable extent corresponding to the affected endocardial regions, which in many cases exceeds the extent of endocardial scar. Given the ominous portent of ventricular arrhythmias in these young patients, we tend to manage them aggressively with a combination of device implantation and ablation therapy.

Patients often present with recurrent palpitations and syncope, and have multiple VT morphologies induced at the time of EP study. Many tachycardias demonstrate reentrant circuits near the tricuspid valve and are amenable to entrainment mapping

and ablation. Others require a substrate-based ablation strategy that utilizes pace-mapping or activation mapping. In patients referred for EP study, we routinely perform detailed electroanatomical mapping of the RV (>300 points) and sometimes the LV (if LV function is compromised or right bundle tachycardias are present) (Figure 13.5). We are able to achieve long-term arrhythmia suppression after ablation therapy in the vast majority of these patients, though some require additional procedures.

MRI

The utility of MRI as a diagnostic criterion for RVCM is well established [47–51]. The presence of wall thinning, delayed enhancement in affected regions, and wall motion abnormalities on gated images are commonly seen in these patients. We have used MRI reconstructions with the CARTO Merge system in selected patients referred for ablation. Although the anatomical detail is quite good, we have found that this strategy, adds little incremental benefit in facilitating the procedure.

ICE

We do not routinely use ICE during endocardial RVCM ablations; however, we have used ICE in cases that required epicardial mapping. In addition to facilitating pericardial access and monitoring for complications, we are able to detect RV wall motion abnormalities and scar, which correlate with low bipolar voltage areas. Ensuring adequate lesion creation in the basal RV can be challenging due to difficult catheter positioning and motion of the tricuspid annulus, and we have utilized ICE to ensure appropriate tissue contact in some cases.

VT in the setting of congenital heart disease

Electroanatomical mapping

The complex intracardiac anatomy in patients with adult congenital heart disease (ACHD) presents a unique challenge in arrhythmia therapy. Prior operative reports and preprocedural imaging with either MR or CT are critically important in planning an ablation strategy. The most common ventricular arrhythmia in ACHD patients is VT in the setting of surgically corrected Tetralogy of Fallot (TOF). TOF patients typically present with macroreentrant VT involving the infundibular patch and to a lesser extent the VSD patch [52–57].

ICE

ICE can be a valuable adjunct to electroanatomical mapping in defining arrhythmia substrate. In surgically corrected TOF patients with infundibular resection or VSD repairs, the location and extent of the patches can often be visualized with ICE. As postoperative changes and artifact often limit detailed assessment of native or prosthetic valvular function with standard transthoracic echo views in these patients, we find ICE valuable as a diagnostic tool in some cases (Figure 13.6).

Guiding lesion formation

Successful VT ablation requires the elimination of tissue critical to the maintenance of the tachycardia. Inherent in this process is the identification of these critical elements and achieving the required tissue destruction. The endpoint of noninducibility of VT is a useful but indirect method of assessing procedural success.

The paradigm of real-time assessment of lesion creation is not possible with our current tools. Inadequate lesion depth and size clearly result in diminished procedure success. The most common reasons for inadequate lesion creation include poor tissue contact with the ablation catheter and inadequate power delivery due to resistive heating at the tissue interface (especially with nonirrigated catheters).

Assuring adequate contact with the ablation catheter can be challenging for all operators, and our traditional tools for assessing contact with fluoroscopy and electroanatomical mapping systems can be misleading. In the left ventricle, there is continuous movement of the endocardium relative to the ablation catheter. This often provides a false sense of adequate contact via the mapping system since the catheter impacts the same location with each cardiac cycle; however, it is not continuously opposed to the endocardial surface. We frequently observe this phenomenon using ICE. With experience, it is possible to reliably image the tip of the ablation catheter with ICE. Figure 13.7 demonstrates a case in which ICE provided valuable information regarding tissue contact and catheter tip location in a patient with an inferobasilar LV aneurysm. Accurately defining the aneurysm cavity with fluoroscopy alone proved challenging in this case; however, we were able to easily define the border of the aneurysm with ICE.

The image quality varies and is often inadequate to visualize individual ablation lesions, especially when imaging from an adjacent chamber. This limitation was explored in an elegant study by Khoury and colleagues [58]. Endocardial lesion geometry was imaged using ICE after coronary arterial microbubble injection in dogs. The depth and diameter of the lesions as measured with ICE after microbubble injection correlated well with pathology (Figure 13.8). Lesion characterization in patients with structural heart disease remains untested.

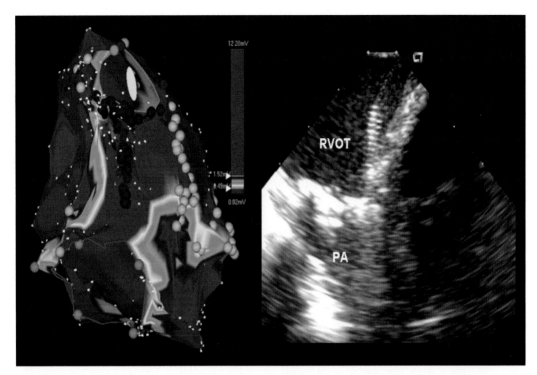

Figure 13.6 Images obtained during ablation in a 38-year-old man with surgically corrected Tetralogy of Fallot presenting with repetitive, monomorphic VT. The electroanatomical map on the left is oriented in a right posterior superior view and demonstrates extensive low voltage involving the superior RV septum and septal RVOT corresponding to the surgical patch of the ventricular septal defect. The gray dots correspond to a line of double potentials along the posterior extent of the infundibular patch. The patient's tachycardia was macroreentrant, involving the septal RVOT at the level of the pulmonic valve. The large low-voltage area in the RVOT creates uncertainty in defining the orientation of the pulmonic valve. Intracardiac echo provided excellent views of both the pulmonic valve and the surgical patch, which facilitated creating an accurate electroanatomical map. The right panel is an ICE image from that procedure which shows the ablation catheter at the level of the pulmonic valve.

We have also utilized ICE during ablation in the LV outflow tract and coronary cusps. We can easily visualize the location of the ablation catheter tip relative to the aortic valve and coronary vessels both in short axis and long axis, thus avoiding inadvertent injury to critical structures and obviating the need for coronary angiography (Figure 13.9).

Monitoring for complications during VT ablation

Pericardial effusion

ICE

The development of a pericardial effusion during ablation can lead to rapid hemodynamic compromise and morbidity. The diagnosis is often delayed until significant fluid accumulation compromises left ventricular filling. The concomitant administration of intravenous heparin during left ventricular ablation can increase bleeding in the setting of an otherwise modest cardiac perforation. Arrhythmia induction and administration of sedative and analgesic agents can reduce systemic blood pressure and confound the diagnosis of pericardial effusion. Given that our average patient undergoing VT ablation is increasingly older and has multiple comorbidities, we find that using ICE fortifies our clinical assessment of patients during ablation procedures.

Using multiple imaging places, the operator can easily scan the entire epicardial surface to detect even small, loculated effusions. We most commonly image the ventricles from the inferior right ventricular outflow tract. Scanning the probe in a clockwise

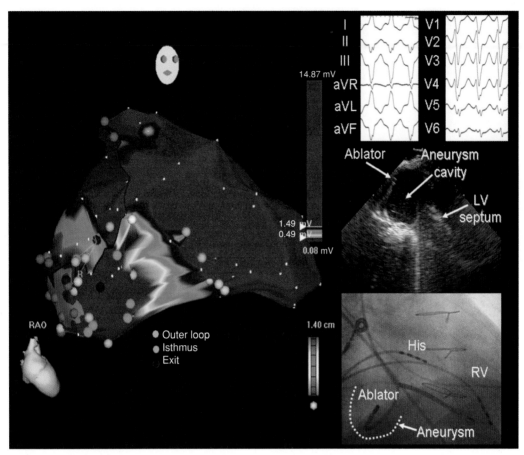

Figure 13.7 Images obtained during ablation in a 70-year-old man with ischemic cardiomyopathy and a posterobasilar LV aneurysm presenting with incessant ventricular tachycardia. The left panel is an electroanatomical bipolar voltage map showing the aneurysm as well as components of the arrhythmia circuit assessed with entrainment mapping. The top right panel is the clinical VT morphology. Given the complex topography of the border of the aneurysm cavity and the normal myocardium, we found it difficult to assess both location and degree of contact of the ablation catheter with respect to the myocardium. We found ICE very useful in localizing the tip of the ablation catheter throughout the aneurysm. The middle right panel is an ICE image from the case showing the tip of the ablation catheter at the superior septal border of the aneurysm. The lower right panel is a corresponding fluoroscopic image in the RAO projection.

direction after passing through the tricuspid valve gives excellent views of the entire epicardial space. We often leave the imaging probe in the right ventricle for the duration of the procedure to facilitate detection of fluid (Figure 13.10).

The increasing utilization of epicardial mapping provides another useful application of ICE in guiding percutaneous pericardial access. We can reliably image the apical septum with ICE and visualize the guidewire and epicardial sheath as they enter the epicardial space (Figure 13.11). This technique is especially useful in the setting of intrapericardial adhesions, when fluoroscopic localization of the guidewire is difficult. Inadvertent introduction of the Touhy needle or guidewire into the right ventricle is also readily seen with ICE.

Intracardiac thrombus

ICE

Our group has previously reported the utility of ICE in demonstrating catheter-associated thrombus during pulmonary vein isolation. The incidence of clinically manifest thromboembolic complications

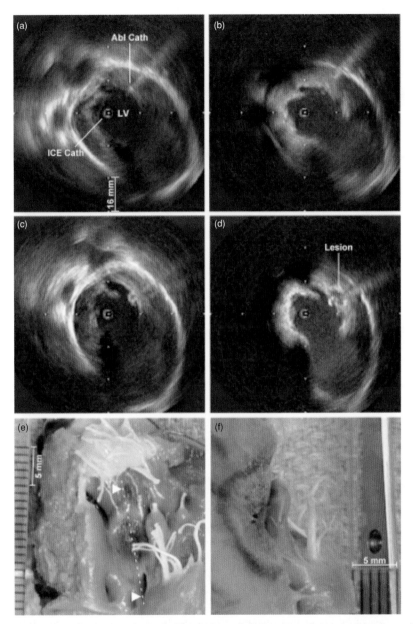

Figure 13.8 (a) Baseline images of the LV obtained with a 9-MHz radial ICE catheter demonstrating a 4-mm ablation catheter along the lateral LV. (b) Baseline images obtained during intracoronary injection of microbubbles. (c) Image obtained after application of radiofrequency lesion in lateral LV. (d) Image obtained after application of radiofrequency lesion in lateral LV with intracoronary microbubble injection. (e) Endocardial pathologic view of ablation lesion. (f) Cross-sectional pathologic view of ablation lesion. Reprinted with permission from [58].

during VT ablation is as high as 2.7% [59]. The high incidence of embolism despite anticoagulation is likely related to the significant endothelial disruption that occurs with irrigated ablation catheters. The true incidence of intracardiac thrombus during VT ablation is not known; presumably, many occur that are not clinically relevant. Although unproven, it is reasonable to expect that early detection

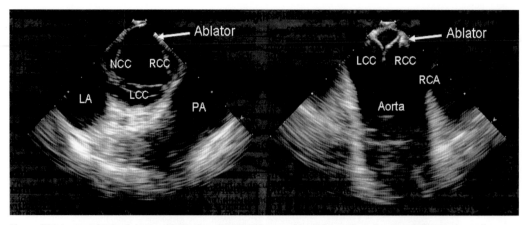

Figure 13.9 Images obtained during ablation in a 47-year-old man with mild systolic dysfunction felt to be due to frequent premature ventricular contractions. The site of origin of the clinical PVC was localized to the right coronary cusp. We use intracardiac echo to facilitate mapping the coronary cusps as well as to localize the tip of the ablation catheter relative to the coronary ostium. The left panel is a short-axis ICE view showing the tip of the ablation catheter in the right coronary cusp. The right panel shows a longitudinal view of the aortic root clearly localizing the catheter tip against the cusp.

of catheter-associated thrombosis with ICE during VT ablation procedures may prevent clinical events.

Ventricular function

ICE
Transient, regional LV dysfunction of previously normal myocardium adjacent to RF lesions frequently occurs during VT ablation, and is easily demonstrable with ICE. Acute increases in wall thickness at the site of RF can also be seen with ICE, and are helpful in verifying tissue injury with RF [60].

We have noted rare cases of global left ventricular systolic dysfunction or pulseless electrical activity following conversion of ventricular arrhythmias. In

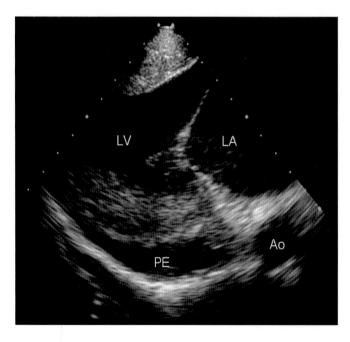

Figure 13.10 Intracardiac echo image obtained during ablation in a 52-year-old man with hypertrophic cardiomyopathy and multiple episodes of VT. He underwent a combined endocardial and epicardial ablation approach. He was known to have a chronic pericardial effusion, and ICE imaging confirmed a moderate sized, loculated posterolateral fluid collection. The fluid collection was drained when epicardial access was obtained during the case. ICE is very useful for detecting even trace amounts of pericardial fluid which may develop during ablation procedures, and allows rapid intervention before hemodynamic compromise occurs.

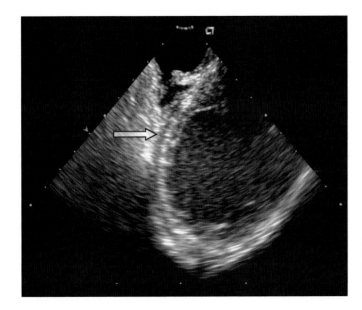

Figure 13.11 Intracardiac echo image obtained during percutaneous pericardial access. The arrow points to the apical septum, which is the preferred site of entry.

circumstances when invasive blood pressure monitoring is not available, significant delay may occur before this diagnosis is made. ICE allows both the rapid assessment of impaired ventricular function and its differentiation from pericardial tamponade.

References

1 Callans DJ, Zado E, Sarter BH, Schwartzman D, Gottlieb CD, Marchlinski FE. Efficacy of radiofrequency catheter ablation for ventricular tachycardia in healed myocardial infarction. Am J Cardiol 1998;82(4):429–432.

2 Hsia HH, Marchlinski FE. Characterization of the electroanatomic substrate for monomorphic ventricular tachycardia in patients with nonischemic cardiomyopathy. Pacing Clin Electrophysiol 2002;25(7):1114–1127.

3 Marchlinski FE, Zado E, Dixit S, et al. Electroanatomic substrate and outcome of catheter ablative therapy for ventricular tachycardia in setting of right ventricular cardiomyopathy. Circulation 2004;110(16):2293–2298.

4 Hsia HH, Lin D, Sauer WH, Callans DJ, Marchlinski FE. Anatomic characterization of endocardial substrate for hemodynamically stable reentrant ventricular tachycardia: identification of endocardial conducting channels. Heart Rhythm 2006;3(5):503–512.

5 Pope JE, Wagner NB, Dubow D, Edmonds JH, Wagner GS, Haisty WK Jr. Development and validation of an automated method of the Selvester QRS scoring system for myocardial infarct size. Am J Cardiol 1988;61(10):734–738.

6 Fuchs RM, Achuff SC, Grunwald L, Yin FC, Griffith LS. Electrocardiographic localization of coronary artery narrowing: studies during myocardial ischemia and infarction with one-vessel disease. Circulation. 1982;66(6):1168–1176.

7 Wagner GS. Clinical usefulness of quantitative ECG methods for evaluating ischemic and infarcted myocardium. Cardiol Clin 1987;5(3):447–454.

8 De Sutter J, Van de Wiele C, Gheeraert P, et al. The Selvester 32-point QRS score for evaluation of myocardial infarct size after primary coronary angioplasty. Am J Cardiol 1999;83(2):255–257.

9 Miller JM, Marchlinski FE, Buxton AE, Josephson ME. Relationship between the 12-lead electrocardiogram during ventricular tachycardia and endocardial site of origin in patients with coronary artery disease. Circulation 1988;77(4):759–766.

10 Daniels DV, Lu YY, Morton JB, et al. Idiopathic epicardial left ventricular tachycardia originating remote from the sinus of Valsalva: electrophysiological characteristics, catheter ablation, and identification from the 12-lead electrocardiogram. Circulation 2006;113(13):1659–1666.

11 Berruezo A, Mont L, Nava S, Chueca E, Bartholomay E, Brugada J. Electrocardiographic recognition of the epicardial origin of ventricular tachycardias. Circulation 2004;109(15):1842–1847.

12 Bazan V, Bala R, Garcia FC, et al. Twelve-lead ECG features to identify ventricular tachycardia arising from the epicardial right ventricle. Heart Rhythm 2006;3(10):1132–1139.

13 Lindvall K, Hamsten A, Landou C, Szamosi A, de Faire U. Comparative study of echo- and angiocardiographically determined regional left ventricular wall motion in recent myocardial infarction. Eur Heart J 1984;5(7):533–544.

14 Presti CF, Gentile R, Armstrong WF, Ryan T, Dillon JC, Feigenbaum H. Improvement in regional wall motion after percutaneous transluminal coronary

angioplasty during acute myocardial infarction: utility of two-dimensional echocardiography. Am Heart J 1988;115(6):1149–1155.

15 Senior R, Sridhara BS, Basu S, et al. Comparison of radionuclide ventriculography and 2D echocardiography for the measurement of left ventricular ejection fraction following acute myocardial infarction. Eur Heart J 1994;15(9):1235–1239.

16 Callans DJ, Ren JF, Michele J, Marchlinski FE, Dillon SM. Electroanatomic left ventricular mapping in the porcine model of healed anterior myocardial infarction. Correlation with intracardiac echocardiography and pathological analysis. Circulation 1999;100(16):1744–1750.

17 Horowitz BN, Vaseghi M, Mahajan A, et al. Percutaneous intrapericardial echocardiography during catheter ablation: a feasibility study. Heart Rhythm 2006;3(11):1275–1282.

18 Marchlinski F, Callans D, Gottlieb C, Rodriguez E, Coyne R, Kleinman D. Magnetic electroanatomical mapping for ablation of focal atrial tachycardias. Pacing Clin Electrophysiol 1998;21(8):1621–1635.

19 Stevenson WG, Delacretaz E, Friedman PL, Ellison KE. Identification and ablation of macroreentrant ventricular tachycardia with the CARTO electroanatomical mapping system. Pacing Clin Electrophysiol 1998;21(7):1448–1456.

20 Nademanee K, Kosar EM. A nonfluoroscopic catheter-based mapping technique to ablate focal ventricular tachycardia. Pacing Clin Electrophysiol 1998;21(7):1442–1447.

21 Nakagawa H, Jackman WM. Use of a three-dimensional, nonfluoroscopic mapping system for catheter ablation of typical atrial flutter. Pacing Clin Electrophysiol 1998;21(6):1279–1286.

22 Gepstein L, Evans SJ. Electroanatomical mapping of the heart: basic concepts and implications for the treatment of cardiac arrhythmias. Pacing Clin Electrophysiol 1998;21(6):1268–1278.

23 Krum D, Goel A, Hauck J, et al. Catheter location, tracking, cardiac chamber geometry creation, and ablation using cutaneous patches. J Interv Card Electrophysiol 2005;12(1):17–22.

24 Gnoatto M, Abello M, Merino JL. Ablation guided by digital anatomic reconstruction (NavX). Rev Esp Cardiol 2004;57(12):1233.

25 Ventura R, Rostock T, Klemm HU, et al. Catheter ablation of common-type atrial flutter guided by three-dimensional right atrial geometry reconstruction and catheter tracking using cutaneous patches: a randomized prospective study. J Cardiovasc Electrophysiol 2004;15(10):1157–1161.

26 Yue AM, Paisey JR, Robinson S, Betts TR, Roberts PR, Morgan JM. Determination of human ventricular repolarization by noncontact mapping: validation with monophasic action potential recordings. Circulation 2004;110(11):1343–1350.

27 Thiagalingam A, Wallace EM, Boyd AC, et al. Noncontact mapping of the left ventricle: insights from validation with

transmural contact mapping. Pacing Clin Electrophysiol 2004;27(5):570–578.

28 Okishige K, Kawabata M, Umayahara S, et al. Radiofrequency catheter ablation of various kinds of arrhythmias guided by virtual electrograms using a noncontact, computerized mapping system. Circ J 2003;67(5):455–460.

29 Schneider MA, Schmitt C. Non-contact mapping: a simultaneous spatial detection in the diagnosis of arrhythmias. Z Kardiol 2000;89(Suppl 3):177–185.

30 Yue AM, Franz MR, Roberts PR, Morgan JM. Global endocardial electrical restitution in human right and left ventricles determined by noncontact mapping. J Am Coll Cardiol 2005;46(6):1067–1075.

31 Thiagalingam A, Wallace EM, Campbell CR, et al. Value of noncontact mapping for identifying left ventricular scar in an ovine model. Circulation 2004;110(20):3175–3180.

32 Dong J, Dickfeld T, Dalal D, et al. Initial experience in the use of integrated electroanatomic mapping with three-dimensional MR/CT images to guide catheter ablation of atrial fibrillation. J Cardiovasc Electrophysiol 2006;17(5):459–466.

33 Tops LF, Bax JJ, Zeppenfeld K, et al. Fusion of multislice computed tomography imaging with three-dimensional electroanatomic mapping to guide radiofrequency catheter ablation procedures. Heart Rhythm 2005;2(10):1076–1081.

34 Fahmy TS, Mlcochova H, Wazni OM, et al. Intracardiac echo-guided image integration: optimizing strategies for registration. J Cardiovasc Electrophysiol 2007;18(3):276–282.

35 Anderson KP, Swerdlow CD, Mason JW. Entrainment of ventricular tachycardia. Am J Cardiol 1984;53(2):335–340.

36 MacLean WA, Plumb VJ, Waldo AL. Transient entrainment and interruption of ventricular tachycardia. Pacing Clin Electrophysiol 1981;4(4):358–366.

37 Almendral JM, Gottlieb CD, Rosenthal ME, et al. Entrainment of ventricular tachycardia: explanation for surface electrocardiographic phenomena by analysis of electrograms recorded within the tachycardia circuit. Circulation 1988;77(3):569–580.

38 Stevenson WG, Khan H, Sager P, et al. Identification of reentry circuit sites during catheter mapping and radiofrequency ablation of ventricular tachycardia late after myocardial infarction. Circulation 1993;88(4 Pt 1):1647–1670.

39 Callans DJ, Hook BG, Josephson ME. Comparison of resetting and entrainment of uniform sustained ventricular tachycardia. Further insights into the characteristics of the excitable gap. Circulation 1993;87(4):1229–1238.

40 Morady F, Kadish A, Rosenheck S, et al. Concealed entrainment as a guide for catheter ablation of ventricular tachycardia in patients with prior myocardial infarction. J Am Coll Cardiol 1991;17(3):678–689.

41 Arenal A, del Castillo S, Gonzalez-Torrecilla E, et al. Tachycardia-related channel in the scar tissue in patients

with sustained monomorphic ventricular tachycardias: influence of the voltage scar definition. Circulation 2004; 110(17):2568–2574.

42 Jacobson JT, Afonso VX, Eisenman G, et al. Characterization of the infarct substrate and ventricular tachycardia circuits with noncontact unipolar mapping in a porcine model of myocardial infarction. Heart Rhythm 2006;3(2):189–197.

43 Bello D, Kipper S, Valderrabano M, Shivkumar K. Catheter ablation of ventricular tachycardia guided by contrast-enhanced cardiac computed tomography. Heart Rhythm 2004;1(4):490–492.

44 Orlov MV, Hoffmeister P, Chaudhry GM, et al. Three-dimensional rotational angiography of the left atrium and esophagus – A virtual computed tomography scan in the electrophysiology lab? Heart Rhythm 2007;4(1):37–43.

45 Marcus FI, Fontaine GH, Guiraudon G, et al. Right ventricular dysplasia: a report of 24 adult cases. Circulation 1982;65(2):384–398.

46 Nasir K, Bomma C, Tandri H, et al. Electrocardiographic features of arrhythmogenic right ventricular dysplasia/cardiomyopathy according to disease severity: a need to broaden diagnostic criteria. Circulation 2004;110(12):1527–1534.

47 Wolf JE, Rose-Pittet L, Page E, et al. Detection of parietal lesions using magnetic resonance imaging in arrhythmogenic dysplasia of the right ventricle. Arch Mal Coeur Vaiss 1989;82(10):1711–1717.

48 Tandri H, Castillo E, Ferrari VA, et al. Magnetic resonance imaging of arrhythmogenic right ventricular dysplasia: sensitivity, specificity, and observer variability of fat detection versus functional analysis of the right ventricle. J Am Coll Cardiol 2006;48(11):2277–2284.

49 Tandri H, Saranathan M, Rodriguez ER, et al. Noninvasive detection of myocardial fibrosis in arrhythmogenic right ventricular cardiomyopathy using delayed-enhancement magnetic resonance imaging. J Am Coll Cardiol 2005;45(1):98–103.

50 Bomma C, Rutberg J, Tandri H, et al. Misdiagnosis of arrhythmogenic right ventricular dysplasia/cardiomyopathy. J Cardiovasc Electrophysiol 2004; 15(3):300–306.

51 Tandri H, Calkins H, Nasir K, et al. Magnetic resonance imaging findings in patients meeting task force criteria for arrhythmogenic right ventricular dysplasia. J Cardiovasc Electrophysiol 2003;14(5):476–482.

52 Rostock T, Willems S, Ventura R, Weiss C, Risius T, Meinertz T. Radiofrequency catheter ablation of a macroreentrant ventricular tachycardia late after surgical repair of tetralogy of Fallot using the electroanatomic mapping (CARTO). Pacing Clin Electrophysiol 2004;27(6 Pt 1):801–804.

53 Rojel U, Cuesta A, Mont L, Brugada J. Radiofrequency ablation of late ventricular tachycardia in patients with corrected Tetralogy of Fallot. Arch Cardiol Mex 2003;73(4):275–279.

54 Hebe J. Role of catheter and surgical ablation in congenital heart disease. Cardiol Clin 2002;20(3):469–486.

55 Chinushi M, Aizawa Y, Kitazawa H, Takahashi K, Washizuka T, Shibata A. Clockwise and counter-clockwise circulation of wavefronts around an anatomical obstacle as one mechanism of two morphologies of sustained ventricular tachycardia in patients after a corrective operation of tetralogy of Fallot. Pacing Clin Electrophysiol 1997;20(9 Pt 1):2279–2281.

56 Horton RP, Canby RC, Kessler DJ, et al. Ablation of ventricular tachycardia associated with tetralogy of Fallot: demonstration of bidirectional block. J Cardiovasc Electrophysiol 1997;8(4):432–435.

57 Stevenson WG, Delacretaz E, Friedman PL, Ellison KE. Identification and ablation of macroreentrant ventricular tachycardia with the CARTO electroanatomical mapping system. Pacing Clin Electrophysiol 1998;21(7): 1448–1456.

58 Khoury DS, Rao L, Ding C, et al. Localizing and quantifying ablation lesions in the left ventricle by myocardial contrast echocardiography. J Cardiovasc Electrophysiol 2004;15(9):1078–1087.

59 Calkins H, Epstein A, Packer D, et al. Catheter ablation of ventricular tachycardia in patients with structural heart disease using cooled radiofrequency energy: results of a prospective multicenter study. Cooled RF Multi Center Investigators Group. J Am Coll Cardiol 2000;35(7):1905–1914.

60 Callans DJ, Ren JF, Narula N, Michele J, Marchlinski FE, Dillon SM. Effects of linear, irrigated-tip radiofrequency ablation in porcine healed anterior infarction. J Cardiovasc Electrophysiol 2001;12(9):1037–1042.

CHAPTER 14

Epicardial ablation of ventricular tachycardia

Mauricio Scanavacca, & Eduardo Sosa

Introduction

Electrophysiologists have shown interest increasingly in improving the results of ventricular tachycardia (VT) catheter ablation as use of this therapy has increased over the last several years. This has led to the incorporation of many new strategies in such procedures. Mapping the epicardial surface of the ventricles is now feasible in the electrophysiologic laboratory. Depending on the VT presentation and the patient clinical characteristics, epicardial mapping and ablation can be performed in addition to endocardial mapping by using currently available systems. The aim of this chapter is to review the role of epicardial mapping and ablation to treat patients with VT.

Subepicardial fibers as substrate for ventricular tachycardia

Ischemic ventricular tachycardia

Most ventricular macroreentrant circuits occurring in the setting of structural heart diseases are related to the arrangement of the surviving myocites within dense ventricular scars [1,2] (Figure 14.1). In ischemic heart disease, left ventricular subendocardial reentry has been the paradigm for treatment of VT using RF ablation. However, sometimes, critical fibers of the VT circuit can be located in the subepicardial layer. In these cases, it is not unusual that VT cannot be terminated by delivering RF pulses

from the endocardial surface, even if deep lesions are generated using an irrigated tip electrode.

The role of subepicardial fibers as substrate for VT reentry was investigated in post-MI patients submitted to epicardial mapping during surgical VT procedures. Littmann et al. [3] prospectively evaluated the functional role of the epicardium in 10 post-MI patients undergoing intraoperative mapping. They described three global activation VT patterns based on computed electrical activation obtained by an epicardial multielectrode array: figure-eight activation in five; circular macroreentry in three, and monoregional spread in two. Epicardial photocoagulation terminated five of the five figure-eight VT, two of three circular macroreentry but not the focal activation pattern VTs, which probably reflected epicardial breakthroughs of reentry substrate originating from subendocardial layers. Kaltenbrunner et al. [4] studied, simultaneously, the role of subendocardial and subepicardial fibers with soft epicardial shock and transatrial left ventricular endocardial balloon electrode arrays in 28 patients with chronic myocardial infarction (inferior, 14 patients; anteroseptal, 14 patients). Epicardial and left ventricular endocardial isochronal maps of 47 induced VTs were constructed and the mapping characteristics of the tachycardias suggested five types of activation patterns: (1) complete subendocardial reentry circuits in seven VTs (15%); (2) complete subepicardial reentry circuits in four VTs (9%); (3) incompletely mapped circuits with a left ventricular endocardial breakthrough preceding the epicardial breakthrough in 25 VTs (53%); (4) incompletely mapped circuits with a left ventricular epicardial breakthrough preceding the endocardial breakthrough in three VTs (6%); and (5) a right

Ventricular Arrhythmias and Sudden Cardiac Death, 1st edition. Edited by P.J. Wang, A. Al-Ahmad, H. Hsia, and P.C. Zei © 2008 Blackwell Publishing, ISBN: 978-1-4051-6114-5.

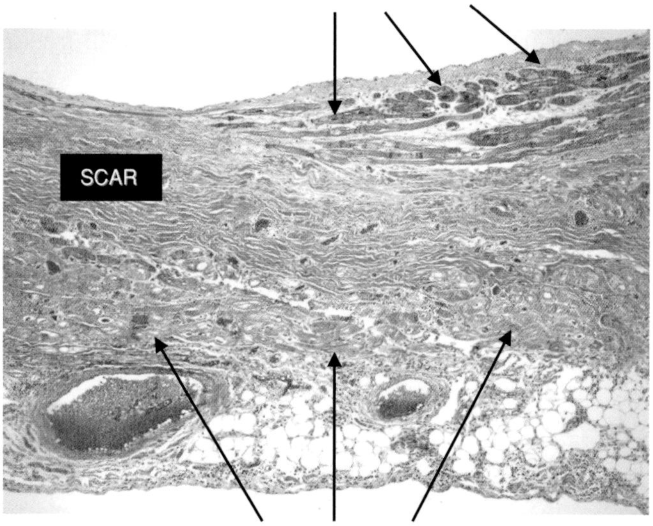

Subendocardial myocardial fibers

SCAR

Figure 14.1 Histopathological examination showing an intramural scar in dilated cardiomyopathy. Note that scar split subendocardial and subepicardial fibers that run in parallel propitiating anatomic conditions for reentry. Masson trichrome stain.

Subepicardial myocardial fibers

ventricular epicardial breakthrough preceding the left ventricular endocardial breakthrough and suggesting deep septal reentry in eight VTs (17%). All patients had at least one of 68 VTs mapped from the endocardium, 25% of patients had also one subepicardial reentry substrate, and 25% sustained VT related with deep septal reentry. Thus, simultaneous epicardial and endocardial mapping showed that most of the substrate for reentry in post-MI VT patients is related to subendocardial myocardial fibers, but in substantial number of patients (25%) VT had a left ventricle epicardial substrate that required specific intervention. Svenson et al. [5] also confirmed that the critical anatomic substrates supporting reentry in post-MI VT might occur at epicardial sites, particularly in patients with right or circumflex coronary artery-related infarction. They performed electrical activation-guided laser photocoagulation intraoperatively to terminate 85 VTs in 30 patients with ischemic heart disease. Seventy-two (84.7%) VTs were terminated by endocardial photocoagulation and, 13 (15.3%) required epicardial photocoagulation. However, these 13 VTs occurred in 10 (33%) of the 30 patients. An interesting observation was that aneurysms were present in 70% of patients with successful endocardial ablation, but in only 10% of patients requiring epicardial ablation. They also observed that epicardial activation data

were similar to those described for VT with an endocardial origin including delayed potentials during sinus rhythm and presystolic or mid-diastolic activation sequences during VT.

More recently, percutaneous epicardial catheter instrumentation in the electrophysiologic laboratory has been performed by electrophysiologists to explore the subepicardial fibers as potential site of VT origin. Sosa et al. [6] performed epicardial and endocardial mapping in 14 patients with VT with an inferior wall myocardial infarction and found electrophysiologic evidence of an epicardial circuit in seven (23%) of 30 sustained VT and four (28%) of 14 patients. Schweikert et al. [7] studied seven patients with post-MI sustained VT after unsuccessful endocardial ablation referred to percutaneous epicardial mapping. The procedure was performed with a nonfluoroscopic electroanatomic system and in six of the seven VTs, the essential part of the reentry circuit was identified on the epicardial surface of the heart. In five of these six VTs, the epicardial sites showed mid-diastolic potentials never seen endocardially. Brugada et al. [8] performed epicardial RF ablation in 10 patients (eight ischemic VT; mean ejection fraction of 0.28 ± 0.1) with incessant VT and eight with failed endocardial ablation. The epicardial ablation effectively terminated the incessant tachycardia in eight patients.

Substrate mapping is a useful strategy to perform RF ablation in patients with unstable VT and involves electroanatomic delineation of channels of surviving myocites in scarred tissue during sinus rhythm. Reddy et al. [9] studied the epicardial extension of healed anterior wall myocardial infarction in a porcine model by using electroanatomic mapping in 13 animals. The area of epicardial scar defined by abnormal bipolar voltage correlated well with the dimensions measured on pathological examination. Radiofrequency lesions created along the endocardial and epicardial scar borders based on the electroanatomic map also presented a good correlation comparing electroanatomic mapping and pathological examination. Cesario et al. [10] combined epicardial and endocardial electroanatomic high-density voltage maps to delineate the myocardial substrate for recurrent ischemic VT in 12 patients. Catheter ablation was performed on the endocardium in all patients; additional epicardial lesions were required in five (40%) patients for successful ablation. Soejima and Stevenson [11] also observed that although successful VT ablation in ischemic VT patients can be obtained by endocardial approach in most patients, epicardial mapping and ablation are needed in selected patients.

Nonischemic ventricular tachycardias

VT mechanism data are more limited in patients with non-ischemic VT. In Chagas disease, a frequent cause of VT in South American countries, epicardial reentry circuits can be frequently found during epicardial mapping and ablation. In those patients, most of the sites of origin are located in the left ventricle basal wall including inferior, posterior, or lateral wall that frequently simulates an inferior or lateral myocardial infarction. Sosa and Scanavacca [12] estimated that in 40% of patients some part of the reentry circuit could be mapped by the epicardial approach obviating the need for endocardial mapping in some patients. Figure 14.2 shows a typical case that can exemplify the potential use of the epicardial approach for VT mapping and ablation in such patients. Figure 14.2(b) shows a section of a patient's heart with Chagas disease and complicated by recurrent sustained VT. The patient was submitted to VT RF catheter ablation before undergoing cardiac transplantation. In this transverse section, we can see the location where an epicardial RF pulse

terminated VT. In this case, there was just a thin intramural scar layer along the anterior-lateral wall of the left ventricle. This scar probably created a line of block isolating a thin layer of subepicardial myocardial fibers. Also note that, there were some gaps in this linear scar that probably propitiated conditions for the reentrant circuit organization. Note that on contrary of ischemic cardiomyopathy where thin myocardial fibers take part in the reentry substrate interspersed through the dense myocardial scar, in this case there was a thin intramural scar that split subendocardial and subepicardial layers propitiating condition for macroreentrant circuits through the holes along the intramural scar. It is important to have in mind how difficult and extensive endocardial lesion delivery would be in order to destroy such epicardial fibers. Figure 14.2(a) shows the epicardial electrogram obtained during sustained VT and Figure 14.2(c) the sustained VT interruption in 6.0 seconds.

Soejima et al. [13] investigated the occurrence, locations, and relationship of VT to low-voltage areas in dilated cardiomyopathy in 28 patients with endocardial (26 patients) and epicardial (eight patients) electroanatomic mapping. They reported that the VT mechanism was caused by focal activation in five, bundle-branch reentry in two, and myocardial reentry in 22 patients (both focal and reentry VTs in one patient). All 20 patients with myocardial reentry had endocardial and/or epicardial (seven patients mapped) scar. Most (63%) endocardial scars were close to the mitral valve annulus. Of the 19 VT circuit isthmuses identified, 12 were associated with a subendocardial scar and seven with a subepicardial scar. Endocardial ablation was effective in six (27%) of 22 patients. Epicardial mapping and ablation led to success in 6 of 10 previously unsuccessful patients, indicating that simultaneous endocardial and epicardial mapping might increase the success rate in this population. They also observed that VT in dilated cardiomyopathy is often the result of intramyocardial reentry associated with scar, often adjacent to a valve annulus, deep in the ventricular wall, and can be greater in extent on the epicardium than on the endocardium. Those data are consistent with the anatomical and pathologic findings, which show that the longitudinal striae of midwall ventricles in patients with dilated cardiomyopathy are clearly different from the

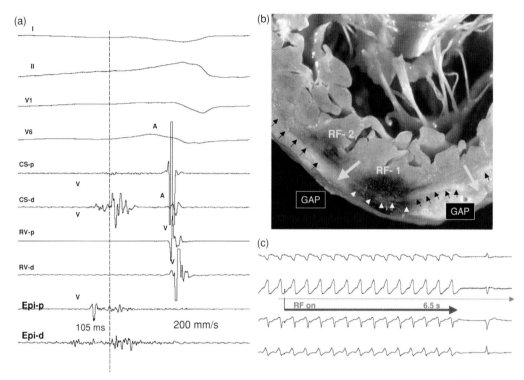

Figure 14.2 This picture shows the pathological and electrophysiological characteristics of a patient with Chagas' heart disease complicated with recurrent sustained ventricular tachycardia (VT). The patient was submitted to VT radiofrequency catheter ablation before undergoing cardiac transplantation. (a) Electrograms obtained on the epicardial surface of the heart where an RF pulse interrupted the sustained VT in 6 seconds (c). (b) macroscopic view of sustained VT site of origin. The small arrows indicate a thin intramural scar that split subendocardial and subepicardial fibers. Note, there are some gaps along the scar that could be involved in the macroreentry circuit. CS: coronary sinus; RV: right ventricle; Epi-p and Epi-d: proximal and distal epicardial electrograms recorded by, respectively, proximal and distal epicardial bipolar electrodes. This figure has been modified from d'Ávila A, Scanavacca M, and Sosa E. Transthoracic epicardial catheter ablation of ventricular tachycardia. Heart Rhythm. 2006;9:1110–1111.

distribution in patients with coronary artery disease who present transmural or predominant endocardial scars. Using MRI with gadolinium injection and late enhancement imaging, the presence, location, and extension of the scars in the human ventricles can be investigated [14]. In 59% of the patients with dilated cardiomyopathy, no scars were visualized using this method. Thirteen percent of patients had subendocardial scars, indistinguishable from that of post-MI. Twenty-eight percent of patients presented with different scar findings when compared to the post-MI patients: there were some patients with intramyocardial localized scars; others with multifocal intramural scars of a patchy pattern and, finally, some presented with long and thin intramural scars, as described previously in this chapter. It is possible that obtaining these MRI images before VT mapping and ablation may be useful for planning the procedure in patients with dilated cardiomyopathy.

Ouyang et al. [15] studied four patients with exercise-induced fast VT with right bundle branch block morphology. ECG showed a small q wave in leads II, III, and aVF during sinus rhythm (SR). Left ventricular angiography showed small inferior-lateral aneurysms in all patients, but with coronary normal arteriogram. Six unstable VTs (cycle length 200–305 ms) and one stable VT (cycle length 370 ms) were reproducibly induced in the four patients. In these patients, during sinus rhythm endocardial mapping, no scar was found. However, epicardial mapping showed fragmented and late potentials in the left inferior-lateral wall. During tachycardia, epicardial mapping showed a macroreentrant VT with focal endocardial activation in the patient with stable VT, whereas in two patients with unstable VT, a diastolic potential was recorded and coincided with the late potential in the same area. This observation suggests that patients with exercise-induced VT with right bundle branch block morphology, left ventricle aneurism, and normal coronary arteriograms may have a subepicardial arrhythmogenic substrate, which may be amenable to epicardial ablation. Another interesting observation was reported by Swarup et al. [16] of successful epicardial mapping and ablation of a patient with idiopathic dilated cardiomyopathy, with two morphologies of recurrent sustained VT originating from the left ventricle, resulting in multiple ICD shocks, and a previously unsuccessful endocardial ablation attempt. Evidence of myocardial scar was limited to the epicardium. Electroanatomic and entrainment mapping defined a figure-of-eight macroreentrant circuit within the epicardial scar. In this case, the VT terminated with radiofrequency application in the central isthmus of the circuit.

Idiopathic ventricular tachycardias

Despite the high success rate of catheter ablation for treatment of idiopathic outflow VT, in a minority of patients, the VT cannot be ablated from the right or left ventricular endocardium or from the aortic cusps, suggesting an epicardial site of origin [17]. Schweikert et al. [7] performed VT epicardial mapping in 20 patients with normal heart and unsuccessful endocardial ablation. In seven patients, the earliest activation time was in the aortic cusps and successful ablation was obtained in those places. But in 11 patients, the earliest activation time was obtained along the main coronary vessels and ablation was successfully performed by the epicardial approach in nine patients; in two patients, the site of origin was under the left atrial appendage and the high impedance in those places precluded RF delivery. Daniels et al. [18] reported 12 patients with idiopathic VT referred for ablation with epicardial left ventricular site of origin identified remote (more than 10 mm) from the aortic cusps. Endocardial ablation was unsuccessful in all 10 patients in whom it was attempted, despite the use of a large-tip or irrigated-tip catheter. Coronary venous

mapping demonstrated that epicardial activation preceded endocardial activation. Ablation through the coronary veins or via percutaneous pericardial approach was successful in nine patients. The initial approach was transvenous in six patients and was successful in five. In the remaining six patients, a percutaneous pericardial approach was used as the initial procedure and after unsuccessful transvenous ablation in one patient. The site of earliest epicardial activation was recorded within 5 mm of the site of earliest venous activation in all seven patients, suggesting a perivascular site of origin. Two patients were referred to epicardial surgical cryoablation as a result of unsuccessful catheter ablation and refractoriness to antiarrhythmic drugs. Such patients had a thick layer of epicardial fat over the site of earliest activation adjacent to the anterior interventricular vein during surgical exploration. Tanner et al. [19] reported five of 33 patients with idiopathic outflow tract tachycardia not amenable to ablation from the left or right ventricular endocardium or the aortic cusps. Three patients underwent successful ablation via a coronary venous approach and two by a percutaneous pericardial approach. Obel et al. [20] also described the successful ablation of idiopathic epicardial outflow VT from within the distal great cardiac vein in five patients who had unsuccessful ablation from endocardial and epicardial sites, including the aortic valve cusps, and in one patient via percutaneous pericardial approach. In all patients, ablation (cryothermal in three, RF in two patients) in the great cardiac vein successfully interrupted the VT without any immediate or long-term complications, confirming the previous observations that the distal great cardiac vein and its branches need to be explored in some patients to successfully ablate idiopathic epicardial outflow VT.

Identification of patients for epicardial mapping and ablation

The 12-lead ECG obtained during spontaneous or induced VT may suggest an epicardial VT origin. Berruezo et al. [21] identified three ECG findings in patients with structural heart disease, important left ventricle dysfunction, and sustained VT with RBBB morphology: (1) a pseudo-delta wave >34 milliseconds (sensitivity 83%, specificity 95%);

(2) an intrinsicoid deflection time >85 milliseconds (sensitivity 87%, specificity 90%); and (3) RS complex duration of $\geq$121 milliseconds (sensitivity 76%, specificity 85%). These findings can be useful in the decision to proceed with epicardial mapping as a first procedure in patients with these clinical and ECG characteristics.

Daniels et al. [18] compared the EKG pattern of idiopathic VT originating from the perivascular sites on the left ventricular epicardium to other locations. They observed that no ECG pattern was specific for epicardial VT recognition; however, a prolonged precordial maximum deflection index (MDI) and early use of transvenous epicardial mapping may be critical to avoiding unsuccessful ablation elsewhere in the ventricles. The precordial MDI (0.61) was significantly longer in patients with epicardial idiopathic left VT relative to other sites of idiopathic VT origin: endocardial idiopathic VT (0.34), endocardial RVOT tachycardia (0.40), and aortic cusp tachycardia (0.46). The MDI $\geq$0.55 was considered the optimal cut point, with 100% sensitivity and 98.7% specificity for detection of nonaortic cusp epicardial origin. Only one aortic cusp VT had a long MDI, and MDI analyzed at lead V2 provided the best discrimination.

Bazan et al. [22] evaluated the usefulness of 12-lead ECG for predicting an epicardial origin for VT arising from the right ventricle by pacing representative sites (134 endocardial and 180 epicardial sites) in patients undergoing endocardial/epicardial mapping. They observed that QRS duration and the reported criteria for epicardial origin of VT in the left ventricle do not identify a probable epicardial origin from the right ventricle. A Q wave or QS in leads that best reflect local activation also suggest an epicardial origin for right ventricle and may help in identifying a probable epicardial site of origin for right ventricle VT. A Q wave in lead II, III, or aVF was more likely noted from inferior epicardial versus endocardial sites (53/73 versus 16/43). A Q wave in lead I was more frequently present from epicardial versus endocardial anterior right ventricle sites (30/82 versus 5/52) and QS in lead V2 was more frequently obtained from epicardial anterior RV sites (22/33 versus 13/33).

The epicardial origin of a VT can also be suspected during intracardiac recording: in case of absence of early endocardial activation sites; when a broad area of earliest endocardial activation is found; when endocardial pace maps are poor, and when there is failure of ablation at the best endocardial sites.

Approaching the epicardial space for epicardial mapping and ablation

At the present, extensive epicardial mapping can be performed by either surgical or nonsurgical technique. Surgical techniques include direct access to open chest or thoracoscopy instrumentation [23]. Although both techniques can be performed in the EP lab, they require a cardiac surgeon. The coronary sinus and great cardiac vein have been usually explored during conventional electrophysiologic studies by 5F and 6F regular multielectrode catheters. However, special microcatheters may be necessary to explore more distal coronary vein branches. de Paola et al. [24] studied the feasibility of distal transvenous epicardial mapping by using microcatheters in 20 consecutive patients with sustained VT and structural heart disease. Presystolic epicardial electrograms were recorded in six patients and concealed entrainment in two, helping as a landmark for endocardial ablation. More recently, the epicardial mapping through the coronary venous system revealed to be useful in patients with idiopathic VT originating remote from the aortic cusp [16–20].

The subxiphoid percutaneous approach allows extensive and unrestricted mapping of the epicardial surface of the heart in the EP Lab and can be performed by electrophysiologists. Although the pericardium is a virtual space, this is not an obstacle for electrophysiologists in accessing this space. Our group developed a simple technique utilizing a *needle* (Figure 14.3) designed to access the epidural space by anesthesiologists. The needle is introduced tangentially to the cardiac border to avoid ventricular perforation. The needle is gently advanced guided by fluoroscopy until the heart movement is felt at the tip of the needle. Then, a few milliliters of contrast is injected to demonstrate the position of the needle tip (if the needle tip is pushing or passing through the tissue). Contrast layering in the pericardial space confirms the space was reached. Then, a guide wire is passed through the needle and an 8 Fr

Anterior access

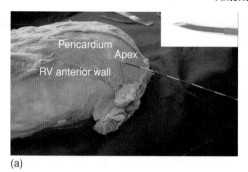

(a)

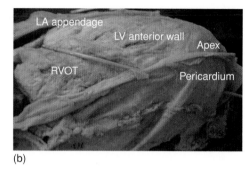

(b)

Posterior access

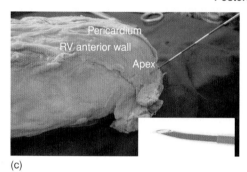

(c)

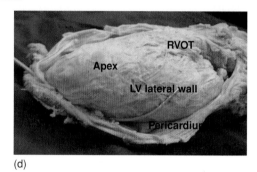

(d)

Figure 14.3 Percutaneoous subxiphoid access to the pericardial space with a Tuhoy needle. The pericardial space can be reached by either the anterior or the posterior access. The needle tip is directed tangentially to the right ventricle wall for obtaining the anterior access, with the opening side of the needle tip anteriorly (a). The anterior access allows the catheter to be moved easily over the RV anterior wall, toward the right ventricle outflow tract (b). If the target is the inferior wall, the posterior access is preferable. In this situation, the needle tip has to be directed toward the inferior and apical aspect of the ventricles with the opening side of the needle posteriorly (c). When the catheter is introduced in this position, it can be easily moved toward the lateral wall of the left ventricle (d).

introducer is advanced. Once the ablation catheter is introduced into the pericardial space, all epicardial surface can be mapped and potentially ablated. When the pericardial approach is performed, two possible access orientations can be chosen: anterior or posterior (Figure 14.4). For the anterior access, the needle tip is directed tangentially to the right ventricle wall, with the opening side of the needle tip anterior (Figure 14.4a). The anterior access allows the catheter to be moved easily over the RV anterior wall, toward the RVOT (Figure 14.4b). If the target is the inferior wall, the posterior access is preferable. In this situation, the needle tip is directed toward the inferior and apical aspect of the ventricles with the opening side of the needle directed posteriorly (Figure 14.4c). When the catheter is introduced in this position, it can be easily moved toward the lateral wall of the left ventricle (Figure 14.4d).

Efficacy and safety of epicardial mapping and ablation

The usefulness of this approach is related to the prevalence of epicardial VT in a given population. In a series of 257 consecutive procedures performed in our institution, epicardial VTs were identified in 28% of the post-MI patients, in 37% of the patients with Chagas' heart disease and in 24% of the patients with idiopathic dilated cardiomyopathy (Figure 14.5). Using RF pulses with a 4-mm-tip catheter and, more recently, with an 8-mm-tip catheter, 60–75% of all epicardial VTs were terminated rendering them noninducible. However, the 3-year

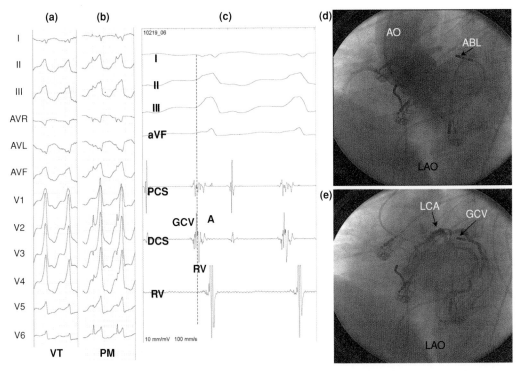

Figure 14.4 Radiofrequency (RF) catheter ablation of an idiopathic epicardial ventricular tachycardia (VT) origination remote from the aortic cusps. Picture (a) shows the 12-lead ECG during sustained VT. Picture (b): 12-lead ECG demonstrating a perfect pace mapping (PM) obtained in the great cardiac vein (GCV), from the place with the earliest activation time (c). Panel (d): fluoroscopic view in

LAO shows the coronary sinus catheter position, further advanced in the GCV. Panel (e): left coronary angiogram in LAO. Note, the RF catheter tip is not too close to the main coronary arteries allowing a safe RF ablation in distal GCV. DCS, distal coronary sinus PCS; proximal coronary sinus; RV, right ventricle.

recurrence rate of arrhythmic events in patients who underwent simultaneously epicardial and endocardial mapping and ablation was 30% (Figure 14.6).

There are some concerns about the safety of the subxiphoid pericardial approach. The first one is related to the possibility of cardiac puncture. In our experience, this occurs in 15% of patients, but termination of the procedure, in general, is not necessary. RV puncture without blood return (dry puncture) occurs in 5% of cases. Pericardial bleeding, drained during the procedure, was observed in 10% of cases. Three procedures (of 257) had to be terminated and the patients required surgical intervention, one because of a peritoneal bleeding caused by an injured diaphragmatic vessel, and two because of a pericardial bleeding.

Another concern is in avoiding coronary artery damage. In this regard, d'Avila et al. [25] reported experimental data in dog models in which linear

and single RF lesions were applied on or near the coronary artery. RF application delivery above the artery may result in intimal hyperplasia and thrombosis. The susceptibility to damage was inversely proportional to the vessel size. Chronic effect of RF lesion on the epicardial coronary artery were analyzed also by Miranda et al. [26] in seven young pigs observed for at least 70 days after RF application and the results suggested that RF pulses delivered in the vicinity of the epicardial vessels do not provoke myocardial infarction or vascular thrombosis. The endothelium was preserved in most of the animals, but intense intimal thickening was seen in a few animals. The presence of fat and veins interposed between the epicardial coronary arteries and the catheter tip was related to much less intimal thickening but the long-term significance of the intimal thickening is still unknown. Kawamura et al. [27] evaluated the efficacy and safety of epicardial radiofrequency

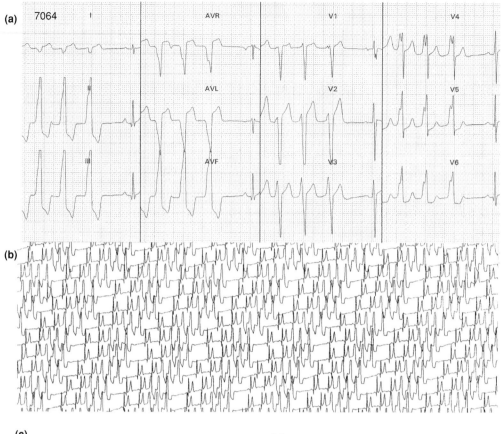

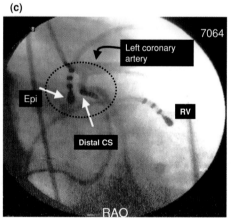

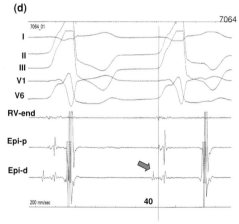

Figure 14.5 (a) 12-lead ECG of a 19-year-old female with idiopathic ventricular tachycardia (VT) and three prior failed RF catheter ablation attempts. (b) ECG monitoring just before the last RF ablation procedure. Figure 14.5(c)–(f): Epicardial RF ablation by the subxiphoid epicardial approach. (c) Fluoroscopic view in RAO showing the epicardial catheter position on the best earliest activation site (d). Note the close proximity of the epicardial RF catheter and the main coronary arteries. (e) ECG just before the RF delivery. (f) ECG following RF ablation. (g) and (h) 12-lead ECG, respectively, from sustained VT and pace mapping recording on the earliest activation site.

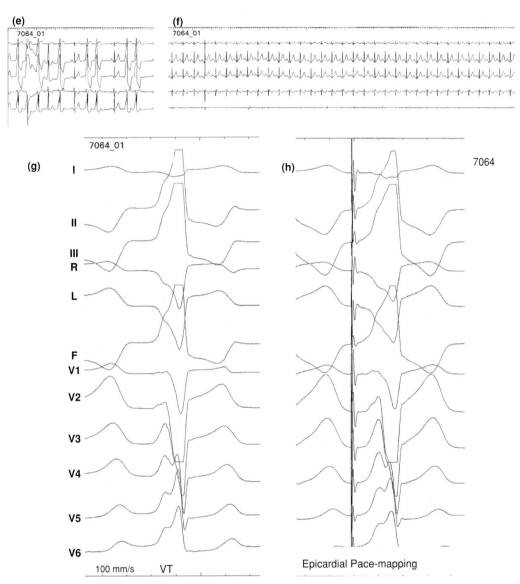

Figure 14.5 (contnued).

ablation close to the anterior descending artery more than or equal to 15 mm and farther from the coronary artery. No damage to major epicardial arteries was detected when the catheter tip was positioned 5 mm away from the coronary artery. Our current approach regarding the risk of damaging the coronary vessels is to obtain an angiogram prior to ablation in all patients. Based on the analysis of the anatomy of coronary arteries, areas can be selected for epicardial ablation. If a critical site of the tachycardia circuit can only be identified

close to a coronary artery, a risk–benefit analysis should be undertaken. RF application caused coronary artery occlusion of a marginal branch causing non-Q-wave MI in only one of 257 consecutive patients.

Phrenic nerve injury is a potential complication during epicardial catheter ablation. Although we have never seen this complication, Bai et al. [28] reported one case during epicardial VT ablation with late recovery. We have used high-output pacing at the eventual ablation site prior to RF delivery to

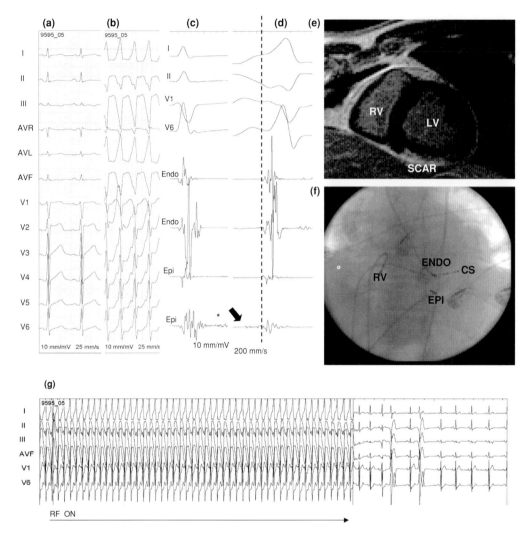

Figure 14.6 Epicardial RF ablation by the percutaneous epicardial approach in a 51-year-old man with mild dilated cardiomyopathy and recurrent sustained ventricular tachycardia (VT). The basal ECG in sinus rhythm (a) was unremarkable and during sustained VT (b) suggested an inferior, septal and basal origin. Fractionated and late potential electrogram (*) were obtained just from the epicardial mapping during sinus rhythm (c). The arrow indicates the fractioned earliest activation site during VT obtained by the epicardial catheter in the inferior, septal and basal wall (E). That area was related to the intramural scar confirmed by late enhanced Gadolinium MRI (d). Part (g) shows the VT interruption during RF delivering from the epicardial catheter in that place.

search phrenic nerve location. Buch et al. [29] suggests interposing a catheter balloon between the RF catheter and phrenic nerve area when the site of origin is close to the phrenic nerve area. Fenelon et al. [30] studied the factors affecting epicardial RF lesion formation in dog's normal ventricular myocardium. In this study they observed that thermally shielded electrodes (50% tip surface along its 4-mm length) promoted similar epicardial lesion compared to conventional 4-mm electrodes, but damage to parietal pericardium and lungs occurred only with conventional electrodes. Thus, thermally shielded catheters could be another alternative to prevent unexpected injuries in cardiac neighbor tissues during epicardial ablation.

Intense postprocedure pericarditis has been observed in animals mapped and ablated intrapericardially at the experimental laboratory; this can be prevented by the pericardial infusion of corticosteroid drugs at the end of the procedure. Intense pericarditis was rarely seen in our patients. Precordial distress and pain were observed in 25% of them. Pericardial effusion was minimal and the symptoms easily controlled with regular anti-inflamatory drugs. Pericardial effusion and pericardial adhesions are also rare, occurring only in one patient who had more than one epicardial procedure ranging from 1 week to 10 months after the first procedure.

Subxiphoide pericardial approach can be limited by epicardial adhesions mainly after surgical procedures. In those cases, most of the epicardial adhesions are restricted to anterior wall; the place where pericardial is incised and frequently left open during cardiac surgery. Despite that, it is possible to reach the pericardial space in some patients by using the inferior access to explore the inferior and lateral wall, when those areas are involved in VT circuit [31].

The epicardial fat can also decrease the effectiveness of ablation success as well as mimic infarct during electroanatomic mapping [32]. The bipolar epicardial ventricular electrogram and epicardial pacing threshold were obtained by 4-mm-tip electrode in 10 patients undergoing cardiac surgery. Comparing 45 areas with and 44 without epicardial fat, we observed that epicardial fat thickness of more than 5 mm significantly decreased bipolar electrogram amplitude and increased pacing threshold. However, in areas with less than 5 mm of fat thickness, there was no significant change in those parameters as compared to areas without epicardial fat [33]. Thus, finding out the distribution and thickness of epicardial fat would be important prior to epicardial ablation so as to understand the possibility of failure in such procedures. Abbara et al. [34] quantitatively assessed the epicardial fat distribution and thickness *in vivo* in 59 patients who underwent multidetector computed tomography for coronary artery assessment using a 16-slice scanner. Epicardial fat diameter was measured in different segments and views. The mean epicardial fat thickness for all cases was 5.3 ± 1.6 mm. The mean total epicardial fat was 22% greater in older patients than in younger patients. Also, women had 17% more total epicardial fat than men for the same matched age. The RV anterior free wall tended to have high epicardial fat, and the LV lateral wall and RV diaphragmatic wall tended to have little to no fat; however, there was significant variation between patients for that. Thus, multidetector computed tomography is a reliable modality for visualizing epicardial fat, and might be considered to be carried out before carrying out epicardial ablation procedures.

The biophysical aspects of epicardial lesions have been studied in animal models using different energy systems and their effectiveness in areas with and without fat [30,33,35,37]. The absence of blood cooling effect in the pericardial space causes the target temperature to be reached at low power delivery thus creating small lesions. In addition, coronary vessels promote a cooling effect protecting the tissue underneath, as well thick epicardial fat prevents deep myocardial lesions. Deep lesions can be obtained by using cooled-tip electrodes, even in areas with epicardial fat [35]. However, the risk of coronary artery injury should also be considered when using these catheters as this risk may increase with a larger lesion size. Epicardial cryoablation is an alternative energy source for creating deep lesions in areas where RF delivery is inadequate. Cryoablation may have a lower risk for coronary artery occlusion [36]. However, the presence of an epicardial fat layer thicker than 5 mm also seems to attenuate epicardial cryolesions [37].

Conclusion

Epicardial mapping allows identification and ablation of subepicardial myocardial fibers related to the focal site of origin or macroreentrant circuits in selected patients with VT. This procedure may be limited by the proximity of coronary vessels, phrenic nerves, epicardial adhesions, and fat tissue.

References

1 Horowitz LN, Josephson ME, Harken AH. Epicardial and endocardial activation during sustained ventricular tachycardia in man. Circulation 1980;61(6):1227–1238.

2 de Bakker JM, Coronel R, Tasseron S, et al. Ventricular tachycardia in the infarcted, Langendorff-perfused human heart: role of the arrangement of surviving cardiac fibers. J Am Coll Cardiol 1990;15(7):1594–1607.

3 Littmann L, Svenson R, Gallagher J, et al. Functional role of epicardium in postinfarction ventricular tachycardia. Circulation 1991;83:1577–1591.

4 Kaltenbrunner W, Cardinal R, Dubuc M, et al. Epicardial and endocardial mapping of ventricular tachycardia in patients with myocardial infarction. Is the origin of the tachycardia always subendocardially localized? Circulation 1991;84(3):1058–1071.

5 Svenson RH, Littmann L, Gallagher JJ, et al. Termination of ventricular tachycardia with epicardial laser photocoagulation: a clinical comparison with patients undergoing successful endocardial photocoagulation alone. J Am Coll Cardiol 1990;15(1):163–170.

6 Sosa E, Scanavacca M, d'Ávila A, Oliveira F, Ramires JA. Nonsurgical transthoracic epicardial catheter ablation to treat recurrent ventricular tachycardia occurring late after myocardial infarction. J Am Coll Cardiol 2000;35(6):1442–1449.

7 Schweikert RA, Saliba WI, Tomassoni G, et al. Percutaneous pericardial instrumentation for endo-epicardial mapping of previously failed ablations. Circulation 2003;108:1329.

8 Brugada J, Berruezo A, Cuesta A, et al. Nonsurgical transthoracic epicardial radiofrequency ablation: an alternative in incessant ventricular tachycardia. J Am Coll Cardiol 2003;41(11):2036–2043.

9 Reddy VY, Wrobleski D, Houghtaling C, Josephson ME, Ruskin JN. Combined epicardial and endocardial electroanatomic mapping in a porcine model of healed myocardial infarction. Circulation 2003;107(25):3236–3242.

10 Cesario DA, Vaseghi M, Boyle NG, et al. Value of high-density endocardial and epicardial mapping for catheter ablation of hemodynamically unstable ventricular tachycardia. Heart Rhythm 2006;3(1):1–10.

11 Soejima K, Stevenson WG. Catheter ablation of ventricular tachycardia in patients with ischemic heart disease. Curr Cardiol Rep 2003;5(5):364–368.

12 Sosa E, Scanavacca M. Epicardial mapping and ablation techniques to control ventricular tachycardia. J Cardiovasc Electrophysiol 2005;16(4):449–452.

13 Soejima K, Stevenson WG, Sapp JL, Selwyn AP, Couper G, Epstein LM. Endocardial and epicardial radiofrequency ablation of ventricular tachycardia associated with dilated cardiomyopathy: the importance of low-voltage scars. J Am Coll Cardiol 2004;43(10):1834–1842.

14 McCrohon JA, Moon JC, Prasad SK, et al. Differentiation of heart failure related to dilated cardiomyopathy and coronary artery disease using gadolinium-enhanced cardiovascular magnetic resonance. Circulation 2003; 108(1):54–59.

15 Ouyang F, Antz M, Deger FT, et al. An underrecognized subepicardial reentrant ventricular tachycardia attributable to left ventricular aneurysm in patients with normal coronary arteriograms. Circulation 2003; 107(21):2702–2709.

16 Swarup V, Morton JB, Arruda M, Wilber DJ. Ablation of epicardial macroreentrant ventricular tachycardia associated with idiopathic nonischemic dilated cardiomyopathy by a percutaneous transthoracic approach. J Cardiovasc Electrophysiol 2002;13(11):1164–1168.

17 Hirasawa Y, Miyauchi Y, Iwasaki YK, Kobayashi Y. Successful radiofrequency catheter ablation of epicardial left ventricular outflow tract tachycardia from the anterior interventricular coronary vein. J Cardiovasc Electrophysiol 2005;16(12):1378–1380.

18 Daniels DV, Lu YY, Morton JB, et al. Idiopathic epicardial left ventricular tachycardia originating remote from the sinus of Valsalva: electrophysiological characteristics, catheter ablation, and identification from the 12-lead electrocardiogram. Circulation 2006;113(13):1659–1666.

19 Tanner H, Hindricks G, Schirdewahn P, et al. Outflow tract tachycardia with r/s transition in lead V3. J Am Coll Cardiol 2005;45(3):418–423.

20 Obel OA, d'Ávila A, Neuzil P, Saad EB, Ruskin JN, Reddy VY. Ablation of left ventricular epicardial outflow tract tachycardia from the distal great cardiac vein. J Am Coll Cardiol 2006;48(9):1813–1817.

21 Berruezo A, Mont L, Nava S, Chueca E, Bartholomay E, Brugada J. Electrocardiographic recognition of the epicardial origin of ventricular tachycardias. Circulation 2004;109(15):1842–1847.

22 Bazan V, Bala R, Garcia FC, et al. Twelve-lead ECG features to identify ventricular tachycardia arising from the epicardial right ventricle. Heart Rhythm 2006;3(10):1132–1139.

23 Soejima K, Couper G, Cooper JM, Sapp JL, Epstein LM, Stevenson WG. Subxiphoid surgical approach for epicardial catheter-based mapping and ablation in patients with prior cardiac surgery or difficult pericardial access. Circulation 2004;110(10):1197–1201.

24 de Paola AA, Melo WD, Tavora MZ, Martinez EE. Angiographic and electrophysiological substrates for ventricular tachycardia mapping through the coronary veins. Heart 1998;79(1):59–63.

25 d' Ávila A, Gutierrez P, Scanavacca M, et al. Effects of radiofrequency pulses delivery in the vicinity of the coronary arteries: implications for nonsurgical transthoracic epicardial catheter ablation to treat ventricular tachycardia. Pacing Clin Electrophysiol 2002;25:1488–1495.

26 D'Avila A, Gutierrez P, Scanavacca M, Reddy V, Lustgarten DL, Sosa E, Ramires JA. Effects of radiofrequency pulses delivered in the vicinity of the coronary arteries: implications for nonsurgical transthoracic epicardial catheter ablation to treat ventricular tachycardia. Pacing Clin Electrophysiol. 2002 Oct;25(10):1488–1495.

27 Kawamura M, Kobayashi Y, Ito H, et al. Epicardial ablation with cooled tip catheter close to the coronary arteries is effective and safe in the porcine heart if the ventricular potential is being monitored in the epicardium and endocardium. Circ J 2006;70(7):926–932.

28 Bai R, Patel D, Di Biase L, et al. Phrenic nerve injury after catheter ablation: should we worry about this complication? J Cardiovasc Electrophysiol 2006;17(9):944–948.

29 Buch E, Vaseghi M, Cesario DA, Shivkumar K. A novel method for preventing phrenic nerve injury during catheter ablation. Heart Rhythm 2007;4(1):95–98.

30 Fenelon G, Pereira KP, de Paola AA. Epicardial radiofrequency ablation of ventricular myocardium: factors

affecting lesion formation and damage to adjacent structures. J Interv Card Electrophysiol 2006;15(1):57–63.

31 Sosa E, Scanavacca M, d'Ávila A, et al. Nonsurgical transthoracic epicardial approach in patients with ventricular tachycardia and previous cardiac surgery. J Interv Card Electrophysiol 2004;10:281–288.

32 Dixit S, Narula N, Callans DJ, Marchlinski FE. Electroanatomic mapping of human heart: epicardial fat can mimic scar. J Cardiovasc Electrophysiol 2003;14(10): 1128.

33 d'Ávila A, Dias R, Scanavacca M, Sosa E. Epicardial fat tissue does not modify amplitude and duration of epicardial electrograms and /or ventricular stimulation threshold [Abstract]. Eur J Cardiol 2002;23:5.

34 Abbara S, Desai JC, Cury RC, Butler J, Nieman K, Reddy V. Mapping epicardial fat with multi-detector computed tomography to facilitate percutaneous transepicardial arrhythmia ablation. Eur J Radiol 2006;57(3):417–422.

35 d'Ávila A, Houghtaling C, Gutierrez P, et al. Catheter ablation of ventricular epicardial tissue: a comparison of standard and cooled-tip radiofrequency energy. Circulation 2004;109(19):2363–2369.

36 Atienza F, Arenal A, Ormaetxe J, Almendral J. Epicardial idiopathic ventricular tachycardia originating within the left main coronary artery ostium area: identification using the LocaLisa nonfluoroscopic catheter navigation system. J Cardiovasc Electrophysiol 2005;16(11):1239–1242.

37 d'Ávila A, Holmvang G, Houghtaling C, et al. Focal and linear endocardial and epicardial catheter-based cryoablation of normal and infracted ventricular tissue [Abstract]. Heart Rhythm 2004;1:1S.

CHAPTER 15

Role of catheter control systems in ablation of ventricular tachycardia

Marco Perez & Amin Al-Ahmad

Introduction

The anatomical complexity and variety of ventricular tachycardias (VTs) require new approaches to catheter ablation. In patients with ischemic reentrant VT, failure and recurrence rates as high as 50% [1,2] also point to the need for novel strategies. In addition, a growing number of adult patients with surgically corrected congenital abnormalities are presenting challenges to the current techniques of catheter control [3].

Manually controlled catheters have several limitations that make VT ablation demanding. The existing catheters have a fixed radius of curvature, often making it difficult to access sites at acute angles. Standard catheter systems utilize a pull-wire system at the handle that can affect the amount of curvature in these fixed-radius systems. While these pull wires allow for deflection, they can add to the thickness and stiffness of the catheters. Transmission of torque via manual rotation is also inefficient, particularly in patients with tortuous vascular systems. Lack of fine control and stability of the catheter tip make it difficult to apply the lesions often needed to achieve successful ablation of VT.

In addition to the limitations of catheter maneuverability, there are other disadvantages to the current system of ablation. The need for manual control of the catheter at the patient's side exposes the operator, staff, and patients to long periods of fluoroscopy which have potential deleterious health consequences [4]. The need to stand with heavy lead protection for prolonged procedures can also lead to operator fatigue and back pain.

Several improvements to the current catheter systems have been proposed. The use of a preformed shaped sheath allows for improved stability at the catheter tip; however, this comes at the cost of restriction in movement. In addition, a long sheath may also pose an increased risk of thrombus formation that can have deleterious effects if it is in the arterial system. Other ideas include the use of multiple lumens for pull wires that permit more contortions of the catheter as well as the use of stabilizing elements at the distal tip [5,6]. These improvements are incremental and leave several properties to be desired.

An ideal catheter control system would minimize risks to patients and operators and provide efficient access to sites that are currently difficult to reach. The ability to make multiple acute angles and maintain control of the catheter tip would allow for better navigation through tortuous paths in the three-dimensional space. Novel systems should have rapid learning curves and result in shorter procedure times. They should also improve the precision and stability of the catheter. This would allow for better tissue contact and diminished catheter movement during ablation which can lead to brush lesions and unnecessary destruction of tissue.

Several advances in catheter control systems have been made that strive to overcome these limitations. Remote magnetic navigation (RMN) introduces a myriad of catheter manipulations that are facilitating the ablation of circuits at anatomically complex sites. Robotic catheter manipulation promises fine catheter precision and removes the operator from exposures. Although

Ventricular Arrhythmias and Sudden Cardiac Death, 1st edition. Edited by P.J. Wang, A. Al-Ahmad, H. Hsia, and P.C. Zei © 2008 Blackwell Publishing, ISBN: 978-1-4051-6114-5.

much of the experience with these systems has been with supraventricular arrhythmias, these technologies are increasingly being applied in the ventricle. These technologies and their use in VT mapping and ablation will be reviewed here. With the advent of new materials and techniques, the success of VT ablation will continue to grow.

Remote magnetic navigation

Introduction to remote magnetic navigation

Remote magnetic navigation is a novel catheter control system that functions by manipulating a magnetically tipped catheter with the use of external magnetic force. The use of intravascular catheter manipulation with magnets was initially reported in 1951 by Tillander [7] who used external magnets to control a catheter with a steel tip in the aorta. The relatively poor strength of the magnets, lack of detailed imaging modalities, and absence of precise three-dimensional direction of the magnetic fields limited this early work. The advent of large, powerful magnets with computer-controlled vectors opened the door to the practical use of magnetic catheter control in the medical field.

Early experience in the field of neurosurgery demonstrated the feasibility of maneuvering magnetically controlled catheters through more challenging intravascular paths. It was first demonstrated that a magnet-controlled catheter could be used to successfully perform brain biopsies in pigs with an accuracy of within 1.5 mm of the targeted tissue [8]. Subsequent studies in humans showed that neuroendovascular magnetic navigation could be used for the embolic therapy of intracranial aneurysms [9].

Applications of this technology in the realm of cardiac electrophysiology were a natural progression. A magnetic guidance system (MGS) was initially developed consisting of three electromagnets cooled by liquid helium in conjunction with fluoroscopic imaging (Niobe, Stereotaxis, St Louis, MO, USA). A 7F ablation catheter with a magnetic tip could then be introduced and directed via magnetic fields generated by electric currents applied by control computers to the superconducting electromagnets. The initial report demonstrated in animal models that such a catheter could be navigated to

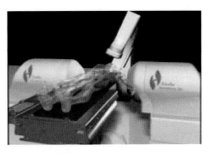

Figure 15.1 Stereotaxis niobe system's permanent magnets. Printed with permission from Stereotaxis.

predefined targets in the ventricles, atria, and pulmonary veins with an accuracy within 1 mm [10]. The system was able to move the catheter in increments of 1° and 1 mm within the heart chambers. This feasibility study was followed shortly by demonstration of safety and efficacy in human subjects. MGS proved successful in navigating to 200 of 202 predetermined sites which included 47 right ventricular apex, free wall, outflow tract, and septal sites [11] without a single episode of perforation or other major adverse side effect.

Several enhancements to the magnetic system have been incorporated. The electromagnets have been replaced by two large, permanent magnets of a neodymium–iron–boron compound able to create a uniform magnetic field of 0.08 Tesla at a distance of approximately 15 cm (Figure 15.1). The addition of a system capable of advancing and retracting the catheter (Cardiodrive, Stereotaxis) (Figure 15.2) allowed for complete remote control of the catheter. Software enhancements and an intuitive computer interface (Navigant, Stereotaxis)

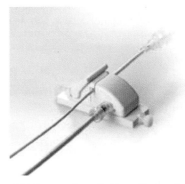

Figure 15.2 Stereotaxis cardiodrive catheter advancement system. Printed with permission from Stereotaxis.

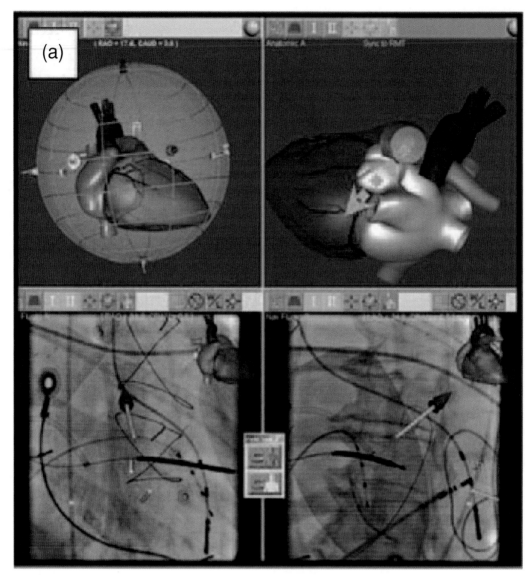

Figure 15.3 (a) Fluoroscopic view of the stereotaxis Navigant system interface with magnetic field vectors. Adapted from Aryana et al., Circulation, 2001. 115(10): p. 1191–1200. Courtesy of Lippincott, Williams & Wilkins (b) Synchronized view of CARTO-RMT map adjacent to the navigant system interface. Adapted from Aryana et al., Circulation, 2001. 115(10): p. 1191–1200. Courtesy of Lippincott, Williams & Wilkins.

added features such as the ability to record and return to positions in three-dimensional space. The entire system can be controlled with a joystick or mouse in a control room shielded from fluoroscopic exposure. The desired magnetic field vector can be drawn and displayed on orthogonal fluoroscopic views (Figure 15.3a). The appropriate orientation of each magnet needed to produce the desired magnetic field is calculated and executed by the control computer. The lag time between movements of magnets to produce changes in field vectors is on the order of a few seconds. In addition, three-dimensional electroanatomic mapping techniques (CARTO-RMT, Biosense Webster) have been adapted to function with this magnetic system (Figure 15.3b).

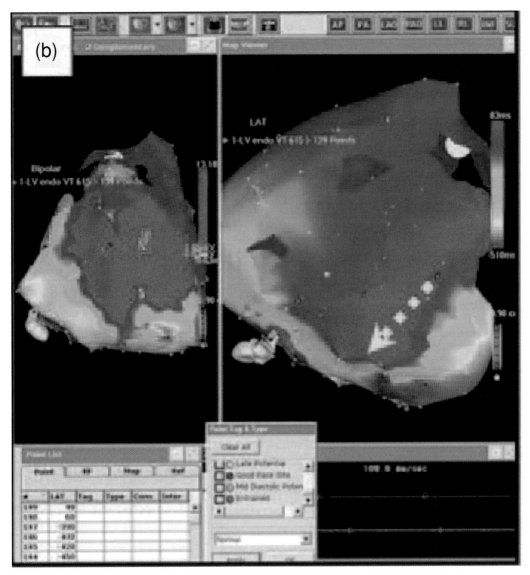

Figure 15.3 (*Continued*).

With the integration of these technologies, one is able to simply identify points in space on the three-dimensional cardiac map and instruct the computer to navigate the real catheter to these points for ablation. These features, plus the ability of RMN to simultaneously record electrocardiographic tracings, pace and perform radiofrequency current catheter ablation on myocardial tissue, solidified this as a technology with great potential in electrophysiology.

Remote magnetic navigation in supraventricular ablation

Most of the experience with RMN has been in the mapping and ablation of supraventricular arrhythmias. In a recent study, a series of 42 patients with documented common-type (slow/fast) or uncommon-type (slow/slow) atrioventricular nodal reentry tachycardia (AVNRT) underwent ablation with RMN [12]. Fifteen patients had successful slow pathway ablation while the remaining 27

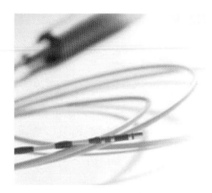

Figure 15.4 Stereotaxis magnetic gentle touch catheter. Printed with permission from Stereotaxis.

patients achieved slow pathway modulation with no complications. The total average procedure time was 145 minutes and mean fluoroscopy time was 8.9 minutes, which means less radiation than that used in a typical conventional procedure. The operating physicians, after having inserted and positioned the catheters under fluoroscopy, spent the remaining time in the control room with only an average of 3.4 minutes of radiation exposure. A similar study reported successful AVNRT ablation in 18 out of 20 procedures with mean fluoroscopic time of 12 minutes without any complications [13]. These case series were attestations that the novel magnetic system provided the precision and safety required for these ablation procedures. The authors were able to adapt quickly to the new equipment and were pleased to report reductions in fluoroscopy exposure to the patients and operators.

Successes in ablation of accessory pathways (AP) using RMN have also been reported [14–16]. One study documented a series of ablations in 59 patients with 19 right-sided APs and 41 left-sided APs using retrograde access in seven patients and transseptal access in 33 patients. During the course of this study, the catheter used evolved from a unipolar, single-magnet-tipped catheter to a quadripolar, triple-magnet-tipped catheter (Figure 15.4). The advanced catheter and greater operator experience led to success rates of 92% with down to 4.9 minutes of median fluoroscopy time using the quadripolar catheter. Again, no complications were reported in any of these procedures.

A further test of the flexibility of this system came when atrial fibrillation (AF) ablation was attempted. AF ablation using conventional approaches can be notoriously time consuming, typically exposing patients and physicians to a significant amount of radiation and requires long training periods. In addition, stable tissue contact becomes more difficult as the catheter is navigated to complex anatomical targets in the left atrium. Given the recent surge in demand for AF ablation, a more efficient method of pulmonary vein isolation is required for universal adoption of this intricate procedure.

Pappone and his group [17,18] have recently reported successful use of RMN in circumferential pulmonary vein ablation (CPVA). The group studied 40 patients with AF, 63% of which had paroxysmal AF and compared ablation with RMN to conventional ablation in a group of 28 patients matched for similar clinical characteristics. After atrial transseptal puncture, the magnetic-tipped catheter was guided into the left atrium using fluoroscopy and the remaining navigation needed to perform the CPVA was performed using RMN from the control room. Successful ablation was achieved in 38 of 40 patients with a median mapping and ablation time of 152.5 minutes, which was slightly longer than that in the control group. Although mapping times were similar in both groups, ablation time, particularly of the right pulmonary veins which can be difficult to reach, was shorter in the RMN group. This was thought to be due to better catheter stability which also allowed for many more mapping points in the RMN group. It was pointed out that procedure times dramatically improved as more experience was gained in the latter phase of the study. Also of note, there were no complications reported in any of the cases.

The experiences gathered in ablation of supraventricular tissue have opened the door to the use of RMN in the ablation of VT. Although reports of mapping and ablation of VT are not as extensive, the fact that the prior studies reported high success rates and rapid learning curves makes translation to VT ablation highly encouraging.

Remote magnetic navigation in ventricular ablation

As noted earlier, there is a wide variety of VTs, each presenting their own set of navigational challenges. Catheter manipulation in the ventricle can be more challenging due to the need to traverse valvular structures and to position the catheter across multiple curves. In addition, the valvular leaflets, trabecular system, and myocardial contraction can make fine catheter movement and stability more complicated.

The right ventricular outflow tract (RVOT), a sometimes challenging area to map and ablate, is the origin of the majority of nonischemic, idiopathic VTs [19]. Ablation strategies with simple activation and pace-mapping techniques have demonstrated success rates between 80% and 100% [20]. However, since small changes within the RVOT can lead to marked changes in the paced ECG, it has been argued that the spatial resolution at the RVOT is currently insufficient [21]. Given the thin nature of the right ventricular free wall, the risk of tamponade from perforation or late rupture is ever present.

RMN would allow for the finer catheter control needed to more precisely pace map in the RVOT and would reduce the risk of rupture of the right ventricle because of the soft, highly flexible catheter tip used. One recent series attempted RVOT tachycardia ablation in a group of seven patients using RMN [22]. In these patients, a 64-polar-basket catheter was first used to locate the area in the RVOT of earliest activation. A three-magnet-tipped catheter was then inserted and placed in the general area of the RVOT identified by the basket catheter. Pace mapping was performed and the optimal pace map was found using RMN, which allowed for fine catheter manipulation. Success, defined as inability to induce the tachycardia with isoproterenol and burst pacing, was achieved in all seven patients. The mean procedural time was 151 minutes, with a mean patient fluoroscopy time of 12.5 minutes. The physicians, however, only had an average of 3.5 minutes of exposure to fluoroscopy during the introduction of sheaths and positioning of the catheters. Pace mapping and ablations were all performed remotely and there were no complications reported. After a mean follow up of 366 days, only one of the seven patients had recurrence of VT necessitating a repeat ablative procedure. Although success rates in this study are comparable to those done using traditional techniques, the significant reduction in radiation exposure and the ability of the operators to sit comfortably during most of the procedure were major advantages noted in this study.

Where larger differences in success rates may begin to emerge are in the ablation of more complex left-sided VTs. Although one might think that the enlarged left ventricle would make navigation with a flexible catheter more difficult, early experience demonstrated the utility of magnetic control in these areas of the heart [10]. To demonstrate that the delivery of ablative therapy in the left ventricle with RMN could be accomplished using a retrograde approach, a case of refractory left fascicular VT was first reported in 2006 [23]. Radiofrequency ablation had already been attempted using conventional means, where 43 applications were given with a total of 70 minutes of radiation time and the procedure time was 258 minutes. Recurrence followed shortly and eventually became incessant. The patient subsequently underwent ablation using a more advanced mapping system; however, stability of the catheter became a major problem during repeated runs of VT. RMN was therefore employed which made navigation to the point of interest much more feasible. After 17 ablative applications in the mid-posterior septal region over a total procedure time of 225 minutes and patient radiation time of 50 minutes, the tachycardia was no longer inducible. The patient failed to reveal any further episodes of VT on subsequent Holter monitoring and follow-up over 12 months.

In a test of the true flexibility and precision of the RMN system, a case of left coronary cusp VT ablation was reported [24]. Navigation in the region of the coronary cusps requires a high degree of precision due to the proximity of the coronary artery ostia. In this case, activation mapping revealed the left coronary cusp, as evident by intracardiac echocardiography and fluoroscopy, to be the site of earliest activation and confirmed by pace mapping. Catheter manipulation and ablation was performed with RMN in a total procedure time of 170 minutes and fluoroscopy time of 22 minutes resulting in complete cessation of ectopy.

Although these reports of successful ablation of nonischemic VT are promising uses of this technology, the vast majority of VT remains scar-related, ischemic VT. Widespread use of RMN for VT ablation will require further experience in this group of patients. The move toward a substrate-based catheter ablation approach [25] has created a demand for improved mapping accuracy and careful,

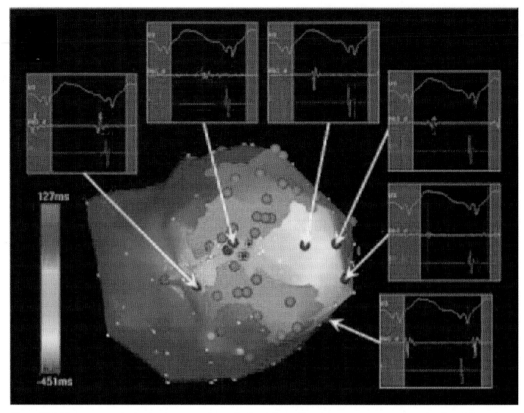

Figure 15.5 Electroanatomical activation map of ventricular tachycardia using remote magnetic navigation. Adapted from Aryana et al., Circulation, 2001. 115(10): p. 1191–1200. Courtesy of Lippincott, Williams & Wilkins.

precise catheter manipulation often requiring skilled operators.

In a recently published series on cases of patients with scar-related monomorphic VT, 27 mapping procedures on 24 patients were performed using RMN [26]. The etiology of the VT was varied and included myocardial infarction (62%), dilated cardiomyopathy (13%), arrhythmogenic right ventricular cardiomyopathy (13%), hypertrophic cardiomyopathy (8%), and sarcoidosis (4%). A combination of endocardial and epicardial electroanatomical mapping using RMN revealed a total of 77 inducible VTs (Figure 15.5), requiring less than 1 minute of fluoroscopy time in most mapping procedures. In those with hemodynamically stable inducible VT, entrainment mapping, late potential mapping, and pace mapping were used. Of the 77 VTs identified, 21 ablations were attempted with RMN and 17 (81%) were successfully terminated. The manual catheter was used in the remainder of cases for safety and efficacy and resulted in total success in 75 of 77 VTs.

Experience gained with such a series of patients proves valuable. Whereas it was previously thought that the magnetization would prohibit the procedure in patients with implantable devices, 19 patients with ICDs underwent RMN with no reports of interference with the device. This was also the first study to show the feasibility of using RMN to map in the epicardium (Figure 15.6). The authors' remark that the number of PVCs observed using RMN were substantially lower than those typically seen with manual catheter control, making entrainment and pace mapping much more feasible. Although only a small subset of these patients underwent ablation with RMN, irrigated catheters and other ablative energy sources compatible with the magnetic system will potentially open the door to completely remote ablation of a larger number of VTs. Once again, magnetically controlled catheter navigation

(a)

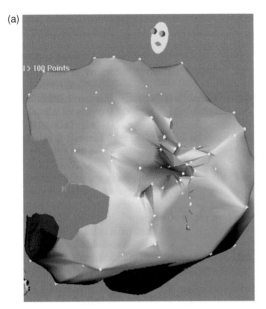

(b)

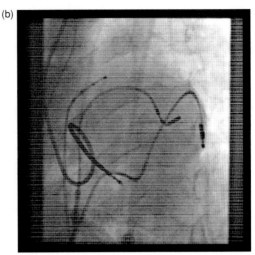

Figure 15.6 (a) Electroanatomical epicardial map of ventricular tachycardia using remote magnetic navigation. Courtesy John Burkhardt, The Cleveland Clinic Foundation. (b) Fluoroscopic view during epicardial mapping of ventricular tachycardia using remote magnetic navigation. (Courtesy John Burkhardt, The Cleveland Clinic Foundation.)

was able to produce the high degree of flexibility and accuracy needed to perform the complex maneuvers to accurately map VT.

Limitations of RMN

Although the advantages offered by RMN are numerous and the results obtained from the techniques have been very promising, there are several limitations worth noting. First and foremost is the cost and upfront investment in equipment and modifications to the operating room that must be made. Magnetic shielding must be incorporated to protect from interference with adjacent rooms and the floors may need to be reinforced to handle the 8000 pounds of weight. Another limitation is that due to the size of the magnets, the fluoroscopic windows are limited to approximately 30° on the left and right anterior oblique angles, which limits visualization of the entire ventricular cavity. Although currently 3D CT or MRI anatomical imaging is not incorporated into the software, this limitation will soon be overcome. Of note, most human studies thus far are feasibility studies and randomized trials demonstrating improved safety and higher success rates will need to be performed.

The promise of shorter procedure times, minimal radiation exposure and higher success rates appear to outweigh the costs and is leading to a relatively quicker adoption of this technology with over 40 systems installed worldwide and over 100 new orders placed. In addition, the ability to use the system to perform procedures remotely has recently been demonstrated (procedure in Italy and operator in the United States) which may become a useful feature of this technology. Early studies showing RMN used in placement or left ventricular leads for biventricular pacing and in complex percutaneous coronary intervention will also help speed the adoption of this system.

Emerging technologies

Although magnetic navigation holds great promise in the field of VT ablation, some alternative technologies, such as robotics, are begging to emerge.

Robotic catheter control system

The surgical field has employed robotic surgery in many applications with great success and has benefited from minimizing incision sizes and recovery periods. It was again neurosurgery that led

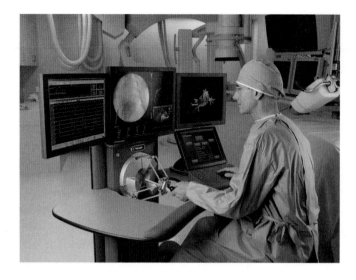

Figure 15.7 Hansen Sensei robotic catheter system master console. (Printed with permission from Hansen Medical.)

the field with the first application in precise robot-assisted brain biopsies in 1985 [27]. However, it was the surge in laparoscopic surgery and the need to precisely control small surgical tools with camera guidance that has brought surgical robotics to the forefront [28]. Some of the major advantages reported are improved dexterity and stability with increased degrees of freedom, better hand–eye coordination, and compensation for tremors. Robotic surgery has expanded to areas such as urologic, orthopedic, and minimally invasive cardiothoracic surgery [29] and has even allowed for truly remote, transcontinental operation [30].

A novel remote robotic catheter control system (RCCS) has been developed (Hansen Medical) for use in percutaneous catheter manipulation. In this system, the operator uses an instinctive "master" console consisting of multiple video monitors and a perceptive motion controller joystick (Figure 15.7) to electromechanically control a remote "slave" device attached to standard steerable guide catheters and optional sheaths (Figure 15.8). Once the catheters are inserted, the operator can sit comfortably at a remote location shielded from fluoroscopy and perform the necessary mapping and ablation.

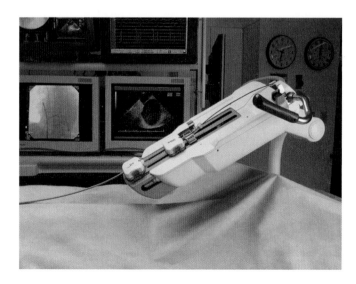

Figure 15.8 Hansen Medical artisan control catheter. (Printed with permission from Hansen Medical.)

Table 15.1 Major differences between remote magnetic navigation and robotic catheter control systems

Property	Magnetic navigation	Robotic navigation
Equipment cost	Significant	Moderate
Room modification	Lead shielding	None
Catheter reaction time	5–20 s per degree change	Immediate
Fluoroscopic windows	30° RAO to 30° LAO	Complete field
Compatible catheters	Proprietary, soft-tipped 8-mm tip recently approved	Standard steerable catheters
Disposable catheters	Not available	Artisan control catheter (Hansen Medical)

Although the experience with these systems in electrophysiology is not as extensive as with RMN, the experiences thus far are encouraging. One of the first reports by Al-Ahmad et al. [31] compared intracardiac navigation times using the RCCS to standard manual catheter system in *ex vivo* porcine hearts. The RCCS was able to reduce the time needed for both navigation and precision targeting in the right and left atrium by more than half compared to manual manipulation. It was subsequently shown that the RCCS in combination with 3D CT image integration could be used to perform left atrial mapping and pulmonary vein isolation in a porcine *in vivo* model [32]. In one human study, six patients successfully underwent AF ablation with a mean procedure time of 166 minutes and fluoroscopy time of 82 minutes and six patients underwent atrial flutter ablation with mean respective times of 145 and 43 minutes [33]. The only complication was tamponade noted during the second trans-septal puncture in one patient requiring pericardiocentesis. To date, however, no experience with ventricular mapping or ablation has been reported with this technology. There are several potential advantages of RCCS over RMN, such as lower initial cost, faster catheter reaction times and wider fluoroscopic windows (Table 15.1). However, future studies comparing the two technologies will need to be performed to assess for real differences in procedure times and success rates.

Future technologies

The preliminary studies mentioned demonstrate the promise of robotic catheter manipulation and with enhancements on the horizon, this technology will continue to progress. As has been done in robotic surgery, the addition of pressure sensors and force feedback to the control of these robotic catheters will allow the operator to "feel" the resistance encountered by the catheter and to more precisely manipulate the tip. Recently, the ability to measure the catheter tissue interface pressure with the robotic system has led to visual feedback to the operator so that pressure can be modulated for good lesion size, while minimizing the risk of perforation [34]. Another progression of robotic technology will be the ability to perform ablation procedures from locations as distant as other continents, as has been done in the surgical field.

Novel materials will also make way for catheters that can be manipulated in ways that are not currently possible. Catheters constructed with electroactive polymers that can conform to different configurations based on the voltage applied [35] may deliver the right balance between stiffness and flexibility needed. The curvatures on such catheters could be adjusted in real time and allow for precise control of the catheter tip. Although currently available electroactive polymers do not provide sufficient deflection force necessary for clinical application, it is only a matter of time before this technology is introduced.

Summary

There are a wide variety of VTs that present challenges to current mapping and ablation techniques. Procedures using manual catheter control are time consuming and expose operators and patients to excessive radiation and fatigue. Technologies such as remote magnetic catheter navigation and robotic catheter control systems offer the ability to manipulate catheters remotely with better flexibility and may result in shorter procedure times and higher success rates. Regardless of which technologies prevail, the goals of finding mapping and ablation techniques that reduce radiation exposure, are more efficient, and minimize adverse outcomes, will remain. As newer, more challenging procedures such as ventricular substrate mapping and ablation are introduced, technologies to meet these demands will continue to evolve.

References

1 Calkins H, A Epstein, D Packer, et al. Catheter ablation of ventricular tachycardia in patients with structural heart disease using cooled radiofrequency energy: results of a prospective multicenter study. Cooled RF Multi Center Investigators Group. J Am Coll Cardiol 2000;35(7):1905–1914.

2 Soejima, K, E Delacretaz, M Suzuki, et al. Saline-cooled versus standard radiofrequency catheter ablation for infarct-related ventricular tachycardias. Circulation 2001;103(14):1858–1862.

3 Moodie DS. Adult congenital heart disease. Curr Opin Cardiol 1994;9(1):137–142.

4 Theocharopoulos N, J Damilakis, K Perisinakis, E Manios, P Vardas, N Gourtsoyiannis. Occupational exposure in the electrophysiology laboratory: quantifying and minimizing radiation burden. Br J Radiol 2006;79(944):644–651.

5 Gambale R, S Forucci, C Shah, M Weiser, S Forde. *Catheter Positioning Systems*, in *United States Patent Office*. 1999, C.R. Bard, Inc., USA.

6 Gibson C and H Seang. *Steerable catheter*, in *United States Patent Office*. 1999, C.R. Bard, Inc., USA.

7 Tillander H. Magnetic guidance of a catheter with articulated steel tip. Acta Radiol 1951;35:62–65.

8 Grady MS, MA Howard, III, RG Dacey, Jr, et al. Experimental study of the magnetic stereotaxis system for catheter manipulation within the brain. J Neurosurg 2000;93(2):282–288.

9 Dabus G, RJ Gerstle, DT Cross, III, CP Derdeyn, and CJ Moran. *Neuroendovascular magnetic navigation: clinical experience in ten patients.* Neuroradiology, 2007;49(4):351-355.

10 Faddis MN, W Blume, J Finney, et al. Novel, magnetically guided catheter for endocardial mapping and radiofrequency catheter ablation. Circulation 2002;106(23):2980–2985.

11 Faddis MN, J Chen, J Osborn, M Talcott, ME Cain, BD Lindsay. Magnetic guidance system for cardiac electrophysiology: a prospective trial of safety and efficacy in humans. J Am Coll Cardiol 2003;42(11):1952–1958.

12 Ernst S, F Ouyang, C Linder, et al. Initial experience with remote catheter ablation using a novel magnetic navigation system: magnetic remote catheter ablation. Circulation 2004;109(12):1472–1475.

13 Thornton AS, P Janse, DA Theuns, MF Scholten, LJ Jordaens. Magnetic navigation in AV nodal re-entrant tachycardia study: early results of ablation with one- and three-magnet catheters. Europace 2006;8(4):225–230.

14 Chun JK, S Ernst, S Matthews, et al. Remote-controlled catheter ablation of accessory pathways: results from the magnetic laboratory. Eur Heart J 2007;28(2):190–195.

15 Chun JK, B Schmidt, KH Kuck, S Ernst. Remote-controlled magnetic ablation of a right anterolateral accessory pathway-The superior caval vein approach. J Interv Card Electrophysiol 2006;16(1):65–68.

16 Ernst S, H Hachiya, JK Chun, F Ouyang. Remote catheter ablation of parahisian accessory pathways using a novel magnetic navigation system—a report of two cases. J Cardiovasc Electrophysiol 2005;16(6):659–662.

17 Pappone C, G Vicedomini, F Manguso, et al. Robotic magnetic navigation for atrial fibrillation ablation. J Am Coll Cardiol 2006;47(7):1390–1400.

18 Pappone C, V Santinelli. Remote navigation and ablation of atrial fibrillation. J Cardiovasc Electrophysiol 2007;18(Suppl 1):S18–S20.

19 Lemery R, P Brugada, J Janssen, E Cheriex, T Dugernier, HJ Wellens. Nonischemic sustained ventricular tachycardia: clinical outcome in 12 patients with arrhythmogenic right ventricular dysplasia. J Am Coll Cardiol 1989;14(1):96–105.

20 Klein LS, HT Shih, FK Hackett, DP Zipes, WM Miles. Radiofrequency catheter ablation of ventricular tachycardia in patients without structural heart disease. Circulation 1992;85(5):1666–1674.

21 Gerstenfeld EP, S Dixit, DJ Callans, Y Rajawat, R Rho, FE Marchlinski. Quantitative comparison of spontaneous and paced 12-lead electrocardiogram during right ventricular outflow tract ventricular tachycardia. J Am Coll Cardiol 2003;41(11):2046–2053.

22 Thornton AS, LJ Jordaens. Remote magnetic navigation for mapping and ablating right ventricular outflow tract tachycardia. Heart Rhythm 2006;3(6):691–696.

23 Thornton AS, J Res, JM Mekel, LJ Jordaens. Use of advanced mapping and remote magnetic navigation to ablate left ventricular fascicular tachycardia. Pacing Clin Electrophysiol 2006;29(6):685–688.

24 Burkhardt JD, WI Saliba, RA Schweikert, J Cummings, A Natale. Remote magnetic navigation to map and ablate left coronary cusp ventricular tachycardia. J Cardiovasc Electrophysiol 2006;17(10):1142–1144.

25 Marchlinski FE, DJ Callans, CD Gottlieb, E Zado. Linear ablation lesions for control of unmappable ventricular tachycardia in patients with ischemic and nonischemic cardiomyopathy. Circulation 2000;101(11):1288–1296.

26 Aryana A, A d'Avila, EK Heist, et al. Remote magnetic navigation to guide endocardial and epicardial catheter mapping of scar-related ventricular tachycardia. Circulation 2007;115(10):1191–1200.

27 Kwoh YS, J Hou, EA Jonckheere, S Hayati. A robot with improved absolute positioning accuracy for CT guided stereotactic brain surgery. IEEE Trans Biomed Eng 1988;35(2):153–160.

28 Cadiere GB, J Himpens, O Germay, et al. Feasibility of robotic laparoscopic surgery: 146 cases. World J Surg 2001;25(11):1467–1477.

29 Falcone T, JM Goldberg, H Margossian, L Stevens. Robotic-assisted laparoscopic microsurgical tubal anastomosis: a human pilot study. Fertil Steril 2000;73(5):1040–1042.

30 Marescaux J, J Leroy, F Rubino, et al. Transcontinental robot-assisted remote telesurgery: feasibility and potential applications. Ann Surg 2002;235(4):487–492.

31 Al-Ahmad A, JD Grossman, PJ Wang. Early experience with a computerized robotically controlled catheter system. J Interv Card Electrophysiol 2005;12(3):199–202.

32 Reddy VY, ZJ Malchano, S Abbarra, et al. Porcine pulmonary vein ablation using a novel robotic catheter control system and real-time integration of CT imaging with electroanatomical mapping. In: *Heart Rhythm*. Boston, MA; 2006.

33 Saliba WI, RA Schweikert, J Cummings, et al. Human pulmonary vein and flutter ablation using the robotic catheter control system and real-time integration of CT imaging with electroanatomical mapping. In: *Heart Rhythm*. Boston, MA; 2006.

34 Al-Ahmad A. The use of pressure sensory feedback in robotic catheter control systems. In *Hearth Rhythm*. Denver, CO; 2007.

35 Bar-Cohen Y. Transition of EAP material from novelty to practical applications – are we there yet? In EAPAD, SPIE's 8th Annual International Symposium on Smart Structures and Materials. Newport, CA; 2001.

CHAPTER 16

Current surgical techniques for ischemic ventricular tachycardia

Robert J. Moraca, Marci S. Bailey, & Ralph J. Damiano Jr

Introduction

The success of implantable cardioverter-defibrillators (ICDs) and catheter ablation has diminished the referral for surgery for the treatment of ventricular arrhythmias. However, it is important to understand the historically important role of surgery and the present indication for operation in the management of ventricular tachycardia (VT). Although ICDs have demonstrably improved survival by preventing sudden death, they fail to treat the underlying arrhythmogenic substrate. Thus, frequent discharges can impair quality of life [1]. Additionally, a population of patients surviving myocardial infarction with ventricular aneurysms, akinetic segments, and ischemic cardiomyopathies develop ventricular arrhythmias and also require surgical intervention for treatment of congestive heart failure. These patients would benefit from concomitant surgery for their VT.

Historical aspects of ventricular tachycardia surgery

In 1961, Estes and Izler from Duke University [2] reported a number of patients who underwent sympathectomy for ventricular tachycardia with reasonable success. However, in the late 1960s, it became apparent that myocardial ischemia initiated many ventricular arrhythmias, and that they were related to areas of infarction and scar. This led to the

development of two surgical approaches to address this problem: infarctectomy and coronary artery bypass grafting [3,4]. Unfortunately, these initial approaches to the surgical treatment of VT had high mortality rates, and relatively poor long-term success. They failed because they were not based on an understanding of the mechanisms involved in ischemic ventricular tachycardia [5] (Table 16.1).

Advances in our understanding of ischemic ventricular tachycardia during the 1970s led to a new surgical approach. Wellens and others [6–9] introduced intraoperative cardiac mapping techniques that for the first time were able to precisely identify myocardial activation during dysrhythmias. Ventricular tachycardia was found to be a reentrant arrhythmia, able to be initiated in the electrophysiology lab. It also became apparent that VT often arose from the border zone between infarcted and normal myocardium, and that the reentrant circuit was often subendocardial in origin [10–15]. This led to new surgical techniques that were guided by both preoperative and intraoperative electrophysiologic studies. The first directed surgical cure of refractory ventricular tachycardia was reported in 1975 [8]. This was a 54-year-old gentleman who presented with refractory ventricular tachycardia following two myocardial infarctions. Epicardial mapping was used to localize the site of earliest epicardial activity to the margin of the aneurysm. Subsequent resection of this area abolished the VT. In 1978, Dr Guiraudon [16] introduced the encircling endocardial ventriculotomy. This operation was designed to isolate the entire border zone from normal myocardium. A near-transmural incision was made from the endocardial surface of the left ventricle down to the epicardial surface (Figure 16.1). While

Ventricular Arrhythmias and Sudden Cardiac Death, 1st edition.
Edited by P.J. Wang, A. Al-Ahmad, H. Hsia, and P.C. Zei
© 2008 Blackwell Publishing, ISBN: 978-1-4051-6114-5.

Table 16.1 Results of nondirected ventricular tachycardia procedures

Procedure	n =	OP mortality	Failure	Success
Sympathectomy	12	25%	17%	58%
CABG	45	22%	22%	56%
Resection	95	24%	17%	59%
CABG and Resection	27	41%	4%	55%
Total (% is of mean group total)	179	26%	16%	58%

CABG, coronary artery bypass graft; OP, operative.

this technique met with clinical success, it caused significant ventricular dysfunction. In 1979, Harken and colleagues from the University of Pennsylvania [17] introduced a new technique involving endomyocardial resection directed by intraoperative mapping in 12 patients. They reported one operative mortality, with the remaining 11 patients having no recurrent arrhythmias at 1 year. In 1982, Moran [18] modified the endomyocardial resection by advocating an extended resection of all visible scar, which would obviate the need for intraoperative

mapping (Figure 16.2). These new procedures resulted in operative mortalities of between 10% and 20%. The success rates improved in some series to over 70%, and 5-year survival was approximately 60% (Table 16.2) [19–24]. Importantly, this surgical experience in the 1980s revealed that intraoperative mapping was not necessary to achieve good results if you did an extended endomyocardial resection. When examining almost 500 patients having either map-guided or nonguided extended resections, Hargrove and Miller [19] determined that the number of patients inducible at the postoperative electrophysiological study was not significantly different between groups.

With the introduction of the implantable cardioverter defibrillator into clinical practice, first as a surgically implanted device and then, beginning in the early 1990s, as a nonthoracotomy transvenous device, referrals of patients for ventricular tachycardia surgery decreased markedly. Thus, many physicians have overlooked the role that surgery continues to play in selected patients. Most worrisome, there has been a new generation of electrophysiologists and cardiac surgeons unfamiliar with

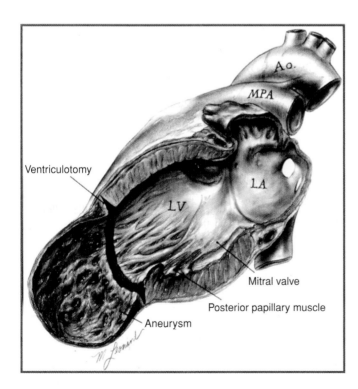

Figure 16.1 Encircling endocardial ventriculotomy.

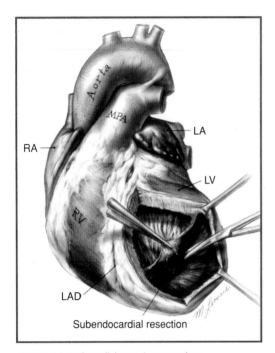

Subendocardial resection

Figure 16.2 Endocardial resection procedure.

ventricular tachycardia surgery. This chapter documents the present techniques and indications for the surgical treatment of ventricular tachycardia in the ICD era.

Table 16.2 Operative results in series with 50 or more patients

Series	n =	OP mortality	Post-OP inducibility
Pennsylvania [19]	314	16%	30%*
Alabama [20]	123	23%	21%†
Stanford [21]	98‡	17%	32%
Dusseldorf [19]	93	5%	19%
Northwestern [22]	79	13%	23%§
Virginia [23]	70	12%	16%
Duke/Barnes [24]	65	14%	2%

* 254 of 264 operative survivors underwent a postoperative electrophysiology study.

† 87 of 95 operative survivors underwent a postoperative electrophysiology study.

‡ Patients with ventricular tachycardia secondary to ischemic heart disease in a total series of 105 patients.

§ 61 of 69 operative survivors underwent a postoperative electrophysiology study.

OP, operative.

Surgical treatment of ventricular tachycardia

There are a number of very important points that need to be emphasized regarding surgical options for ventricular tachycardia. First of all, the surgical mortality in the ICD era has been significantly lower than that historically reported in the early clinical experience with direct ventricular tachycardia surgery. This is because high-risk patients (i.e., poor left ventricular function, no discrete aneurysm, polymorphic ventricular tachycardia) are no longer referred for surgery, but are preferentially treated with ICD. In a small series of patients reported from University of Virginia and from our institution, hospital mortality dropped to <5%, with surgical success rates over 70% [25].

Our experience at Washington University over the last 20 years has numbered 74 patients. In the last 10 years, 11 patients underwent direct VT surgery with no operative mortality. In this most recent era, the median ICU stay was 3 days and the median hospital length of stay was 11 days. While 27% of patients (3/11) had a recurrence of their ventricular tachycardia at a mean follow-up of 5.8 years, there have been no late deaths in this group due to the liberal use of adjunctive ICD therapy. The overall survival of the group over the last 20 years has been excellent, with a 5-year survival of 65%. Thus, in properly selected patients, a low operative mortality can be expected, with good late results.

The second important point regarding surgery is that the underlying left ventricular dysfunction can be addressed. This is not the case with catheter ablation, which simply takes care of the arrhythmogenic substrate. Coronary bypass grafting, left ventricular reconstruction or remodeling, and mitral valve repair—all can have a significant impact on late survival in appropriate patients [26,27]. It is critical that patients who are referred for surgery for their left ventricular dysfunction be offered a concomitant procedure to treat their ventricular tachycardia where indicated, due to the good success rates of preventing recurrent ventricular tachycardia [26,27]. This can improve patient's quality of life by decreasing the number of defibrillator shocks.

Finally, VT surgery can play a role in patients who are receiving frequent discharges from their device.

Quality of life of these patients is poor [1,28]. In patients who have failed catheter ablation or are poor candidates for this procedure, surgery can play an important role if the patients have an appropriate substrate. The different procedures for the treatment of ventricular tachycardia are discussed below.

Revascularization

Surgical coronary revascularization (coronary artery bypass graft, CABG) alone has not been highly effective at treating VT [29–31]. However, ischemia is a primary trigger for some ventricular arrhythmias and there has been ample evidence to suggest that CABG can alter the arrhythmic substrate in selected patients to reduce ventricular arrhythmias [32,33]. Several groups have documented that 40–60% of patients undergoing CABG with a preoperative clinical history of ventricular arrhythmias or fibrillation had no inducible ventricular arrhythmias at postoperative electrophysiological testing [29,30]. Folsom [34] demonstrated only 25% of patients after CABG and ICD implantation for preoperative ventricular arrhythmias had inducible arrhythmias postoperatively. Additionally, in the selected subset of patients with exercise-induced ischemia resulting in ventricular arrhythmias, surgical revascularization has been very effective. However, in the majority of patients with chronic ischemic VT, the results of CABG have been too unpredictable and most patients required concomitant ICD therapy. In patients with poor LV function, ICD plays a role even without a history of VT. The Multi-center Automatic Defibrillator Trial II (MADIT II) found that prophylactic ICD implantation improved survival in patients with prior MI and poor LV function [35–37].

The only candidates for CABG alone are patients with significant coronary artery disease, no ventricular dilation or aneurysm, and who suffer from documented exercise (or ischemia-induced) ventricular arrhythmias. Postoperative exercise testing and electrophysiological studies are used to determine whether implantation of an ICD is warranted.

Endocardial resection

The surgical approach entails the resection of all endocardial scar (Figure 16.2). This procedure, introduced by Harken in 1979 [17], has become the gold standard and the most commonly performed surgery for VT. The amount of ventricular tissue involved or its location near the posterior papillary muscle may limit a complete resection. In these instances, alternative ablation techniques are used either adjunctively or as the sole therapy. Although many groups have reported using energy sources such as laser, radiofrequency ablation, bipolar, and microwave, the most commonly used and well-studied ablation technology is cryoablation. Popularized in the 1980s, the cryoablation probe is applied to the scar and typically cooled to −60° C for 2–3 minutes, resulting in lesions up to 1 cm in depth.

Although intraoperative mapping has yielded a wealth of information into the mechanisms of ventricular arrhythmias, its clinical practicality and questionable added efficacy to VT surgery has prevented its widespread adoption. Virtually all surgeons have adopted a technique of resecting all visible endocardial scars without the use of intraoperative mapping.

Since 1986, 74 patients at Washington University, Barnes-Jewish Hospital, have undergone endocardial resection with adjunctive cryotherapy (ERP) for ventricular arrhythmias. The mean age was 57 ± 14 years, and 81% of patients were male. One-quarter of patients were either in New York Heart Association (NYHA) Class III or IV heart failure, and the mean left ventricular ejection fraction was 34 ± 9%. Ninety-two percent of patients underwent ERP with a concomitant procedure while 8% underwent ERP alone. The spectrum of other procedures included ERP + left ventricular aneurysm repair (26%), ERP + CABG (5%), ERP + CABG + left ventricular aneurysm repair (46%), and ERP + left ventricular aneurysm + other cardiac procedure (15%). The overall operative mortality was 15%, with a median intensive care unit (ICU) length of stay of 4 days and a median hospital length of stay at 12 days. As stated previously, there has been no operative mortality over the last 10 years. Late follow-up was complete in 89% of patients. A Kaplan–Meier survival analysis was performed and absolute survival for all patients in this series was 74% at 1 year and 65% at 5 years. Eighty-eight percent of the cases were performed during the first decade (1986–1996), reflecting the diminishing role of surgical management in this disease (Figure 16.3).

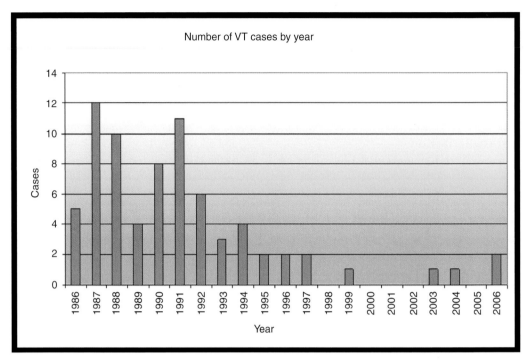

Figure 16.3 Washington University School of Medicine experience with VT surgery.

Left ventricular reconstruction

In 1985, Vincent Dor [38,39] described a surgical technique to restore a dilated left ventricle or ventricular aneurysm to its normal elliptical shape by reducing the volume. The Dor procedure uses an endoventricular circular patch to reduce ventricular volume, which subsequently reduces wall tension and ischemia. Good surgical candidates for left ventricular reconstruction will typically present with heart failure (ejection fraction <40%), coronary artery disease, large areas of myocardial akinesis (ventricular dilation), or a left ventricular aneurysm. These patients commonly have associated ventricular arrhythmias. Currently, Dor emphasizes the importance of complete revascularization (CABG), repair of any mitral pathology, and endocardial resection with cryoablation at the same setting. Several groups [10–15] have demonstrated that the triggers for ventricular arrhythmias occur at the scar border zone in patients with ischemic cardiomyopathy. Thus, the Dor procedure addresses ventricular arrhythmias by removing the anatomic substrate during resection of the postinfarct scar/aneurysm. In 1994, Dor and associates

[39] reported a 90% freedom from inducible ventricular tachycardia at 1 year following endocardial resection and left ventricle reconstruction in 106 patients. In 2004, Mickleborough [40] reported her long-term outcomes following LV reconstruction and coronary revascularization for patients with hypokinesis or akinesis and coronary artery disease with poor LV function. Results demonstrated freedom from ventricular tachycardia; sudden death at 1, 5, and 10 years was 99%, 97%, and 94%, respectively. In a study by Sartipy and colleagues [41], 53 patients with inducible VT preoperatively underwent the Dor procedure. With a mean follow-up of 3.7 ± 2.0 years, the freedom from postoperative spontaneous VT was 90%. In another study by Sartipy and colleagues [42], quality of life was assessed before operation and following the Dor procedure. The results demonstrated that quality of life, assessed by the physical component summary score of the Medical Outcome Study 36-Item Short Form, improved significantly ($P = 0.04$) at 6 months postoperatively. A significant and clinically relevant improvement in both physical aspects (+25%; $P < 0.001$) and mental aspects (+37%;

$P = 0.003$) of quality of life was found at late follow-up. In 2004, Maxey [43] demonstrated that the Dor procedure restores the left ventricle geometry, resulting in a mean ejection fraction increase of 12.5%. Ventricular function continues to improve over the patient's lifetime. The RESTORE [26] group experience examined a registry of 1198 postinfarction patients between 1998 and 2003 who underwent left ventricular restoration and found that 5-year freedom from hospital readmission for CHF was 78%. Additionally, 67% of patients were Class III or IV preoperatively while 85% were Class I or II postoperatively.

The efficacy of left ventricular restoration alone has been controversial. As discussed previously, the MADIT II trial has demonstrated that patients with poor left ventricular function benefit from prophylactic ICD implantation. LV restoration reduces the mechanical ventricular stretch, wall tension, and subsequent ischemia, which may have an effect on ventricular arrhythmogenicity. In addition, surgical removal of the infarct/scar can eliminate the ventricular reentrant circuits. However, the Cleveland Clinic experience [44] illustrated the lack of efficacy of the Dor procedure alone without endocardial resection surgery. In their series, 42% (48/113) of patients who had a postoperative electrophysiology study had inducible VT after the Dor procedure. In patients with ICDs, 15% either had sudden cardiac death or appropriate shocks. With early EPS, ICD implantation, or both, the overall incidence of sudden cardiac death was <1%. In 2004, DiDonato [27] demonstrated in 382 patients that left ventricular restoration with endocardial resection reduced the inducible ventricular tachycardia from 41 to 8%; suggesting that many patients may not need a postoperative ICD.

In our experience, it is recommended that all patients following the Dor procedure undergo postoperative EPS and/or implantation of an ICD if they have had a history of ventricular arrhythmias or inducible VT preoperatively.

Cardiac assist devices and heart transplantation

Rarely, patients will present with uncontrolled ventricular arrhythmias refractory to conventional surgical, ICD or medical therapy. Typically, these patients will have an end-stage cardiomyopathy resulting in incessant VT. If the patients are not amenable to conventional cardiac revascularization or other procedures, these malignant arrhythmias may be effectively palliated with a cardiac assist device, either as a bridge to transplantation or as destination therapy [45–47]. The cardiac assist device effectively reduces myocardial oxygen demand and can abate the ischemia-induced arrhythmias [48].

Conclusions

Implantable cardioverter defibrillators and catheter ablation have significantly reduced the role of surgery in the treatment of ventricular arrhythmias. When indicated, however, current surgical techniques can be quite successful. The surgical approach should be individualized to each patient. The current indications for surgery include the following:

1 In patients with ischemic VT requiring revascularization with poor left ventricular function and no significant wall thinning, CABG and ICD placement is the recommended treatment. If significant wall thinning or a discrete aneurysm is present, ventricular remodeling, extended endomyocardial resection, and cryoablation should be performed.

2 Surgery for VT should be considered for patients suffering from frequent ICD discharges that are poorly tolerated and have an amenable anatomic substrate. In the presence of frequent ICD shocks with a discrete LV aneurysm and/or wall thinning, ventricular remodeling, extended endomyocardial resection, and cryoablation should be considered.

References

1 Godemann F, Butter C, Lampe F, Linden M, Schlegl M, Schultheiss H-P. Panic disorders and agoraphobic: side effects of treatment with an implantable cardioverter/defibrillator. Clin Cardiol 2004;27:321–326.

2 Estes EH, Izlar HL. Recurrent ventricular tachycardia: a case successfully treated by bilateral cardiac sympathectomy. Am J Med 1961;31:493–497.

3 Ecker RR, Mullins CB, Grammer JC, Rea WJ, Atkins JM. Control of intractable ventricular tachycardia by coronary revascularization. Circulation 1971;44:666–670.

4 Heimbecker RO, Lemire G, Chen C. Surgery for massive myocardial infarction. An experimental study of emergency infarctectomy with a preliminary report on the clinical application. Circulation 1968;37(Suppl 4):II3–II11.

5 Ungerleider RM, Holman WL, Stanley TE, et al. Encircling endocardial ventriculotomy for refractory ischemic ventricular tachycardia. I. Electrophysiological effects. J Thorac Cardiovasc Surg 1982;83:840–849.

6 Wellens HJ, Schuilenburg RM, Durrer D. Electrical stimulation of the heart in patients with ventricular tachycardia. Circulation 1972;46:216–226.

7 Josephson M, Horowitz L, Farshidi A, Spear JF, Kastor JA, Moore EN. Recurrent sustained ventricular tachycardia: 2. Endocardial mapping. Circulation 1978;57:440–447.

8 Gallagher JJ, Oldham HN, Wallace AG, Peter RH, Kasell J. Ventricular aneurysm with ventricular tachycardia—Report of a case with epicardial mapping and successful resection. Am J Cardiol 1975;35:696–700.

9 Wittig JH, Boineau JP. Surgical treatment of ventricular arrhythmias using epicardial transmural and endocardial mapping. Ann Thorac Surg 1975;20:117–126.

10 Cox JL, McLaughlin VW, Flowers NC, Horan LG. The ischemic zone surrounding acute myocardial infarction. Its morphology as detected by dehydrogenase staining. Am Heart J 1968;76:650–659.

11 Fenoglio J, Pham T, Harken A, et al. Recurrent sustained ventricular tachycardia: structure and ultrastructure of subendocardial regions in which tachycardia originates. Circulation 1983;68:518–533.

12 Scherlag BJ, El-Sheriff N, Hopen RR, Lazzara R. Characterization and localization of ventricular arrhythmias resulting from myocardial ischemia and infarction. Circ Res 1974;35:372–383.

13 Gardner P, Ursell P, Fenoglio J, Wit AL. Electrophysiologic and anatomical basis for fractionated electrograms recorded from healed myocardial infarcts. Circulation 1985;72:596–611.

14 Dillon SM, Allessie MA, Ursell PC, Wit AL. Influences of anisotropic tissue structure on reentrant circuits in the epicardial border zone of subacute canine infarcts. Circ Res 1988;63:182–206.

15 Cox JL, Daniel TM, Sabiston DC Jr, Boineau JP. Desynchronized activation in myocardial infarction: a reentry basis for ventricular arrhythmias. Circulation 1969;39(Suppl 3):63.

16 Guiraudon G, Fontaine G, Frank R, Escande G, Etievent P, Cabrol C. Encircling endocardial ventriculotomy: a new surgical treatment for life-threatening ventricular tachycardias resistant to medical treatment following myocardial infarction. Ann Thorac Surg 1978;26:438–444.

17 Harken AH, Josephson ME, Horowitz LN. Surgical endocardial resection for the treatment of malignant ventricular tachycardia. Ann Surg 1979;190:456–460.

18 Moran JM, Kehoe RF, Loeb JM, Lichtenthal PR, Sanders JH, Michaelis LL. Extended endocardial resection for the treatment of ventricular tachycardia and ventricular fibrillation. Ann Thorac Surg 1982;34:538–552.

19 Hargrove WC, Miller JM. Endocardial ablation for ischemic ventricular tachycardia. Cardiac Surg State of the Art Rev 1990;4:247–253.

20 McGiffin DC, Kirklin JK, Plumb VJ, et al. Relief of life-threatening ventricular tachycardia and survival after direct operations. Circulation 1987;76:V93–V103.

21 Swerdlow CD, Mason JW, Stinson EB, Oyer PE, Winkle RA, Derby GC. Results of operations for ventricular tachycardia in 105 patients. J Thorac Cardiovasc Surg 1986;92:105–13.

22 Moran JM, Kehoe RF, Loeb JM, Sanders JH, Tommaso CL, Michaelis LL. Operative therapy of malignant ventricular rhythm disturbances. Ann Surg 1983;198:479–486.

23 Kron IL, Lerman BB, Nolan SP, Flanagan TL, Haines DE, DiMarco JP. Sequential endocardial resection for the surgical treatment of refractory ventricular tachycardia. J Thorac Cardiovasc Surg 1987;94:843–847.

24 Ferguson TB, Smith JM, Cox JL, Cain ME, Lindsay BD. Direct operation versus ICD therapy for ischemic ventricular tachycardia. Ann Thorac Surg 1994;58:1291–1296.

25 Johnson D, Cox J. Ventricular arrhythmias. In: Buxton B, ed. *Ischemic Heart Disease Surgical Management.* London: Mosby International 1999:327–335.

26 Athanasuleas CL, Buckberg GD, Stanley AW, et al. (RESTORE Group). Surgical ventricular restoration: the RESTORE Group experience. Heart Fail Rev 2004;9:287–297.

27 DiDonato M, Sabatier M, Dor V, Buckberg G (RESTORE Group). Ventricular arrhythmias after LV remodelling: surgical ventricular restoration or ICD? Heart Fail Rev 2004;9:299–306.

28 Wallace RL, Sears SF, Lewis TA, Griffis JT, Curtis A, Conti J. Predictors of quality of life in long-term recipients of implantable cardioverter defibrillators. J Cardiopulm Rehabil 2002;22:278–281.

29 Garan H, Ruskin JN, DiMarco JP, et al. Electrophysiologic studies before and after myocardial revascularization in patients with life-threatening ventricular arrhythmias. Am J Cardiol 1983;51:519–524.

30 Manolis AS, Rastegar H, Estes NA III. Effects of coronary artery bypass grafting on ventricular arrhythmias: results with electrophysiological testing and long-term follow-up. Pacing Clin Electrophysiol 1993;16:984–991.

31 Bigger JT Jr. Prophylactic use of implanted cardiac defibrillators in patients at High risk for ventricular arrhythmias after coronary-artery bypass graft surgery. N Engl J Med 1997;337:1569–1575.

32 Can L, Kayikçioğlu M, Halil H, et al. The effect of myocardial surgical revascularization on left ventricular late potentials. Ann Noninvasive Electrocardiol 2001;6:84–91.

33 Takami Y, Ina H. Quantitative improvement in signal-averaged electrocardiography after coronary artery bypass grafting. Circ J 2003;67:146–148.

34 Lee JH, Folsom DL, Biblo LA, et al. Combined internal cardioverter-defibrillator implantation and myocardial revascularization for ischemic ventricular arrhythmias: optimal cost-effective strategy. Cardiovasc Surg 1995;3:393–397.

35 Moss AJ, Zareba W, Hall WJ, et al. (Multicenter Automatic Defibrillator Implantation Trial II Investigators).

Prophylactic implantation of a defibrillator in patients with myocardial infarction and reduced ejection fraction. N Engl J Med 2002;346:877–883.

36 Moss A, Cannom D, Daubert J, et al. Multi-center automatic defibrillator implantation trial II (MADIT II): design and clinical protocol. Ann Noninvasive Electrocardiol 1999;4:83–91.

37 Manolis AS, Rastegar H, Estes NA III. Prophylactic automatic implantable cardioverter-defibrillator patches in patients at high risk for postoperative ventricular tachyarrhythmias. J Am Coll Cardiol 1989;13:1367–1373.

38 Dor V, Saab M, Coste P, Kornaszewska M, Montiglio F. Left ventricular aneurysm: a new surgical approach. Thorac Cardiovasc Surg 1989;37:11–19.

39 Dor V, Sabatier M, Montiglio F. Results of non-guided subtotal endocardiectomy associated with left ventricular reconstruction in patients with ischemic ventricular arrhythmias. J Thorac Cardiovasc Surg 1994;107:1301–1308.

40 Mickleborough LL, Merchant N, Ivanov J, Rao V, Carson S. Left ventricular reconstruction: early and late results. J Thorac Cardiovasc Surg 2004;128:27–37.

41 Sartipy U, Albage A, Straat E, Insulander P, Lindblom D. Surgery for ventricular tachycardia in patients undergoing left ventricular reconstruction by the Dor procedure. Ann Thorac Surg 2006;81:65–71.

42 Sartipy U, Albage A, Lindblom D. Improved health-related quality of life and functional status after surgical ventricular restoration. Ann Thorac Surg 2007;83:1381–1387.

43 Maxey TS, Reece TB, Ellman PI, et al. Coronary artery bypass with ventricular restoration is superior to coronary artery bypass alone in patients with ischemic cardiomyopathy. J Thorac Cardiovasc Surg 2004;127:428–434.

44 O'Neill JO, Starling RC, Khaykin Y, et al. Residual high incidence of ventricular arrhythmias after left ventricular reconstructive surgery. J Thorac Cardiovasc Surg 2005;130:1250–1256.

45 Fasseas P, Kutalek SP, Samuels FL, Holmes EC, Samuels LE. Ventricular assist device support for management of sustained ventricular arrhythmias. Tex Heart Inst J 2002;29:33–36.

46 Kulick DM, Bolman RM, Salerno CT, Bank AJ, Park SJ. Management of recurrent ventricular tachycardia with ventricular assist device placement. Ann Thorac Surg 1998;66:571–573.

47 Ziv O, Dizon J, Thosani A, Naka Y, Magnano AR, Garan H. Effects of left ventricular assist device therapy on ventricular arrhythmias. J Am Coll Cardiol 2005;45:1428–1434.

48 Wadia Y, Delgado RM, Odegaard P, Frazier OH. Jarvik 2000 FlowMaker axial-flow left ventricular assist device support for management of refractory ventricular arrhythmias. Congest Heart Fail 2004;10:195–196.

CHAPTER 17

Epidemiology and etiologies of sudden cardiac death

Keane K. Lee, Amin Al-Ahmad, Paul J. Wang, &
Robert J. Myerburg

Prevention of sudden cardiac death

Sudden cardiac death is one of the most significant and challenging problems facing modern medicine today. The magnitude of the problem and the sudden nature of its occurrence make the problem of sudden cardiac death particularly difficult to overcome. As shown in Table 17.1, there is a large range of the strategies to prevent sudden death. A combination of these preventative strategies may be used to reduce the incidence of sudden cardiac death. For a complex challenge such as sudden cardiac death, these efforts include public education, screening programs to identify patients at risk, and preventative medicine strategies to prevent the underlying diseases leading to sudden death. In patients with prior cardiac arrest or at higher risk, secondary prevention strategies include implantable defibrillators or pharmacological therapy to treat life-threatening ventricular arrhythmias. Lastly, community intervention strategies are important for the emergency care and rescue of patients with cardiac arrest and may involve strategies to increase the access of the automatic external defibrillator.

Definition

Sudden cardiac death (SCD) can be defined strictly as death from a rapid termination of heart pump

Ventricular Arrhythmias and Sudden Cardiac Death, 1st edition.
Edited by P.J. Wang, A. Al-Ahmad, H. Hsia, and P.C. Zei
© 2008 Blackwell Publishing, ISBN: 978-1-4051-6114-5.

function due to a primary cardiac cause [1]. However, because the exact timing and cause of death is difficult to determine, authors have used various surrogate definitions. A commonly used definition is natural and unanticipated death associated with the abrupt loss of consciousness less than 1 hour after the start of acute symptoms [2]. This definition, which includes the key elements of rapid progression, unexpected nature, and natural cause, does not distinguish between cardiac and noncardiac causes. Therefore, another proposed criterion is the lack of evidence of a noncardiac cause, such as airway obstruction or intracranial hemorrhage [3]. In patients who have an arrest out of the hospital without any witness, the chronicity of symptoms and lack of a noncardiac cause can be difficult to establish. Because two-thirds of cardiac deaths occur outside of the hospital and only a small percentage of these are resuscitated, there is some uncertainty in the diagnosis and estimation of the incidence of SCD [3,4].

Trends over time

The age- and sex-adjusted incidence of SCD has declined steadily over the two decades since 1979. Although the incidence of ventricular fibrillation has followed the overall trend of decline in SCD, the incidence of asystole and pulsus electrical activity have remained stable. (Figure 17.1) The decline in the incidence of SCD has paralleled the decline in the incidence of coronary artery disease and other cardiovascular and vascular diseases such as hypertension and stroke.

Table 17.1 Range of preventative strategies for sudden cardiac death

Primary prevention
    Public education
    Screening programs
    Preventative medicine
Secondary prevention
    Prophylaxis against fatal arrhythmias
    Management of cardiac arrest survivors
Community intervention
    Emergency rescue
    Strategic automatic external defibrillator access

Incidence

General population

Estimates of the incidence of SCD in the United States per year vary between about 200,000 and 400,000 [5,6]. The most widely accepted estimate is 300,000 SCDs per year, which corresponds to about 120/100,000 people per year or approximately 1 per 1000 adults per year. This revised estimate made in 2001 from the American Heart Association Statistical Update is based on adjudicated death certificate information. Table 17.2 provides the primary and secondary conditions used to determine the incidence of SCD based on death certificate information. In Table 17.3, the Florida Department of Health statistics indicate the range of conditions with reported SCD. Atherosclerotic coronary artery disease is the most prevalent condition associated with SCD.

About 20% of all the deaths in the United States are classified as SCD [7]. The estimate of deaths from SCD varies due to the different definitions of SCD used by different sources. There may be geo-graphic differences in SCD, likely related to differences in incidences of coronary artery disease [8]. One study showed that out-of-hospital cardiac arrest attended by emergency medical services ranged between 36/100,000 and 128/100,000 per year in different communities [9]. In addition, how the temporality of SCD is defined changes the estimate of incidence significantly. For instance if the definition of "sudden" is "within 24 hours of symptoms," the number of SCDs increases, but the proportion due to cardiac causes becomes lower [10].

About 65% of patients with SCD have some coronary artery disease [11]. Conversely, 50% of coronary artery disease deaths are sudden, defined as less than 1 hour of symptom onset [12]. Among consecutive resuscitated patients, of whom all received coronary angiograms, 48% had a coronary artery occlusion while 71% had clinically significant coronary artery disease [13]. These statistics confirm that the incidence of SCD in any population depends on the incidence of coronary artery disease.

People who are at high risk for SCD, such as those with severely impaired left ventricular systolic function, have been identified through various studies. Implantation of defibrillators in those with severely depressed left ventricular ejection fraction have been shown in randomized control trials to increase survival [14,15]. However, the absolute number of patients who suffer from SCD in these high-risk subgroups is significantly smaller than those who have SCD in the general population without these risk factors (Figure 17.2). Therefore, the effect of implantable defibrillators on the total incidence of SCD has not been large [16,17]. The challenge in the future is to find screening markers

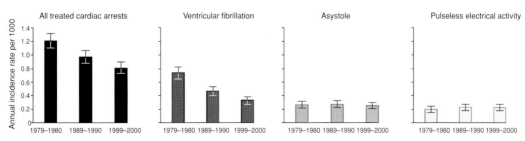

Figure 17.1 Age- and sex-adjusted incidence of treated out-of-hospital cardiac arrest. (Adapted from Cobb, et al., JAMA 2002;288:3008–3013 [111].)

Table 17.2 Sudden cardiac death estimates out of hospital death certificate data

Reported primary cause		Reported secondary cause		Edited primary cause		Adjudication
ICD-9	Condition	ICD-9	Condition	ICD-9	Condition	SCD count
410–414	ASHD	427.5	SCA	—	—	Yes
427.5	SCA	410–414	ASHD	410–414	ASHD	Yes
427.5	SCA	None provided		—	—	No
425	CM	427.5	SCA	—	—	No
428	HF	427.5	SCA	—	—	No
427.5	SCA	425	CM	425	CM	No

ASHD, atherosclerotic heart disease; SCA, sudden cardiac arrest.

Table 17.3 Edited death certificate data on sudden cardiac death, State of Florida, Department of Health, 1999

ICD-9	Number (%)	ICD-9	Number (%)
410	13,032 (35.1%)	410	13,032 (30.0%)
411	92 (0.3%)	411	92 (0.2%)
412	30 (0.1%)	412	30 (0.1%)
413	53 (0.1%)	413	53 (0.1%)
414	22,322 (60.1%)	414	22,322 (51.3%)
427	1644 (4.4%)	427	1644 (3.8%)
428	1033 (2.4%)	429	5307 (12.2%)

Modified from: Myerburg RJ, J Cardiovasc Electrophysiol 2002 [110].

that can identify high-risk patients in the at-large population.

Risk factors

Age

The incidence of SCD increases with age with the peak risk in men being in the 55–64-year age group. The Framingham study data show a peak of 6.75:1 risk in men in the 55–64-year age group, as compared to 2.17:1 in the 65–74-year age group [4]. These findings may be attributed to the increase in coronary artery disease with age, which is usually manifested by the late middle-age period [18]. The incidence is 100 times less in people younger than 30 years as compared to people older than 35 years [19–21]. The estimated incidence of SCD in those younger than 30 years is 1 in 100,000 per year. However, the proportion of sudden deaths that are cardiac in nature is higher among the younger population [6]. Among people who die from heart disease, 76% in the 20–39 year age group were sudden compared to 62% in the 45–54 year age group in men and 58% in the 55–64 year age group [4,22,23]. These studies indicate that although young people are less likely to have SCD, a higher proportion of deaths in the young tend to be sudden and from a cardiac etiology.

Heredity

Because of the strong correlation between coronary artery disease and SCD, hereditary factors that influence coronary artery disease will indirectly predict SCD. Acute coronary syndrome, which is a subset of coronary artery disease, involves atherogenesis, plaque destabilization and rupture, and thrombosis. This cascade may then lead to arrhythmogenesis. Genetic studies have identified mutations and polymorphisms in this pathway that may predispose individuals to SCD by acute coronary syndrome [24–27]. Two population studies show a clustering of SCD as a manifestation of coronary artery disease in certain families [28,29]. In the future, genetic tests may become potent predictors for SCD in the setting of coronary artery disease. Already, in congenital ion channel syndromes, such as congenital long-QT syndromes and the Brugada syndrome, genetic studies have identified multiple gene defects that explain clustering of symptoms in families [30,31].

Gender

Males have a higher incidence of SCD as compared to females up until the middle-age years, because women are significantly less likely to have coronary artery disease in the premenopausal period [32–34]. In the Framingham study, 89% of SCDs were in men [4]. Other prospective studies have shown

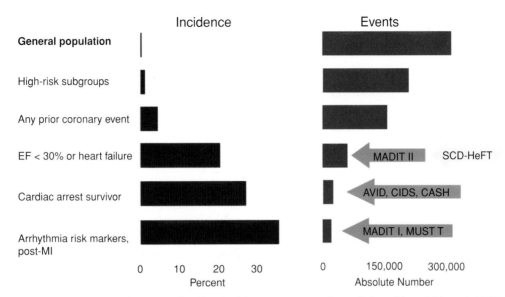

Figure 17.2 Subgroup risk and incidence of sudden death in coronary artery disease. (Adapted from Cobb, et al., JAMA 2002;288:3008–3013 [111].)

similar percentages, ranging from 75% to 89%, of SCD occurring in males. Even though females are less likely to have SCD, their risk of SCD also increases with the typical coronary artery disease risk factors [32,33,35]. Specifically, smoking, diabetes, and oral contraceptive use are causes most strongly associated with SCD in women [33,36].

Race

There have been multiple studies comparing the incidence of SCD in Caucasians versus African-Americans [10,34,37,38]. One large study of all SCDs in Chicago, Illinois in the 2-year period of 1987 and 1988, showed a higher incidence among African-Americans as compared to Caucasians in all age groups [38]. More recent randomized control trials of implantable cardioverter-defibrillators (ICDs) showed that African-Americans are more likely to suffer SCD even after ICD placement. In the MADIT-II study [39], the benefit of ICDs in reducing the incidence of SCD was found to be more evident in Caucasians than in African-Americans. Another study [40] showed that African-Americans with nonsustained ventricular tachycardia were significantly more likely than Caucasians to suffer from cardiac arrest or arrhythmic death, even in the setting of antiarrhythmic medication and ICDs. The etiology of these disparities may be due

to differences in environment, genetics, or access to care.

Medical, environmental, and lifestyle risk factors

Traditional coronary artery disease risk factors identify population subgroups that are at increased risk of ischemic heart disease and, thus, also SCD. However, these risk factors do not discriminate among the high-risk coronary artery disease population, in which individuals are more likely to have SCD [41]. The presence of traditional risk factors in people with SCD versus those who have any manifestation of coronary artery disease are relatively similar [22]. Moving from predicting population risk to accurately assessing individual risk of SCD is an active research goal. Genetic risk factors to identify individuals susceptible to vulnerable plaque and other pathology in the mechanistic chain of SCD may be keys to assessing risk.

Among coronary artery disease risk factors, cigarette smoking and obesity are associated with an increased proportion of coronary artery disease deaths that are sudden. Cigarette smokers in the Framingham study had a twofold to threefold increase in SCD risk [4]. Obesity in the same study was also predictive of a higher proportion of cardiac deaths being sudden. The Framingham study shows no significant relation between a sedentary lifestyle and SCD [4]. However, SCD was more likely to occur during acute physical exertion, demonstrated by a relative risk of 17. Among those with a sedentary lifestyle, the relative risk of SCD during acute physical exertion rose to 74. A study of patients with ICDs shows that the relative risk of a ventricular tachyarrhythmia was 7.5 during physical activity [42]. Even though SCD tends to occur more often during physical exertion, habitual exercise decreases the risk of SCD [43,44].

Psychosocial stressors are associated with myocardial infarction and SCD [45–48]. For instance, after the earthquake in the Los Angeles, California area in 1994, there was a sharp rise in cases of SCDs in the subsequent 6-day period as compared to control periods in the years before [49]. In another study of people with ICDs, the relative risk of a ventricular tachyarrhythmia was 9.5 during periods of mental stress [42]. A third study showed that ventricular tachyarrhythmic events recorded by ICDs were more likely to be preceded by periods of anger [50].

Underlying cardiac diseases associated with SCD

The majority of individuals experiencing SCD have coronary artery disease as an underlying condi-

Table 17.4 Causes of out-of-hospital and emergency-department deaths: USA, 1998

Attributed cause (ICD-9)	Deaths (%) [n = 456,076]
Acute ischemic HD (410–411)	26.9%
Chronic ischemic HD (412–414)	35.3%
Cardiovascular disease, unspecified (429.2)	12.1%
Cardiomyopathy/arrhythmias (425–427)	9.3%
Hypertensive HD (402, 404)	5.1%
Heart failure (428)	6.7%
Carditis, valvular HD (420–424, 429.1–429.2)	2.2%
Pulmonary HD (415–417)	1.0%
All others (390–398, 429.3–429.9)	1.4%

HD, heart disease.
Modified from Zheng Z-J, Croft JB, Giles WH, et al., Circulation, 2001 [11].

Table 17.5 Etiological bases of sudden cardiac death

Coronary artery disease	80%
Cardiomyopathies	10–15%
Valvular/inflammatory/infiltrative	±5%
Subtle, poorly defined lesions	≤ 1%
Molecular lesions	
Functional abnormalities	
"Normal hearts"—idiopathic VF	

tion, representing approximately 80% of all patients (Tables 17.4 and 17.5). The second most common cause of SCD is the range of cardiomyopathies, including nonischemic and hypertrophic categories. Valvular, inflammatory, and infiltrative diseases represent approximately 5% of patients having SCD. A wide range of other lesions are responsible the remaining 1% or less of patients with SCD. These include the ion channel abnormalities such as long-QT syndrome and Brugada syndrome and idiopathic ventricular fibrillation.

Coronary artery disease

About 60–80% of SCD is attributed to coronary artery disease [51–54]. The clinical presentation of sudden death in this large group of patients with SCD is quite varied (Figure 17.3) About one-third of patients have known coronary artery diseases and may have nonspecific markers of sudden death. Nearly one-third of patients present with SCD as the first clinical presentation. About 20% of patients present with acute myocardial infarction or an unstable syndrome. A much smaller proportion of patients have hemodynamic risk markers such as decreased ejection fraction or arrhythmic risk markers. The proportion of these presentations will greatly impact the success of various strategies to reduce SCD and guide the development of future successful techniques (Table 17.8).

More than 50% of people with SCD have some evidence of acute changes in coronary artery plaque morphology leading to plaque rupture and thrombosis, seen on autopsy [6]. In one study of autopsies in people with SCD caused by acute coronary occlusion, 44% had superficial erosions of plaque, but showed no plaque rupture [55]. Figure 17.4 illustrates the cascade of events that may lead to SCD in ischemic heart disease. Coronary

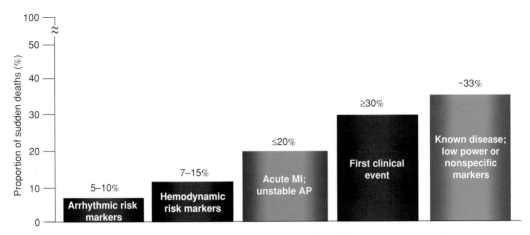

Figure 17.3 Distribution of sudden death among clinical subgroups. (Adapted from Myerburg RJ, J Cardiovasc Electrophysiol 2002 [110].)

risk factors play a role in atherogenesis, which creates a conditional risk for cardiovascular events. Changes in plaque anatomy may result in a transition from the quiescent state to a less stable transitional state. Further disruption in plaque structure may lead to an acute coronary syndrome. These events may serve as triggers of life-threatening ventricular arrhythmias, particularly in the presence of an underlying electrophysiological predisposition. The sudden blockage of an epicardial coronary artery, leading to acute myocardial ischemia, causes a shift of many ions across the cardiomyocyte membrane [51]. This change in electrophysiological activity initiates a cascade of activity on ion channels and transporters, the details of which are not fully known. In a canine model, intracellular K^+ shifts extracellularly, thereby slowing conduction, changing refractoriness, and leading to ventricular tachycardia/fibrillation [56,57]. Intracellular K^+ loss is accompanied by intracellular Na^+ and Ca^{2+} gain, which trigger delayed afterdepolarization [58]. These depolarizations may propagate action potentials that ultimately cause ventricular tachycardia.

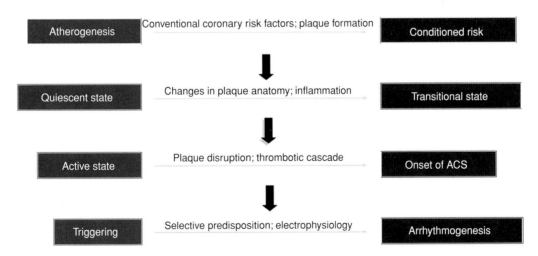

Figure 17.4 Cascade for sudden cardiac death in coronary artery disease. Adapted from Myerburg RJ, J Cardiovasc Electrophysiol 2002 [110].

Genetic Imprints on the Coronary Heart Disease SCD Cascade

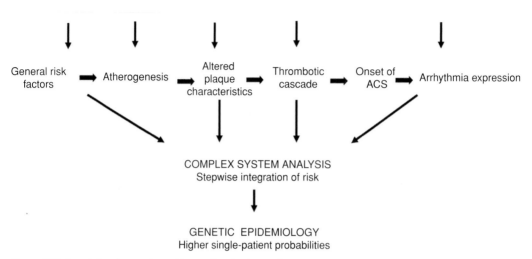

Figure 17.5 Genetic imprints on the sudden cardiac death cascade in coronary artery disease. (Adapted from Myerburg RJ, J Cardiovasc Electrophysiol 2002 [110].)

Even though sudden coronary artery occlusion is the most common trigger for SCD, not all people who have had such an event have SCD. A case–control study of ST-elevation myocardial infarction patients compared those with and without cardiac arrest from ventricular fibrillation. Patient variables that were analyzed included traditional coronary artery disease risk factors, along with infarct location, family history of SCD, and amount of ST elevation. Family history of SCD had the largest odds ratio of 2.7 [59]. This finding supports the hypothesis that a genetic substrate for SCD in addition to a triggering event, such as acute myocardial ischemia, ultimately leads to SCD. In people with congenital long-QT syndrome and the Brugada syndrome, multiple single-nucleotide polymorphisms have been shown to alter ion channel activity, thereby increasing the risk of SCD [31,60]. Genetic polymorphisms could also serve as the basis to explain predilections for SCD in the setting of acute myocardial ischemia. Figure 17.5 illustrates the genetic factors that may play a role in arrhythmogenesis from many influences. Genetic factors may separately influence the general risk factors such as hypertension, diabetes, etc. as well as the process of atherogenesis itself. In addition, genetic influences may play a role in determining plaque characteristics

Cardiomyopathies
Dilated and other cardiomyopathies
Cardiomyopathy, including ischemic, idiopathic, and hypertrophic types, is the primary etiology in 10–15% of SCDs [2]. Cardiomyopathy accounts for the second largest number of SCDs from cardiac causes behind coronary artery disease [54]. The absolute risk of SCD increases with worsening left ventricular function and impairment of functional capacity [61,62]. Therefore, it makes sense that implantation of defibrillators in patients with low left ventricular ejection fraction confers a survival benefit [14,15]. With increasingly severe cardiomyopathy, the proportion of deaths due to SCD decreases even though the absolute number of SCDs increases (Figure 17.6) [63,64]. This paradoxical finding can be attributed to the fact that the risk of nonarrhythmic death supersedes that of arrhythmic death with worsening heart failure. Thus, the degree of heart failure lacks specificity in identifying patients at risk for SCD. The high risk of SCD in people with cardiomyopathy applies regardless of etiology. Increased incidences of SCD are noted in those with ischemic, idiopathic, alcoholic, viral myopathic, and peripartum cardiomyopathies [65–69].

Acute heart failure from any cause increases risk of SCD. During periods of decompensated

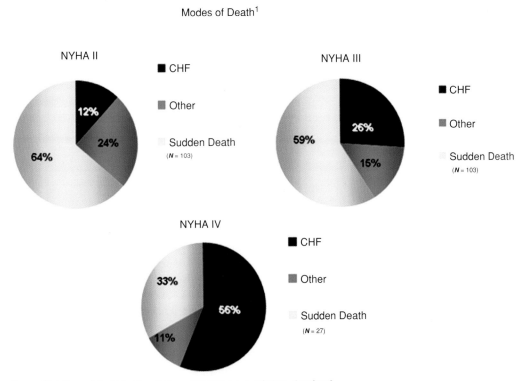

Figure 17.6 Type of death in Class II, III, and IV NYHA heart failure class [109].

heart failure and fluid overload, the myocardial fibers are stretched dramatically. Stretching of the myocardium has been experimentally shown to increase arrhythmogenesis [70]. Another animal model has shown that myocardial stretching accelerates and increases the complexity of ventricular fibrillation [71]. Electrolyte disturbances and neurohormonal changes in the setting of acute heart failure also likely contribute to SCD. During decompensated heart failure, the sympathetic nervous system and catecholamines are upregulated, which has been hypothesized to play an important role in SCD [72].

Hypertrophic cardiomyopathy

Hypertrophic cardiomyopathy (HCM) is a genetic cardiac disorder that is primarily manifested by thickening of the ventricular septum and in some cases left ventricular outflow tract obstruction. HCM, the most common genetic cardiac disorder, is found in one out of every 500 people in the general population [73]. The majority of people with

HCM are asymptomatic, but some develop dyspnea, angina, syncope, and sudden death from arrhythmias [73]. Even though the overall mortality of people with HCM is less than 1% per year, HCM is the most common cause of sudden death in young athletes (Table 17.6) [74–76]. SCD can occur in anyone with HCM, but those with SCD tend to be younger. About 70% of people with SCD associated with HCM are younger than 35 years [77]. Therefore, risk stratification has been an area of intense interest.

About 10–20% of the HCM population have an increased risk for SCD [78]. No single test or disease feature captures the risk profile of an HCM patient. Therefore, a set of criteria have been developed to better define the high-risk population. Risk factors for sudden death include cardiac arrest from ventricular fibrillation, sustained ventricular tachycardia, family history of SCD, syncope, ventricular septal wall thickness greater than 30 mm, abnormal blood pressure with exercise, nonsustained ventricular tachycardia, and possibly malignant genetic

Table 17.6 Sudden cardiac death
in adolescents and young adults

Cardiomyopathies
  Dilated
  Hypertrophic
Right ventricular dysplasia
Electrical abnormalities
  Long-QT syndromes
  Brugada syndrome
  W-P-W syndrome
Viral myocarditis
Abnormal coronary arteries
Drug-induced arrhythmias
Inflammatory/infiltrative diseases
Idiopathic ventricular fibrillation
Diseases of heart valves
Undefined causes

Table 17.7 Risk factors for sudden cardiac death: familial
clustering in the Paris Prospective Study I

Hx of parental	SCD	Fatal MI	Controls	p
Sudden death events	[n = 118] 22 [18.6%]	[n = 192] 19 [9.9%]	[n = 6762] – [718, 10.6%]	0.02
Relative risk	1.95 [P = 0.005]	0.97 [P = NS]		
Absolute risk w/(+) Hx	2.90% [22/759]	2.50% [19/759]	— [718/759]	

From Jouven X, et al., Circulation 1999 [29].

defect [79]. To establish the SCD risk profile, HCM patients should have a careful history and physical examination, two-dimensional echocardiography, ambulatory Holter monitoring, and an exercise test. Although some mutations such as those related to β-myosin heavy chains and troponin T may be associated with higher frequency of early death compared to other mutations, genetic testing is primarily used to identify family members with the disease rather than for risk stratification [80].

Inflammatory, infiltrative, neoplastic cardiomyopathy

There are a large number of cardiac diseases in this category and they are all associated with increased SCD with or without heart failure. The disease spectrum includes viral myocarditis, myocardial vasculitis, sarcoidosis, systemic sclerosis, amyloidosis, hemochromatosis, arrhythmogenic right ventricular dysplasia (ARVD), intramural tumors, and intracavitary tumors [2]. In one study, 67% of cardiac sarcoid disease deaths were attributed to SCD [81]. The incidence of SCD in cardiac amyloidosis has been reported to be about 30% [82].

ARVD is manifested by the fibrofatty infiltration of the right ventricular, thereby causing right ventricular dysfunction and ventricular arrhythmias [83–85]. In the United States, up to 20% of SCD in young people is attributed to ARVD [85,86]. A case series of 100 people with ARVD showed that the most common symptoms presented are palpitations (27%), syncope (26%), and SCD (23%) [87]. In another study of ARVD patients who received ICDs, 39% of primary prevention patients and 85% of secondary prevention patients received appropriate shocks [88]. Strenuous exercise and acute mental stress have been shown to be triggers of SCD in ARVD [89–92]. Risk factors for SCD in the ARVD population include history of SCD, ventricular tachycardia not responsive to antiarrhythmic

Table 17.8 Cascade of indicators of risk of SCD

Variables	Examples	Measures
Conventional evolution risk factors	Framingham risk index	Predict of disease
Anatomic Disease screening	Electron beam tomography	Identify abnormal coronary arteries
Clinical marker	EF; stress test Angiography	Extent of disease
Transient risk predictors	Inflammatory markers	Prediction of unstable plaques
Individual risk predictors	familial/genetic profiles	Specific SCD expression

medication, and poor right ventricular function [93].

Electrophysiological abnormalities

SCD in the structurally normal heart is not common, accounting for about 5% of patients with SCD. Primary electrophysiological abnormalities can cause SCD in structurally normal hearts. Electrophysiological diseases that increase the risk of SCD can be classified into those disturbing the conduction system and those affecting repolarization. Conduction system abnormalities include His–Purkinje system fibrosis and anomalous pathways, such as Wolff–Parkinson–White syndrome [94]. Repolarization abnormalities include congenital and acquired long-QT syndromes and the Brugada syndrome.

Congenital long-QT interval syndromes

The congenital long-QT syndrome is caused by a range of genetic defects of the molecular structure in ion channel proteins that delay ventricular repolarization. Syncope and SCD, the manifestations of long-QT syndrome, occur most commonly during adolescence [95]. The major risk factor for syncope or SCD in adolescents is a QTc interval greater than 500 milliseconds [96–98]. Three genotypes (LQT1, LQT2, and LQT3) have been established, corresponding to the KCNQ1 and KCNH2 potassium channels and the SCN5A sodium channel, respectively. LQT1 and LQT2 patients have a higher lifetime risk of cardiac events compared to those with LQT3 [99]. Gender and age also contribute to risk stratification. Males have a higher risk of cardiac events in the preadolescent group, while females have a higher risk in the adolescent period and afterwards [95]. β-Blockers decrease the risk of SCD in the LQT1 and LQT2 groups, but not in those with the LQT3 genotype [100].

Brugada syndrome

The Brugada syndrome is an inherited disorder of sodium ion channels that is marked by ECG characteristics of right bundle branch block and ST segment elevation in the precordial leads [101]. People with the Brugada syndrome have a high incidence of SCD despite having structurally normal hearts. The initial symptom presented is usually syncope from rapid polymorphic ventricular tachycardia or SCD. Patients usually have ventricular tachycardia or fibrillation episodes at night or in the early morning hours [102]. The ECG may be normal in many individuals with the Brugada syndrome. The typical ECG abnormalities can be triggered by hyperthermia, potassium abnormalities, sodium channel blockers, β-blockers, α-adrenergic agonists, or alcohol and cocaine use [103]. In endemic areas, such as southeast Asia, the syndrome has a prevalence of 5 in 10,000 people and is the leading cause of death in men under the age of 40 years [102]. Mutations in the SCN5A sodium channel gene have been found in 18–30% of families with the Brugada syndrome [104]. The high-risk characteristics of the Brugada syndrome that may justify ICD implantation include SCD, syncope, family history of SCD, and positive electrophysiological study [104].

Accessory pathways

SCD can rarely occur in people with A-V accessory pathways, such as in the Wolff–Parkinson–White syndrome. The mechanism for SCD is rapid conduction through the accessory pathway during atrial fibrillation. In the setting of a short antegrade refractory period of the accessory pathway, rapid ventricular stimulation can lead to ventricular tachycardia degenerating into ventricular fibrillation [94,105,106]. The incidence of SCD in those with Wolff–Parkinson–White syndrome is estimated to be 0.15–0.39% over a follow-up period of 3–10 years [106]. Cardiac arrest is thus an uncommon manifestation of the syndrome. However, because of the concern for risk of SCD in young individuals with Wolff–Parkinson–White syndrome, a low threshold exists for electrophysiological testing to assess the risk of SCD in symptomatic patients. Factors increasing the risk of SCD include: the shortest pre-excited R–R interval during spontaneous or induced atrial fibrillation of less than 250 milliseconds, symptomatic tachycardia, multiple accessory pathways, and Ebstein's anomaly [107].

Conclusions

Sudden cardiac death is one of the most important and challenging public health problems facing modern medicine today [108]. The magnitude of the problem and its sudden nature make it particularly difficult to overcome. The diversity of causes and factors makes a single strategy an unlikely solution. Instead, multiple methods of addressing the manifold risk factors and influences are warranted.

References

1 Survivors of out-of-hospital cardiac arrest with apparently normal heart. Need for definition and standardized clinical evaluation. Consensus Statement of the Joint Steering Committees of the Unexplained Cardiac Arrest Registry of Europe and of the Idiopathic Ventricular Fibrillation Registry of the United States. Circulation 1997;95(1):265–272.

2 Bruanwald E, Zipes DP, Libby P. *Heart Disease: A Textbook of Cardiovascular Medicine*, 6th ed. New York: WB Saunders Company; 2001.

3 Cummins RO, Chamberlain DA, Abramson NS, et al. Recommended guidelines for uniform reporting of data from out-of-hospital cardiac arrest: the Utstein Style. A statement for health professionals from a task force of the American Heart Association, the European Resuscitation Council, the Heart and Stroke Foundation of Canada, and the Australian Resuscitation Council. Circulation 1991;84(2):960–975.

4 Kannel WB, Thomas HE Jr. Sudden coronary death: the Framingham Study. Ann N Y Acad Sci 1982;382:3–21.

5 Podrid PJ, Myerburg RJ. Epidemiology and stratification of risk for sudden cardiac death. Clin Cardiol 2005;28(11 Suppl 1):I3–I11.

6 Zipes DP, Camm AJ, Borggrefe M, et al. ACC/AHA/ESC 2006 Guidelines for Management of Patients With Ventricular Arrhythmias and the Prevention of Sudden Cardiac Death: a report of the American College of Cardiology/American Heart Association Task Force and the European Society of Cardiology Committee for Practice Guidelines (writing committee to develop Guidelines for Management of Patients With Ventricular Arrhythmias and the Prevention of Sudden Cardiac Death): developed in collaboration with the European Heart Rhythm Association and the Heart Rhythm Society. Circulation 2006;114(10):e385–e484. Epub, August 25, 2006.

7 Yamada Y, Izawa H, Ichihara S, et al. Prediction of the risk of myocardial infarction from polymorphisms in candidate genes. N Engl J Med 2002;347(24):1916–1923.

8 Gillum RF, Engdahl J, Bang A, Karlson BW, Lindqvist J, Herlitz J. Geographic variation in sudden coronary death characteristics and outcome among patients suffering from out of hospital cardiac arrest of non-cardiac aetiology. Am Heart J 1990;119(2 Pt 1):380–389.

9 Engdahl J, Bang A, Karlson BW, Lindqvist J, Herlitz J. Characteristics and outcome among patients suffering from out of hospital cardiac arrest of non-cardiac aetiology. Resuscitation 2003;57(1):33–41.

10 Kuller L, Lilienfeld A, Fisher R. An epidemiological study of sudden and unexpected deaths in adults. Medicine (Baltimore) 1967;46(4):341–361.

11 Zheng ZJ, Croft JB, Giles WH, et al. Sudden cardiac death in the United States, 1989 to 1998 Precursors of sudden coronary death. Factors related to the incidence of sudden death. Circulation 2001;104(18):2158–2163.

12 Kannel WB, Doyle JT, McNamara PM, Quickenton P, Gordon T. Precursors of sudden coronary death. Factors related to the incidence of sudden death. Circulation 1975;51(4):606–613.

13 Spaulding CM, Joly LM, Rosenberg A, et al. Immediate coronary angiography in survivors of out-of-hospital cardiac arrest. N Engl J Med 1997;336(23):1629–1633.

14 Bardy GH, Lee KL, Mark DB, et al. Amiodarone or an implantable cardioverter-defibrillator for congestive heart failure. N Engl J Med 2005;352(3):225–237.

15 Moss AJ, Zareba W, Hall WJ, et al. Prophylactic implantation of a defibrillator in patients with myocardial infarction and reduced ejection fraction. N Engl J Med 2002;346(12):877–883.

16 Myerburg RJ, Interian A Jr, Mitrani RM, Kessler KM, Castellanos A. Frequency of sudden cardiac death and profiles of risk. Am J Cardiol 1997;80(5B):10F–19F.

17 Myerburg RJ, Mitrani R, Interian A Jr, Castellanos A. Interpretation of outcomes of antiarrhythmic clinical trials: design features and population impact. Circulation 1998;97(15):1514–1521.

18 Holmberg M, Holmberg S, Herlitz J. Incidence, duration and survival of ventricular fibrillation in out-of-hospital cardiac arrest patients in Sweden. Resuscitation 2000;44(1):7–17.

19 Wren C, O'Sullivan JJ, Wright C, et al. Sudden death in children and adolescents. Paediatric out-of-hospital cardiac arrests—epidemiology and outcome. Causes of sudden unexpected cardiac death in the first two decades of life. Heart 2000;83(4):410–413.

20 Kuisma M, Suominen P, Korpela R, et al. Paediatric out-of-hospital cardiac arrests—epidemiology and outcome. Causes of sudden unexpected cardiac death in the first two decades of life. Resuscitation 1995;30(2):141–150.

21 Steinberger J, Lucas RV Jr, Edwards JE, Titus JL. Causes of sudden unexpected cardiac death in the first two decades of life. Am J Cardiol 1996;77(11):992–995.

22 Holmes DR Jr, Davis K, Gersh BJ, et al. Risk factor profiles of patients with sudden cardiac death and death from other cardiac causes: a report from the Coronary Artery Surgery Study (CASS). Sudden and unexpected deaths in young adults. An epidemiological study. J Am Coll Cardiol 1989;13(3):524–530.

23 Kuller L, Lilienfeld A, Fisher R. Sudden and unexpected deaths in young adults. An epidemiological study. JAMA 1966;198(3):248–252.

24 Boerwinkle E, Ellsworth DL, Hallman DM, et al. Genetic analysis of atherosclerosis: a research paradigm for the common chronic diseases. Identification of genes potentially involved in rupture of human atherosclerotic

plaques. Single nucleotide polymorphisms in multiple novel thrombospondin genes may be associated with familial premature myocardial infarction. Hum Mol Genet 1996;5(Spec No):1405–1410.

25 Faber BC, Cleutjens KB, Niessen RL, et al. Identification of genes potentially involved in rupture of human atherosclerotic plaques. Single nucleotide polymorphisms in multiple novel thrombospondin genes may be associated with familial premature myocardial infarction. Circ Res 2001;89(6):547–554.

26 Topol EJ, McCarthy J, Gabriel S, et al. Single nucleotide polymorphisms in multiple novel thrombospondin genes may be associated with familial premature myocardial infarction. Circulation 2001;104(22):2641–2644.

27 Spooner PM, Albert C, Benjamin EJ, et al. Sudden cardiac death, genes, and arrhythmogenesis: consideration of new population and mechanistic approaches from a National Heart, Lung, and Blood Institute workshop, Part II. Circulation 2001;103(20):2447–2452.

28 Friedlander Y, Siscovick DS, Weinmann S, et al. Family history as a risk factor for primary cardiac arrest. Predicting sudden death in the population: the Paris Prospective Study I. Circulation 1998;97(2):155–160.

29 Jouven X, Desnos M, Guerot C, Ducimetiere P. Predicting sudden death in the population: the Paris Prospective Study I. Circulation 1999;99(15):1978–1983.

30 Schott JJ, Charpentier F, Peltier S, et al. Mapping of a gene for long QT syndrome to chromosome 4q25-27. Am J Hum Genet 1995;57(5):1114–1122.

31 Makita N, Sumitomo N, Watanabe I, Tsutsui H. Novel SCN5A mutation (Q55X) associated with age-dependent expression of Brugada syndrome presenting as neurally mediated syncope. Heart Rhythm 2007;4(4):516–519. Epub, November 10, 2006.

32 Schatzkin A, Cupples LA, Heeren T, et al. The epidemiology of sudden unexpected death: risk factors for men and women in the Framingham Heart Study. Sudden death in the Framingham Heart Study. Differences in incidence and risk factors by sex and coronary disease status. Sudden cardiac death in Hispanic Americans and African Americans. Am Heart J 1984;107(6):1300–1306.

33 Schatzkin A, Cupples LA, Heeren T, Morelock S, Kannel WB, Gillum RF. Sudden death in the Framingham Heart Study. Differences in incidence and risk factors by sex and coronary disease status. Sudden cardiac death in Hispanic Americans and African Americans. Am J Epidemiol 1984;120(6):888–899.

34 Gillum RF. Sudden cardiac death in Hispanic Americans and African Americans. Am J Public Health 1997;87(9):1461–1466.

35 Krueger DE, Ellenberg SS, Bloom S, et al. Risk factors for fatal heart attack in young women. Am J Epidemiol 1981;113(4):357–370.

36 Jick H, Dinan B, Herman R, Rothman KJ. Myocardial infarction and other vascular diseases in young women. Role of estrogens and other factors. JAMA 1978;240(23):2548–2552.

37 Hagstrom RM, Federspiel CF, Ho YC, et al. Incidence of myocardial infarction and sudden death from coronary heart disease in Nashville, Tennessee. Racial differences in the incidence of cardiac arrest and subsequent survival. The CPR Chicago Project. Circulation 1971;44(5):884–890.

38 Becker LB, Han BH, Meyer PM, et al. Racial differences in the incidence of cardiac arrest and subsequent survival. The CPR Chicago Project. N Engl J Med 1993;329(9):600–606.

39 Vorobiof G, Goldenberg I, Moss AJ, Zareba W, McNitt S. Effectiveness of the implantable cardioverter defibrillator in blacks versus whites (from MADIT-II). Am J Cardiol 2006;98(10):1383–1386. Epub, October 2, 2006.

40 Russo AM, Hafley GE, Lee KL, et al. Racial differences in outcome in the Multicenter UnSustained Tachycardia Trial (MUSTT): a comparison of whites versus blacks. Circulation 2003;108(1):67–72. Epub, June 23, 2003.

41 Grundy SM, Balady GJ, Criqui MH, et al. Primary prevention of coronary heart disease: guidance from Framingham. A statement for healthcare professionals from the AHA Task Force on Risk Reduction. American Heart Association. Circulation 1998;97(18):1876–1887.

42 Fries R, Konig J, Schafers HJ, Bohm M. Triggering effect of physical and mental stress on spontaneous ventricular tachyarrhythmias in patients with implantable cardioverter-defibrillators. Clin Cardiol 2002;25(10):474–478.

43 Mittleman MA, Maclure M, Tofler GH, Sherwood JB, Goldberg RJ, Muller JE. Triggering of sudden death from cardiac causes by vigorous exertion. Triggering of acute myocardial infarction by heavy physical exertion. Protection against triggering by regular exertion. Determinants of Myocardial Infarction Onset Study Investigators. N Engl J Med 1993;329(23):1677–1683.

44 Albert CM, Mittleman MA, Chae CU, Lee IM, Hennekens CH, Manson JE. Triggering of sudden death from cardiac causes by vigorous exertion. N Engl J Med 2000;343(19):1355–1361.

45 Rozanski A, Blumenthal JA, Kaplan J, et al. Impact of psychological factors on the pathogenesis of cardiovascular disease and implications for therapy. Effects of mental stress in patients with coronary artery disease: evidence and clinical implications. Social and psychosocial influences on sudden cardiac death, ventricular arrhythmia and cardiac autonomic function. Psychological factors and survival in the cardiac arrhythmia suppression trial (CAST): a reexamination. Circulation 1999;99(16):2192–2217.

46 Krantz DS, Sheps DS, Carney RM, et al. Effects of mental stress in patients with coronary artery disease: evidence and clinical implications. Social and psychosocial influences on sudden cardiac death, ventricular arrhythmia and cardiac autonomic function. Psychological factors and survival in the cardiac arrhythmia suppression trial (CAST): a reexamination. JAMA 2000;283(14):1800–1802.

47 Hemingway H, Malik M, Marmot M, et al. Social and psychosocial influences on sudden cardiac death, ventricular arrhythmia and cardiac autonomic function. Psychological factors and survival in the cardiac arrhythmia suppression trial (CAST): a reexamination. Eur Heart J 2001;22(13):1082–1101.

48 Thomas SA, Friedmann E, Wimbush F, Schron E. Psychological factors and survival in the cardiac arrhythmia suppression trial (CAST): a reexamination. Am J Crit Care 1997;6(2):116–126.

49 Leor J, Poole WK, Kloner RA. Sudden cardiac death triggered by an earthquake. N Engl J Med 1996;334(7):413–419.

50 Lampert R, Joska T, Burg MM, Batsford WP, McPherson CA, Jain D. Emotional and physical precipitants of ventricular arrhythmia. Circulation 2002;106(14):1800–1805.

51 Rubart M, Zipes DP. Mechanisms of sudden cardiac death. J Clin Invest 2005;115(9):2305–2315.

52 Myerburg RJ, Kessler KM, Castellanos A. Sudden cardiac death: epidemiology, transient risk, and intervention assessment. Ann Intern Med 1993;119(12):1187–1197.

53 Myerburg RJ, Interian A Jr, Mitrani RM, et al. Frequency of sudden cardiac death and profiles of risk. Sudden cardiac death: epidemiology, transient risk, and intervention assessment. Am J Cardiol 1997;80(5B):10F–19F.

54 Zipes DP, Wellens HJ. Sudden cardiac death. Circulation 1998;98(21):2334–2351.

55 Farb A, Tang AL, Burke AP, Sessums L, Liang Y, Virmani R. Sudden coronary death. Frequency of active coronary lesions, inactive coronary lesions, and myocardial infarction. Circulation 1995;92(7):1701–1709.

56 Wu J, Zipes DP. Transmural reentry triggered by epicardial stimulation during acute ischemia in canine ventricular muscle. Am J Physiol Heart Circ Physiol 2002;283(5):H2004–H2011.

57 Takahashi T, van Dessel P, Lopshire JC, et al. Optical mapping of the functional reentrant circuit of ventricular tachycardia in acute myocardial infarction. Heart Rhythm 2004;1(4):451–459.

58 Shivkumar K, Deutsch NA, Lamp ST, Khuu K, Goldhaber JI, Weiss JN. Mechanism of hypoxic K loss in rabbit ventricle. J Clin Invest 1997;100(7):1782–1788.

59 Dekker LR, Bezzina CR, Henriques JP, et al. Familial sudden death is an important risk factor for primary ventricular fibrillation: a case-control study in acute myocardial infarction patients. Circulation 2006;114(11):1140–1145. Epub, August 28, 2006.

60 Rubart M, Zipes DP. Genes and cardiac repolarization: the challenge ahead. Circulation 2005;112(9):1242–1244.

61 Myerburg RJ, Kessler KM, Castellanos A. Sudden cardiac death. Structure, function, and time-dependence of risk. Circulation 1992;85(Suppl 1):I2–I10.

62 Bigger JT Jr, Fleiss JL, Kleiger R, Miller JP, Rolnitzky LM. The relationships among ventricular arrhythmias, left ventricular dysfunction, and mortality in the 2 years after myocardial infarction. Circulation 1984;69(2):250–258.

63 Luu M, Stevenson WG, Stevenson LW, Baron K, Walden J. Diverse mechanisms of unexpected cardiac arrest in advanced heart failure. Circulation 1989;80(6):1675–1680.

64 Packer M. Lack of relation between ventricular arrhythmias and sudden death in patients with chronic heart failure. Circulation 1992;85(Suppl 1):I50–I56.

65 Kjekshus J. Arrhythmias and mortality in congestive heart failure. Am J Cardiol 1990;65(19):42I–48I.

66 Packer M. Sudden unexpected death in patients with congestive heart failure: a second frontier. Circulation 1985;72(4):681–685.

67 Huang SK, Messer JV, Denes P. Significance of ventricular tachycardia in idiopathic dilated cardiomyopathy: observations in 35 patients. Am J Cardiol 1983;51(3):507–512.

68 Meinertz T, Hofmann T, Kasper W, et al. Significance of ventricular arrhythmias in idiopathic dilated cardiomyopathy. Am J Cardiol 1984;53(7):902–907.

69 Poll DS, Marchlinski FE, Buxton AE, Doherty JU, Waxman HL, Josephson ME. Sustained ventricular tachycardia in patients with idiopathic dilated cardiomyopathy: electrophysiologic testing and lack of response to antiarrhythmic drug therapy. Circulation 1984; 70(3):451–456.

70 Surawicz B. Ventricular fibrillation. J Am Coll Cardiol 1985;5(Suppl 6):43B–54B.

71 Chorro FJ, Canoves J, Guerrero J, et al. Opposite effects of myocardial stretch and verapamil on the complexity of the ventricular fibrillatory pattern: an experimental study. Pacing Clin Electrophysiol 2000;23(11 Pt 1):1594–1603.

72 Hara H, Ogihara T, Nakamaru M, Rakugi H, Tateyama H. Changes in the levels of plasma atrial natriuretic peptide, hemodynamic measurements, and the levels of vasoactive hormones during the clinical course of congestive heart failure. Clin Cardiol 1988;11(11):743–747.

73 Maron BJ, Gardin JM, Flack JM, Gidding SS, Kurosaki TT, Bild DE. Prevalence of hypertrophic cardiomyopathy in a general population of young adults. Echocardiographic analysis of 4111 subjects in the CARDIA Study. Coronary Artery Risk Development in (Young) Adults. Circulation 1995;92(4):785–789.

74 Braunwald E, Lambrew CT, Rockoff SD, Ross J Jr, Morrow AG. Idiopathic hypertrophic subaortic stenosis. I. A description of the disease based upon an analysis of 64 patients. Circulation 1964;30:(Suppl 4):3–119.

75 Spirito P, Seidman CE, McKenna WJ, Maron BJ. The management of hypertrophic cardiomyopathy. N Engl J Med 1997;336(11):775–785.

76 Maron BJ, Moller JH, Seidman CE, et al. Impact of laboratory molecular diagnosis on contemporary diagnostic criteria for genetically transmitted cardiovascular diseases: hypertrophic cardiomyopathy, long-QT syndrome, and marfan syndrome. A statement for healthcare professionals from the councils on clinical cardiology, cardiovascular disease in the young, and basic science, American Heart Association. Circulation 1998;98(14):1460–1471.

77 Maron BJ, McKenna WJ, Danielson GK, et al. American College of Cardiology/European Society of Cardiology Clinical Expert Consensus Document on Hypertrophic Cardiomyopathy. A report of the American College of Cardiology Foundation Task Force on Clinical Expert Consensus Documents and the European Society of Cardiology Committee for Practice Guidelines. Eur Heart J 2003;24(21):1965–1991.

78 Elliott PM, Poloniecki J, Dickie S, et al. Sudden death in hypertrophic cardiomyopathy: identification of high risk patients. J Am Coll Cardiol 2000;36(7):2212–2218.

79 Nishimura RA, Holmes DR Jr. Clinical practice. Hypertrophic obstructive cardiomyopathy. N Engl J Med 2004;350(13):1320–1327.

80 Maron BJ. Hypertrophic cardiomyopathy: a systematic review. JAMA 2002;287(10):1308–1320.

81 Silverman KJ, Hutchins GM, Bulkley BH. Cardiac sarcoid: a clinicopathologic study of 84 unselected patients with systemic sarcoidosis. Circulation 1978;58(6):1204–1211.

82 Wright JR, Calkins E. Clinical-pathologic differentiation of common amyloid syndromes. Medicine (Baltimore) 1981;60(6):429–448.

83 Marcus FI, Fontaine G, Marcus FI, et al. Arrhythmogenic right ventricular dysplasia/cardiomyopathy: a review right ventricular dysplasia: a report of 24 adult cases. Pacing Clin Electrophysiol 1995;18(6):1298–1314.

84 Marcus FI, Fontaine GH, Guiraudon G, et al. Right ventricular dysplasia: a report of 24 adult cases. Circulation 1982;65(2):384–398.

85 Thiene G, Nava A, Corrado D, Rossi L, Pennelli N. Right ventricular cardiomyopathy and sudden death in young people. N Engl J Med 1988;318(3):129–133.

86 Shen WK, Edwards WD, Hammill SC, Bailey KR, Ballard DJ, Gersh BJ. Sudden unexpected nontraumatic death in 54 young adults: a 30-year population-based study. Am J Cardiol 1995;76(3):148–152.

87 Dalal D, Nasir K, Bomma C, et al. Arrhythmogenic right ventricular dysplasia: a United States experience. Circulation 2005;112(25):3823–3832. Epub, December 12, 2005.

88 Piccini JP, Dalal D, Roguin A, et al. Predictors of appropriate implantable defibrillator therapies in patients with arrhythmogenic right ventricular dysplasia. Heart Rhythm 2005;2(11):1188–1194.

89 Leclercq JF, Coumel P. Characteristics, prognosis and treatment of the ventricular arrhythmias of right ventricular dysplasia. Eur Heart J 1989;10(Suppl D): 61–67.

90 Leclercq JF, Potenza S, Maison-Blanche P, Chastang C, Coumel P. Determinants of spontaneous occurrence of sustained monomorphic ventricular tachycardia in right ventricular dysplasia. J Am Coll Cardiol 1996;28(3):720–724.

91 Fornes P, Ratel S, Lecomte D. Pathology of arrhythmogenic right ventricular cardiomyopathy/dysplasia—an autopsy study of 20 forensic cases. J Forensic Sci 1998;43(4):777–783.

92 Furlanello F, Bertoldi A, Dallago M, et al. Cardiac arrest and sudden death in competitive athletes with arrhythmogenic right ventricular dysplasia. Pacing Clin Electrophysiol 1998;21(1 Pt 2):331–335.

93 Priori SG, Aliot E, Blomstrom-Lundqvist C, et al. Task force on sudden cardiac death of the European Society of Cardiology. Eur Heart J 2001;22(16):1374–1450.

94 Klein GJ, Bashore TM, Sellers TD, Pritchett EL, Smith WM, Gallagher JJ. Ventricular fibrillation in the Wolff-Parkinson-White syndrome. N Engl J Med 1979;301(20):1080–1085.

95 Sauer AJ, Moss AJ, McNitt S, et al. Long QT syndrome in adults. J Am Coll Cardiol 2007;49(3):329–337. Epub, January 4, 2007.

96 Moss AJ, Schwartz PJ, Crampton RS, et al. The long QT syndrome. Prospective longitudinal study of 328 families. Circulation 1991;84(3):1136–1144.

97 Schwartz PJ, Moss AJ, Vincent GM, Crampton RS. Diagnostic criteria for the long QT syndrome. An update. Circulation 1993;88(2):782–784.

98 Vincent GM, Timothy KW, Leppert M, Keating M. The spectrum of symptoms and QT intervals in carriers of the gene for the long-QT syndrome. N Engl J Med 1992;327(12):846–852.

99 Zareba W, Moss AJ, Schwartz PJ, et al. Influence of genotype on the clinical course of the long-QT syndrome. International Long-QT Syndrome Registry Research Group. N Engl J Med 1998;339(14):960–965.

100 Moss AJ, Zareba W, Hall WJ, et al. Effectiveness and limitations of beta-blocker therapy in congenital long-QT syndrome. Circulation 2000;101(6):616–623.

101 Brugada J, Brugada R, Brugada P. Right bundle-branch block and ST-segment elevation in leads V1 through V3: a marker for sudden death in patients without demonstrable structural heart disease. Circulation 1998;97(5):457–460.

102 Nademanee K, Veerakul G, Nimmannit S, et al. Arrhythmogenic marker for the sudden unexplained death syndrome in Thai men. Circulation 1997;96(8):2595–2600.

103 Herbert E, Chahine M. Clinical aspects and physiopathology of Brugada syndrome: review of current concepts. Can J Physiol Pharmacol 2006;84(8–9):795–802.

104 Antzelevitch C, Brugada P, Borggrefe M, et al. Brugada syndrome: report of the second consensus conference: endorsed by the Heart Rhythm Society and the European Heart Rhythm Association. Circulation 2005;111(5):659–670. Epub, January 17, 2005.

105 Dreifus LS, Haiat R, Watanabe Y, Arriaga J, Reitman N. Ventricular fibrillation. A possible mechanism of sudden death in patients and Wolff-Parkinson-White syndrome. Circulation 1971;43(4):520–527.

106 Munger TM, Packer DL, Hammill SC, et al. A population study of the natural history of Wolff-Parkinson-White syndrome in Olmsted County, Minnesota, 1953–1989. Circulation 1993;87(3):866–873.

107 Blomstrom-Lundqvist C, Scheinman MM, Aliot EM, et al. ACC/AHA/ESC guidelines for the management of

patients with supraventricular arrhythmias—executive summary. A report of the American college of cardiology/American heart association task force on practice guidelines and the European society of cardiology committee for practice guidelines (writing committee to develop guidelines for the management of patients with supraventricular arrhythmias) developed in collaboration with NASPE-Heart Rhythm Society. J Am Coll Cardiol 2003;42(8):1493–1531.

108 Huikuri HV, Castellanos A, Myerburg RJ. Sudden death due to cardiac arrhythmias. N Engl J Med 2001;345(20):1473–1482.

CHAPTER 18

Non-invasive tests for risk stratification in ischemic and non-ischemic cardiomyopathy

J. Thomas Bigger, Mark C. Haigney, & Robert E. Kleiger

In this chapter we discuss noninvasive tests that have value for selecting patients for prophylactic implantable cardioverter defibrillators (ICD). The criteria used to select patients for ICD prophylaxis for the Sudden Cardiac Death in Heart Failure Trial (SCD-HeFT) [1], i.e., left ventricular ejection fraction (LVEF) <0.36 and New York Heart Association Class II or III heart failure symptoms, are evidence-based and commonly used to select patients in clinical practice. This group of patients has a moderate risk for cardiac death and has significant benefit from ICD therapy. Unfortunately, fewer than 80% of patients selected using these criteria have an appropriate ICD shock and the absolute reduction in deaths is 7.2% during 5 years of follow-up. Thus, most patients bear the inconvenience of ICD therapy as well as risk of physical and psychological complications without deriving benefit from their implanted device. Furthermore, the health care system bears substantial expenses for prophylactic ICDs that never give therapy for ventricular tachyarrhythmias. The low rate of ICD usage in patients who receive them prophylactically motivates a continuing effort to improve risk stratification. Currently, it is our view that there is no mandate for ICD prophylaxis, but every patient eligible for coverage should be evaluated and an individualized assessment and decision should be made.

Ventricular Arrhythmias and Sudden Cardiac Death, 1st edition. Edited by P.J. Wang, A. Al-Ahmad, H. Hsia, and P.C. Zei © 2008 Blackwell Publishing, ISBN: 978-1-4051-6114-5.

Formerly, risk stratification focused on combining tests to improve the positive predictive accuracy, at the expense of selecting a smaller and smaller high-risk group. Currently, a new concept is being explored: to find tests that identify, among the group with a low LVEF, a subgroup of patients that has such a low mortality rate that ICD prophylaxis is unlikely to improve survival. Because SCD-HeFT criteria identify patients with ischemic or nonischemic cardiomyopathy who are not only at risk, but who, as a group, also benefit from ICD prophylaxis, further risk stratification in patients with reduced LVEF should have high negative predictive accuracy (low false negative rate) to avoid excluding patients who would benefit from having ICD therapy using current indications. In this chapter, we do not consider the diagnosis and treatment of myocardial ischemia because these issues are usually addressed before patients are evaluated for prophylactic ICD.

Risk factors for sudden death in cardiomyopathy

The majority of sudden deaths in cardiomyopathy patients are due to tachyarrhythmias (VT or VF) that result from an unhappy interaction between abnormal myocardial substrate and transient "triggering" factors [2]. These fixed and transient elements can be evaluated with many parameters, but Coumel and, more recently, Zareba [3] have categorized tests into three domains that appear critical to the initiation of tachyarrhythmias: myocardial substrate, autonomic nervous system (ANS), and

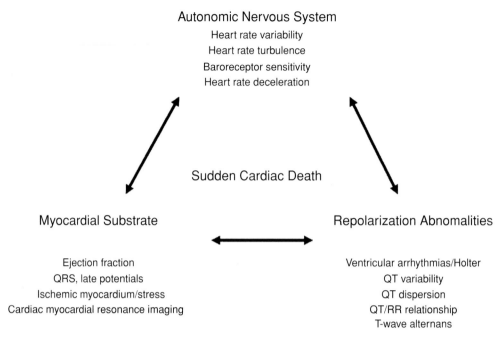

Figure 18.1 The modified Coumel model depicting three critical domains contributing to sudden cardiac death and their representative noninvasive measures. (From reference [8], with permission.)

repolarization abnormalities (see Figure 18.1). While this construct makes certain arbitrary allocations, it is a helpful model of our present understanding, and we used it to structure this chapter. This conceptual model derives indirect support from previous randomized controlled trial experience. The MADIT II trial randomized postinfarction patients on the basis of an LVEF < 0.31; the trial's success underscores the important contribution of abnormal substrate to subsequent cardiac arrest [4]. Nevertheless, using LVEF as the main criterion for selecting patients for ICD prophylaxis was associated with a relatively high number needed to treat (17 at 2-yr follow up) to save one life in MADIT II compared to MADIT (4 at 2.4 yr) and the Multicenter Unsustained Tachycardia Trial (MUSTT) (3 at 5 yr) [5]. In these early primary prevention trials, patients had to have inducible sustained ventricular tachyarrhythmias as well as reduced LVEF to participate [6,7]. While this stringent approach identified a high-risk population, an unacceptably high proportion of uninducible participants in the MUSTT registry experienced cardiac arrest during follow up (12% at 2 yr and 24% at 5 yr) [7], suggesting that their risk stratification procedure was too restrictive. Echocardiography and electrophysiologic testing may fail as adequate risk stratifiers because they do not assess the role of potential triggers of arrhythmogenesis, e.g., autonomic nervous activity and transient repolarization abnormalities. In this chapter we will consider the evidence for novel and established strategies for risk stratification in cardiomyopathy patients. Although the ideal approach for selecting patients for ICD prophylaxis risk stratification has not been established, no single test is likely to be ideal, given the complexity of mechanisms responsible for sudden death. The model illustrated in Figure 18.1 represents one attempt to categorize mechanisms of sudden death and organize a variety of tests that can be employed to predict sudden death. It seems likely that successful identification of patients who are likely or unlikely to benefit from ICD prophylaxis will require more than one of the three domains depicted in the model.

Left ventricular ejection fraction

LVEF is one of the oldest and most used tests for cardiovascular risk stratification. The Multicenter

Table 18.1 Variables used for risk stratification in ICD prophylaxis trials

Trial	Year	N	Etiology	LVEF	Other risk stratifier(s)
MADIT	1996	196	I-CM	<0.36	VTu and EPS, and EPS (on procainamide)
CABG Patch	1997	900	I-CM	<0.36	SAECG
MUSTT	1999	704	I-CM	<0.41	VTu and EPS
MADIT II	2002	1232	I-CM	<0.31	None
DEFINITE	2004	458	NI-CM	<0.36	VPC $\geq$ 10/h or VTu
COMPANION	2004	1520	I- or NI-CM	<0.36	NYHA Class III/IV and QRS $\geq$120 ms
DINAMIT	2004	674	I-CM	<0.36	SDNN $\leq$ 70 ms or 24-h heart rate > 80/min
SCD-HeFT	2005	2521	I- or NI-CM	<0.36	NYHA Class II/III

EPS, electrophysiologic studies; I-CM, ischemic cardiomyopathy; N, number randomized; NI-CM, nonischemic cardiomy-opathy; NYHA, New York Heart Association; SAECG, signal averaged ECG; SDNN, standard deviation of normal RR intervals; VPC, ventricular premature complexes; VTu, unsustained ventricular tachycardia.

Post Infarction Program (MPIP) described the inverse relationship between LVEF, measured by radionuclide ventriculography, and cardiac mortality in patients with recent acute myocardial infarction [8,9]. As LVEF falls below 0.41, there is a progressive increase in the 1-year cardiac mortality rate; as LVEF falls below 0.31, the mortality rate rises steeply.

At the time of discharge after hospitalization for acute myocardial infarction, about 33% of the patients have an LVEF < 0.41 and 15% have an LVEF < 0.31 [10]. Studies before and during the thrombolytic era have shown the breakpoint separating patients at relatively low, versus higher, mortality risk is similar across nearly 30 years of study [8,9,11]. In patients with a previous myocardial infarction, approximately half of all cardiac deaths are sudden, using a 1-hour definition for sudden death. LVEF does not selectively predict the mechanism of cardiac death; it predicts both arrhythmic and nonarrhythmic cardiac deaths [12]. As LVEF falls below 0.31, the fraction of deaths that are sudden (arrhythmic) decreases, but the sudden death rate increases.

A reduced LVEF was a major eligibility criterion for enrolling patients in all randomized clinical trials of ICD prophylaxis (Table 18.1). Six randomized trials enrolled patients with LVEF < 0.36 along with one or more additional risk-stratifying characteristics; one trial, Multicenter Automatic Defibrillator Implantation Trial (MADIT) II used LVEF < 0.31 alone to select coronary heart disease patients for ICD prophylaxis [4]. In addition, a study of electrophysiologically guided antiarrhyth-mic therapy, the Multicenter UnSustained Tachycardia Trial (MUSTT), required participants to have an LVEF < 0.41, as well as coronary heart disease, unsustained VT, and sustained VT/VF induced by programmed ventricular stimulation [13]. Because patients with reduced LVEF were selected for all ICD prophylaxis trials, LVEF is a prominent feature of guidelines for ICD therapy and a cornerstone of patient selection for ICD prophylaxis in clinical practice.

However, LVEF alone is not an optimal criterion for implanting ICD prophylactically. The sensitivity, specificity, and negative predictive accuracy of LVEF have all been criticized [12]. The Maastricht Circulatory Arrest Registry reported that only 19% of patients with coronary heart disease had an LVEF < 0.31 before their cardiac arrest [14]. This remarkably small sensitivity suggests that a large fraction of cardiac arrests in the community are caused by an acute coronary event. Only about one-third of the survivors of cardiac arrest who participated in secondary prevention ICD trials had LVEF < 0.31 [15–17]. Buxton and Moss [12] also criticized LVEF for low specificity. The negative predictive accuracy of LVEF is also modest. Nevertheless, it is clear that, however measured, LVEF identifies a moderately high-risk group; thus, LVEF has earned the trust of cardiologists as a useful test for selecting patients for ICD prophylaxis. Every ICD prophylaxis trial has used LVEF, usually values <0.36, as an inclusion criterion. During the past 25 years, many other tests have been combined with LVEF to improve identification of high-risk patients. Some of these combinations will be discussed in upcoming sections about other tests for risk stratification.

QRS duration and signal-averaged ECG

Intraventricular conduction defects with QRS duration ≥120 milliseconds due to complete LBBB, RBBB, or nonspecific IVCD have been found to be associated with increased mortality in postmyocardial infarct patients and in patients with congestive heart failure due to both ischemic and nonischemic etiologies. It is clear that a widened QRS is found more often in patients with greater structural heart damage and lower LVEF. There is some controversy whether a prolonged QRS is an independent predictor of cardiac mortality and whether it predicts arrhythmic death as well as nonsudden death. In a large Italian study of over 5000 patients with heart failure, LBBB was detected in 1391 patients (25%) and this group had both an increased total mortality and an increased sudden death rate with a hazard ratio of 1.58 [18]. The etiologies of heart failure included ischemia, hypertensive heart disease, and nonischemic dilated cardiomyopathy.

Shamim et al. [19] studied 241 patients with congestive heart failure. They found the best predictors of mortality were LVEF, MVO_2, and intraventricular conduction delay. Mortality, both sudden and nonsudden, increased as conduction delay increased. Shamim et al. [20] also showed in a group of 112 elderly patients with heart failure that an increase in QRS duration on ECG recorded at least 12 months apart was associated with increased mortality. Those patients with a QRS increase > 20% had a worse prognosis than those with an increase between 5% and 20%.

In the VALIANT Trial, QRS duration was measured in 403 postinfarct patients with either heart failure or significant left ventricular dysfunction [21]. The cohort was divided into quartiles of QRS duration. Increased QRS duration was found to be a predictor of heart failure, cardiac mortality, and sudden death, but on multivariate analysis did not remain an independent predictor. Bauer et al. [22] evaluated the significance of QRS duration in > 1400 survivors of acute myocardial infarction, 98% of whom had revascularization therapy. QRS duration > 120 milliseconds was found in 6% of the patients. Other variables studied included age, clinical features, LVEF, mean heart rate, and heart rate turbulence. Seventy patients died during the follow-up period. The strongest univariate predictor of mortality was QRS duration followed by heart rate turbulence. In multivariate analysis, QRS duration remained an independent predictor for total mortality, but not for sudden death.

In summary, QRS duration in patients with heart failure and/or left ventricular dysfunction is a powerful univariate predictor of total mortality and, in some studies, an independent predictor of total mortality and/or sudden death. A retrospective study from MADIT II suggests that QRS duration used with other risk variables might be useful for predicting the benefit of ICD prophylaxis [23].

The signal-averaged ECG "averages" sequential highly amplified QRS complexes acquired from bipolar, orthogonal X, Y, and Z leads, reducing noise and permitting identification of low-frequency signals consistent with areas of slow conduction. An abnormal signal-averaged electrocardiogram (SAECG) predicts VT inducible by programmed ventricular stimulation in both ischemic and nonischemic subjects, and predicts spontaneous arrhythmic events in patients with ischemic cardiomyopathy [24,25], but is inconsistent in nonischemic patients [26,27]. In The CABG Patch Trial, subjects with coronary artery disease and an abnormal SAECG failed to benefit from prophylactic ICD implantation after complete revascularization by coronary bypass surgery [28]. However, an abnormal SAECG appears to be a significant predictor of sudden death in the presence of other arrhythmic risk predictors, i.e., unsustained ventricular tachycardia and substantially reduced LVEF, and when revascularization is not systematically employed. In MUSTT, all participants had coronary heart disease, unsustained VT, and an LVEF < 0.41 [29]. Among 1268 participants eligible for the SAECG substudy, 553 (44%) had an abnormal SAECG, i.e., a filtered QRS complex > 114 milliseconds in duration; the median LVEF was 0.30; and 230 (18%) experienced arrhythmic death or nonfatal cardiac arrest. Patients with an LVEF < 0.30 and a filtered QRS > 114 milliseconds had a 36% 5-year incidence of arrhythmic death or nonfatal cardiac arrest, while those with an EF 0.30–0.40 and a normal SAECG (filtered QRS < 114) had a 13% 5-year incidence of arrhythmic

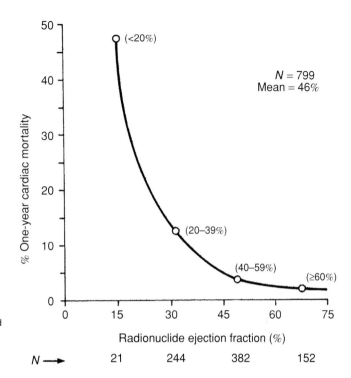

Figure 18.2 One-year cardiac mortality rate as a function of radionuclide left ventricular ejection fraction determined before hospital discharge after acute myocardial infarction. (From Reference [8], with permission.)

death or cardiac arrest [29]. Hohnloser et al. [30] suggest that since the advent of early revascularization during acute ischemia and infarction has become more commonly employed, the SAECG has become less helpful in predicting arrhythmic events.

Other echocardiographic measures

Echocardiography is a useful noninvasive method to risk stratify patients with depressed left ventricular function. Its major use has been to determine LVEF. Like other methods used to measure LVEF, echocardiography has technical limitations. However, there are many echocardiographic or Doppler features other than LVEF, which have an impact on cardiovascular mortality. Among the most important of these are significant mitral or tricuspid regurgitation [31,32], pulmonary hypertension [33], diastolic abnormalities, particularly pseudonormalized or restrictive left ventricular filling patterns [34], inter- or intraventricular dyssynchrony [35], decreased right ventricular function [36], and left ventricular hypertrophy or increased LV mass [37,38]. Almost all the studies showing increased mortality associated with these abnormal echocardiographic

findings are small and cardiovascular mortality has not been subclassified as sudden or due to increasing heart failure. It seems likely that, like depressed ejection fraction, these findings are better predictors of pump failure than sudden death, yet their association with a poor prognosis might lead to device therapies, such as cardiac resynchronization therapy (CRT) or a left ventricular assist device as a bridge to a cardiac transplant. Currently, echocardiographic features to evaluate patients suitable for CRT or to evaluate the degree of improvement on CRT are an area of active investigation.

Cardiac magnetic resonance imaging

Although cardiac magnetic resonance (CMR) imaging will be explored in greater depth in other chapters, it should be pointed out that CMR with gadolinium enhancement appears to be very promising as a means for detecting potentially proarrhythmic substrate. The presence of infarcted tissue increases the volume of distribution of gadolinium, and the contrast agent has slower uptake and efflux kinetics in areas of fibrosis versus normal muscle [39]. The infusion of gadolinium allows the assessment of myocardial delayed enhancement, in which the mass of noninfarcted, infarcted, and peri-infarct regions can be quantified based on the timing and intensity of contrast enhancement.

Border regions that might be substrate for reentry have intermediate intensity of myocardial delayed enhancement. Bello et al. [40] found that infarct mass and surface area predicted the inducibility of VT better than LVEF, and Yan et al. [41] found that the percentage of myocardial delayed enhancement predicted cardiovascular mortality. The presence of midwall fibrosis in subjects with nonischemic cardiomyopathy conferred a fivefold risk for sudden death or VT [42]. Due to its extraordinary anatomic detail and pathophysiological implications, CMR with gadolinium appears likely to become an important method for assessing the presence of arrhythmogenic substrate.

Autonomic nervous system

Multiple experimental studies, as well as clinical observation of patients with coronary heart disease and/or with severely depressed left ventricular function, have documented that alterations in the autonomic nervous system profoundly affect the risk of malignant ventricular arrhythmias or sudden death [43–46]. In general, maneuvers that increase parasympathetic modulation of the heart decrease the risk of malignant ventricular arrhythmias, whereas increased sympathetic activity or decreased parasympathetic modulation reduces ventricular fibrillation threshold and results in more spontaneous episodes of ventricular fibrillation when animals have an ischemic challenge [47–54]. Thus, low-dose atropine, scopolamine, or exercise training, which increase parasympathetic nervous activity or direct vagal stimulation, protect ischemic animals from ventricular fibrillation; sympathetic stimulation or the administration of catecholamines increase the risk of cardiac arrest secondary to malignant ventricular arrhythmias [55–57].

In humans, direct measurement of vagal or sympathetic modulation is not practical, but neural modulation of RR intervals may be inferred by a variety of noninvasive or nearly noninvasive tests. These include the measurement of heart rate variability usually from 24-hour ambulatory ECG

recordings, heart rate turbulence, also from 24-hour ECG recordings, determination of baroreceptor sensitivity utilizing phenylephrine injection, and deceleration capacity, also from 24-hour ECG recordings [58–68].

Heart rate variability can be assessed by a variety of methods. Time domain measurements are statistical measures utilizing the RR intervals recorded from ECG recordings or the differences between intervals. The most commonly used measures are SDNN, the standard deviation of all normal-to-normal RR intervals in the record; SDANN, the standard deviation of all 5-minute average RR intervals; pNN50, the proportion of beats varying by more than 50 milliseconds from the preceding QRS; and rMSSD, the square root of the squares of successive differences between the RR intervals [61,67]. Heart rate variability is also evaluated by spectral measures. Either fast Fourier transforms or autoregressive techniques partition RR variability into the component frequencies responsible for cyclic variation of RR intervals [65,69–71]. Over 24 hours, high frequency, low frequency, and total power can be calculated. These measures are strongly correlated with time domain measures and offer insights into the relative balance between sympathetic and parasympathetic modulation. Power spectral measures predict both mortality and malignant ventricular arrhythmias in patients with ischemic heart disease and in nonischemic heart disease with reduced LVEF.

Geometric measures of heart rate variability have been used extensively at St George's Hospital in London [72–74]. By making histograms of the normal RR intervals, either an index or a measurement of the width of the base of the RR histogram in milliseconds can be calculated. These geometric measurements are strongly correlated to traditional time and frequency domain measurements, but are less affected by noisy recordings (Figure 18.3).

The first large clinical study demonstrating the predictive value of heart rate variability (HRV) measurements after myocardial infarction was the MPIP study [59,60]. In this study, 808 survivors of acute myocardial infarction had a 24-hour continuous ambulatory ECG recording; 127 died during 31 months of follow up. SDNN was a stronger univariate ECG predictor of outcome than heart rate, ventricular premature contraction (VPC)

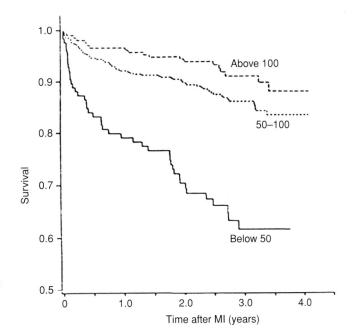

Figure 18.3 Cumulative (Kaplan–Meier) survival curves as a function of heart rate variability (SDNN) groups: < 50 ms, 50 to < 100 ms, > 100 ms. (From Reference [59], with permission.)

frequency or unsustained VT (see Table 18.4). Approximately one-third of the deaths occurred in the group with SDNN < 50 milliseconds and approximately one-third of this group died. Thus, both sensitivity and positive predictive accuracy were approximately the same, 33%. This study was done prior to the advent of reperfusion or β-blocker therapy for acute myocardial infarction. However, multiple studies done after the development of reperfusion therapy show that decreased heart rate variability is still associated with a poor survival after myocardial infarction. A series of studies from the St George's Hospital group showed that decreased heart rate index or other geometrical measures of HRV not only are associated with increased mortality rates, but also are better predictors of arrhythmic death than decreased LVEF, late potentials, or VPC quantified by ambulatory ECG recordings [72–75]. Moreover, as was shown in MPIP, the combination of HRV and other adverse predictors such as frequent VPC, decreased ejection fraction, or unsustained VT identifies subgroups of post-MI patients with very low or high mortalities. GISSI-2, a large study of thrombolytic therapy during acute myocardial infarction conducted an HRV substudy in 576 patients who had a 24-hour continuous ECG recording before discharge from hospital [76]. They found that low HRV (SDNN, rMSSD, and NN50) remains a strong risk predictor after thrombolysis and after statistical adjustment for other risk predictors using Cox regression models.

There is at present no consensus as to when and how heart rate variability should be measured after myocardial infarction. Several studies have utilized nonlinear measurements such as Poincare plots, fractal dimensions, such as detrended fractal scaling, power law slope etc., in post myocardial infarction populations and have reported superior predictive accuracy compared to traditional time and spectral measurements [77–82]. In general, all measures of HRV are good predictors.

Heart rate turbulence

Heart rate turbulence is a novel analytic method that evaluates the perturbation (shortening then lengthening) in RR intervals following a VPC. Two parameters quantify the response to VPC: turbulence onset (TO) and turbulence slope (TS). Turbulence onset, a decrease in the first two normal RR intervals following a VPC compared with two normal RR intervals just before the VPC, presumably reflects baroreflex activity induced by a decreased stroke volume for the VPC and low blood pressure during the compensatory pause. Normally, the two RR intervals after a VPC are shorter than the two normal RR intervals immediately preceding the VPC. Turbulence slope quantifies the degree of lengthening of RR intervals following the shortening of RR intervals immediately after a VPC, again reflecting baroreflex activity [63,82,83]. It is calculated by determining the maximum slope of any five-beat sequence of normal RR intervals during the 15–20 RR intervals after a VPC. Turbulence onset (TO) and turbulence slope (TS) are calculated from all single VPC in a 24-hour ECG recording.

Heart rate turbulence was studied in the digitized Holter archives of MPIP, European Myocardial Infarct Amiodarone Trial (EMIAT), and Autonomic Tone and Reflexes after Myocardial Infarction (ATRAMI) study [63]. In these studies abnormal TO and TS values were better predictors of outcome than conventional HRV measures. Barthel et al. [83] prospectively studied over 1400 survivors of acute myocardial infarction utilizing HRT measures categorizing them: 0 if both TS and TO were normal, 1 if one was abnormal, and 2 if both were abnormal. HRT was evaluated in a Cox regression model along with other variables, i.e., age, diabetes, previous myocardial infarction, LVEF, HRV, and ventricular arrhythmias. HRT category 2 was the most powerful univariate predictor of mortality with a hazard ratio of 5.9. The next most powerful univariate predictor of mortality was LVEF. In a multivariate analysis, HRT category 2 remained the strongest predictor of mortality (hazard ratio 2.8).

Baroreflex sensitivity

Baroreflex sensitivity (BRS) has been used to stratify risk after MI. BRS is measured by determining the response of RR intervals to alterations in blood pressure. Although BRS can be measured either by decreasing blood pressure with vasodilators or increasing blood pressure by injecting phenylephrine, an α-adrenergic agonist, the latter has been used most often [64,65]. Farrell et al. [84] in a small post-MI sample of 68 patients found that an abnormal BRS response predicted mortality better than HRV measurements. ATRAMI Investigators [64] studied the predictive value of SDNN and BRS (phenylephrine injection method) in 1284 relatively low-risk survivors of acute myocardial infarction. Depressed values of either SDNN or BRS were associated with

an increase in mortality during 21 months of follow up. Patients with depressed BRS (< 3 ms/mm Hg) and depressed HRV (SDNN < 70 ms) had a 17% versus 2% mortality risk in the subgroup with normal values for both tests. In 2001, ATRAMI Investigators [65] reported a database study to explore the possible utility of LVEF, BRS, unsustained VT, and SDNN to select patients for ICD prophylaxis. Various combinations of these tests identified small subgroups with high-risk (hazard ratios from 10 to 20), improving on the positive predictive accuracy of LVEF alone. Also, some of these tests identified high-risk patients among patients with LVEF > 0.35. These results suggest that autonomic testing, e.g., SDNN and BRS, along with unsustained VT can not only identify patients with recent MI who are at higher risk among those with LVEF ≤ 0.35, but also find high-risk patients among those with LVEF > 0.35. It remains to be seen whether this latter finding can be developed into a clinically useful tool for selecting patients for ICD prophylaxis.

Deceleration capacity

Bauer et al. [66] proposed deceleration capacity as a risk stratifier following acute myocardial infarction. They studied more than 1400 postinfarct patients in Germany and then validated their results in large post-MI groups from Finland and St George's Hospital in London. They were able to separate the contribution to heart rate variability due to vagally mediated deceleration of heart rate from that variability due to sympathetically mediated acceleration of rate. Loss of deceleration capacity was associated with a poor prognosis and, in conjunction with LVEF, had both high sensitivity and specificity for arrhythmic events and was more accurate than the combination of LVEF and SDNN. However, no comparison was made with heart rate turbulence findings [66]. More recently, Schmidt and coworkers studied a postinfarct population utilizing both HRT and deceleration capacity. They defined a subgroup of patients with both category 2 HRT and deceleration capacity less than 4.5 milliseconds as severe autonomic failure (SAF). They found that total mortality, cardiac mortality, and sudden death rates were essentially equal in patients with LVEF > 0.30 and SAF, and in patients with ejection fractions < 0.31.

Nonischemic cardiomyopathy

As is clear from the previous discussion, most studies utilizing HRV, BRS, and HRT and its variants as predictors of adverse arrhythmic events, have examined postinfarct survival; there are relatively few such studies in nonischemic dilated cardiomyopathy. Aronson et al. [85] reported that depressed HRV predicted mortality in patients hospitalized for severe heart failure. One-half of his patients had nonischemic etiologies for their heart failure. Ponikowski et al. [86] reported similar results for outpatients with chronic congestive heart failure. Seventy-eight patients had ischemic heart disease, 24 had nonischemic dilated cardiomyopathy. SDNN, SDANN, and the mean of 5-minute standard deviations were all independent predictors of mortality even after controlling for NYHA class, LVEF, peak oxygen consumption, and ventricular tachycardia recorded on 24-hour ambulatory ECG. These studies did not adjudicate the mechanisms of death, but it is likely that many were due to heart failure, not arrhythmias.

Rashba et al. [87] reported the results of a substudy of the DEFINITE trial (Defibrillators in Nonischemic Cardiomyopathy); 274 (60%) of the 458 patients in DEFINITE had a 24-hour ECG recording, 23% of whom did not have HRV (SDNN) measured because of atrial fibrillation or frequent VPC. These investigators applied the two-tiered screening method first used for microvolt T-wave alternans (read below) to SDNN. In a 3-year follow up, the results of HRV analysis demonstrated that the 70 low-risk patients whose SDNN was > 113 milliseconds had no deaths or arrhythmic events irrespective of ICD placement. The mortality rate for the 69 patients whose SDNN was between 81 and 113 milliseconds was 7%, and for the 72 patients with an SDNN < 81 10%. The authors suggest that patients with nonischemic cardiomyopathy, LVEF less than < 0.36 but with preserved HRV may not require an ICD implant despite their eligibility by LVEF and heart failure criteria.

Unsustained ventricular arrhythmias

Ventricular premature complexes (VPC) have attracted attention since the earliest days of electrocardiography because the large, wide, bizarre QRS complexes are so striking. When coronary care units (CCU) developed in the early 1960s, patients had continuous ECG monitoring for arrhythmia surveillance. Observations in the CCU prompted the concept of "warning arrhythmias," i.e., certain unsustained ventricular arrhythmias are a prelude to sustained, potentially lethal, ventricular arrhythmias. Also, a strategy of treating warning arrhythmias to prevent more serious arrhythmias was explored with mixed results, i.e., the adverse effects of Class I antiarrhythmic drugs offset their benefit; β-blockers showed significant benefit.

Continuous ambulatory (Holter) ECG recording also was developed in the 1960s and 1970s. Early use of this technology documented the causes of symptoms that suggested arrhythmias. In the 1970s several groups quantified ventricular arrhythmias after myocardial infarction using 1–24-hour continuous ECG recordings and related these to vital status during 1–4 years of follow up [88–93]. A relationship between asymptomatic or minimally symptomatic ventricular arrhythmias and death was soon apparent. But, a new question was raised: did spontaneous ventricular arrhythmias detected and quantified a few weeks after myocardial infarction represent a primary threat to survival or were they an epiphenomenon related to left ventricular damage and scarring [94,95]. Many investigators thought that VPCs were so closely linked to left ventricular dysfunction and fibrosis that treating them was futile [95]. This question was debated actively and was the motivating force for additional studies. Four large studies addressed this question: two used clinical features of heart failure to represent left ventricular dysfunction [89,90] and the other two used radionuclide LVEF [96,97]. These studies are summarized in Table 18.2. These studies indicated strongly that VPC in patients with a previous myocardial infarction had a strong association with death independent of left ventricular dysfunction (Figure 18.4).

Table 18.3 shows hazard ratios from MPIP adjusted for the other factors so that they can be multiplied to estimate the risks associated with various combinations of these variables. For example, the instantaneous probability of dying in patients with LVEF below 0.30, more than three VPCs per hour, and unsustained VT was 13 times ($3.5 \times 2.0 \times 1.9$)

Table 18.2 Independent relationship between ventricular arrhythmias or left ventricular dysfunction and mortality in coronary heart disease

	Ruberman et al. [89]	Moss et al. [90]	MILIS [97]	MPIP [96]
Number of patients	1739	940	533	766
Enrollment (weeks after infarction)	12	2–3	1–2	1–2
Measure of LVD	Clinical	Clinical	RNEF	RNEF
Duration of ECG recording (h)	1	6	24	24
Ventricular arrhythmia	Complex VPCs	Complex VPCs	Frequent VPCs	Frequent or repetitive VPCs
Follow up (yr)	3	4	1.5	2
Number of deaths	208	115	66	101
Mortality effect of ventricular arrhythmias independent of LVD	Yes	Yes	Yes	Yes

Complex ventricular arrhythmias: R-on-T VPC, ≥2 consecutive VPCs, multiform VPC, or bigeminy; frequent VPCs: ≥10 per hour; LVD, left ventricular dysfunction; repetitive VPC, ≥ 2 consecutive VPCs; RNEF, radionuclide ejection fraction; VPC, ventricular premature complexes.

that in patients with none of these predictors of high risk.

Also, MPIP investigators found that the instantaneous probability of dying any time during the first 6 months after the index infarction was, on the average, 3.3 times that of dying during the subsequent 6–36 months [96].

The evidence from MPIP and from MILIS indicated an independent association between ventricular arrhythmias and death in the early years after myocardial infarction [96,97]. Since ventricular arrhythmias posed a risk independent of other important postinfarction risk predictors, it was reasonable to hypothesize that antiarrhythmic treatment could improve survival. However, MPIP investigators noted that a randomized clinical trial should be done to determine if antiarrhythmic drug treatment does reduce mortality after myocardial infarction before recommending this approach in clinical practice [96]. Despite this advice, many physicians were already using antiarrhythmic drugs to treat ventricular arrhythmias after myocardial infarction [98]. Although several preliminary or feasibility studies had been done, many questions

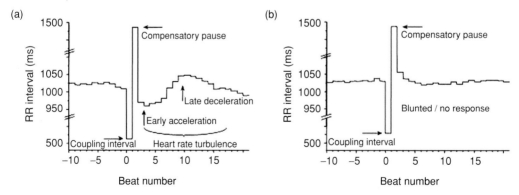

Figure 18.4 Heart rate turbulence patterns in two patients with recent myocardial infarction. Panel (a) shows transient acceleration after a VPC (TO) with subsequent deceleration (TS). Panel (b) shows a blunted response to a VPC with no appreciable acceleration or deceleration of heart rate. During follow up, patient A survived and patient B died. (From Reference [62], with permission.)

Table 18.3 Independent association of LVEF and ventricular arrhythmias to death after myocardial infarction

Variable	Hazard ratio	P value
LVEF < 0.30 vs. ≥0.30	3.5	< 0.001
VPC/h ≥3 vs. < 3	2.0	< 0.05
Unsustained VT (yes, no)	1.9	< 0.05
Time after infarction first 6 mo vs. 6–30 mo	3.3	< 0.001

Note: Hazard ratio, ratio of the instantaneous probability of dying for patients in one category to that for patients in the other, calculated from Cox regression analysis; LVEF, left ventricular ejection fraction; VPC, ventricular premature complexes; VT, ventricular tachycardia.

remained about the feasibility of a trial to evaluate treatment of postmyocardial infarction ventricular arrhythmias.

As the next step, the National Heart, Lung, and Blood Institute (NHLBI) conducted the Cardiac Arrhythmia Pilot Study (CAPS) at 10 centers to answer the following primary question: can any of several treatment strategies suppress VPC frequency by at least 70% and maintain suppression for a 1-year period [99]? CAPS enrolled 502 patients between July 1983 and July 1985 and randomized 100 of them to each of five treatment arms: a placebo arm and four active treatment arms [100]; three drugs, encainide, flecainide, and moricizine adequately suppressed VPC and were well tolerated [100].

The Cardiac Arrhythmia Suppression Trial (CAST) was a definitive NHLBI-sponsored follow-up to CAPS. Patients with previous myocardial infarction with reduced LVEF and unsustained ventricular arrhythmias were recruited to test the suppression hypothesis, i.e., suppressing ventricular arrhythmias will improve survival [101,102]. Arrhythmia suppression was defined as ≥80% reduction in the total number of VPCs plus ≥90% suppression of unsustained VT.

On April 18, 1989, NHLBI stopped CAST recruitment because of increased mortality on encainide and flecainide (relative risk of 3.6 [95% confidence interval 1.7–8.5]) [101]. The moricizine arm continued until July 30, 1991 when the moricizine arm satisfied a prespecified futility criterion, i.e., very small chance of finding drug benefit if the trial continued [103].

CAST showed that VPC suppression or aggravation by encainide or flecainide identified low- or high-risk patients, respectively [104,105]. CAST also found that ischemic episodes were three times as likely to be fatal if they occurred during encainide or flecainide treatment [106].

We still have no idea what the pathogenesis of postinfarction VPCs is even though they have a strong and independent association with mortality. Ventricular arrhythmias after myocardial infarction continue to be an important risk predictor, but not a therapeutic target for Class I antiarrhythmic drugs.

Microvolt T-wave alternans

Research on microvolt T-wave alternans (MTWA) has been very active over the past 5 years and a critical mass of information has accrued. Because MTWA has very high negative predictive accuracy (NPA), it has generated an innovative two-tiered strategy of risk stratification. As a result of accumulating research results, we think that MTWA is ready for wider applications in clinical practice, particularly at the heart failure venue.

Early observations

Sir Thomas Lewis [107] first recognized electrical alternans in electrocardiograms as a pathophysiological manifestation that occurred in serious heart

Table 18.4 Association of Holter variables with 3-year all-cause mortality

Variable	N	Relative risk*	P value†
SDNN < 50 ms	125	3.4	< 0.0001
VPC ≥ 10/h	158	2.6	< 0.0001
Unsustained VT (no, yes)	91	2.7	< 0.001
Mean RR interval < 750 ms	211	2.0	< 0.01

*From Cox model with variables dichotomized at the cut point indicated in the first column.

†P values for Chi-square with 1 degree of freedom from Cox models with variables treated as continuous univariate predictors.

N, number of patients; SDNN, standard deviation of all normal RR intervals; VPC, ventricular premature complexes; VT, ventricular tachycardia.

disease or, in normal persons, when the heart rate was very rapid. Alternans of ST-T waves has a strong association with serious ventricular arrhythmias in a wide variety of conditions. Richard Cohen's laboratory at the Massachusetts Institute of Technology (MIT) developed a method for quantifying MTWA that is not apparent by visual inspection of the ECG. T-wave alternans was studied in a series of laboratory experiments using ischemia, hypoxia, etc. [108,109]. During ischemia, as the T-wave alternans voltage progressively increased, the ventricular fibrillation threshold progressively decreased [109]. In 1988, a small pilot study was published showing a relationship between MTWA and inducibility of sustained ventricular tachyarrhythmias during programmed ventricular stimulation in patients [109]. In 1994, Rosenbaum et al. [110] reported studies in 83 patients who were referred to the cardiac electrophysiology laboratory at the Massachusetts General Hospital. MTWA was detected and quantified using atrial pacing to increase heart rate and evoke MTWA; the MIT spectral method was used to quantify MTWA. The MTWA test result was found to be associated with two endpoints—induced sustained ventricular tachyarrhythmias and spontaneous ventricular tachyarrhythmias—during an average follow up of 20 months. The probability of inducing sustained ventricular tachyarrhythmias was proportional to the magnitude of MTWA. Bundle branch block and antiarrhythmic drugs did not prevent accurate detection of MTWA. Of the 66 patients followed long term, 13 had sustained ventricular tachycardia, ventricular fibrillation, or sudden cardiac death. Programmed ventricular stimulation and MTWA had very similar predictive value for arrhythmic events that occurred during follow up.

Meta-analysis of studies done between 1990 and 2004

In 2005, Gehi et al. [111] reported a meta-analysis of MTWA cohort studies published between January 1990 and December 2004. Studies were included if (1) they were prospective cohort studies of ≥10 human subjects who had exercise-based MTWA testing; (2) they provided a clear definition of normal or abnormal MTWA tests; (3) the had ≥6 months follow-up; and (4) they provided primary data on clinical outcomes, including sudden cardiac death, ventricular arrhythmias, and/or implantable cardioverter-defibrillator (ICD) shocks. The quality of publications was evaluated and prespecified data items were extracted from them. All studies used the Cambridge Heart, Inc. spectral method to determine whether MTWA was present or absent. Outcomes were presented as positive predictive accuracy (PPA), negative predictive accuracy (NPA), and univariate relative risk with 95% confidence intervals. Summary estimates of the overall predictive accuracy of MTWA for the outcomes were computed and sensitivity analyses were conducted. After applying these criteria and procedures, 19 prospective studies and 2608 participants were included in the meta-analysis; average follow up was 21 months. Summary estimates of MTWA data are shown in Table 18.5. Overall, patients with an abnormal MTWA test had 3.8 times the risk of patients with a normal test. The PPA for sustained arrhythmic events varied strikingly, 6–30%, with the pretest probability. PPA did not vary much if "indeterminate" tests (read below) were included or excluded in the MTWA abnormal group. Patients with a normal MTWA had only a 3% chance of an arrhythmic event during an average follow up of 21 months

Table 18.5 Summary estimates of PPA, NPA, and univariate relative risk in 19 prospective studies of microvolt T-wave alternans for the prediction of cardiac arrhythmic events

	All studies	Ischemic CM	Nonischemic CM	After MI
Number of studies	19	2	7	3
Mean follow up (mo)	21	19	20	18
PPA	19% (18–21%)	30% (24–36%)	21% (18–25%)	6% (5–7%)
NPA	97% (97–98%)	92% (88–95%)	95% (94–97%)	99% (99–100%)
Relative risk	3.8 (2.4–5.9)	2.4 (1.3–4.5)	3.7 (1.5–9.0)	4.7 (1.1–20.2)

CM, cardiomyopathy; MI, myocardial infarction; NPA, negative predictive accuracy; PPA, positive predictive accuracy.

(NPA of 97%) and NPA varied much less with pretest probability than PPA. In studies that compared MTWA with other tests used for risk stratification, MTWA was always among the best predictors and added to predictive accuracy in multivariate analyses. The authors of the meta-analysis recommended (1) further studies of "indeterminate" MTWA, (2) studies that use all-cause mortality as an end point, and (3) studies that combined MTWA with other tests to improve selection of patients for ICD prophylaxis.

Two-tiered screening for ICD prophylaxis

In 2003, Hohnloser et al. [112] published the results of a retrospective study of 129 patients similar to those who participated in MADIT II. They suggested that death or arrhythmic events were so infrequent in patients who had a normal MTWA that ICD prophylaxis could be safely withheld in this subgroup. This two-tiered screening approach was a new concept in risk stratification: a high-risk group was identified by reduced LVEF, but a low-risk subgroup was identified by an additional test, e.g., MTWA. In 2006, two large studies ($n = 549$ and 768) published prospective evaluations of the two-tiered approach in a total of 1317 patients who had reduced LVEF (< 0.41 or < 0.36), and no history of sustained ventricular arrhythmias [113,114]. Both studies found that two-thirds of the participants had an abnormal (positive or indeterminate) MTWA test and that the NPA of MTWA was very high. These studies supported the suggestion that a normal MTWA test could be used to exclude otherwise eligible patients from ICD prophylaxis. The data were not strong enough to mandate withholding ICD prophylaxis in patients with a normal MTWA, but the results of MTWA tests do importantly inform individualized decisions about ICD prophylaxis. The prevalence and significance of abnormal MTWA tests is similar in patients with either ischemic or nonischemic cardiomyopathy (Figure 18.5).

In a 11-center study with 549 participants, Bloomfield et al. [113] showed that NPA of MTWA testing was greater in nonischemic than ischemic cardiomyopathy (LVEF < 0.41), similar to the meta-analysis findings and the recently completed ALPHA study. The NPA of MTWA tests was very high ($\geq 98\%$ at 2–3 yr of follow up) in patients with nonischemic heart failure.

"Indeterminate" MTWA

Chow et al. [114] and Kaufman et al. [115] showed that "indeterminate" MTWA tests predict death or sustained ventricular tachyarrhythmias at least as well as a test that is positive for MTWA. About 90% of "indeterminate" MTWA tests are due to chronotropic incompetence (inability to attain a heart rate of ≥ 105 beats/min), exercise-induced VPC, or unsustained MTWA [115]. Because all these conditions are strongly associated with death, ICD prophylaxis should not be withheld when a MTWA test is "indeterminate" for one of these reasons. If a technical deficiency (noise or too rapid rise in heart rate) is the cause of an "indeterminate" result, the MTWA test should be repeated.

MTWA and ICD benefit

Chow et al. [116] also showed that patients with a normal MTWA test did not benefit from ICD prophylaxis. About half ($n = 392$) of their 768 patients with ischemic cardiomyopathy (LVEF < 0.36) received a prophylactic ICD based on a recommendation by their primary physician, most often due to the results of an electrophysiologic study. Although this study was not randomized, careful statistical adjustment (propensity scores in Cox models) was done to control variables likely to influence the decision to implant a prophylactic ICD. As mentioned above, a controlled trial that randomizes patients who are eligible for a prophylactic ICD, but have negative MTWA tests is probably not feasible, given the effort and expenses of screening and enrolling the huge number of patients such a trial would require. Sample size calculations indicate that, if patients with nonischemic cardiomyopathy and a normal MTWA test were randomized to ICD or medical therapy, over 20,000 patients would have to be randomized to have 80% power to detect a 25% reduction in all-cause mortality.

MTWA for risk stratification after myocardial infarction

Use of MTWA after acute MI is still not well defined. Large, multicenter studies were done in Japan and a few single-center epidemiologic studies were done

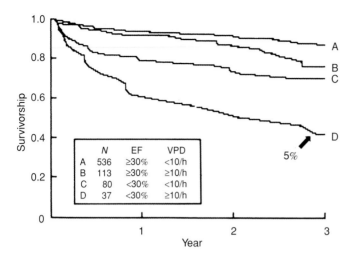

Figure 18.5 Survival as a function of left ventricular dysfunction and ventricular arrhythmias. Survival curves were calculated by the Kaplan–Meier method. EF = left ventricular ejection fraction, VPD = ventricular premature depolarizations. 15% of the patients had LVEF < 0.30, 20% had ≥10 VPC per hour, and 5% had both (curve D). The small group who were high risk on both variables (curve D) had a 3-year mortality rate > 50%. (From reference [10], with permission.)

Table 18.6 Microvolt T-wave after acute myocardial infarction (MI)

	Schwab et al. [117]	Ikeda et al. [118]	Tapanainen et al. [119]	Ikeda et al. [120]	Ikeda et al. [121]
Patient group	Acute MI	Acute MI	After MI	After MI	After MI
Number of patients	140	102	379	834	1003
End point(s)	—	VT/VF	Death of any cause	SCD/VF	SCD/CA/VF
Months of follow up	15 ± 7	13 ± 6	14 ± 8	25 ± 13	32 ± 14
Age	60 ± 13	60 ± 10	62 ± 10	63 ± 11	64 ± 11
Male	76%	83%	72%	84%	79%
LVEF < 0.40	—	27%	—	18%	0%
Mean LVEF	0.56 ± 0.14	0.49 ± 0.09	0.45 ± 0.10	0.51 ± 0.10	0.55 ± 0.10
Revascularization	45%	98%	45%	91%	99%
β-Blocker	85%	33%	97%	13%	21%
			MTWA		
Days after MI	15 ± 6	20 ± 6	8 ± 2	80 ± 160	48 ± 66
Exercise mode	Bicycle	Bicycle	Bicycle	Bicycle	Bicycle/treadmill
Positive	20%	49%	15%	36%	18%
Indeterminate	26%	17%	32%*	12%	9%
Negative	54%	34%	38%	52%	74%
Incomplete	—	—	15%	—	—
Hazard ratio	—	17	15	11	24
95% CI	—	2–128	1.6–43	3.4–38	7–81
Sensitivity	—	93%	96%	92%	83%
Specificity	—	59%	41%	61%	83%
PPA	—	28%	11%	7%	9%
NPA	—	98%	99%	99%	99.6%

*We moved patients with heart rate < 105 beats/min from the incomplete category to the indeterminate category in accordance with current definitions.

CA, cardiac arrest; CI, confidence interval; LVEF, left ventricular ejection fraction; NPA, negative predictive accuracy; PPA, positive predictive accuracy; SCD, sudden cardiac death; VF, ventricular fibrillation; VT, ventricular tachycardia.

in Europe. No large North American studies have been published (see Table 18.6).

In 2001, Schwab et al. [117] reported a single-center study of 140 patients who performed bicycle exercise 15 ± 6 days after acute MI to determine the prevalence of positive MTWA tests and their association with other risk-stratifying variables. MTWA tests were positive in 27% of patients; positive tests were associated with older age and reduced LVEF, but not with VPC, unsustained VT, or HRV in a 24-hour ECG recording, or late potentials in a signal-averaged ECG.

In 2000, Ikeda et al. [118] reported a single-center study of patients with recent acute MI to determine whether combining a marker of repolarization abnormalities (MTWA) and a marker of depolarization abnormality (late potentials) improves prediction of arrhythmic events during long-term follow up. This study screened 142 patients, 98% of whom had percutaneous transluminal coronary angioplasty during the acute MI. Of those screened, 119 were assessed with MTWA, SAECG, and LVEF just before hospital discharge (7–30 days, 20 ± 6 days after MI) and all three tests were interpretable in 102 patients. Of the 102 patients, 50 (49%) had MTWA, 21 (21%) had late potentials, and 28 (27%) had an LVEF < 0.40. During 13 ± 6 months of follow up, 15 episodes of sustained VT or VF (the primary end point) occurred. MTWA had the highest sensitivity (93%) and negative predictive accuracy (98%) for VT/VF, but the specificity (59%) and positive predictive accuracy (28%) were lower for MTWA tests than for late potentials or LVEF < 0.40. There were 16 patients with a positive MTWA test who also had late potentials identified in their SAECG; this group had a 50% PPA, a sensitivity of 53%, an NPA of 92%, and a hazard ratio of 20 (95% confidence interval of 3–125; $P < 0.001$).

In 2001, Tapanainen et al. [119] reported a single-center study done in Oulu, Finland to evaluate non-invasive risk-stratifying tests in 379 patients who survived the acute phase of MI. Predischarge bicycle exercise tests were done 8 ± 2 days after acute MI to determine MTWA; other risk-stratifying tests included 24-hour ECG recordings, HRV, unsustained VT, BRS, SAECG, QTc interval, QT dispersion, and wall motion index by two-dimensional echocardiography; for these tests, the cutoff for high risk was selected prospectively based on previous studies. Of the 379 participants, 323 (85%) had an MTWA test done: 56 (17%) were positive, 144 (45%) were negative, and 46 (14%) were indeterminate. The MTWA test was incomplete in 133 patients (35%), i.e., 77 (20%) did not reach a heart rate of 105 per minute for ≥ 1 minute and 56 (15%) could not perform bicycle exercise. Follow-up data were available in 378 participants; 26 patients died during a mean of 14 ± 8 months follow up. Although a positive MTWA was not associated with increased mortality, an incomplete MTWA test (inability to exercise or inability to attain a heart rate ≥ 105 per minute with MTWA absent) was the strongest univariate predictor of all-cause mortality (hazard ratio 25, 95% confidence interval 6–105, $P < 0.001$); several other noninvasive tests (signal averaged ECG, BRS, QT dispersion and wall motion score) also provided significant univariate prognostic information. These same tests were significant predictors of all-cause or cardiac mortality in multivariate analyses.

In 2002, Ikeda et al. [120] reported the predictive value of MTWA, alone or combined with other risk predictors, for sudden cardiac death or nonfatal ventricular fibrillation during a mean follow-up of 25 ± 6 months in patients with recent MI. This prospective study enrolled 850 MI survivors at seven Japanese centers; 83% had been revascularized by percutaneous coronary intervention and 8% by coronary artery bypass graft surgery during the acute phase of MI. Notably, only 13% of the participants were on β-blocking drugs at the time of recruitment. Most patients (82%) underwent an MTWA test between 2 and 10 weeks (mean of 80 days) after an acute MI; the remaining 149 patients (18%) underwent the test several months or years later. MTWA alone had a sensitivity of 92% (twice as high as LVEF < 0.40), but a positive predictive accuracy of only 7%. Combining MTWA with one or more additional tests (LVEF < 0.40, unsustained VT, or late potentials), increased positive predictive accuracy from 7% to 42%, whereas the sensitivity decreased from 92% to 23%. Because MTWA, as a single test, identified nearly all patients who died during 25 ± 13 months of follow up, these investigators suggested that MTWA was the best candidate for initial screening of patients for sudden cardiac death after MI. If health policy for prophylactic ICD therapy requires a high level of cost effectiveness, greater PPA can be achieved by combining MTWA with other noninvasive risk predictors, e.g., reduced LVEF or late potentials in a SAECG. These findings suggest that MTWA measured in the late phase of MI is a strong risk stratifier for sudden cardiac death during follow up.

The prevalence of MTWA and its prognostic significance were much greater in the Japanese multicenter study [120] that performed the MTWA test a mean of 80 days after MI than in the Finnish study that performed the test a mean of 8 days after MI [119]. Accordingly, it has been recommended that MTWA tests should be performed 3 weeks or more after MI to improve the tests' prognostic power. This issue needs further study.

In 2006, Ikeda et al. reported an eight-center cohort study that enrolled 1041 post-MI Japanese patients with preserved LVEF, i.e., ≥ 0.40, (mean LVEF 0.55 ± 0.10) [121]. Nearly all patients were revascularized in the acute phase of MI; 94% had percutaneous coronary interventions and 5% had coronary artery bypass grafting. MTWA testing was performed 48 ± 66 days after acute MI, along with LVEF, 24-hour ECG recordings, and signal-averaged ECGs. MTWA was positive in 169 patients (17%), indeterminate in 87 (9%), and negative in 747 (74%). A positive MTWA test, unsustained VT, and ventricular late potentials were predictors of serious arrhythmic events (sudden cardiac death, cardiac arrest, or resuscitated ventricular fibrillation); 38 patients died nonarrhythmic deaths and 18 had serious arrhythmic events during 32 ± 14 months of follow up. On multivariate analysis, a positive microvolt TWA test was the strongest predictor of total or arrhythmic death, with a hazard ratio of 19.7 (95% confidence intervals 5.5–70.4, $P < 0.0001$), compared to multivariate hazard ratios of 3.3 and 1.8 for unsustained VT and ventricular late potentials. MTWA also had the highest sensitivity (83%), i.e., it identified nearly all patients who died or developed nonfatal sustained ventricular tachyarrhythmias during follow up, and had very high negative predictive accuracy (99.6%) for arrhythmic events. Notably, patients with preserved cardiac function had a low, 9%, incidence of indeterminate MTWA tests. Microvolt TWA is useful for risk stratification in this low-risk population, but the false positive rate is too high (91%) to use this test alone to select patients for ICD prophylaxis.

There are still many issues to be addressed to fully develop MTWA testing after acute MI. First, there is the issue of how long after MI to do MTWA tests. Also, we need to understand better what processes are responsible for the delayed development of MTWA after acute MI. Some have postulated that MTWA is a consequence of left ventricular remodeling, a process that also takes weeks to months after MI. The delay in development of MTWA is not necessarily a limitation since early deployment of ICD in high-risk patients has not been shown to reduce sudden cardiac death rates. Also, how to use MTWA tests needs refinement of goals and empirical evidence to support implementation. Patients screened with MTWA alone and testing negative have extraordinarily low risk. Among the patients who test positive early after MI are many false positives. Theoretically, this problem could be overcome by combining MTWA with another test with high NPA that reflects another risk mechanism, e.g., a measure of HRV such as SDNN, but the utility of this strategy has not been tested.

Summary of MTWA

The MTWA test is a safe, inexpensive outpatient test in which patients typically walk on a treadmill at a mild level of effort to raise the heart rate to about 110 beats per minute. Drugs, including β-blocking drugs, do not have to be held for the test [113]. The test has outstanding NPA in patients with heart failure/reduced LVEF of either ischemic or nonischemic etiology [113,114]. When compared directly with other risk predictors, the MTWA test usually ranks among the best [111]. Ninety percent of "indeterminate" MTWA tests are highly predictive of outcomes (death or sustained ventricular tachyarrhythmias) [114,115]. One study showed that ICD therapy had no significant benefit in patients with a normal MTWA test [116]. The information that MTWA test results give is crucial to deciding about prophylactic ICD implants; it also helps substantially to individualize responses to ICD recalls or advisories [122]. Use of MTWA after acute MI is under development. In recognition of its utility, ACC/AHA/ESC 2006 Guidelines for Management of Patients With Ventricular Arrhythmias and the Prevention of Sudden Cardiac Death gave MTWA a Class IIa indication (reasonable to use T-wave alternans for improving the diagnosis and risk

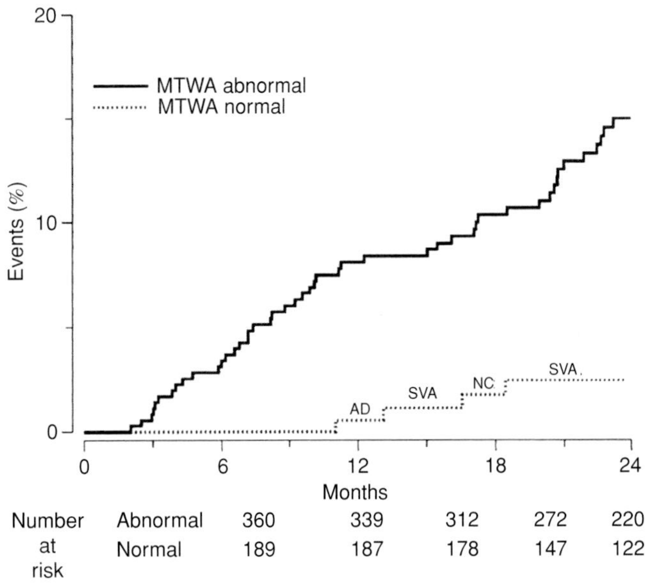

Figure 18.6 The primary end point (death [$n = 40$] or sustained ventricular arrhythmia [$n = 11$]) for patients with normal or abnormal microvolt T-wave alternans (MTWA) test results. In 2 years of follow up, only four end point events (one arrhythmic death [AD], one noncardiac [cancer] death [NC], two nonfatal sustained ventricular arrhythmias [SVA]) occurred in the 189 patients with a normal MTWA test; 47 outcomes occurred in the 360 patients with an abnormal test (From reference [113], with permission.)

Number at risk					
	Abnormal	360	339	312	272	220
	Normal	189	187	178	147	122

stratification of patients with ventricular arrhythmias or who are at risk for developing life-threatening ventricular arrhythmias), level of evidence A. Early in 2006, CMS determined that MTWA diagnostic testing is reasonable and necessary for the evaluation of patients at risk of sudden cardiac death, only when the spectral analytic method is used. National coverage was approved.

QT interval as a measure of myocardial vulnerability

The QT interval reflects the duration of ventricular depolarization and repolarization, and abnormal QT prolongation has been identified as a marker of increased risk for sudden death [123] (hazard ratio 2.17, 95% confidence interval 0.67–7.45) [124]. Ischemic and nonischemic cardiomyopathies have been found to be associated with prolongation of the rate-related QT interval, increased slope of the QT/RR relationship, and increased beat-to-beat variability in the QT duration. As expected, cardiomyopathy has also been shown to manifest prolongation of the repolarization phase of the action potential in myocytes from humans and animal models [125]. The electrophysiologic mechanism of delayed repolarization is complex and multifactorial, involving (at the least) a decrease in

repolarizing current (I_{K1}, I_{To}) [126], perhaps an increase in depolarizing current (I_{NCX} and late I_{Na}) [127], and a reduction in the amplitude and slowed pumping of cytosolic calcium into the sarcoplasmic reticulum [128]. Using arterially perfused ventricular wedge preparations from the pacing dog heart failure model, Akar and Rosenbaum [129] demonstrated an increase in both the duration of repolarization and the transmural dispersion or difference in repolarization duration from epicardium to midmyocardium (see Figure 18.7). In this model, prolongation of the action potential was greatest in the midmyocardial layer, and the termination of these potentials was simultaneous with the end of the T wave. Prolongation of the QT interval in heart failure, then, appears to reflect prolongation of M cell action potentials and appears to be associated with an increase in transmural dispersion of repolarization. Similarly, variability in the QT interval appears to reflect changing durations of repolarization in the M cell layer (read what follows).

QT dispersion

QT dispersion is the difference between the longest and shortest QT interval measured on a 12-lead ECG [130], and has been proposed as a measure of regional dispersion of repolarization. In

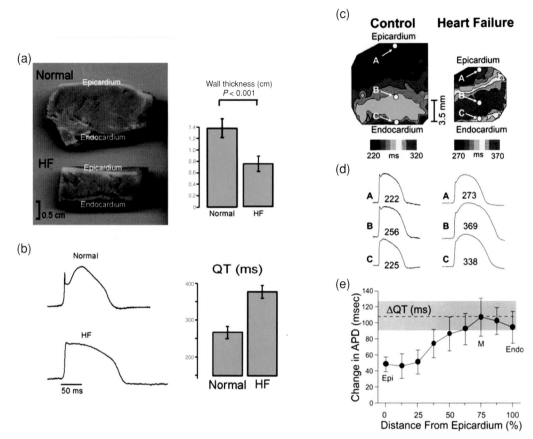

Figure 18.7 Effect of heart failure on ventricular repolarization in dogs. Panel (a): Chronic pacing for 4–6 weeks resulted in significant thinning of the left ventricular wall in failing (HF) compared to control dogs. Panel (b): HF dogs demonstrated significant prolongation of the QT interval in wedges taken from the left ventricle. Panel (c): Arterially perfused ventricular wedges were loaded with the voltage sensitive dye (di-4-ANEPPS) and action potential recorded using 256 detectors at 1-mm intervals. HF dogs manifested greater heterogeneity in action potential duration across the ventricular wall. Panel (d): The action potentials were prolonged to the greatest extent in the midmyocardial ("M") cell layer. Panel (e): Prolongation of the QT interval was driven by prolongation of action potential duration in the M cell layer. (From reference [129], with permission.)

the DIAMOND-CHF trial, QT dispersion failed to predict arrhythmic death [131]. The validity of the claim that differences in the precordial QT reflect spatial heterogeneity of repolarization has been challenged by Malik and Batchvarov [132], and, given its inconsistent performance in clinical trials, enthusiasm for this metric has waned. Analysis of the "T-wave residua," i.e., residual nondipolar component of the T wave from digitized 12-lead ECGs, appears promising as an alternative approach. Zabel et al. [133] found that increased "T-wave residua" was associated with significantly higher mortality in a 10-year prospective study of 813 patients with car-

diovascular disease. This approach appears promising, but these data need to be replicated, preferably in an ICD-eligible population, before routine measurement of T-wave residua can be advocated as a risk stratifier for ICD prophylaxis.

QT/RR relationship

The duration of repolarization is proportional to the previous diastolic interval, so that action potential and QT duration shorten as heart rate increases. Action potential restitution is the relationship between action potential duration and the preceding diastolic interval, and the steeper the slope of restitution, the greater the change in action potential duration with a change in heart period. The "Restitution Hypothesis" maintains that the slope of restitution is a powerful determinant of arrhythmia risk, with slopes > 1 being associated with increasing oscillations in action potential duration leading to "wavebreak," and drugs which flatten the slope (i.e. verapamil and bretylium) reduce the risk of fibrillation [134,135]. While Franz [136] has challenged the validity of this hypothesis by showing that the slope of AP restitution at very short diastolic intervals is frequently > 1 in healthy hearts, observational data seem to support the notion that a "flatter" relationship of repolarization to RR interval is less arrhythmogenic. The linear relation between QT and RR interval ("QT dynamicity") has been investigated retrospectively in several moderate-sized studies using 24-hour ECG (Holter) recordings a significant increase in mortality was found in patients with higher slopes. In a model that contained age, LVEF, SDNN, and creatinine, Pathak et al. [137] studied 175 heart failure patients and found that a QT/RR slope > 0.28 over 24-hours was associated with a multivariate hazard ratio of 3.4 (95% CI 1.43–8.4, $P = 0.0058$) for sudden death, while in the EMIAT study [138] an increased QT/RR slope during daytime hours, but not overnight or over 24 hours, was an independent predictor of sudden death in a retrospective comparison of 188 nonsurvivors with matched controls. Although QT dynamicity's simplicity and ease of measurement are attractive, questions remain regarding the reproducibility of these findings, which reduce its clinical utility. In Pathak's study only 24-hour dynamicity was predictive while in EMIAT, only daytime measures predicted sudden death [137].

QT variability

While MTWA measures variability in the amplitude of the T wave at the alternans frequency only, heart failure is associated with variability in repolarization duration at other frequencies. Shusterman and co-workers [139] found that episodes of VT recorded on Holter recordings were preceded by an increase in T-wave variability at both the alternans and other frequencies. Using a semiautomated, template-matching algorithm, Berger et al.

[140] have shown that cardiomyopathy is associated with an increase in beat-to-beat variability of the duration of the QT interval, reflecting increased lability of repolarization out of proportion to heart rate variability. Since QT variability in normal subjects is driven to a large degree by heart rate variability, the measure defined by Berger (QT variability index or "QTVI") incorporates an assessment of heart rate variability. A heart rate time series is constructed from the sequence of RR intervals using short-term, high-fidelity ECG recordings. The heart rate mean (HRm) and variance (HRv) and QT interval mean (QTm) and variance (QTv) are computed from the respective time series. A normalized QT variability index (QTVI) is then computed:

$$QTVI = \log 10 \frac{(QTv/QTm^2)}{(HRv/HRm^2)}.$$

The QTVI therefore is the log ratio between the QT interval and heart rate variability, each normalized by the squared mean of the respective time series. Atiga et al. [141] reported that elevated QTVI identified cardiac arrest survivors more accurately than TWA or EPS in a group of 98 patients with arrhythmic complaints, whereas Hohnloser and Cohen [142] came to the opposite conclusion, finding that TWA was a better predictor of ICD-treated VT/VF than QTVI. Following the Berger approach, QT variability (with and without normalization to heart rate variability) was measured in supine 10-minute Holter recordings in 476 patients enrolled in the MADIT II study who also received an ICD [143]. The primary endpoint was the occurrence of appropriate ICD therapy for VT/VF determined by device interrogation. The 2-year risk of VT/VF (by Kaplan–Meier analysis) was 37% (top quartile) versus 22% (lower three quartiles, $P = 0.01$). In a Cox regression model that included race, time after myocardial infarction, NYHA class, and LVEF, QTVI was an independent predictor of VT/VF; hazard ratio 1.80, 95% CI: 1.09–2.60, $P = 0.018$). Interestingly, there was no significant difference in HRV (measured as SDNN) between either the high-risk and low-risk quartiles or the VT/VF present and absent groups. When HRV was removed from the metric ("QTVN"), prediction improved, with a hazard ratio for VT/VF of 2.18 (95% CI 1.34–3.55, $P = 0.002$). Although most of the arrhythmic events in these patients were VT, those in the

Table 18.7 Summary of clinical studies of QT interval duration, slope or variability

Author	Test	Population (N)	Mean follow up (yr)	End points (N)	Hazard ratio (95% CI)
de Bruyne et al. [123]	QTc > 460 ms 12-lead ECG	> 55 yr 2093 men 3176 women	4	Death	2.4 (1.5–3.8) men 2.1 (1.4–3.2) women
Zabel et al. [133]	T wave residua (median) 12-lead ECG	Heart disease (772)	10.4 ± 3.8	Death (252)	1.47 (1.14–1.92)
Pathak et al. [137]	QT/RR slope > 0.28 on 24-h Holter	Heart failure (175)	2.5	Death (48)	3.14 (1.43–8.4)
Milliez et al. [138]	QT/RR slope > 0.272 morning on 24-h Holter	Post-MI LVEF < 0.40 (274)	NR	Arrhythmic deaths (59)	1.15 per 0.025 increase in slope (1.01–1.31)
Haigney et al. [143]	QTVI > −0.52 QTVN > 0.257 10 min Holter	Post-MI LVEF < 0.31 (476)	2	VT/VF detected on ICD	QTVI 1.80 (1.09–2.60) QTVN 2.2 (1.34–3.55)
Piccirillo et al. [144]	QTVI > 80% 5 min Holter	Nonischemic LVEF 0.35–0.40 (396)	5	Death and sudden death	Death 2.4 (1.2–4.9) SCD 4.6 (1.5–13.4)
Jensen et al. [145]	SD QT/SDNN 24-h Holter	Post-MI (311)	3	Death (70)	1.9 per 0.1 (1.5–2.4)

LVEF, left ventricular ejection fraction; NR, Not reported; "QTc", heart rate corrected QT (Bazett); QT/RR slope, the regression between QT interval and RR interval; QTVI, QT variability index; QTVN, QT variance normalized for mean QT interval; SD QT/SDNN, standard deviation of QT divided by standard deviation of normal RR (NN) intervals.

top quartile for QTVN were also more likely to experience VF compared to those in the lower quartiles ($P = 0.046$, by Kaplan–Meier analysis). Neither LVEF < 0.25 nor a positive electrophysiologic study was associated with a significant increase in the risk for VT/VF: hazard ratio for LVEF < 0.25, 1.21, 95% CI 0.77–1.87, ($P = 0.41$); hazard ratio for a positive electrophysiologic study 1.26, 95% CI 0.86–1.86 ($P = 0.24$). The importance of normalizing QT variability to HRV may depend on the study population under consideration. In 396 nonischemic patients with LVEF between 0.35 and 0.40, Piccirillo et al. [144] found that QTVI (but not QTVN) dichotomized at the 80th percentile was a significant predictor of both total mortality (hazard ratio 2.4, 95% CI 1.2–4.9) and sudden death (hazard ratio 4.6, 95% CI 1.5–13.4) in a multivariate comparison. In 481 postinfarction patients with a high proportion of noncardiomyopathic patients, Jensen and co-workers [145] examined a broad spectrum of measures derived from 24-hour Holter recordings. In a multivariate comparison, they found that the ratio of the standard deviation of QT to the standard deviation of RR intervals was the most powerful predictor of total mortality and cardiovascular mortality, that it was the only significant predictor of sudden death, outperforming QT/RR slope, LVEF, SDNN, VPCs per hour, and QRS duration (see Table 18.7) [145]. However, their study did not compare QTVI as defined by Berger, i.e., with normalization to mean QT and heart rate, to their ratio. Furthermore, they did not compare the predictive power of short-term to 24-hour recordings. Therefore the optimum method for assessing QT variability still remains undefined.

The mechanism linking QT variability to arrhythmogenesis is incompletely understood. Based on Akar and Rosenbaum's [129] investigations in the heart failure dog, QT variability appears to reflect instability in the duration of repolarization in the M cell layer. One would hypothesize that such M cell variability would be associated with transient increases in transmural dispersion of repolarization that would increase vulnerability to ventricular arrhythmias. At present, QT variability has not been evaluated as part of a two-tiered risk stratification strategy so its utility for selecting patients for ICD prophylaxis cannot be compared with T-wave alternans. However, in MADIT II, the lowest risk quartile for QTVN still had a 17% incidence of VT/VF (i.e., negative predictive accuracy is too low), indicating that QT variability alone is unlikely to be sufficient to identify a low-risk group, but it may prove complementary to MTWA. The ongoing NHLBI-sponsored M2Risk Study may provide an answer. This observational study will follow 700 patients who have LVEF < 0.35 with prophylactic ICDs. At enrollment, each participant will undergo a battery of noninvasive tests; including HRV, SAECG, T-wave alternans, and QT variability to determine which test (or combination of tests) best predict appropriate ICD therapy.

Summary

There is a great need for ICD prophylaxis because cardiac arrest is relatively common and nearly always fatal. The current criteria for selecting candidates for prophylaxis are imperfect, i.e., produce too many false positives and false negatives. A new two-tiered selection process using LVEF and MTWA has proven successful. The two-tiered method was also successful in one study that used LVEF and SDNN. Progress is being made in identifying high-risk patients among postinfarction patients with LVEF > 0.30. The authors hope that risk stratification will continue to be refined until most patients who will benefit will get a prophylactic ICD and patients who will not benefit will not.

References

1 Bardy GH, Lee KL, Mark DB, et al. (for the Sudden Cardiac Death in Heart Failure Trial (SCD-HeFT) Investigators). Amiodarone or an implantable cardioverter defibrillator for congestive heart failure. N Engl J Med 2005;352:225–237.

2 Zipes D, Wellens H. Sudden cardiac death. Circulation 1998;98:2334–2351.

3 Zareba W. QT-RR slope: dynamics of repolarization in the risk stratification. J Cardiovasc Electrophysiol 2003;14:234–235.

4 Moss AJ, Zareba W, Hall WJ, et al. (Multicenter Automatic Defibrillator Implantation Trial II Investigators). Prophylactic implantation of a defibrillator in patients with myocardial infarction and reduced ejection fraction. N Engl J Med 2002;346:877–883.

5 Camm J, Klein H, Nisam S. The cost of implantable defibrillators: perceptions and reality. Eur Heart J 2007;28:392–397.

6 Moss AJ, Hall WJ, Cannom DS, et al. Improved survival with an implanted defibrillator in patients with coronary disease at high risk for ventricular arrhythmia. Multicenter Automatic Defibrillator Implantation Trial Investigators. N Engl J Med 1996;335:1933–1940.

7 Buxton AE, Lee KL, DiCarlo L, et al. Electrophysiologic testing to identify patients with coronary artery disease who are at risk for sudden death. Multicenter Unsustained Tachycardia Trial Investigators. N Engl J Med 2000;342:1937–1945.

8 The Multicenter Postinfarction Research Group. Risk stratification and survival after myocardial infarction. N Engl J Med 1983;309:331–336.

9 Rouleau JL, Talajic M, Sussex B, et al. Myocardial infarction patients in the 1990s—their risk factors, stratification and survival in Canada: the Canadian Assessment of Myocardial Infarction (CAMI) Study. J Am Coll Cardiol 1996;27:1119–1127.

10 Bigger JT Jr. Relation between left ventricular dysfunction and ventricular arrhythmias after myocardial infarction. Am J Cardiol 1986;57:8b–14b.

11 Solomon SD, Zelenkofske S, McMurray JJV, et al. (for the Valsartan in Acute Myocardial Infarction Trial (VALIANT) Investigators). Sudden death in patients with myocardial infarction and left ventricular dysfunction, heart failure, or both. N Engl J Med 2005;352:2581–2588.

12 Buxton AE, Moss AJ. Should everyone with an ejection fraction less than or equal to 30% receive an implantable cardioverter-defibrillator? Circulation 2005;111:2537–2549.

13 Buxton AE, Lee KL, Fisher JD, Josephson ME, Prystowsky EN, Hafley G. (Multicenter Unsustained Tachycardia Trial Investigators). A randomized study of the prevention of sudden death in patients with coronary artery disease. N Engl J Med 1999;341:1882–1890.

14 Gorgels AP, Gijsbers C, de Vreede-Swagemakers J, Lousberg A, Wellens HJ. Out-of-hospital cardiac arrest-the relevance of heart failure. The Maastricht Circulatory Arrest Registry. Eur Heart J 2003;24:1204–1209.

15 The Antiarrhythmics Versus Implantable Defibrillators (AVID) Investigators. A comparison of antiarrhythmic-drug therapy with implantable defibrillators in patients resuscitated from near-fatal ventricular arrhythmias. N Engl J Med 1997;337:1576–1583.

16 Connolly S, Gent M, Roberts R, et al. Canadian Implantable Defibrillator Study (CIDS): a randomized trial of the implantable cardioverter defibrillator against amiodarone. Circulation 2000;101:1297–1302.

17 Kuck K-H, Cappato R, Siebels J, Ruppel R. Randomized comparison of antiarrhythmic drug therapy with implantable defibrillators in patients resuscitated from cardiac arrest: the cardiac arrest study Hamburg (CASH). Circulation 2000;102:748–754.

18 Baldasseroni S, Opasich C, Gorini M, et al. (Italian Network on Congestive Heart Failure Investigators). Left bundle-branch block is associated with increased 1-year sudden and total mortality rate in 5517 outpatients with congestive heart failure: a report from the Italian network on congestive heart failure. Am Heart J 2002;143:398–405.

19 Shamim W, Francis DP, Yousufuddin M, et al. Intraventricular conduction delay: a prognostic marker in chronic heart failure. Int J Cardiol 1999;70:171–178.

20 Shamim W, Yousufuddin M, Cicoria M, Gibson DG, Coats AJS, Henein MY. Incremental changes in QRS duration in serial ECGs over time identify high risk elderly patients with heart failure. Heart 2002;88:47–51.

21 Yerra L, Anavekar N, Skali H, et al. Association of QRS duration and outcomes after myocardial infarction: the VALIANT Trial. Heart Rhythm 2006;3:313–316.

22 Bauer A, Watanabe MA, Barthel P, Schneider R, Ulm K, Schmidt G. QRS duration and late mortality in unselected post-infarction patients of the revascularization era. Eur Heart J 2005;27:427–433.

23 Zareba W, Moss AJ, Noninvasive risk stratification in post-infarction patients with severe LV dysfunction and methodology of the MADIT II noninvasive electrocardiology substudy. J Electrocardiol 2003;36(Suppl):101–108.

24 Gomes JA, Winters SL, Martinson M, Machac J, Stewart D, Targonski A. The prognostic significance of quantitative signal-averaged variables relative to clinical variables, site of myocardial infarction, ejection fraction and ventricular premature beats: a prospective study. J Am Coll Cardiol 1989;13:377–384.

25 Farrell TG, Bashir Y, Cripps T, et al. Risk stratification for arrhythmic events in postinfarction patients based on heart rate variability, ambulatory electrocardiographic variables and the signal-averaged electrocardiogram. J Am Coll Cardiol 1991;18:687–697.

26 Turitto G, Ahuja RK, Caref EB, el-Sherif N. Risk stratification for arrhythmic events in patients with nonischemic dilated cardiomyopathy and nonsustained ventricular tachycardia: role of programmed ventricular stimulation and the signal-averaged electrocardiogram. J Am Coll Cardiol 1994;24:1523–1528.

27 Mancini DM, Wong KL, Simson MB. Prognostic value of an abnormal signal-averaged electrocardiogram in patients with nonischemic congestive cardiomyopathy. Circulation 1993;87:1083–1092.

28 Bigger JT. Prophylactic use of implanted cardiac defibrillators in patients at high risk for ventricular arrhythmias after coronary-artery bypass graft surgery. Coronary Artery Bypass Graft (CABG) Patch Trial Investigators. N Engl J Med 1997;337:1569–1575.

29 Gomes JA, Cain ME, Buxton AE, Josephson ME, Lee KL, Hafley GE. Prediction of long-term outcomes by signal-averaged electrocardiography in patients with unsustained ventricular tachycardia, coronary artery disease, and left ventricular dysfunction. Circulation 2001;104:436–441.

30 Hohnloser SH, Franck P, Klingenheben T, Zabel M, Just H. Open infarct artery, late potentials, and other prognostic factors in patients after acute myocardial

infarction in the thrombolysis era. A prospective trial. Circulation 1994;90:1747–1756.

31 Koelling TM, Aaronson KD, Cody RJ, Bach DS, Armstrong WF. Prognostic significance of mitral regurgitation and tricuspid regurgitation in patients with left ventricular systolic dysfunction. Am Heart J 2002;144: 524–529.

32 Salukhe TV, Henein MY, Sutton R. Ischemic mitral regurgitation and its related risk after myocardial infarction. Circulation 2005;111:254–256.

33 Ristow B, Ali S, Ren X, Whooley MA, Schiller NB. Elevated pulmonary artery pressure by Doppler echocardiography predicts hospitalization for heart failure and mortality in ambulatory stable coronary artery disease. The Heart and Soul Study. J Am Coll Cardiol 2007;49:43–49.

34 Møller JE, Søndergaard E, Poulsen SH, Egstrup K. Pseudonormal and restrictive filling patterns predict left ventricular dilation and cardiac death after a first myocardial infarction: a serial color M-mode Doppler echocardiographic study. J Am Coll Cardiol 2000;36:1841–1846.

35 Agler DA, Adams DB, Waggoner AD. Cardiac resynchronization therapy and the emerging role of echocardiography (part 2): the comprehensive examination. J Am Soc Echocardiogr 2007;20:76–90.

36 Skali H, Zornoff LA, Pfeffer MA, et al. Survival and Ventricular Enlargement (SAVE) Investigators. Prognostic use of echocardiography 1 year after a myocardial infarction. Am Heart J 2005;150:743–749.

37 Ghali JK, Liao Y, Cooper RS. Influence of left ventricular geometric patterns on prognosis in patients with or without coronary artery disease. J Am Coll Cardiol 1998;31:1635–1640.

38 Milani RV, Lavie CJ, Mehra MR, Ventura HO, Kurtz JD, Messerli FH. Left ventricular geometry and survival in patients with normal left ventricular ejection fraction. Am J Cardiol 2006;97:959–963.

39 Decking UK, Pai VM, Wen H, Balaban RS. Does binding of Gd-DTPA to myocardial tissue contribute to late enhancement in a model of acute myocardial infarction? Magn Reson Med 2003;49:168–171.

40 Bello D, Fieno DS, Kim RJ, et al. Infarct morphology identifies patients with substrate for sustained ventricular tachycardia. J Am Coll Cardiol 2005;45:1104–1108.

41 Yan AT, Shayne AJ, Brown KA, et al. Characterization of the peri-infarct zone by contrast-enhanced cardiac magnetic resonance imaging is a powerful predictor of post-myocardial infarction mortality. Circulation 2006;114:32–39.

42 Assomull RG, Prasad SK, Lyne J, et al. Cardiovascular magnetic resonance, fibrosis, and prognosis in dilated cardiomyopathy. J Am Coll Cardiol 2006;48:1977–1985.

43 Eckberg DW. Parasympathetic cardiovascular control in human disease: a critical review of methods and results. Am J Physiol 1980;241:H581–H593.

44 Bigger JT, Albrecht P, Steinman RC, Rolnitzky LM, Fleiss JL, Cohen RJ. Comparison of time- and frequency

domain-based measures of cardiac parasympathetic activity in Holter recordings after myocardial infarction. Am J Cardiol 1989;64:536–538.

45 Corr PB, Yamada KA, Witkowski FX. Mechanisms controlling cardiac autonomic function and their relation to arrhythmogenesis. In: Fozzard HA, Haber E, Jenning RB, Katz AM, eds. *The Heart and Cardiovascular System.* New York: Raven Press; 1986:1343–1403.

46 Ewing DJ. Heart rate variability: an important new risk factor in patients following myocardial infarction. Clin Cardiol 1991;14:683–685.

47 Hinkle LE, Carver ST, Plakun A. Slow heart rates and increased risk of cardiac death in middle-aged men. Arch Intern Med 1972;129:732–748.

48 Kent KM, Smith ER, Redwood DR, Epstein SE. Electrical stability of acutely ischemic myocardium. Influence of heart rate and vagal stimulation. Circulation 1973;47:291–298.

49 Lown B. Sudden cardiac death: the major challenge confronting contemporary cardiology. Am J Cardiol 1979;43:313–328.

50 Malliani A, Schwartz PJ, Zanchetti MD. Neural mechanisms in life-threatening arrhythmias. Am Heart J 1980;100:705–715.

51 Schwartz PJ. The autonomic nervous system and sudden death. Eur Heart J 1998;19(Suppl F):F72–F80.

52 Webb SW, Adgey AAJ, Pantridge JF. Autonomic disturbance at onset of acute myocardial infarction. Br Med J 1972;3:89–92.

53 Zipes DP. Influence of myocardial ischemia and infarction on autonomic innervation of heart. Circulation 1990;82:1095–1105.

54 Billman GE, Hoskins RS. Time-series analysis of heart rate variability during submaximal exercise. Evidence for reduced cardiac vagal tone in animals susceptible to ventricular fibrillation. Circulation 1989;80:146–157.

55 Vybiral T, Bryg RJ, Maddens ME, et al. Effects of transdermal scopolamine on heart rate variability in normal subjects. Am J Cardiol 1990;65:604–608.

56 Lown B, Verrier RL. Neural factors and sudden death. In: Schwartz PJ, Brown AM, Malliani A, Zancheii A, eds. *Neural Mechanisms in Cardiac Arrhythmias.* New York: Raven Press; 1978:87–98.

57 Schwartz PJ, Stone HL. The analysis and modulation of autonomic reflexes in the prediction and prevention of sudden death. In: Zipes DP, Jalife J, eds. *Cardiac Electrophysiology and Arrhythmias.* Orlando, FL: Grune & Stratton; 1985:166–176.

58 Kleiger RE, Stein P, Bosner M, Rottman J. Time domain measurements of heart rate variability. Cardiol Clin 1992;10:487–498.

59 Kleiger RE, Miller JP, Bigger JT, Moss AJ, The Multicenter Post-Infarction Research Group. Decreased heart rate variability and its association with increased mortality after acute myocardial infarction. Am J Cardiol 1987;59:256–262.

60 Kleiger RE, Miller JP, Krone RJ, Bigger JT. The independence of cycle length variability and exercise testing on

predicting mortality of patients surviving acute myocardial infarction. Am J Cardiol 1990;65:408–411.

61 Kleiger RE, Stein PK. Heart rate variability in ischaemic disease. In: Marek Malik, John Camm, eds. *Dynamic Electrocardiography,* Chapter 12. Futura Blackwell; 2004:112–121.

62 Bauer A, Schmidt G. Heart rate turbulence in ischemic heart disease. In: Marek Malik, John Camm, eds. *Dynamic Electrocardiography,* Chapter 23. Futura; 2004:211–213.

63 Schmidt G, Malik M, Barthel P, et al. Heart-rate turbulence after ventricular premature beats as a predictor of mortality after acute myocardial infarction. Lancet 1999;353:1390–1396.

64 La Rovere MT, Bigger JT, Marcus FI, Mortara A, Schwartz PJ (ATRAMI (Autonomic Tone and Reflexes After Myocardial Infarction) Investigators). Baroreflex sensitivity and heart rate variability in prediction of total cardiac mortality after myocardial infarction. Lancet 1998;351:478–484.

65 La Rovere MT, Pinna GD, Hohnloser SH, et al. (on behalf of the ATRAMI Investigators). Baroreflex sensitivity and heart rate variability in the identification of patients at risk for life-threatening arrhythmias. Implications for clinical trials. Circulation 2001;103:2072–2077.

66 Bauer A, Kantelhardt JW, Barthel P, et al. Deceleration capacity of heart rate as a predictor of mortality after myocardial infarction: cohort study. Lancet 2006;367:1674–1681.

67 Kleiger R. Heart rate variability and mortality and sudden death post infarction. J Cardiovas Electrophysiol 1995;6:365–367.

68 Kleiger RE, Stein PK, Bigger JT. Heart rate variability: measurement and clinical utility. Ann Noninv Electrocard 2005;10:1–14.

69 Bigger JT, Fleiss JL, Steinman RC, Rolnitzky LM, Kleiger RE, Rottman JN. Frequency domain measures of heart period variability and mortality after myocardial infarction. Circulation 1992;85:164–171.

70 Bigger JT, Fleiss JL, Steinman RC, Rolnitzky LM, Kleiger RE, Rottman JN. Correlations among time and frequency domain measures of heart period variability 2 weeks after acute myocardial infarction. Am J Cardiol 1992;69:891–898.

71 Bigger JT, Kleiger RE, Fleiss JL, Rolnitzky LM, Steinman RC, Miller JP. Components of heart rate variability measured during healing of acute myocardial infarction. Am J Cardiol 1988;61:208–215.

72 Farrell TG, Bashir Y, Cripps T, et al. Risk stratification for arrhythmic events in postinfarction patients based on heart rate variability, ambulatory electrocardiographic variables and the signal-averaged electrocardiogram. J Am Coll Cardiol 1991;18:687–697.

73 Malik M, Cripps T, Farrell T, Camm AJ. Prognostic value of heart rate variability after myocardial infarction: a comparison of different data-processing methods. Med Biol Eng Comput 1989;27:603–611.

74 Malik M, Farrell TG, Camm AJ. Evaluation of receiver operator characteristics. Optimal time of day for the assessment of heart rate variability after acute myocardial infarction. Int J Biomed Comput 1991;29:175–192.

75 Odemuyiwa O, Malik M, Farrell T, Bashir Y, Poloniecki J, Camm J. Comparison of the predictive characteristics of heart rate variability index and left ventricular ejection fraction for all-cause mortality, arrhythmic events and sudden death after acute myocardial infarction. Am J Cardiol 1991;68:434–439.

76 Zuanetti G, Neilson JM, Latini R, Santoro E, Maggioni AP, Ewing DJ. On behalf of behalf of GISSI-2 investigators. Prognostic significance of heart rate variability in post myocardial infarction patients in the fibrinolytic era. The GISSI 2 results. Circulation 1996;94:432–436.

77 Makikallio TH, Hoiber S, Kober L, et al. Fractal analysis of heart rate dynamics as a predictor of mortality in patients with depressed left ventricular function after acute myocardial infarction. TRACE Investigators. TRAndolapril Cardiac Evaluation. Am J Cardiol 1999;83:836–839.

78 Tapanainen JM, Thomsen PE, Kober L, et al. Fractal analysis of heart rate variability and mortality after an acute myocardial infarction. Am J Cardiol 2002;90:347–352.

79 Voss A, Hnatkova K, Wessel N, et al. Multiparametric analysis of heart rate variability used for risk stratification among survivors of acute myocardial infarction. PACE 1998;21:186–192.

80 Bigger JT Jr, Steinman RC, Rolnitzky LM, Fleiss JL, Albrecht P, Cohen RJ. Power law behavior of RR-interval variability in healthy middle-aged persons, patients with recent myocardial infarction, and patients with heart transplants. Circulation 1996;93:2142–2151.

81 Makikallio TH, Perkiomaki JS, Huikuri HV. Nonlinear dynamics of RR intervals. In: Malik M, Camm AJ, eds. *Dynamic Electrocardiography.* Chapter 3. Futura; 2004:22–30.

82 Huikuri HV, Mäkikallio TH, Peng C-K, Goldberger AL, Hintze U, Møller M (for the DIAMOND Study Group). Fractal correlation properties of R-R interval dynamics and mortality in patients with depressed left ventricular function after an acute myocardial infarction. Circulation 2000;101:47–53.

83 Barthel P, Schneider R, Ing D, et al. Risk stratification after acute myocardial infarction by heart rate turbulence. Circulation 2003;108:1221–1226.

84 Farrell TG, Paul V, Cripps TR, et al. Baroreflex sensitivity and electrophysiological correlates in patients after acute myocardial infarction. Circulation 1991;83:945–952.

85 Aronson D, Mittleman MA, Burger AJ. Measures of heart period variability as predictors of mortality in hospitalized patients with decompensated congestive heart failure. Am J Cardiol 2004;93:59–63.

86 Ponikowski P, Anker SD, Chua TP, et al. Depressed heart rate variability as an independent predictor of death in

chronic congestive heart failure secondary to ischemic or idiopathic dilated cardiomyopathy. Am J Cardiol 1997;79:1645–1650.

87 Rashba EJ, Estes NAM, Wang P, et al. (for the Defibrillators in Non-Ischemic Cardiomyopathy Treatment Evaluation (DEFINITE) Investigators). Preserved heart rate variability identifies low-risk patients with nonischemic dilated cardiomyopathy: results from the DEFINITE trial. Heart Rhythm 2006; 3:281–286.

88 Kotler MN, Tabatznik B, Mower MM, Tominaga S. Prognostic significance of ventricular ectopic beats with respect to sudden death in the late post-infarction period. Circulation 1973;47:959–966.

89 Ruberman W, Weinblatt E, Goldberg JD, Frank CW, Shapiro S. Ventricular premature beats and mortality after myocardial infarction. N Engl J Med 1977;297:750–757.

90 Moss AJ, Davis HT, DeCamilla J, Bayer LW. Ventricular ectopic beats and their relation to sudden and nonsudden cardiac death after myocardial infarction. Circulation 1978;60:998–1003.

91 Anderson KP, DeCamilla J, Moss AJ. Clinical significance of ventricular tachycardia (3 beats or longer) detected during ambulatory monitoring after myocardial infarction. Circulation 1978;57:890–897.

92 Rehnqvist N, Lundman T, Sjogren A. Prognostic implications of ventricular arrhythmias registered before discharge and one year after acute myocardial infarction. Acta Med Scand 1978;204:203–209.

93 Ruberman W, Weinblatt E, Goldberg JD, Frank CW, Chaudhary BS, Shapiro S. Ventricular premature complexes and sudden death after myocardial infarction. Circulation 1981;64:297–305.

94 Schulze RA Jr, Strauss HW, Pitt B. Sudden death in the year following myocardial infarction: relation to ventricular premature contractions in the late hospital phase and left ventricular ejection fraction. Am J Med 1977;62:192–199.

95 Califf R, Burks J, Behar V, Margolis J, Wagner G. Relationships among ventricular arrhythmias, coronary artery disease, and angiographic and electrocardiographic indicators of myocardial fibrosis. Circulation 1978;57:725–732.

96 Bigger JT, Fleiss JL, Kleiger RE, Miller JP, Rolnitzky LM. The relationships among ventricular arrhythmias, left ventricular dysfunction, and mortality in the 2 years after myocardial infarction. Circulation 1984;69:250–258.

97 Mukharji J, Rude RE, Poole WK, et al. (MILIS Study Group). Risk factors for sudden death after acute myocardial infarction: two year follow up. Am J Cardiol 1984;54:31–36.

98 Morganroth J, Bigger JT Jr, Anderson JL. Treatment of ventricular arrhythmias by United States cardiologists: a survey before the Cardiac Arrhythmia Suppression Trial results were available. Am J Cardiol 1990;65:40–48.

99 The CAPS investigators. The cardiac arrhythmia pilot study. Am J Cardiol 1986;54:91–95.

100 The Cardiac Arrthythmia Pilot Study (CAPS) Investigators. Effects of encainide, flecainide, imipramine and moricizine on ventricular arrthythmias during the year after acute myocardial infarction: the CAPS. Am J Cardiol 1988;61:501–509.

101 The Cardiac Arrhythmia Suppression Trial (CAST) Investigators. Preliminary report: effect of encainide and flecainide on mortality in a randomized trial of arrhythmia suppression after myocardial infarction. N Engl Med 1989;321:406–412.

102 Echt DS, Liebson PR, Mitchell LB, et al., CAST Investigators. N Eng J Med 1991;324:781–788.

103 The Cardiac Arrhythmia Suppression Trial II Investigators. Effect of the antiarrhythmic agent moricizine on survival after myocardial infarction. N Engl J Med 1992;327:227–233.

104 Wyse DG, Hallstrom A, McBride R, Cohen JD, Steinberg JS, Mahmarian J, CAST Investigators. Events in the Cardiac Arrhythmia Suppression Trial (CAST): mortality in patients surviving open label titration but not randomized to double-blind therapy. J Am Coll Cardiol 1991;18:20–28.

105 Goldsmith S, Brooks MM, Ledingham R, et al. Association between ease of suppression of ventricular arrhythmia and survival. Circulation 1995;91:79–83.

106 Greenberg HM, Dwyer EM, Hochman JS, Steinberg JS, Echt DS, Peters RW. Interaction of ischaemia and encainide/flecainide treatment: a proposed mechanism for the increased mortality in CAST 1. Br Heart J 1995;74:631–635.

107 Lewis T. Notes upon alternation of the heart. Quart J Med 1910;4:141–144.

108 Adam DR, Smith JM, Akselrod SM, Nyberg S, Powell AO, Cohen RJ. Fluctuations in T-wave morphology and susceptibility to ventricular fibrillation. J Electrocardiol 1984;17:209–218.

109 Smith JM, Clancy EA, Valeri CR, Ruskin JN, Cohen RJ. Electrical alternans and cardiac electrical instability. Circulation 1988;77:110–121.

110 Rosenbaum DS, Jackson LE, Smith JM, Garan H, Ruskin JN, Cohen RJ. Electrical alternans and vulnerability to ventricular arrhythmias. N Engl J Med 1994;330:235–241.

111 Gehi AK, Stein RH, Metz LD, Gomes JA. Microvolt T-wave alternans for the risk stratification of ventricular tachyarrhythmic events: a meta-analysis. J Am Coll Cardiol 2005;46:75–82.

112 Hohnloser SH, Ikeda T, Bloomfield DM, Dabbous OH, Cohen RJ. T-wave alternans negative coronary patients with low ejection and benefit from defibrillator implantation. Lancet 2003;362:125–126.

113 Bloomfield DM, Bigger JT, Steinman RC, et al. Microvolt T-wave alternans and the risk of death or sustained ventricular arrhythmias in patients with left ventricular dysfunction. J Am Coll Cardiol 2006;47: 456–463.

114 Chow T, Kereiakes DJ, Bartone C, et al. Prognostic utility of microvolt T-wave alternans in risk stratification of patients with ischemic cardiomyopathy. J Am Coll Cardiol 2006;47:1820–1827.

115 Kaufman ES, Bloomfield DM, Steinman RC, et al. "Indeterminate" microvolt T-wave alternans tests predict high risk of death or sustained ventricular arrhythmias in patients with left ventricular dysfunction. J Am Coll Cardiol 2006;48;1399–1404.

116 Chow T, Kereiakes DJ, Bartone C, et al. Microvolt T-wave alternans identifies patients with ischemic cardiomyopathy who benefit from implantable cardioverter-defibrillator therapy. J Am Coll Cardiol 2007;49:50–58.

117 Schwab JO, Weber S, Schmitt H, et al. Incidence of T wave alternation after acute myocardial infarction and correlation with other prognostic parameter: results of a prospective study. Pacing Clin Electrophysiol 2001;24:957–961.

118 Ikeda T, Sakata T, Takami M, et al. Combined assessment of T-wave alternans and late potentials used to predict arrhythmic events after myocardial infarction. A prospective study. J Am Coll Cardiol 2000;35:722–730.

119 Tapanainen JM, Still A-M, Airaksinen KEJ, Huikuri HV. Prognostic significance of risk stratifiers of mortality, including T wave alternans, after acute myocardial infarction: results of a prospective follow-up study. J Cardiovasc Electrophysiol 2001;12:645–652.

120 Ikeda T, Saito H, Tanno K, et al. T-wave alternans as a predictor for sudden cardiac death after myocardial infarction. Am J Cardiol 2002;89:79–82.

121 Ikeda T, Yoshino H, Sugi K, et al. Predictive value of microvolt T-wave alternans for sudden cardiac death in patients with preserved cardiac function after acute myocardial infarction: results of a collaborative cohort study. J Am Coll Cardiol 2006;48:2268–2274.

122 Bigger JT, Kleiger RE. Individualizing decisions for patients with prophylactic implantable cardiac defibrillators subject to device advisories: a commentary. Am J Cardiol 2006;98:1291–1293.

123 de Bruyne MC, Hoes AW, Kors JA, Hofman A, van Bemmel JH, Grobbee DE. Prolonged QT interval predicts cardiac and all-cause mortality in the elderly: the Rotterdam Study. Eur Heart J 1999;20:278–282.

124 Karjalainen J, Raunanen A, Ristola P, Viitasalo M. QT interval as a cardiac risk factor in a middle aged population. Heart 1997;77:543–548.

125 Tomaselli GF, Beuckelmann DJ, Calkins HG, et al. Sudden cardiac death in heart failure: the role of abnormal repolarization. Circulation 1994;90:2534–2539.

126 Beuckelmann DJ, Nabauer M, Erdmann E. Alterations of K$^+$ currents in isolated human ventricular myocytes from patients with terminal heart failure. Circ Res 1993;73:379–385.

127 Maltsev VA, Silverman N, Sabbah HN, Undrovinas AI. Chronic heart failure slows late sodium current in human and canine ventricular myocytes: implications for

repolarization variability. Eur J Heart Fail 2007;9:219–227.

128 Gwathmey JK, Copelas L, MacKinnon R, et al. Abnormal intracellular calcium handling in myocardium from patients with end-stage heart failure. Circ Res 1987;61:70–76.

129 Akar FG, Rosenbaum DS. Transmural electrophysiological heterogeneities underlying arrhythmogenesis in heart failure. Circ Res 2003;93:638–645.

130 Day CP, McComb JM, Campbell RW. QT dispersion: an indication of arrhythmia risk in patients with long QT intervals. Br Heart J 1990;63:342–344.

131 Brendorp B, Elming H, Jun L, et al. QT dispersion has no prognostic information for patients with advanced congestive heart failure and reduced left ventricular systolic function. Circulation 2001;103:831–835.

132 Malik M, Batchvarov VN. Measurement, interpretation and clinical potential of QT dispersion. J Am Coll Cardiol 2000;36:1749–1766.

133 Zabel M, Malik M, Hnatkova K, et al. Analysis of T-wave morphology from the 12-lead electrocardiogram for prediction of long-term prognosis in male US veterans. Circulation 2002;105:1066–1070.

134 Nolasco JB, Dahlen RW. A graphic method for the study of alternation in cardiac action potentials. J Appl Physiol 1968;25:191–196.

135 Weiss JN, Garfinkel A, Karagueuzian HS, Qu Z, Chen PS. Chaos and the transition to ventricular fibrillation: a new approach to antiarrhythmic drug evaluation. Circulation 1999;99:2819–2826.

136 Franz MR. The electrical restitution curve revisited: steep or flat slope—which is better? J Cardiovasc Electrophysiol 2003;14:S140–S147.

137 Pathak A, Curnier D, Fourcade J, et al. QT dynamicity: a prognostic factor for sudden cardiac death in chronic heart failure. Eur J Heart Fail 2005;7:269–275.

138 Milliez P, Leenhardt A, Maisonblanche P, et al. (EMIAT Investigators). Usefulness of ventricular repolarization dynamicity in predicting arrhythmic deaths in patients with ischemic cardiomyopathy (from the European Myocardial Infarct Amiodarone Trial). Am J Cardiol 2005;95:821–826.

139 Shusterman V, Goldberg A, London B. Upsurge in T-wave alternans and nonalternating repolarization instability precedes spontaneous initiation of ventricular tachyarrhythmias in humans. Circulation 2006;113:2880–2887.

140 Berger RD, Kasper EK, Baughman KL, Marban E, Calkins H, Tomaselli GF. Beat-to-beat QT interval variability: novel evidence for repolarization lability in ischemic and nonischemic dilated cardiomyopathy. Circulation 1997;96:1557–1565.

141 Atiga WL, Calkins H, Lawrence JH, Tomaselli GF, Smith JM, Berger RD. Beat-to-beat repolarization lability identifies patients at risk for sudden cardiac death. J Cardiovasc Electrophysiol 1998;9:899–908.

142 Hohnloser S, Cohen RJ. T wave alternans and left ventricular ejection fraction, but not QT variability index,

predict appropriate ICD discharge. J Cardiovasc Electrophysiol 1999;10:626–627.

143 Haigney MC, Zareba W, Gentlesk PJ, et al. (Multicenter Automatic Defibrillator Implantation Trial II investigators). QT interval variability and spontaneous ventricular tachycardia or fibrillation in the Multicenter Automatic Defibrillator Implantation Trial (MADIT) II patients. J Am Coll Cardiol 2004;44:1481–1487.

144 Piccirillo G, Magri D, Matera S, et al. QT variability strongly predicts sudden cardiac death in asymptomatic subjects with mild or moderate left ventricular systolic dysfunction: a prospective study. Eur Heart J 2006 [Epub, November 13, 2006; 28:1344–1350.

145 Jensen BT, Abildstrom SZ, Larroude CE, et al. QT dynamics in risk stratification after myocardial infarction. Heart Rhythm 2005;2:357–364.

CHAPTER 19

Risk stratification: where we are and where do we go from here

Jeffrey J. Goldberger

Abbreviations

ABCD, Alternans Before Cardioverter Defibrillator Trial; CABG-Patch, Coronary Artery Bypass Graft – Patch (ICD) Trial; DETERMINE, *DE*fibrillators *T*o *RE*duce *R*isk by *M*agnet*I*c Reso*N*ance Imaging *E*valuation; DINAMIT, Defibrillator in Acute Myocardial Infarction Trial; MADIT, Multicenter Automatic Defibrillator Implantation Trial; MADIT-II, Multicenter Automatic Defibrillator Implantation Trial II; MUSTT, Multicenter Unsustained Tachycardia Trial; SCD-HeFT, Sudden Cardiac Death in Heart Failure Trial; ICD, implantable cardioverter defibrillator.

The number of sudden cardiac deaths reported to occur per year in the United States shows a wide range, from approximately 180,000 to over 400,000 [1–5]. Most sudden cardiac deaths are attributable to underlying cardiovascular disease. In the United States, the cardiovascular disease associated most frequently is coronary artery disease. As such, much attention has been focused on developing techniques to identify such patients with coronary artery disease who are at risk for sudden cardiac death. With the advent of advanced pharmacologic and device therapies for prevention of sudden cardiac death, the significance of developing risk stratification strategies to implement clinical decisions has increased. It is important to note that the field of risk stratification is full of individual techniques, many of which have been shown to identify patients at risk for sudden cardiac death. Specifically, those with

positive results have a higher rate of sudden death than those with negative results. However, there are few (if any) individual techniques that reliably separate those at risk versus those at very low risk for sudden death. As such, combinations of techniques and approaches will need to be integrated into a risk stratification strategy to achieve better discrimination. Yet, few studies have tested and implemented risk stratification strategies in which treatment is determined by the results of combinations of tests. This leaves ample opportunity for further studies to assess the utility of risk stratification strategies. In this chapter, the focus will be on patients with coronary artery disease as these do account for most sudden deaths and this has been the most studied structural heart disease in the risk stratification area.

There are some general statements that apply to our current risk stratification strategies. First, the most widely used risk stratification strategy employs a low ejection fraction as a main criterion. While such a strategy has been shown to be effective, it is also clear that most patients who experience sudden cardiac death do not fall within the low ejection fraction criteria used in such a strategy. Furthermore, it has also been demonstrated that there may be gradations of risk even within this low ejection fraction group, such that those with a high risk for sudden cardiac death can be differentiated from those with a very low risk for sudden cardiac death. Thus, ejection fraction provides a prime example of a risk stratification technique that is useful for identifying high-risk patients, but also does not discriminate well between those at risk and those at low risk for sudden death. While medical therapy with β-blockers, ACE inhibitors, and statins, among others [6] is virtually uniformly recommended across

Ventricular Arrhythmias and Sudden Cardiac Death, 1st edition. Edited by P.J. Wang, A. Al-Ahmad, H. Hsia, and P.C. Zei © 2008 Blackwell Publishing, ISBN: 978-1-4051-6114-5.

the spectrum of ejection fraction and coronary artery disease, particularly those with prior myocardial infarction, the major current therapy that is much more dependent on the risk stratification strategy results is the implantable cardioverter-defibrillator (ICD). The goal of risk stratification strategies should therefore be (1) to better identify patients who are at risk for sudden cardiac death but are yet to be identified and (2) to identify those patients with low ejection fraction who are currently classified as high risk, but with appropriate evaluation may be reclassified as having low risk for sudden cardiac death and therefore may not need an ICD. If this is achievable, ICD therapy can be deployed to those who need it and not to those who do not need it. This is both a challenge and an opportunity.

Understanding risk stratification

In order to make advances in risk stratification, it is important to understand some basic issues that are particularly relevant to the development of a risk score or strategy. Although the events or combinations of events that lead to sudden cardiac death are deterministic, our ability to specifically identify the timing and sequence of these events is limited. Furthermore, it is likely that the etiology of sudden cardiac death is multifactorial. Given that the goal of risk stratification for sudden cardiac death is to identify patients who might die an arrhythmic death that could be prevented (in 2007 by an ICD, but it could be other therapies in the future), it is important to incorporate as many of these factors as are necessary to obtain good risk prediction.

A more fundamental issue with regard to risk prediction is the lack of a true gold standard. This contrasts with the evaluation of the clinical utility of a diagnostic test, where the results of the test are generally compared to a gold standard diagnosis. When one approaches the topic of sudden death, it is important to first acknowledge that there are nonarrhythmic causes of sudden death [7]. In addition, while risk within a population is a continuous function, risk stratification strategies are used clinically in a dichotomous fashion—an intervention (i.e., ICD) is either recommended or not. The dichotomous classification creates high- and low-risk groups, each of which includes patients who will and those who will not experience sudden cardiac

death (but in different proportions). In evaluating a new test or technique, it is not possible to correctly "classify" all the future events of the cohort. Typically, the evaluation of a risk stratification technique involves obtaining the results of a test or score at some initial time in a cohort of patients, following this cohort for some period of time, and at the end of the observation period determining whether the event of interest has occurred or not. Thus, at the end of the evaluation period for a particular risk stratification strategy for sudden cardiac death, there will be two groups—those who did and those who did not die suddenly. Given this finite duration of evaluation, there will be patients who are considered survivors, yet might die suddenly soon after the period of observation or analysis. Yet, for the purpose of the analysis, these individuals were considered survivors. Inclusion of a slightly longer monitoring period would cause the classification of these patients to change (from survivors to nonsurvivors). This may affect the calculated predictive value of the test. Similarly, there may be competing causes of mortality—both cardiac and noncardiac, some of which are associated with the same risk factors as those for sudden cardiac death—that cause a patient to experience nonsudden death when the risk profile should have placed them in the high-risk sudden death group (had they not died of lung cancer caused by smoking on Tuesday, they would have died suddenly on Wednesday).

What exactly does the clinician need from a risk stratification scheme? Given that an intervention will be recommended or not based on this risk stratification scheme, it should have high discrimination ability [8]. This is most appropriately assessed by the receiver operating characteristic (ROC) curve. It has been well demonstrated that for an individual risk factor *alone* to substantially affect the ROC curve, the hazard ratio associated with that risk factor must be quite large (>10–20). The relative risk or hazard ratios for several known risk factors for sudden cardiac death are generally in the 2–6 range. This holds true even for left ventricular ejection fraction [9], considered to be one of the strongest risk factors for sudden death. Pepe et al. [10] note that extremely strong associations are required for meaningful classification accuracy. They further note that it is common for a marker to have independent association with outcome that is considered strong by epidemiologic standards, but does not contribute meaningfully to improved risk discrimination. Many risk factors are continuous variables that display substantial overlap in distribution between those who will and those who will not experience sudden cardiac death. Because of the substantial overlap, these tests applied singly cannot provide good discrimination. However, when combinations of risk factors are used for risk prediction, clinically meaningful discrimination can be achieved, as has been demonstrated by the Framingham study group [11].

One should also be cautious of attempts to evaluate only individual components of a test's performance. For example, in both MADIT-II [12] and SCD-HeFT [13] the arrhythmic sudden death rate at 2–3 years was <10% (the treatment effect defined as the difference in survival between those treated and those not treated with an ICD). If one introduced a coin toss as a risk stratification tool (HEADS indicates High risk) to identify arrhythmic sudden death in a similar population (10% rate of arrhythmic sudden deaths), the negative predictive value of this test would be 90% (out of 100 patients, 10 would die an arrhythmic sudden death and 90 would not; 5 of the former 10 and 45 of the latter 90 would get TAILS. The negative predictive value is the true negatives (45) divided by the total number of negatives (50)). This risk stratification test with no discrimination ability has a high negative predictive value (90%).

Also, as noted previously, for clinical decision making, tests are often stratified dichotomously. Ejection fraction less than or greater than 35% is often used as a separator of high versus low risk for the purposes of considering an ICD implant. This process results in a potential loss of information on risk. Thus, the patient with an ejection fraction of 34% and the patient with an ejection fraction of 14% may both be classified in the same group, but have quite different risk for sudden cardiac death. Similarly, the patient with an ejection fraction of 36% and the patient with an ejection fraction of 54% would also both be classified in the same group, but could have quite different risk for sudden cardiac death. Remaining cognizant of the factors that affect the discrimination capacity of a risk stratification strategy will allow for better application of the currently available techniques.

Risk stratification techniques

Individual risk stratification techniques focus on identification of substrate, triggers, or modulating factors for development of life-threatening ventricular tachyarrhythmias. While sudden cardiac death may be attributable to other causes, the ICD is most specifically effective for the treatment of primary ventricular tachyarrhythmias and this is therefore the focus of the risk stratification techniques. However, many of the techniques that predict sudden cardiac death also predict nonsudden cardiac death, an issue for the specificity of the technique. The role of many of these techniques has been reviewed recently [14]. There is no technique that individually has a high discrimination ability.

The substrate for ventricular tachyarrhythmias refers specifically to the morphology and/or topology of the myocardial infarction that allows the ventricle to be predisposed to reentrant ventricular tachycardia and/or ventricular fibrillation. Both animal and human studies have demonstrated the importance of infarction size and border zone characteristics in the pathophysiology of ventricular tachyarrhythmias. Until recently, clinical determination of myocardial infarct size was highly imprecise. As the left ventricular ejection fraction is easily measurable and is somewhat related to infarct size, among many other parameters, this has emerged as an important risk stratification technique. However, contrast-enhanced MRI has recently allowed more precise delineation of infarct size. It has also been used to provide an index of the border zone of the myocardial infarction [15,16]. Infarct characteristics by MRI have been related to the inducibility of ventricular tachycardia [16,17]. Although electrophysiologic testing is not a direct measurement of anatomic substrate, the inducibility of monomorphic ventricular tachycardia provides information regarding the presence of substrate for this reentrant arrhythmia. Specifically, a potential circuit related to the myocardial infarction must exist if monomorphic ventricular tachycardia is induced.

Risk stratification techniques have also focused on abnormalities of depolarization. This includes the standard QRS duration on electrocardiogram and the signal-averaged electrocardiogram. Slow conduction may exist in areas near the myocardial infarction, and manifest in prolonged QRS duration or the presence of late potentials. These abnormalities are also likely related to substrate for ventricular tachyarrhythmias. Abnormalities in repolarization have also been tested as risk stratification techniques. Because of the difficulty in quantifying repolarization abnormalities, a number of different techniques have emerged. This includes measurement of the QT interval using correction formulae for different heart rates, evaluation of T-wave morphology, measurement of T-wave alternans, and evaluation of the QT–RR relationship. Each of these techniques has proven to identify patients at high risk.

Abnormalities in autonomic tone or responsiveness also seem to be critically related to the development of ventricular tachyarrhythmias. While the precise relationship between abnormalities in autonomic tone and ventricular tachyarrhythmias is unclear, multiple studies have demonstrated a clear relationship between abnormalities in autonomic tone and subsequent mortality. Most recently, results of the DINAMIT study [18] raised the question whether the abnormalities in heart rate variability might be more predictive of nonsudden death than sudden death. Nevertheless, the role of adrenergic activation in arrhythmogenesis has a long history. Furthermore, it has been well demonstrated that the period of exercise and the postexercise recovery period are times of enhanced risk for sudden cardiac death with up to 20-fold increase in risk of sudden cardiac death at these times compared to sedentary periods [19,20]. In addition, ICD discharges are also frequently associated with other types of adrenergic activation, including anger and other emotional distress [21,22]. It is therefore likely that there is a pathophysiologic link between sympathetic activation and sudden death.

Risk stratification strategies

As noted previously, most studies on risk stratification techniques generally compare the utility of different techniques to identify the most predictive technique. While this is certainly helpful, this has not resulted in risk stratification strategies that could be called excellent. The combination of low ejection fraction and abnormal signal-averaged electrocardiogram was tested in the CABG–Patch Trial [23], which revealed no survival advantage to those treated with an ICD. The combination of low ejection fraction and abnormal heart variability immediately following myocardial infarction was tested in the DINAMIT Trial [18] and this revealed no benefit to the ICD. The combination of low ejection fraction and inducible ventricular tachycardia was tested in the MADIT [24] and MUSTT [25] studies, which did demonstrate an improved survival with the ICD. Finally, the combination of low ejection fraction ($\leq$35%) and New York Heart Association class (SCD-HeFT) [13] or ejection fraction <30% (MADIT–II) [12] have been shown to identify patients who have improved survival with an ICD. Table 19.1 lists several clinical trials done in patients with coronary artery disease that

Table 19.1 Summary of selected studies utilizing ICD therapy and identified risk predictors in patients with coronary artery disease

	Year published	NYHA	NSVT	LVEF	Other tests	Other issues
MADIT	1996	I-III	Yes	$\leq$ 35%	EPS	
CABG–Patch*	1997	I-III		$\leq$ 35%	SAECG	At time of CABG
MUSTT	1999	I-III	Yes	$\leq$ 40%	EPS	
MADIT-II	2002	I-III		$\leq$ 30%		
DINAMIT*	2004	I-III		$\leq$ 35%	HRV	6–40 days post-MI
SCD-HeFT	2005	II-III		$\leq$ 35%		
ABCD	Presented AHA 2006	I-III	Yes	$\leq$ 40%	TWA, EPS	

∗ No benefit demonstrated for ICD versus medical therapy.
NYHA, New York Heart Association class for congestive heart failure; NSVT, nonsustained ventricular tachycardia; LVEF, left ventricular ejection fraction; EPS, electrophysiology study; CABG, coronary artery bypass graft surgery; SAECG, signal averaged ECG; MI, myocardial infarction; HRV, heart rate variability; TWA, T wave alternans.

incorporated ICD therapy and some risk stratification technique(s). It is very difficult to draw any specific conclusions regarding risk stratification from these trials, though many do provide information on ICD efficacy. Specifically, even a trial that demonstrates ICD efficacy does not necessarily demonstrate good discrimination between the two groups. Even low ejection fraction does not always identify a group of patients that benefits from an ICD.

Bailey et al. [9] performed an analysis of existing techniques to identify a strategy for identifying patients at risk for sudden cardiac death. The strategy employs the results of multiple testing. Bailey et al. [9] proposed that Stage 1 testing include the signal-averaged electrocardiogram and measurement of left ventricular ejection fraction. If both are positive, the risk for a major arrhythmic event is 38.7%. If one is positive, the probability of a major arrhythmic event over 2 years was predicted to be 10.6% and would justify further testing. However, if both are negative the risk is 2.2% and no further testing would be recommended. Stage 2 would be performed on the patients with only one positive test result; this would include a Holter monitor for assessment of serious ventricular arrhythmias and heart rate variability. If both are negative then the probability of a major arrhythmic event over 2 years is 4.7%, if only one is positive it is 17.5% and if both are positive the risk is 48%. Finally, Stage 3 consists of performing electrophysiologic studies on the Stage 2 patients in whom only one is positive. If the electrophysiologic study is negative the risk of a major arrhythmic event over 2 years is 8.9% and if it is positive the risk is 45.1%. Importantly, they calculated the number of patients that would be classified into a low-risk group, high-risk group, and an unstratified group. Eighty percent of the population would be classified as low risk with a 2.9% probability of a major arrhythmic event, while 11.8% would be classified as high risk with a 41.4% risk of a major arrhythmic event. Finally, 8.2% of the population would be unstratified with an 8.9% probability of a major arrhythmic event over 2 years. This compares to the use of the original MADIT criteria, which included a low left ventricular ejection fraction, spontaneous nonsustained ventricular tachycardia, and inducible ventricular tachycardia during electrophysiologic testing. Bailey et al. observed

that this strategy only identifies 1.9% of the population with a risk of 66.5% of a major arrhythmic event over 2 years. The limitation of this analysis is that this was a statistical analysis based on numerous studies reporting sensitivities and specificities and not an actual tested strategy. It is interesting that since 2001, no such study has been performed despite the strong theoretical basis for this kind of approach.

Risk stratification: where do we go from here?

Given the multiple risk stratification techniques that are available, the first major advance in the field of risk stratification would be to identify which techniques should be employed in the strategy for risk stratification. There are emerging data that suggest clinical variables can be very important in risk stratification. The SCD-HeFT study [13] included New York Heart Association class 2 or 3 in their paradigm. *Post hoc* analyses of both the MADIT-II and the MUSTT [26] have shown that clinical parameters such as creatinine, QRS duration/left bundle branch block, age, and ejection fraction can be used to identify risk of sudden cardiac death. After clinical screening, it may be valuable to perform selected noninvasive tests to identify patients who might warrant further investigation and/or treatment. Finally, the role of electrophysiologic testing remains to be determined. Although this is an invasive test, it does appear to provide important risk stratification. This is evident from the MUSTT [25], in the analysis by Bailey et al. [9], and most recently in the ABCD Trial, presented at the 2006 sessions of the American Heart Association. In this latter prospective trial, an abnormal T-wave alternans in combination with inducible ventricular tachycardia resulted in a 12.6% risk for an arrhythmic event, compared to 2.3% if both were negative, and 5–7.5% if one were positive.

Although ejection fraction is both easy to measure and a very prevalent tool used by clinicians, it is not clear that it is the most useful assessment of substrate to determine risk for sudden cardiac death. Most recently, it has been demonstrated that infarct characteristics such as surface area and mass are better predictors of inducible ventricular tachycardia during electrophysiologic testing than ejection fraction [17]. Further testing in this cohort of patients and in another study demonstrated that the infarct border zone as quantified by intermediate signal intensities on contrast-enhanced MRI, provides even better discrimination of those with inducible ventricular tachycardia [16,27]. As this may be most closely related to the substrate for ventricular tachycardia, it is possible that this anatomic discrimination could be a better predictor for risk of sudden cardiac death. The utility of contrast-enhanced MRI to identify such a population, is being tested in the prospective DETERMINE Trial. In this trial, patients with coronary artery disease whose ejection fraction does not meet criteria for ICD implantation (<30–35%) and who have significant infarct size on contrast-enhanced MRI (>15% of left ventricular mass) will be randomized to receive standard medical therapy or standard medical therapy plus an ICD.

The importance of exercise as a precipitant for sudden cardiac death raises the strong possibility that some sort of exercise-related test might be helpful in identifying risk for sudden cardiac death. Perhaps the predictive value of T-wave alternans, which is measured during exercise, is due, at least in part, to this association. Other evaluations of exercise-induced abnormalities such as delayed heart rate recovery or abnormal QT–RR dynamics could also potentially provide important prognostic information. This framework is analogous to the utility of the electrocardiogram as a tool to detect myocardial ischemia. In susceptible individuals, ischemia occurs more commonly with exertion than at rest. Thus, the exercise electrocardiogram is a much more useful and predictive evaluation than a rest electrocardiogram for detection of ischemia.

The role of genetics and proteomics in prediction of sudden cardiac death is not yet established. In patients with coronary artery disease, it is unlikely that a single gene or small set of genes are uniquely predictive of sudden cardiac death mortality given the multifactorial nature of the disease. Importantly, single genes will probably not have a relative risk high enough to significantly discriminate between those at risk and those not at risk. However, combinations of genetic abnormalities and their use in conjunction with other information could be useful. In addition, the genotype underlying the phenotypic presentation of patients who are at risk for sudden cardiac death may provide complementary information.

Summary

Decades of research on risk stratification for sudden cardiac death have identified multiple clinical characteristics and tests that relate to the pathophysiology of sudden cardiac death. As we learn more about this complex entity, it is likely that further tests and evaluations will be possible. The challenge for research in risk stratification is to focus on the purpose and process of risk stratification to improve discrimination of those at high risk versus those at low risk for sudden cardiac death, rather than searching for the "ultimate" risk stratification technique.

References

1 Centers for Disease Control and Prevention. State-specific mortality from sudden cardiac death—United States, 1999. MMWR 2002;51:123–126.

2 Myerburg RJ. Scientific gaps in the prediction and prevention of sudden cardiac death. J Cardiovasc Electrophysiol 2002;13:709–723.

3 Cobb LA, Fahrenbruch CE, Olsufka M, Copass MK. Changing incidence of out-of-hospital ventricular fibrillation, 1980–2000. JAMA 2002;288:3008–3013.

4 Chugh SS, Jui J, Gunson K, et al. Current burden of sudden cardiac death: multiple source surveillance versus retrospective death certificate-based review in a large U.S. community. J Am Coll Cardiol 2004;44:1268–1275.

5 Rosamond W, Flegal K, Friday G, et al. Heart disease and stroke statistics—2007 update: a report from the American Heart Association Statistics Committee and Stroke Statistics Subcommittee. Circulation 2007;115:e69–e171.

6 Goldberger JJ, Weinberg KM, Kadish AH. Impact of nontraditional antiarrhythmic drugs on sudden cardiac death. In: Zipes D, Jalife J, eds. *Cardiac Electrophysiology: From Cell to Bedside*, 4th ed. Philadelphia: Saunders; 2004:950–958.

7 Pratt CM, Greenway PS, Schoenfeld MH, Hibben ML, Reiffel JA. Exploration of the precision of classifying sudden cardiac death: implications for the interpretation of clinical trials. Circulation 1996;93:519–524.

8 Cook NR. Use and misuse of the receiver operating characteristic curve in risk prediction. Circulation 2007;115:928–935.

9 Bailey JJ, Berson AS, Handelsman H, Hodges M. Utility of current risk stratification tests for predicting major arrhythmic events after myocardial infarction. J Am Coll Cardiol 2001;38:1902–1911.

10 Pepe MS, Janes H, Longton G, Leisenring W, Newcomb P. Limitations of the odds ratio in gauging the performance of a diagnostic, prognostic, or screening marker. Am J Epidemiol 2004;159:882–890.

11 Wilson P, D'Agostino R, Levy D, Belanger A, Silbershatz H, Kannel W. Prediction of coronary heart disease using risk factor categories. Circulation 1998;97:1837–1847.

12 Moss AJ, Zareba W, Hall WJ, et al. (for the Multicenter Automatic Defibrillator Implantation Trial II Investigators). Prophylactic implantation of a defibrillator in patients with myocardial infarction and reduced ejection fraction. N Engl J Med 2002;346:877–883.

13 Bardy GH, Lee KL, Mark DB, et al. (for the Sudden Cardiac Death in Heart Failure Trial (SCD-HeFT) Investigators). Amiodarone or an implantable cardioverter-defibrillator for congestive heart failure. N Engl J Med 2005;352:225–237.

14 Goldberger J. Noninvasive risk stratification. Circulation 2007, in process.

15 Yan A, Shayne A, Brown K, et al. Characterization of the peri-infarct zone by contrast-enhanced cardiac magnetic resonance imaging is a powerful predictor of post-myocardial infarction mortality. Circulation 2006; 114:32–39.

16 Schmidt A, Azevedo CF, Cheng A, et al. Infarct tissue heterogeneity by magnetic resonance imaging identifies enhanced cardiac arrhythmia susceptibility in patients with left ventricular dysfunction. Circulation 2007;115:2006–2014.

17 Bello D, Fieno DS, Kim RJ, et al. Infarct morphology identifies patients with substrate for sustained ventricular tachycardia. J Am Coll Cardiol 2005;45:1104–1108.

18 Hohnloser SH, Kuck KH, Dorian P, et al. (on behalf of the DINAMIT Investigators). Prophylactic use of an implantable cardioverter-defibrillator after acute myocardial infarction. N Engl J Med 2004;351:2481–2488.

19 Albert CM, Mittleman MA, Chae CU, Lee IM, Hennekens CH, Manson JE. Triggering of sudden death from cardiac causes by vigorous exertion. N Engl J Med 2000;343:1355–1361.

20 Mittleman MA, Siscovick DS. Physical exertion as a trigger of myocardial infarction and sudden cardiac death. Cardiol Clin 1996;14:263–270.

21 Fries R, Konig J, Schafers HJ, Bohm M. Triggering effect of physical and mental stress on spontaneous ventricular tachyarrhythmias in patients with implantable cardioverter-defibrillators. Clin Cardiol 2002;25:474–478.

22 Lampert R, Joska T, Burg MM, Batsford WP, McPherson CA, Jain D. Emotional and physical precipitants of ventricular arrhythmia. Circulation 2002;106:1800–1805.

23 Bigger JT Jr (for the Coronary Artery Bypass Graft (CABG) Patch Trial Investigators). Prophylactic use of implanted cardiac defibrillators in patients at high risk for ventricular arrhythmias after coronary artery bypass graft surgery. N Engl J Med 1997;337:1569–1575.

24 Moss AJ, Hall WJ, Cannom DS, et al, (for the Multicenter Automatic Defibrillator Implantation Trial Investigators). Improved survival with an implanted defibrillator in patients with coronary disease at high risk for ventricular arrhythmia. N Engl J Med 1996;335:1933–1940.

25 Buxton AE, Lee KL, Fisher JD, Josephson ME, Prystowsky EN, Hafley G (for the Multicenter Unsustained Tachycardia Trial Investigators). A randomized study of the prevention of sudden death in patients with coronary artery disease. N Engl J Med 1999;341:1882–1890.

26 Buxton AE, Lee KL, Hafley GE, Pires LA, Fisher JD, Gold MR, Josephson ME, Lehmann MH, Prystowsky EN, for the MUSTT Investigators. Limitations of ejection fraction for prediction of sudden death risk in patients with coronary artery disease. J Am Coll Cardiol 2007;50:1150–1157.

27 Rubenstein J, Lee D, Wu E, Kadish A, Passman R, Goldberger J. The prediction of ventricular tachyarrhythmia inducibility by quantification of the peri-infarct border zone by delayed-enhancement cardiac MRI. J Cardiovasc Magn Reson 2007;9:118–119.

CHAPTER 20

Pharmacological management of ventricular arrhythmias

Kevin J. Makati, Munther Homoud, Mark S. Link, Jonathan Weinstock, & N.A. Mark Estes III

Introduction

Therapy for ventricular arrhythmias has evolved considerably over the last two decades. This transformation is largely based on the results of multiple clinical trials that have assessed the risks, benefits, and costs of pharmacologic and nonpharmacologic approaches [1]. In general, therapy for ventricular arrhythmias is indicated to reduce the risk of sudden cardiac death or to treat symptoms related to their presence. Rarely, therapy may be justified to prevent deterioration of left ventricular function. In the case of pharmacotherapy, the clinician must weigh these potential benefits against the risks and costs of pharmaceuticals with an evidence-based yet individualized approach for each patient. Tailoring therapy requires the clinician to identify high-risk clinical parameters such as prior history of myocardial infarction (MI) or symptomatic and compromised left ventricular ejection fraction. When evaluated to decrease the risk of sudden death in these high-risk populations, pharmaceutical agents are considered a primary preventative strategy. By contrast, when used to treat a patient who has survived a prior cardiac arrest or sustained ventricular arrhythmia, pharmaceutical agents are implemented as a secondary preventative measure. When used to improve symptomatic arrhythmia, tachymyopathies (tachyarrhythmia-induced left ventricular dysfunction), or as an agent to reduce device therapy from an implantable cardioverter-defibrillator

Ventricular Arrhythmias and Sudden Cardiac Death, 1st edition. Edited by P.J. Wang, A. Al-Ahmad, H. Hsia, and P.C. Zei © 2008 Blackwell Publishing, ISBN: 978-1-4051-6114-5.

(ICD), pharmaceutical agents are considered adjunctive therapy [1].

While medications, such as antiarrhythmics, treat ventricular arrhythmia by affecting electrophysiologic properties, other pharmacologic agents exist that have antiarrhythmic effects without specific electrophysiologic mechanisms. True antiarrhythmic agents are commonly categorized by the Vaughan Williams classification based on their predominant electrophysiologic effects (Table 20.1) [2]. Agents that affect ion channels, currents, or receptors, the true antiarrhythmics agents, deserve special attention as their basic and clinical effects are well characterized. By contrast, agents that have a salutary effect on ventricular arrhythmias or survival without a known, specific effect on ion channels, currents, or receptors are categorized as nonantiarrhythmics (Table 20.2).

Primary and secondary prevention of sudden cardiac arrest

Treatment of ventricular arrhythmias for the primary and secondary prevention of sudden cardiac arrest has undergone a dramatic evolution from pharmacologic approaches to widespread use of nonpharmacologic therapy, i.e., device therapy and ablation. The "PVC hypothesis" held that suppression of spontaneous ventricular arrhythmias with antiarrhythmic agents would improve survival. Use of these agents was common in selected patient populations to suppress ventricular arrhythmias. Like many other biologically plausible hypotheses, this notion did not withstand the unbiased evaluation

Table 20.1 Vaughan Williams classification of antiarrhythmic agents

Class	General mechanism	Prototypic agents
IA	Moderate Na^+ channel blockade	Quinidine, procainamide, disopyramide
IB	Mild Na^+ channel blockade	Lidocaine*, mexiletine, tocainide[†], phenytoin
IC	Marked Na^+ channel blockade	Flecainide, propafenone
II	β-Blockers	Metoprolol, propranolol, atenolol, carvedilol, acebutolol, betaxolol, bisoprolol, esmolol*, nadolol
III	K^+ channel blockade	Sotalol, amiodarone, bretylium[†], dofetilide, ibutilide*, azimilide[†]
IV	Ca^{2+} channel blockade	Verapamil, diltiazem, and others
V	Adenosine receptor blockade, Na^+/Ca^{2+} pump inhibitor	Adenosine*, Digitalis

*Intravenous form only.
[†]Limited or no availability.

provided by evidence-based medicine. Multiple appropriately designed prospective randomized trials of antiarrhythmic agents in post-MI patients with impaired left ventricular function demonstrated either harmful or neutral effects on total survival (Table 20.3) [3–7].

Similarly, well-designed prospective trials in patients with congestive heart failure (CHF) have made it clear that survival is unchanged with the use of antiarrhythmic agents. While there was some cause for optimism with one initial trial, subsequent investigations could not reproduce these results. Treatment with amiodarone in patients with CHF in the Grupo de Estudio de la Sobrevida en la Insuficiencia Cardiaca en Argentina (GESICA) trial resulted in a trend toward reduction in CHF hospitalizations, sudden death, and total mortality (Table 20.4) [8]. However, these results could not be reproduced in the Congestive Heart Failure Survival Trial of Antiarrhythmic Therapy (CHF-STAT), which in contrast to GESICA, had a high proportion of patients with coronary artery disease (CAD)

Table 20.2 Agents with antiarrhythmic effects

HMG-CoA reductase inhibitors
ω-3 Fatty acids
Antithrombotic and thrombolytic agents
Angiotensin-modifying agents
Aldosterone receptor blockers
Magnesium

[9]. The Danish Investigations of Arrhythmia and Mortality on Dofetilide in Congestive Heart Failure (DIAMOND-CHF) trial showed that dofetilide could be used for the treatment of atrial fibrillation in patients with CHF without excess mortality by following a rigorous protocol that included hospitalization for dofetilide loading [10]. In summary, the evidence does not support the use of antiarrhythmic agents for the primary prevention of sudden cardiac arrest in post-MI or CHF patients.

Trials investigating antiarrhythmic agents in a secondary prevention population were accompanied by high recurrence rates of ventricular arrhythmias when guided by pharmacologic suppression of spontaneous or induced arrhythmias (Table 20.5) [11–17]. While clinical investigations using antiarrhythmic agents failed to demonstrate their clinical utility for the primary and secondary prevention of sudden cardiac arrest (SCA), comparative trials of antiarrhythmics and the ICD are being designed.

Although clinical trial data do not support the use of drug therapy as a means of improving survival in patients who have a history of MI, CHF, or prior cardiac arrest, pharmacologic therapy remains useful as adjunctive therapy for the treatment of symptomatic ventricular arrhythmias. Antiarrhythmic agents, also, have an important role as adjunctive therapy in suppressing spontaneous arrhythmias in individuals with ICDs (Table 20.6) [11,17–22]. Antiarrhythmic agents can reduce the frequency of ICD device therapy by various mechanisms: (1) Increasing the tachycardia cycle length

Table 20.3 Summary of trials for prevention of sudden cardiac arrest in patients with prior myocardial infarction

Trial	Population	Design	Results
Class I antiarrhythmic drugs			
CAST I [3]	6 d–2 yr post-MI, LVEF ≤55% if MI within 90 d, LVEF >40% if MI >90 d, ≥ 6 PVCs/h suppressible by AAD	Encainide or flecainide vs. placebo	Excess arrhythmic (5.7% vs. 2.1% placebo) and all cause mortality (2.6% vs. 1.3% placebo) in patients assigned to AAD arm
CAST II [4]	6 d–2 yr post-MI, LVEF ≤ 40%, ≥6 PVCs/h	Moricizine vs. placebo	No difference in mortality, trend toward increased mortality in AAD arm (*P* = 0.4)
Teo et al. [86]	Recent MI	Meta-analysis of 138 trials in 98,000 patients	Increased mortality in patients on Class I AADs (OR 1.14 *P* = 0.03)
IMPACT [111]	Recent MI	Mexiletine vs. placebo	Trend toward increased mortality in AAD arm (7.6% vs. 4.8% placebo)
The Chamberlain study [80]	6–14 d post-MI (high risk)	Mexiletine vs. placebo	No difference in mortality
Class II antiarrhythmic drugs (see Table 20.8)			
Class III antiarrhythmic drugs			
SWORD [5]	LVEF ≤ 40%, and recent MI (6–42 d) or CHF and remote MI (>42 d)	*d*-Sotalol vs. placebo	Increased mortality in AAD arm (5% vs. 3.1% placebo, RR 1.65)
Julian et al. [112]	Post-MI (5–14 d)	Racemic sotalol	Nonsignificant 18% reduction in overall mortality in AAD arm
EMIAT [88]	Post-MI, LVEF ≤ 40%	Amiodarone vs. placebo	No difference in mortality, 35% RR of arrhythmic death in AAD arm
CAMIAT [7]	6–45 d post-MI, 10 PVCs/h or NSVT	Amiodarone vs. placebo	No difference in mortality, 48.5% RR of resuscitated VF or arrhythmic death in AAD arm

(continued)

Table 20.3 (continued)

Trial	Population	Design	Results
ATMA [99]	Trials enrolling patients post-MI and HF	Meta-analysis of eight post-MI trials and five HF trials comparing amiodarone vs. usual care including 6553 pts	Reduced SCA and arrhythmic death by 29% and all cause mortality by 13% in AAD arm
BASIS [113]	Post-MI and asymptomatic ventricular arrhythmias	Amiodarone vs. OMM	Reduced mortality and arrhythmic events in patients with LVEF ≥40% but not <40% in AAD arm
DIAMOND-MI [114,115]	Post-MI within 7 d, and LVEF ≤ 35%	Dofetilide vs. OMM	No difference in overall mortality, Seven TdP in AAD arm.
Sim et al. [98]	Post-MI including patients with LV dysfunction	Meta-analysis of amiodarone vs. placebo in post-MI patients	Reduced mortality by 10–19% in AAD arm in patients with LV dysfunction or history of CA
Class IV antiarrhythmic drugs			
DAVIT I, II [106]	AMI	Meta-analysis of early and late intervention of AMI with Verapamil	Reduction in SCA in AAD arm

CAST, Cardiac Arrhythmia Suppression Trial; MI, myocardial infarction; LVEF, left ventricular ejection fraction; PVC, premature ventricular contraction; AAD, antiarrhythmic drug; OR, odds ratio; IMPACT, International mexiletine and placebo antiarrhythmic coronary trial; RR, relative risk; SWORD, Survival With Oral d-Sotalol; HF, heart failure; EMIAT, European Myocardial Infarct Amiodarone Trial; CAMIAT, Canadian Amiodarone Myocardial Infarction Trial; NSVT, nonsustained ventricular tachycardia; ATMA, Amiodarone Trials Meta-Analysis Investigators; SCD, sudden cardiac death; BASIS, Basel Antiarrhythmic Study of Infarct Survival; OMM, optimal medical management; DIAMOND-MI, Danish Investigation of Arrhythmias and Mortality on Dofetilide in MI; TdP, torsade de pointes; LV, left ventricular; CA, cardiac arrest; AMI, acute myocardial infarction.

Table 20.4 Summary of randomized controlled trials for prevention of sudden cardiac arrest in patients with congestive heart failure

Trial	Population	Design	Results
SCD-HeFT [61]	LVEF $\leq$ 35%, Class II–III HF	Amiodarone vs. ICD vs. placebo	Reduction in all cause mortality by 23% in ICD arm only
GESICA [8]	LVEF $\leq$ 35%, CXR CT ratio > 0.55, LVEDd $\geq$ 3.2 cm/m^2	Amiodarone vs. placebo	No reduced all cause mortality and trend toward reduced SCA and HF related deaths
CHF-STAT [9]	Symptomatic HF, LVEF $\leq$ 40%, $\geq$10 PVCs/h	Amiodarone vs. placebo	No significant mortality or SCD reduction
DIAMOND-CHF [10]	Symptomatic HF, LVEF $\leq$ 35%, hospitalization for HF within 30 d of enrollment	Dofetilide vs. placebo	No significant survival benefit. HF hospitalization reduction in treatment arm

SCD-HeFT, Sudden Cardiac Death in Heart Failure Trial; LVEF, left ventricular ejection fraction; ICD, implantable cardioverter-defibrillator; GESICA, Grupo de Estudio de la Sobrevida en la Insuficiencia Cardiaca en Argentina; CXR, chest X-ray; LVEDd, left ventricular end diastolic dimension; SCD; sudden cardiac death; HF, heart failure; CHF-STAT, Congestive Heart Failure: Survival Trial of Antiarrhythmic Therapy; PVC, premature ventricular contraction; DIAMOND, Danish Investigation of Arrhythmias and Mortality on Dofetilide.

Table 20.5 Summary of antiarrhythmic drug trials for secondary prevention of sudden cardiac death

AVID [11]	VF, symptomatic VT, or significant hemodynamic sustained VT and LVEF $\leq$ 40%	ICD vs. Class III AADs (primarily amiodarone)	31% reduction in mortality in ICD arm over study period
CIDS [12,13]	VF or out-of-hospital CA or VT with syncope or VT with symptoms, LVEF $\leq$ 35% or syncope with SMVT on EPS	ICD vs. amiodarone	22% RR in all cause mortality in ICD arm. Updated analysis showed higher mortality in AAD arm (5.5%/yr vs. 2.8%/yr ICD arm)
CASH [14]	Survivors of CA secondary to arrhythmia	ICD vs. amiodarone, metoprolol, or propafenone	Excess mortality in propafenone. Trend toward all cause mortality reduction of 23% in ICD arm
Dutch Study [15]	CA with VT/VF, prior MI, and inducible EPS	ICD vs. OMM and Class IA, IC, and III AADs	Reduction in deaths (HR 0.27), hemodynamically significant syncope, and HF requiring transplant in ICD arm
ESVEM [16]	CA or VT/VF and $\geq$10 PVCs/h or syncope and EPS induced VT	EPS or Holter guided sequential AADs; no placebo, ICD, or amiodarone used	Lower recurrence of arrhythmia in sotalol arm but equivalent to Class I AAD +β-blockers
CASCADE [17]	Out-of-hospital VF survivors unrelated to transmural MI, $\geq$10 PVCs/h, or inducible VT/VF on EPS	Amiodarone vs. EPS guided Class I AADs	Reduction in combined endpoint of cardiac death, resuscitated VF, or syncopal ICD shock in amiodarone arm

AVID, Antiarrhythmics versus Implantable Defibrillators; VF, ventricular fibrillation; VT, ventricular tachycardia; LVEF, left ventricular ejection fraction; ICD, implantable cardioverter-defibrillator; AAD, antiarrhythmic drug; CIDS, Canadian implantable defibrillator study; CA, cardiac arrest; SMVT, sustained monomorphic ventricular tachycardia; EPS, electrophysiology study; CASH, Cardiac Arrest Study Hamburg; MI, myocardial infarction; OMM, optimal medical management; HF, heart failure; HR, hazard ratio; ESVEM, Electrophysiologic Study versus Electrocardiographic Monitoring; CASCADE, Cardiac Arrest in Seattle: Conventional Versus Amiodarone Drug Evaluation.

Table 20.6 Trials showing antiarrhythmic agents used as adjunctive therapy with ICDs

Trial	Population	Design	Result
CASCADE [17]	Out-of-hospital VF survivors unrelated to transmural MI, ≥ 10 PVCs/h, or inducible VT/VF on EPS	Amiodarone vs. EPS guided Class I AADs	Reduction in combined endpoint of cardiac death, resuscitated VF, or syncopal ICD shock in amiodarone arm
Pacifico et al. [18]	Recipients of ICDs stratified according EF ($\leq 30\%$ or $>30\%$)	Sotalol 160 mg vs. 320 mg vs. placebo	Significant reduction in all cause ICD shocks
Kuhlkamp et al. [19]	Inducible sustained VT/VF during EPS	d,l-Sotalol vs. placebo	Reduction in VT/VF occurrence by 20.6%
OPTIC study [20]	Recipients of ICDs with sustained VT/VF or CA and LVEF $\leq 40\%$, or inducible VT/VF by EPS and LVEF $\leq 40\%$, or syncope with VT/VF on EPS	Amidarone $+\beta$-blocker vs. Sotalol vs. β-blocker alone	Significant reduction in ICD shock with amiodarone plus β-blocker vs. β-blocker alone. Trend toward ICD shock reduction in sotalol arm
Singer et al. [21]	Recipients of ICDs and mostly NYHA II, III with remote MI	Azimilide 125 mg vs. 75 mg vs. 35 mg vs. placebo	Significant reduction in ICD therapy among all AAD dose groups
SHIELD [22]	Recipients of ICDs with documented spontaneous VT, or CA/VF with LVEF $\leq 40\%$	Azimilide 75 mg vs. 125 mg vs. placebo	Significant reduction in shocks or ATP terminated VT in AAD groups
AVID [11]	VF, symptomatic VT, or hemodynamically significant sustained VT and LVEF $\leq 40\%$	ICD vs. Class III AADs	Reduction in 1 yr arrhythmia event rate by 26% with amiodarone

CASCADE, Cardiac Arrest in Seattle: Conventional Versus Amiodarone Drug Evaluation; VF, ventricular fibrillation; MI, myocardial infarction; EPS, electrophysiology study; AAD, antiarrhythmic drug; ICD, implantable cardioverter-defibrillator; EF, ejection fraction; LVEF, left ventricular ejection fraction; OPTIC, CA, cardiac arrest, Optimal Pharmacological Therapy in Cardioverter Defibrillator Patients; SHIELD, SHock Inhibition Evaluation with azimiLiDe; ATP, antitachycardia pacing; AVID, Antiarrhythmics versus Implantable Defibrillators.

allowing for successful antitachycardia pacing (ATP) while maintaining consciousness; (2) Reducing supraventricular tachycardia causing inappropriate ICD device therapy; (3) Reducing defibrillation thresholds (DFT); and (4) Improving quality of life by reducing the need for ICD device therapy. Antiarrhythmic drugs can also have deleterious effects including proarrhythmia resulting in increased ICD device therapy, slowing of the tachycardia cycle length below the level of detection, and elevation of defibrillation thresholds; all of which result in poor quality of life. Future studies may clarify which agents provide a greater benefit/risk ratio in this regard.

Drug selection

When using medications to manage ventricular arrhythmia, the selection of pharmacologic agent depends on the characteristics of the clinical arrhythmia and the presence of underlying structural heart disease. In each patient, the clinician must carefully weigh the risks and benefits of antiarrhythmic therapy. Clinical characteristics of ventricular arrhythmia that should be factored into the algorithm for clinical decision making include the mechanism of initiation of the ventricular arrhythmia, factors which act to maintain the arrhythmia, the associated mortality risk, and whether the arrhythmia

Table 20.7 Outcomes of major angiotensin-converting enzyme inhibitor trials

Trial	Population	Drug	Mortality reduction	SCA reduction
V-HeFT II [116]	HF	Enalapril	+	+
Hy-C [117]	HF	Captopril	+	+
SOLVD [118]	HF	Enalapril	+	NA
CONSENSUS II	AMI	Enalapril	±	±
SAVE [119]	AMI and LVEF ≤ 40%	Captopril	+	+ + /−
AIRE [120]	AMI and HF	Ramipril	+	+
GISSI 3 [121]	AMI	Lisinopril	+	NA
ISIS-4 [122]	AMI	Captopril	+	NA
SMILE [123]	AMI	Zofenopril	+	+ + /−
TRACE [124]	AMI and LVEF ≤ 35%	Trandolapril	+	+
HOPE [125]	PVD or DM	Ramipril	NA	+ + /−

+, significant benefit; NA, not available; ±, no difference; + + /−, benefit, nonsignificant trend; V-HeFT, Vasodilator-Heart Failure Trial; Hy-C, Effect of direct vasodilation with hydralazine versus angiotensin-converting enzyme inhibition with captopril on mortality in advanced heart failure; SOLVD, Studies of Left Ventricular Dysfunction; HF, heart failure; CONSENSUS, Cooperative New Scandinavian Enalapril Survival Study; AMI, acute myocardial infarction; SAVE, Survival and Ventricular Enlargement Trial; LVEF, left ventricular ejection fraction; AIRE, Acute Infarction Ramipril Efficacy; GISSI, Gruppo Italiano per lo Studio della Sopravvivenza nell'Infarto; ISIS, International Study of Infarct Survival; SMILE, Survival of Myocardial Infarction Long-term Evaluation; TRACE, Trial of the Angiotensin-Converting–Enzyme Inhibitor; HOPE, Heart Outcomes Prevention Evaluation; PVD, peripheral vascular disease; DM, diabetes mellitus.

provokes symptoms. Profiling each arrhythmia by these characteristics and being mindful of the evidence that demonstrates the risks and benefits of each agent will help the clinician make prudent management decisions.

Agents with antiarrhythmic effects

Before considering specific antiarrhythmic drugs that are categorized by the Vaughan Williams classification scheme, a discussion of nonantiarrhythmic agents with antiarrhythmic effects is warranted as these agents have been of particular interest recently (Table 20.2). Agents that have antiarrhythmic effects, while not classified as traditional antiarrhythmic agents, include HMG CoA reductase inhibitors (statins), fish oil, antithrombotic and thrombolytic agents, angiotensin-modifying agents, aldosterone receptor blockers, and magnesium. The mechanisms by which these agents exert electrophysiologic effect are poorly understood. The so-called "nonantiarrhythmics" do not exert direct effects on specialized conduction tissue or modification of myocyte electrophysiologic properties as recognized by the Vaughan Williams classification. However, they have been shown to improve survival in selected patient populations, and in this respect, are believed to have antiarrhythmic properties. Additionally, nonantiarrhythmics have beneficial pleotrophic effects on cardiac function, which frequently makes them a logical initial choice when selecting therapy as it addresses the underlying abnormal and proarrhythmic substrate.

Ace inhibitors

Ace inhibitors have been studied both on a cellular level and in clinical trials (Table 20.7) [23]. At a cellular level, the use of ACE inhibitors has been shown to increase ventricular refractory periods by decreasing I_K currents and enhancing L-type calcium channels [24]. ACE inhibitors may also decrease ventricular arrhythmias by modifying maladaptive cardiac remodeling as seen in hypertensive and cardiomyopathic patients. Results of trials involving ACE inhibitors range from no effect to significant reductions in sudden cardiac arrest (SCA) events. A meta-analysis reveals SCA reductions range from 20% to 50% [25]. Data regarding angiotensin receptor blockade (ARB) are less robust, but suggest similar potential benefits. ARBs act not only to alter remodeling, but also potentially have direct effects on the conduction system as well as refractory periods of myocytes.

Aldosterone antagonist

An optimal medical regimen in patients with advanced, symptomatic heart failure or a history of myocardial infarction with left ventricular dysfunction now includes the addition of aldosterone antagonists. The mechanism of action has been suggested to be modulation of the neuroendocrine axis, although the exact mechanism is unclear. Spironolactone-induced uptake of cardiac norepinephrine has been demonstrated in heart failure patients [26] and may explain reduced arrhythmogenicity in treated subjects, although beneficial effects on vascular endothelium may also contribute to its therapeutic effects [27]. As shown in the RALES [28] and EPHESUS trials [29], patients with structural heart disease on aldosterone antagonists had reduction in total mortality as well as SCA rates.

Statins

The benefits of statins in patients with coronary artery disease are well documented. Statins have direct effects on coronary vasculature by reducing plaque burden, which in turn reduces the substrate for arrhythmia by reducing ischemia. More recent work demonstrates anti-inflammatory properties of statins although the direct mechanism to reduce arrhythmia is poorly understood. Early epidemiologic trials have demonstrated reduction in cardiac mortality and specifically SCA, suggesting a reduction in arrhythmogenicity in patients on statin therapy [30]. More contemporary trials also demonstrated additional SCA reduction in patients already on other medications recognized to reduce arrhythmias [31–36]. Trials that used ICDs further confirmed epidemiologic studies by demonstrating specific reductions of ventricular arrhythmia as recorded by the device [37]. It is well known that statins exert their effect by modifying the vascular endothelium independently of serum cholesterol concentrations. A study in nonischemic cardiomyopathy patients with ICDs exemplified this phenomenon by demonstrating that patients who were treated with statins had fewer ICD therapies for ventricular arrhythmia than in the control arm [38,39].

ω-3 fatty acids

Oils containing either plant-based (α-linoleic acid) and fish-based (eicosapentaenoic acid) ω-3 position fatty acids have previously been shown to reduce SCA and mortality in patients with CAD in both epidemiologic studies and clinical trials [40–45]. The proposed mechanism of action may act through cell membrane stabilization, lowering of plasma triglyceride levels, inhibition of platelet aggregation, and maintenance of L-type calcium channels preventing cellular calcium overload [46]. Results obtained in recent trials investigating the effects of fish oil on ventricular arrhythmias as recorded by ICDs are controversial. The SOFA trial investigated fish oil usage in patients with prior histories of ventricular arrhythmia and ICDs and showed no difference in arrhythmia when compared to control [47]. Another study showed no improvement in ventricular arrhythmia incidence and the potential for proarrhythmia [48]. Fish oil consumption as a means of attenuating ventricular arrhythmia occurrence requires further investigation before it can be recommended on a consistent basis, although fish consumption in moderation is recommended as part of a heart healthy diet.

Magnesium

Magnesium use in ventricular arrhythmias has been justified by several trials documenting benefits in hypomagnesemic patients and acquired torsade de pointes (TdP) [49], although the benefit of magnesium is also seen independently of magnesium levels [50]. The MAGIC trial investigated magnesium in the setting of SCA and did not show a significant benefit in patients presenting with cardiac arrest [51]. More recent studies have had mixed outcomes when looking at patients experiencing myocardial infarctions [52–55].

Antiarrhythmic drug therapy

Antiarrhythmic drug therapy for ventricular arrhythmia has generally been used for primary prevention, secondary prevention, and more recently as adjunctive therapy to ICDs. High-risk populations including patients experiencing MIs and CHF were the focus of investigations, although literature is emerging on how to manage special populations with inherited disorders as well. It is critical to realize that with the development of the ICD, antiarrhythmics have fallen out of favor as a primary or secondary prophylactic agent for the management

Table 20.8 Summary of ICD trials for primary prevention of sudden cardiac death

Trial	Population	Design	Results
MADIT [56]	Prior MI, NYHA I–II HF, LVEF ≤ 35%, NSVT, nonsuppressible VT/VF on EPS	ICD vs. optimal medical management	All cause mortality reduction in ICD arm
MUSTT [59]	CAD, LVEF ≤ 40%, NSVT	EPS directed AAD or ICD therapy based on efficacy vs. OMM	Reduction in CA, or arrhythmic death in EPS guided arm attributed to ICD
MADIT II [57]	LVEF ≤ 30%, post MI	ICD vs. OMM	All cause mortality reduction in ICD arm
DEFINITE [58]	NYHA I–III, NICMP LVEF ≤ 35%, >10 PVCs/h or NSVT	ICD vs. OMM	Significant reduction in arrhythmic deaths, trend toward reduction in all cause mortality
COMPANION [60]	NYHA III–IV, QRS >120 ms, LVEF ≤ 35%	CRT vs. CRT-D vs. OMM	Reduction in all cause mortality in CRT-D arm, and death or HF hospitalization in CRT-D or CRT
SCD-HeFT [61]	NYHA II–III HF, LVEF ≤ 35%	ICD vs. OMM vs. amiodarone	Reduction in all cause mortality and arrhythmic death in ICD arm only

MADIT, Multicenter Automatic Defibrillator Implantation Trial; MI, myocardial infarction; NYHA, New York heart association; HF, heart failure; LVEF, left ventricular ejection fraction; NSVT, nonsustained ventricular tachycardia; VT, ventricular tachycardia; VF, ventricular fibrillation; EPS, electrophysiology study; ICD, implantable cardioverter-defibrillator; MUSTT, Multicenter Unsustained Tachycardia Trial; CAD, coronary artery disease; AAD, antiarrhythmic drug; DEFINITE, Defibrillators in Non-Ischemic Cardiomyopathy Treatment Evaluation; NICMP, nonischemic dilated cardiomyopathy; PVC, premature ventricular contraction; OMM, optimal medical management; COMPANION, Comparison of Medical Therapy, Pacing, and Defibrillation in Heart Failure tachycardia; CRT, cardiac resynchronization therapy; CRT-D, CRT/defibrillator; SCD-HeFT, Sudden Cardiac Death in Heart Failure Trial.

of ventricular arrhythmia (Table 20.8) [56–61]. Instead, concomitant therapy with ICDs is promising and has many beneficial effects as previously mentioned. The benefits imparted by combined device/antiarrhythmic therapy must be balanced against the potential for proarrhythmia, undersensing of ventricular arrhythmias, and potentially elevating DFTs or pacing thresholds. In addition to pharmacologic therapy used for long-term prevention of shocks or arrhythmia, antiarrhythmic agents have a role in acute ventricular arrhythmia management. For recommendations related to the use of antiarrhythmic agents for acute management of ventricular arrhythmias, the reader is referred to the recent revision of the American Heart Association Guidelines for Cardiopulmonary Resuscitation and Emergency Cardiovascular Care [62].

Class I agents

Primary prevention

Antiarrhythmic prophylaxis was first investigated prospectively in the Cardiac Arrhythmia Suppression Trial where flecainide and encainide (CAST I) and moricizine (CAST II) were used in patients experiencing MIs to suppress premature ventricular contractions (PVCs) (Table 20.3) [3,4]. It was thought that suppression of PVCs would reduce mortality by reduction of arrhythmic deaths. The trials were both stopped prematurely after interim statistical analysis showed a higher mortality or no benefit in the antiarrhythmic arms. Class I antiarrhythmics are no longer indicated for the management of ventricular arrhythmias in patients with structural heart disease.

Secondary prevention

Several studies examined Class I agents in patients experiencing cardiac arrest. The Dutch Study compared Class IA, IC, and III antiarrhythmics to ICD therapy (Table 20.5) [11–17]. The antiarrhythmic agent was selected based on its ability to suppress induction of ventricular arrhythmias during programmed electrical stimulation. Patients with arrhythmias that could not be suppressed with antiarrhythmics were randomized to an ICD. The trial showed that ICDs were superior to antiarrhythmics in reducing total mortality and syncope with circulatory arrest. The CASH trial investigated propafenone, amiodarone, and metoprolol with ICDs. The Class IC arm was prematurely terminated after interim analysis revealed an increased mortality. In a pooled analysis of secondary prevention studies, patients randomized to Class I antiarrhythmics had an all cause mortality of 40–45% over a 2-year period suggesting a proarrhythmic effect [63]. Class II antiarrhythmics are not recommended as a secondary preventative strategy in managing patients with SCA. Appropriate usage for other emergent ventricular arrhythmias are governed by the current Advanced Cardiac Life Support guidelines and are not discussed here.

Adjunctive therapy

Class I antiarrhythmics have varying effects on ICDs. Consistent DFT elevation has been seen with Class IA and IB agents in both animal and human studies [64–66]. In contrast, effects of Class IC agents on DFTs are less consistent and have been found to be unpredictable depending on the clinical model studied. It is well known that Class IC agents, specifically flecainide, can raise pacing thresholds and need to be monitored if this agent is chosen as adjunctive therapy. Other classes of antiarrhythmics should be entertained first before selecting a Class I agent as its effect on DFTs are variable, and suppression of arrhythmia in some studies has been shown to be inferior when compared to other agents [16].

Special populations

Class IA

In patients with Brugada syndrome, quinidine may help in terminating incessant arrhythmias [67–69]. The QT prolonging effects of quinidine have been suggested to be beneficial in short-QT syndromes; however, further investigations are necessary before making formal recommendations [70]. Procainamide, although an older-generation antiarrhythmic, is still used for the management of sustained, repetitive, and incessant ventricular tachycardia (VT) in patients with normal ejection fractions and may be more appropriate than amiodarone when early slowing and termination are desired [71,72]. It has also been used in addition to other sodium channel blockers as a provocative test for Brugada syndrome and may have prognostic value [73–75]. This agent is preferred over amiodarone in pregnant patients with ventricular arrhythmias needing chronic therapy due to birth defects caused by the latter agent. Intravenous procainamide must be used judiciously because transient hypotension might occur. Procainamide can prolong the QT interval causing TdP and must be used cautiously or not at all in patients with baseline QT prolongation. Disopyramide has been useful in patients with hypertrophic cardiomyopathy, more for its favorable negative inotropic effects than its ability to suppress arrhythmia.

Class IB

Lidocaine has largely been replaced by amiodarone as an antiarrhythmic drug of choice for many ventricular arrhythmias both in efficacy and mortality data [76]. It is versatile as it can be used intravenously, and in a variety of patients including those with low ejection fractions, prolonged baseline QT intervals, and when VT is thought to be related to ischemia [77,78]. Patients who present with TdP may be managed with intravenous lidocaine; it has been found to be effective in not only drug-associated TdP [79] but also in patients with LQT3 genetic mutations. Lidocaine can also be used in pregnant patients with non-QT-related ventricular arrhythmias. Patients with digitalis toxicity should not be managed with lidocaine or phenytoin. A single study in animals suggested a slight increase in DFT; however, this effect may have been caused by an interaction with anesthetic agents [65]. Phenytoin can also be used in patients with prolonged baseline QT intervals; however, the occurrence of transient hypotension may limit its application in

Table 20.9 Outcome of major β-blocker trials

Trial	Population	Drug	Mortality reduction	SCD reduction
MDC [126]	HF	Metoprolol tartrate	±	±
CIBIS [127]	HF	Bisoprolol	+ + /−	±/NA
US Carvedilol Trial [128]	HF	Carvedilol	+	+/NA
ANZ [129]	HF	Carvedilol	+ + /−	+/NA
MERIT-HF [130]	HF	Metoprolol succinate	+	+
CIBIS II [131]	HF	Bisoprolol	+	+
CAPRICORN [132]	AMI and LVEF ≤ 40%	Carvedilol	+	+ + /−
COPERNICUS [133]	HF	Carvedilol	+	+
COMET [134]	HF	Carvedilol	+	+

+, significant benefit; + + /−, benefit, nonsignificant trend; +/NA benefit, statistical data unavailable; ±/NA, no difference, statistical data unavailable; MDC, Metoprolol in Dilated Cardiomyopathy; HF, heart failure; CIBIS, Cardiac Insufficiency Bisoprolol Study; ANZ, Australia/New Zealand Heart Failure Collaborative Group; MERIT-HF, Metoprolol CR/XL Randomized Intervention Trial in Congestive Heart Failure; CAPRICORN, Carvedilol Post-Infarct Survival Control in LV Dysfunction; AMI, acute myocardial infarction; LVEF, left ventricular ejection fraction; COPERNICUS, Carvedilol Prospective Randomized Cumulative Survival; COMET, Carvedilol Or Metoprolol European Trial.

an emergent setting. Tocainide, marketed as tonocard, is no longer manufactured.

Class IC
As mentioned, Class IC agents have varying effects on DFTs; they predictably raise pacing thresholds. These agents are specifically contraindicated for patients who are recovering from MIs or have structural heart disease as shown in the CAST trial, although similar adverse effects were also seen in trials using mexiletine [80] and disopyramide [81]. Advanced age has also been shown to increase adverse events in patients using Class IC agents. Flecainide, as with other sodium channel blocking antiarrhythmics, can cause arrhythmias related to toxic levels and manifest as resistant ventricular arrhythmias, 1:1 conducting atrial flutter, and incessant ICD shocks. Some of these toxic drug syndromes can be treated with β-blockade, and sodium chloride or bicarbonate. Given that flecainide has a considerably long list of adverse effects, it is predominantly used for atrial arrhythmias in structurally normal hearts in conjunction with atrioventricular nodal blocking agents to prevent rapid conduction. Flecainide has been used as a provocative agent to detect occult Brugada syndrome; however, a formal guideline dictating its exact role does not exist. Propafenone has been shown in multiple trials to increase ventricular arrhythmias and

mortality in patients with structural heart disease [82,83].

Class II agents
Of all the antiarrhythmics studied, β-blockers are overrepresented in a variety of CHF and acute coronary syndrome trials investigating SCA (Table 20.9) [84]. It is the only agent to consistently reduce SCA and potentially modify the underlying arrhythmogenic substrate by complementary effects on coronary vasculature and myocyte function. Direct electrophysiologic effects of β-blockers have been well studied and are known to be effective in suppressing ventricular arrhythmias when induction has been attempted in the electrophysiology lab [85]. β-Blockers have been shown to be the single causative agent in antiarrhythmic drug trials to drive reductions in SCA [86]. It cannot be overstated that β-blockers should be there in most medical regimens as part of an optimal heart failure treatment plan or as an adjunctive agent to ICDs if reductions in SCA and device therapy are the desired endpoints.

Primary prevention
β-Blockers are the only antiarrhythmic drug to consistently improve survival by decreasing arrhythmic mortality in primary prevention studies. A review of post-MI patients showed a decreased incidence of

SCA in over 25,000 patients studied (Table 20.9) [87]. This effect persists when used in conjunction with other antiarrhythmics and may suggest a beneficial interaction as in the case with amiodarone [88]. In addition to coronary disease populations, trials investigating SCA in acute coronary syndromes and CHF patients also report significant SCA reduction when β-blockers are used as primary prophylaxis for ventricular arrhythmia [89,90]. It is noteworthy that β-blockers remain inferior to ICDs as a means of primary SCA prevention and should be prescribed as an adjunct to device therapy rather than a replacement if protection from SCA is desired [91,92].

Secondary prevention

β-Blockers as secondary prophylaxis in SCA has been studied, but modern trials investigating these agents against controls are rare even as it forms the basis of an optimal medical regimen for all patients being randomized. The AVID trial examined patients who suffered a cardiac arrest and randomized them to amiodarone or ICDs [11]. Patients who only received a β-blocker as an antiarrhythmic agent showed a mortality benefit in cardiac arrest survivors, which reflects earlier work by Brodsky et al. [93] showing improved survival in SCA survivors who were young and had left ventricular dysfunction. As in primary prevention studies, β-blocker therapy was associated with inferior survival when compared with ICD therapy in various patient populations [93,94].

Adjunctive therapy

The benefit of adding β-blockers to ICD therapy has been studied in the OPTIC trial [20]. The investigators sought to define an optimal antiarrhythmic regimen to reduce ICD therapy in patients who have experienced cardiac arrest either spontaneously or by programmed electrical stimulation. Patients treated with amiodarone plus β-blocker or sotalol had significantly less appropriate and inappropriate ICD therapy when compared to patients treated with β-blocker alone. The independent effect of β-blockers on ICD therapy has been previously studied and has been shown to increase the time to first shock [95], and reduce the frequency of appropriate shock in a dose-dependent fashion [96].

Special populations

Data supports β-blockade in CHF and CAD populations for primary prevention, secondary prevention, and adjunctive therapy with ICDs. β-Blockers have a defined role in long-QT syndrome as well. It is believed that β-blockers act to decrease adrenergic tone, thereby decreasing arrhythmogenicity of the abnormal substrate. β-Blockers may decrease ventricular arrhythmia in hypertrophic cardiomyopathy patients and also have a beneficial role in relieving outflow obstruction. β-Blockers and other agents that slow the ventricular rate should be avoided for patients who demonstrate pause-dependent ventricular arrhythmias.

Class III agents

Class III agents were hoped to provide protection from SCA after the failure observed with Class I agents. Class III agents affect membrane repolarization, prolong action potential duration, and refractory periods and act mainly through potassium channels, although amiodarone exhibits sodium and calcium channel blocking properties as well as β- and α-receptor blocking effects. Whereas sotalol and dofetilide produce these effects through blockade of the rapidly activating outward K^+ current I_{Kr}, amiodarone and azimilide block both I_{Kr} and the slowly activating component of the delayed rectifier K^+ current I_{Ks}. Sotalol is a nonselective β-blocking agent available as a racemate of both the *d*- and *l*-rotary forms. The *d*-isomer has less than 2% β-blocking activity of the *l*-isomer [97]. Azimilide is a relatively new Class III agent not yet approved that shares similar effects on cardiac conduction tissue as amiodarone. Bretylium, also a Class III agent, is no longer manufactured (Table 20.1).

Primary prevention

Early meta-analyses suggested a potential benefit on SCA prevention [86,98,99]. When studied in a prospective fashion, however, these benefits were not seen as much as demonstrated in SCD-HeFT [61]. Multiple prospectively designed trials showed either no benefit or a higher mortality when compared with ICD therapy (Table 20.10) [61,100]. Electrophysiology study guided antiarrhythmic therapy not only failed to identify patients who did not need ICDs, but demonstrated a higher mortality when compared to patients who received

Table 20.10 Outcome of trials using amiodarone in sudden cardiac death prevention

Trial	Population	Design	Result
Ceremuzynski et al. [135]	Post-MI patients intolerant to β-blocker	Amiodarone vs. placebo	Reduction in cardiac mortality and ventricular arrhythmia
AMIOVIRT [100]	NICMP, LVEF ≤ 35%, asymptomatic NSVT, NYHA I–III HF	ICD vs. amiodarone	No difference between mortality and arrhythmic death; however, no control arm
SCD-HeFT [61]	LVEF ≤ 35%, Class II–III HF	Amiodarone vs. ICD vs. placebo	Reduction in all cause mortality and arrhythmic death in ICD arm only
GESICA [8]	LVEF ≤ 35%, CXR CT ratio >0.55, LVEDd ≥ 3.2 cm/m^2	Amiodarone vs. placebo	Reduced mortality and trend toward SCD and HF reductions
CHF-STAT [9]	Symptomatic HF, LVEF ≤ 40%, ≥10 PVCs/h	Amiodarone vs. placebo	No significant mortality or SCD reduction
Sim et al. [98]	Post MI including pts with LV dysfunction	Meta-analysis of amiodarone vs. placebo in post-MI patients	Reduced mortality in AAD arm in patients with LV dysfunction or history CA
ATMA [99]	Trials enrolling patients post-MI and HF	Meta-analysis of eight post-MI trials comparing Amiodarone vs. usual care, five HF trials including 6553 pts	Reduced SCD and arrhythmic death in AAD arm
EMIAT [6]	5–21 d post-MI, LVEF ≤ 40%	Amiodarone vs. placebo	No difference in mortality, decreased arrhythmic death in AAD arm
CAMIAT [7]	6–45 d post-MI, ≥10 PVCs/h or NSVT	Amiodarone vs. placebo	No difference in mortality, decreased resuscitated VF or arrhythmic death in AAD arm

AMIOVIRT, Amiodarone versus implantable cardioverter-defibrillator; NICMP, nonischemic cardiomyopathy; LVEF, left ventricular ejection fraction; NSVT, nonsustained ventricular tachycardia; NYHA, New York heart association; HF, heart failure; SCD-HEFT, sudden cardiac death in heart failure trial; GESICA, Grupo de Estudio de la Sobrevida en la Insuficiencia Cardiaca en Argentina; CXR, chest X-ray; CT, cardiothoracic; LVEDd, left ventricular end diastolic dimension; PVC, premature ventricular contraction; SCD, sudden cardiac death; CHF-STAT, congestive heart failure: survival trial of antiarrhythmic therapy; MI, myocardial infarction; ATMA, amiodarone trials meta-analysis investigators; AAD, antiarrhythmic drug; EMIAT, European Myocardial Infarct Amiodarone Trial; CAMIAT, Canadian Amiodarone Myocardial Infarction Trial.

an ICD [59,101,102]. Class III agents are no longer considered acceptable alternatives to ICDs for the primary prevention of SCA.

Secondary prevention

Several large-scale trials investigated amiodarone in survivors of ventricular arrhythmia (Table 20.5) [11,12,14]. In the AVID trial, patients who survived cardiac arrest, or had sustained ventricular tachycardia with either hemodynamic collapse or LVEF <40%, were randomized to a Class III antiarrhythmic or an ICD. Although the trial sought to compare the efficacy of sotalol against amiodarone, only 2.6% of patients received sotalol at discharge. The CIDS trial evaluated a similar population and randomized patients to ICDs or amiodarone. The

CASH trial also investigated cardiac arrest survivors and randomized them to β-blockers, amiodarone, and propafenone. Although each study had limitations in trial design, they concluded that Class III antiarrhythmics were inferior to ICDs in reducing SCA, that all of them cause mortality.

Adjunctive therapy

Class III drugs have had a unique role as adjunctive agents in patients who have ICDs. In the OPTIC trial, patients randomized to amiodarone and β-blocker had a significant reduction in appropriate and inappropriate shock when compared with β-blocker or sotalol [20]. Patients who received ICDs in the AVID trial and were treated with amiodarone, sotalol, or mexiletine, had a significant reduction in ICD discharges and extension of time to first shock interval. Sotalol has independently been shown to decrease the composite endpoint of death or ICD shock regardless of ejection fraction [18,19]. Azimilide was shown to have a dose-dependent reduction on ICD therapy including ATP without affecting DFTs [21]. The SHIELD trial not only demonstrated reductions in ventricular arrhythmia recurrence, but also documented an acceptable side effect profile when compared to placebo [22]. More studies are necessary to determine whether azimilide consistently affects hard clinical endpoints such as shock frequency or psychological distress.

Special populations

Trials investigating CAD patients demonstrated that amiodarone was safe when used with β-blockers [88]. Amiodarone was shown to be superior to placebo and lidocaine in the management of out-of-hospital shock-resistant ventricular fibrillation (VF) and is now recommended over other antiarrhythmics for shock-refractory VF although no agent has been shown to improve survival at hospital discharge [62,76,103]. Sotalol has been investigated in the early post-MI period [104]. Although no significant benefit was observed, the study did verify its safety in this population. Sotalol has been shown to reduce DFTs and improve responsiveness to shocks [105].

Class IV agents

Verapamil and diltiazem constitute prototypic agents in this class of antiarrhythmic drugs. There is no role for Class IV agents in the primary or secondary prevention of sudden cardiac death. Verapamil has been investigated in the post-MI population without β-blockade and demonstrated a reduction in SCA [106]. The treatment effect was most likely mediated by a reduction in ischemia and would not apply to contemporary patients on modern drug regimens that include β-blockers.

Special populations

Not all ventricular arrhythmias are associated with high rates of SCA. In select groups with low SCA incidence, ventricular arrhythmias may be treated with conventional medications. Verapamil has been used effectively for reentrant fascicular ventricular tachycardias [107]; however, the advent of curative catheter ablation techniques has lessened the importance of this drug therapy. Although potentially lethal, milder forms of long-QT syndromes [108,109] and catecholaminergic VT [110] may be effectively treated with Class IV agents. β-Blockers have largely replaced many Class IV agent indications and are now generally considered to be first-line medical therapy.

Conclusion

The role of antiarrhythmic agents in the contemporary management of ventricular arrhythmia has been modified extensively on the basis of multiple prospective randomized controlled trials. Antiarrhythmic agents now play a very limited role in the primary or secondary prevention of SCA. By contrast, there is an emerging role for these agents as adjunctive therapy to treat symptoms due to arrhythmias or improve outcomes in patients with ICDs. Although newer agents are available, the potential benefits of medical therapy in patients with ventricular arrhythmias will always be compared against nonpharmacologic device therapy, which has set up a new paradigm for SCA prevention and treatment. The development of radiofrequency ablation offers permanent cures to patients with a low risk of SCA who would otherwise require lifelong medications for symptom control. When pharmacologic treatment is desired, nonantiarrhythmics are generally preferred as their adverse side effect profiles are less deleterious than those of the antiarrhythmics. Finally, implantable devices offer superior protection to patients at high risk for SCA and are currently the preferred mode of treatment over pharmacotherapy. However, adjunctive therapy with medications has the added benefit of symptom relief and may redefine how pharmaceuticals are used in managing ventricular arrhythmia.

References

1 Zipes DP, Camm AJ, Borggrefe M, et al. ACC/AHA/ESC 2006 Guidelines for Management of Patients With Ventricular Arrhythmias and the Prevention of Sudden Cardiac Death: a report of the American College of Cardiology/American Heart Association Task Force and the European Society of Cardiology Committee for Practice Guidelines (writing committee to develop Guidelines for Management of Patients With Ventricular Arrhythmias and the Prevention of Sudden Cardiac Death): developed in collaboration with the European Heart Rhythm Association and the Heart Rhythm Society. Circulation 2006;114(10):e385–e484.

2 Estes NAM III, Garan H, McGovern B, Ruskin JN. Class I antiarrhythmic agents: electrophysiological considerations and classification. In: *Mechanisms and Treatment of Cardiac Arrhythmias: Relevance of Basic Studies to Clinical Management.* Vienna: Urban And Schwarzenberg; 1985:183–201.

3 Echt DS, Liebson PR, Mitchell, LB, et al. Mortality and morbidity in patients receiving encainide, flecainide, or placebo. The Cardiac Arrhythmia Suppression Trial. N Engl J Med 1991;324(12):781–788.

4 The Cardiac Arrhythmia Suppression Trial II Investigators. Effect of the antiarrhythmic agent moricizine on survival after myocardial infarction. N Engl J Med 1992;327(4):227–233.

5 Waldo AL, Camm AJ, deRuyter H, et al. Effect of d-sotalol on mortality in patients with left ventricular dysfunction after recent and remote myocardial infarction. The SWORD Investigators. Survival With Oral d-Sotalol. Lancet 1996;348(9019):7–12.

6 Julian DG, Camm AJ, Frangin G, et al. Randomised trial of effect of amiodarone on mortality in patients with left-ventricular dysfunction after recent myocardial infarction: EMIAT. European Myocardial Infarct Amiodarone Trial Investigators. Lancet 1997;349(9053):667–674.

7 Cairns JA, Connolly SJ, Roberts R, Gent M. Randomised trial of outcome after myocardial infarction in patients with frequent or repetitive ventricular premature depolarisations: CAMIAT. Canadian Amiodarone Myocardial Infarction Arrhythmia Trial Investigators. Lancet 1997;349(9053):675–682.

8 Doval HC, Nul DR, Grancelli HO, Perrone SV, Bortman GR, Curiel R. Randomised trial of low-dose amiodarone in severe congestive heart failure. Grupo de Estudio de la Sobrevida en la Insuficiencia Cardiaca en Argentina (GESICA). Lancet 1994;344(8921):493–498.

9 Singh SN, Fletcher RD, Fisher S, Lazzari D, Deedwania P, Lewis D, Massie B, et al. Veterans affairs congestive heart failure antiarrhythmic trial. CHF STAT Investigators. Am J Cardiol 1993;72(16):99F–102F.

10 Torp-Pedersen C, Moller M, Bloch-Thomsen PE, et al. Dofetilide in patients with congestive heart failure and left ventricular dysfunction. Danish Investigations of Arrhythmia and Mortality on Dofetilide Study Group. N Engl J Med 1999;341(12):857–865.

11 The Antiarrhythmics versus Implantable Defibrillators (AVID) Investigators. A comparison of antiarrhythmic-drug therapy with implantable defibrillators in patients resuscitated from near-fatal ventricular arrhythmias. N Engl J Med 1997;337(22):1576–1583.

12 Connolly SJ, Gent M, Roberts RS, et al. Canadian implantable defibrillator study (CIDS): a randomized trial of the implantable cardioverter defibrillator against amiodarone. Circulation 2000;101(11):1297–1302.

13 Bokhari F, Newman D, Greene M, Korley V, Manga I, Dorian P. Long-term comparison of the implantable cardioverter defibrillator versus amiodarone: eleven-year follow-up of a subset of patients in the Canadian Implantable Defibrillator Study (CIDS). Circulation 2004;110(2):112–116.

14 Kuck KH, Cappato R, Siebels J, and Ruppel R. Randomized comparison of antiarrhythmic drug therapy with implantable defibrillators in patients resuscitated from cardiac arrest: the Cardiac Arrest Study Hamburg (CASH). Circulation 2000;102(7):748–754.

15 Wever EF, Hauer RN, van Capelle FL, et al. Randomized study of implantable defibrillator as first-choice therapy versus conventional strategy in postinfarct sudden death survivors. Circulation 1995;91(8):2195–2203.

16 Mason JW. A comparison of seven antiarrhythmic drugs in patients with ventricular tachyarrhythmias. Electrophysiologic Study versus Electrocardiographic Monitoring Investigators. N Engl J Med 1993;329(7):452–458.

17 Greene HL. The CASCADE Study: randomized antiarrhythmic drug therapy in survivors of cardiac arrest in Seattle. CASCADE Investigators. Am J Cardiol 1993;72(16):70F–74F.

18 Pacifico A, Hohnloser SH, Williams JH, et al. Prevention of implantable-defibrillator shocks by treatment with sotalol. d,l-Sotalol Implantable Cardioverter-Defibrillator Study Group. N Engl J Med 1999;340(24):1855–1862.

19 Kuhlkamp V, Mewis C, Mermi J, Bosch RF, and Seipel L. Suppression of sustained ventricular tachyarrhythmias: a comparison of d,l-sotalol with no antiarrhythmic drug treatment. J Am Coll Cardiol 1999;33(1):46–52.

20 Connolly SJ, Dorian P, Roberts RS, et al. Comparison of beta-blockers, amiodarone plus beta-blockers, or sotalol for prevention of shocks from implantable cardioverter defibrillators: the OPTIC Study: a randomized trial. JAMA 2006;295(2):165–171.

21 Singer I, Al-Khalidi H, Niazi I, et al. Azimilide decreases recurrent ventricular tachyarrhythmias in patients with implantable cardioverter defibrillators. J Am Coll Cardiol 2004;43(1):39–43.

22 Dorian P, Borggrefe M, Al-Khalidi HR, et al. Placebo-controlled, randomized clinical trial of azimilide for prevention of ventricular tachyarrhythmias in patients with an implantable cardioverter defibrillator. Circulation 2004;110(24):3646–3654.

23 Siddiqui A, Kowey PR. Sudden death secondary to cardiac arrhythmias: mechanisms and treatment strategies. Curr Opin Cardiol 2006;21(5):517–525.

24 Racke HF, Koppers D, Lemke P, Casaretto H, Hauswirth, O, et al. Fosinoprilate prolongs the action potential: reduction of I_K and enhancement of the L-type calcium current in guinea pig ventricular myocytes. Cardiovasc Res 1994;28(2):201–208.

25 Domanski MJ, Exner DV, Borkowf CB, Geller NL, Rosenberg Y, Pfeffer MA. Effect of angiotensin converting enzyme inhibition on sudden cardiac death in patients following acute myocardial infarction. A meta-analysis of randomized clinical trials. J Am Coll Cardiol 1999;33(3):598–604.

26 Barr CS, Lang CC, Hanson J, Arnott M, Kennedy N, Struthers AD. Effects of adding spironolactone to an angiotensin-converting enzyme inhibitor in chronic congestive heart failure secondary to coronary artery disease. Am J Cardiol 1995;76(17):1259–1265.

27 Farquharson CA, Struthers AD. Spironolactone increases nitric oxide bioactivity, improves endothelial vasodilator dysfunction, and suppresses vascular angiotensin I/angiotensin II conversion in patients with chronic heart failure. Circulation 2000;101(6):594–597.

28 Pitt B, Zannad F, Remme WJ, et al. The effect of spironolactone on morbidity and mortality in patients with severe heart failure. Randomized Aldactone Evaluation Study Investigators. N Engl J Med 1999;341(10):709–717.

29 Pitt B, Remme W, Zannad F, et al. Eplerenone, a selective aldosterone blocker, in patients with left ventricular dysfunction after myocardial infarction. N Engl J Med 2003;348(14):1309–1321.

30 Randomised trial of cholesterol lowering in 4444 patients with coronary heart disease: the Scandinavian Simvastatin Survival Study (4S). Lancet 1994;344(8934):1383–1389.

31 The Long-Term Intervention with Pravastatin in Ischaemic Disease (LIPID) Study Group. Prevention of cardiovascular events and death with pravastatin in patients with coronary heart disease and a broad range of initial cholesterol levels. N Engl J Med 1998;339(19):1349–1357.

32 Sacks FM, Pfeffer MA, Moye LA, et al. The effect of pravastatin on coronary events after myocardial infarction in patients with average cholesterol levels. Cholesterol and Recurrent Events Trial investigators. N Engl J Med 1996;335(14):1001–1009.

33 LaRosa JC, He J, Vupputuri S. Effect of statins on risk of coronary disease: a meta-analysis of randomized controlled trials. JAMA 1999;282(24):2340–2346.

34 De Sutter J, Tavernier R, De Buyzere M, Jordaens L, De Backer G. Lipid lowering drugs and recurrences of

life-threatening ventricular arrhythmias in high-risk patients. J Am Coll Cardiol 2000;36(3):766–772.

35 Makikallio TH, Barthel P, Schneider R, et al. Frequency of sudden cardiac death among acute myocardial infarction survivors with optimized medical and revascularization therapy. Am J Cardiol 2006;97(4):480–484.

36 Sackner-Bernstein J. Reducing the risks of sudden death and heart failure post myocardial infarction: utility of optimized pharmacotherapy. Clin Cardiol 2005;28(11 Suppl 1):I19–II27.

37 Chiu JH, Abdelhadi RH, Chung MK, et al. Effect of statin therapy on risk of ventricular arrhythmia among patients with coronary artery disease and an implantable cardioverter-defibrillator. Am J Cardiol 2005;95(4):490–491.

38 Goldberger JJ, Subacius H, Schaechter A, et al. Effects of statin therapy on arrhythmic events and survival in patients with nonischemic dilated cardiomyopathy. J Am Coll Cardiol 2006;48(6):1228–1233.

39 Vyas AK, Guo H, Moss AJ, et al. Reduction in ventricular tachyarrhythmias with statins in the Multicenter Automatic Defibrillator Implantation Trial (MADIT)-II. J Am Coll Cardiol 2006;47(4):769–773.

40 de Lorgeril M, Salen P, Martin JL, Monjaud I, Delaye J, Mamelle N. Mediterranean diet, traditional risk factors, and the rate of cardiovascular complications after myocardial infarction: final report of the Lyon Diet Heart Study. Circulation 1999;99(6):779–785.

41 Burr ML, Fehily AM, Gilbert JF, et al. Effects of changes in fat, fish, and fibre intakes on death and myocardial reinfarction: diet and reinfarction trial (DART). Lancet 1989;2(8666): 757–761.

42 Gruppo Italiano per lo Studio della Sopravvivenza nell'Infarto miocardico. Dietary supplementation with n-3 polyunsaturated fatty acids and vitamin E after myocardial infarction: results of the GISSI-Prevenzione trial. Lancet 1999;354(9177):447–455.

43 Albert CM, Hennekens CH, O'Donnell CJ, et al. Fish consumption and risk of sudden cardiac death. JAMA 1998;279(1):23–28.

44 Siscovick DS, et al. Dietary intake and cell membrane levels of long-chain n-3 polyunsaturated fatty acids and the risk of primary cardiac arrest. JAMA 1995;274(17):1363–1367.

45 Bucher HC, Hengstler P, Schindler C, Meier G, et al. N-3 polyunsaturated fatty acids in coronary heart disease: a meta-analysis of randomized controlled trials. Am J Med 2002;112(4):298–304.

46 Hallaq H, Smith TW, Leaf A. Modulation of dihydropyridine-sensitive calcium channels in heart cells by fish oil fatty acids. Proc Natl Acad Sci USA 1992;89(5):1760–1764.

47 Brouwer IA, Zock PL, Camm AJ, et al. Effect of fish oil on ventricular tachyarrhythmia and death in patients with implantable cardioverter defibrillators: the Study on Omega-3 Fatty Acids and Ventricular Arrhythmia (SOFA) randomized trial. JAMA 2006;295(22):2613–2619.

48 Raitt MH, Connor WE, Morris C, et al. Fish oil supplementation and risk of ventricular tachycardia and ventricular fibrillation in patients with implantable defibrillators: a randomized controlled trial. JAMA 2005;293(23):2884–2891.

49 Topol EJ, Lerman BB. Hypomagnesemic torsades de pointes. Am J Cardiol 1983;52(10):1367–1368.

50 Tsuji H, Venditti Jr, FJ, Evans JC, Larson MG, Levy D. The associations of levels of serum potassium and magnesium with ventricular premature complexes (the Framingham Heart Study). Am J Cardiol 1994;74(3):232–235.

51 Thel MC, Armstrong AL, McNulty SE, Califf RM, O'Connor CM. Randomised trial of magnesium in inhospital cardiac arrest. Duke Internal Medicine Housestaff. Lancet 1997;350(9087):1272–1276.

52 Antman EM, Anbe DT, Armstrong PW, et al. A comparison of results of meta-analyses of randomized control trials and recommendations of clinical experts. Treatments for myocardial infarction. JAMA 1992;268(2):240–248.

53 Teo KK, Yusuf S. Role of magnesium in reducing mortality in acute myocardial infarction. A review of the evidence. Drugs 1993;46(3):347–359.

54 Woods KL, Fletcher S. Long-term outcome after intravenous magnesium sulphate in suspected acute myocardial infarction: the second Leicester Intravenous Magnesium Intervention Trial (LIMIT-2). Lancet 1994;343(8901):816–819.

55 Antman EM. Randomized trials of magnesium in acute myocardial infarction: big numbers do not tell the whole story. Am J Cardiol 1995;75(5):391–393.

56 Moss AJ, Hall WJ, Cannom DS, et al. Improved survival with an implanted defibrillator in patients with coronary disease at high risk for ventricular arrhythmia. Multicenter Automatic Defibrillator Implantation Trial Investigators. N Engl J Med 1996;335(26):1933–1940.

57 Moss AJ, Zareba W, Hall WJ, et al. Prophylactic implantation of a defibrillator in patients with myocardial infarction and reduced ejection fraction. N Engl J Med 2002;346(12):877–883.

58 Kadish A, Dyer A, Daubert JP, et al. Prophylactic defibrillator implantation in patients with nonischemic dilated cardiomyopathy. N Engl J Med 2004;350(21):2151–2158.

59 Buxton AE, Lee KL, Fisher JD, et al. A randomized study of the prevention of sudden death in patients with coronary artery disease. Multicenter Unsustained Tachycardia Trial Investigators. N Engl J Med 1999;341(25):1882–1890.

60 Bristow MR, Saxon LA, Boehmer J, et al. Cardiac-resynchronization therapy with or without an implantable defibrillator in advanced chronic heart failure. N Engl J Med 2004;350(21):2140–2150.

61 Bardy GH, Lee KL, Mark DB, et al. Amiodarone or an implantable cardioverter-defibrillator for congestive heart failure. N Engl J Med 2005;352(3):225–237.

62 American Heart Association. 2005 American Heart Association Guidelines for Cardiopulmonary Resuscitation and Emergency Cardiovascular Care. Part 7.2: Management of Cardiac Arrest. Circulation 2005;112(Suppl 24):IV 58–IV 66.

63 Cappato R. Secondary prevention of sudden death: the Dutch Study, the Antiarrhythmics Versus Implantable Defibrillator Trial, the Cardiac Arrest Study Hamburg, and the Canadian Implantable Defibrillator Study. Am J Cardiol 1999;83(5B):68D–73D.

64 Echt DS, Black JN, Barbey JT, et al. Evaluation of antiarrhythmic drugs on defibrillation energy requirements in dogs. Sodium channel block and action potential prolongation. Circulation 1989;79(5):1106–1117.

65 Kerber RE, Pandian NG, Jensen SR, et al. Effect of lidocaine and bretylium on energy requirements for transthoracic defibrillation: experimental studies. J Am Coll Cardiol 1986;7(2):397–405.

66 Ujhelyi MR, Schur M, Frede T, et al. Differential effects of lidocaine on defibrillation threshold with monophasic versus biphasic shock waveforms. Circulation 1995;92(6):1644–1650.

67 Mok NS, Chan NY, Chiu AC. Successful use of quinidine in treatment of electrical storm in Brugada syndrome. Pacing Clin Electrophysiol 2004;27(6 Pt 1):821–823.

68 Maury P, Couderc P, Delay M, et al. Electrical storm in Brugada syndrome successfully treated using isoprenaline. Europace 2004;6(2):130–133.

69 Alings M, Dekker L, Sadee A, et al. Quinidine induced electrocardiographic normalization in two patients with Brugada syndrome. Pacing Clin Electrophysiol 2001;24(9 Pt 1):1420–1422.

70 Gaita F, Giustetto C, Bianchi F, et al. Short QT syndrome: pharmacological treatment. J Am Coll Cardiol 2004;43(8):1494–1499.

71 Gorgels AP, van den Dool A, Hofs A, et al. Comparison of procainamide and lidocaine in terminating sustained monomorphic ventricular tachycardia. Am J Cardiol 1996;78(1):43–46.

72 Callans DJ, Marchlinski FE. Dissociation of termination and prevention of inducibility of sustained ventricular tachycardia with infusion of procainamide: evidence for distinct mechanisms. J Am Coll Cardiol 1992;19(1):111–117.

73 Brugada R, Brugada J, Antzelevitch C, et al. Sodium channel blockers identify risk for sudden death in patients with ST-segment elevation and right bundle branch block but structurally normal hearts. Circulation 2000;101(5):510–515.

74 Priori SG, Napolitano C, Gasparini M, et al. Natural history of Brugada syndrome: insights for risk stratification and management. Circulation 2002;105(11):1342–1347.

75 Brugada J, Brugada R, Antzelevitch C, et al. Long-term follow-up of individuals with the electrocardiographic pattern of right bundle-branch block and ST-segment elevation in precordial leads V1 to V3. Circulation 2002;105(1):73–78.

76 Dorian P, Cass D, Schwartz B, et al. Amiodarone as compared with lidocaine for shock-resistant ventricular fibrillation. N Engl J Med 2002;346(12):884–890.

77 Nasir N Jr, Doyle TK, Wheeler SH, et al. Usefulness of Holter monitoring in predicting efficacy of amiodarone therapy for sustained ventricular tachycardia associated with coronary artery disease. Am J Cardiol 1994;73(8):554–558.

78 Lie KI, Wellens HJ, van Capelle FJ, et al. Lidocaine in the prevention of primary ventricular fibrillation. A double-blind, randomized study of 212 consecutive patients. N Engl J Med 1974;291(25):1324–1326.

79 Assimes TL, Malcolm I. Torsade de pointes with sotalol overdose treated successfully with lidocaine. Can J Cardiol 1998;14(5):753–756.

80 Chamberlain DA, Jewitt DE, Julian DG, et al. Oral mexiletine in high-risk patients after myocardial infarction. Lancet 1980;2(8208–8209):1324–1327.

81 U.K. Rythmodan Multicentre Study Group. Oral disopyramide after admission to hospital with suspected acute myocardial infarction. Postgrad Med J 1984;60(700):98–107.

82 Siebels J, Cappato R, Ruppel R, et al. ICD versus drugs in cardiac arrest survivors: preliminary results of the Cardiac Arrest Study Hamburg. Pacing Clin Electrophysiol 1993;16(3 Pt 2):552–558.

83 Wyse DG, Talajic M, Hafley GE, et al. Antiarrhythmic drug therapy in the Multicenter UnSustained Tachycardia Trial (MUSTT): drug testing and as-treated analysis. J Am Coll Cardiol 2001;38(2):344–351.

84 Adamson PB, Gilbert EM. Reducing the risk of sudden death in heart failure with beta-blockers. J Card Fail 2006;12(9):734–746.

85 Duff HJ, Mitchell LB, Wyse DG. Antiarrhythmic efficacy of propranolol: comparison of low and high serum concentrations. J Am Coll Cardiol 1986;8(4):959–965.

86 Teo KK, Yusuf S, Furberg CD. Effects of prophylactic antiarrhythmic drug therapy in acute myocardial infarction. An overview of results from randomized controlled trials. JAMA 1993;270(13):1589–1595.

87 Freemantle N, Cleland J, Young P, et al. beta Blockade after myocardial infarction: systematic review and meta regression analysis. BMJ 1999;318(7200):1730–1737.

88 Boutitie F, Boissel JP, Connolly SJ, et al. Amiodarone interaction with beta-blockers: analysis of the merged EMIAT (European Myocardial Infarct Amiodarone Trial) and CAMIAT (Canadian Amiodarone Myocardial Infarction Trial) databases. The EMIAT and CAMIAT Investigators. Circulation 1999;99(17):2268–2275.

89 Antman EM, Anbe DT, Armstrong PW, et al. ACC/AHA guidelines for the management of patients with ST-elevation myocardial infarction; A report of the American College of Cardiology/American Heart Association Task Force on Practice Guidelines (Committee to Revise the 1999 Guidelines for the Management of patients with acute myocardial infarction). J Am Coll Cardiol 2004;44(3):E1–E211.

90 Priori SG, Aliot E, Blomstrom-Lundqvist C, et al. Task Force on Sudden Cardiac Death, European Society of Cardiology. Europace 2002;4(1):3–18.

91 Ermis C, Zadeii G, Zhu AX, et al. Improved survival of cardiac transplantation candidates with implantable cardioverter defibrillator therapy: role of beta-blocker or amiodarone treatment. J Cardiovasc Electrophysiol 2003;14(6):578–583.

92 Ellison KE, Hafley GE, Hickey K, et al. Effect of beta-blocking therapy on outcome in the Multicenter UnSustained Tachycardia Trial (MUSTT). Circulation 2002;106(21):2694–2699.

93 Brodsky MA, Allen BJ, Luckett CR, et al. Antiarrhythmic efficacy of solitary beta-adrenergic blockade for patients with sustained ventricular tachyarrhythmias. Am Heart J 1989;118(2):272–280.

94 Exner DV, Reiffel JA, Epstein AE, et al. Beta-blocker use and survival in patients with ventricular fibrillation or symptomatic ventricular tachycardia: the Antiarrhythmics Versus Implantable Defibrillators (AVID) trial. J Am Coll Cardiol 1999;34(2):325–333.

95 Hreybe H, Bedi HM, Ezzeddine R, et al. Indications for internal cardioverter defibrillator implantation predict time to first shock and the modulating effect of beta-blockers. Am Heart J 2005;150(5):1064.

96 Brodine WN, Tung RT, Lee JK, et al. Effects of beta-blockers on implantable cardioverter defibrillator therapy and survival in the patients with ischemic cardiomyopathy (from the Multicenter Automatic Defibrillator Implantation Trial-II). Am J Cardiol 2005;96(5):691–695.

97 Link MS, Homound M, Foote CB, et al. Antiarrhythmic drug therapy for ventricular arrhythmias: current perspectives. J Cardiovasc Electrophysiol 1996;7(7):653–670.

98 Sim I, McDonald KM, Lavori PW, et al. Quantitative overview of randomized trials of amiodarone to prevent sudden cardiac death. Circulation 1997;96(9):2823–2829.

99 Amiodarone Trials Meta-Analysis Investigators. Effect of prophylactic amiodarone on mortality after acute myocardial infarction and in congestive heart failure: meta-analysis of individual data from 6500 patients in randomised trials. Lancet 1997;350(9089):1417–1424.

100 Strickberger SA, Hummel JD, Bartlett TG, et al. Amiodarone versus implantable cardioverter-defibrillator: randomized trial in patients with nonischemic dilated cardiomyopathy and asymptomatic nonsustained ventricular tachycardia—AMIOVIRT. J Am Coll Cardiol 2003;41(10):1707–1712.

101 Schlapfer J, Rapp F, Kappenberger L, et al. Electrophysiologically guided amiodarone therapy versus the implantable cardioverter-defibrillator for sustained ventricular tachyarrhythmias after myocardial infarction: results of long-term follow-up. J Am Coll Cardiol 2002;39(11):1813–1819.

102 Lau EW, Griffith MJ, Pathmanathan RK, et al. The Midlands Trial of Empirical Amiodarone versus Electrophysiology-guided Interventions and Implantable Cardioverter-defibrillators (MAVERIC): a multi-centre prospective randomised clinical trial on the

secondary prevention of sudden cardiac death. Europace 2004;6(4):257–266.

103 Kudenchuk PJ, Cobb LA, Copass MK, et al. Amiodarone for resuscitation after out-of-hospital cardiac arrest due to ventricular fibrillation. N Engl J Med 1999;341(12):871–878.

104 Julian DG, Prescott RJ, Jackson FS, et al. Controlled trial of sotalol for one year after myocardial infarction. Lancet 1982;1(8282):1142–1147.

105 Dorian P, Newman D. Effect of sotalol on ventricular fibrillation and defibrillation in humans. Am J Cardiol 1993;72(4):72A–79A.

106 Hansen JF. Review of postinfarct treatment with verapamil: combined experience of early and late intervention studies with verapamil in patients with acute myocardial infarction. Danish Study Group on Verapamil in Myocardial Infarction. Cardiovasc Drugs Ther 1994;8(Suppl 3):543–547.

107 Bhadha K, Marchlinski FE, Iskandrian AS. Ventricular tachycardia in patients without structural heart disease. Am Heart J 1993;126(5):1194–1198.

108 Jacobs A, Knight BP, McDonald KT, et al. Verapamil decreases ventricular tachyarrhythmias in a patient with Timothy syndrome (LQT8). Heart Rhythm 2006;3(8):967–970.

109 Milberg P, Reinsch N, Osada N, et al. Verapamil prevents torsade de pointes by reduction of transmural dispersion of repolarization and suppression of early afterdepolarizations in an intact heart model of LQT3. Basic Res Cardiol 2005;100(4):365–371.

110 Swan H, Laitinen P, Kontula K, et al. Calcium channel antagonism reduces exercise-induced ventricular arrhythmias in catecholaminergic polymorphic ventricular tachycardia patients with RyR2 mutations. J Cardiovasc Electrophysiol 2005;16(2):162–166.

111 Impact Research Group. International mexiletine and placebo antiarrhythmic coronary trial: I. Report on arrhythmia and other findings. J Am Coll Cardiol 1984;4(6):1148–1163.

112 Julian DG, Jackson FS, Szekely P, et al. A controlled trial of sotalol for 1 year after myocardial infarction. Circulation 1983;67(6 Pt 2):I61–I62.

113 Pfisterer M, Kiowski W, Burckhardt D, et al. Beneficial effect of amiodarone on cardiac mortality in patients with asymptomatic complex ventricular arrhythmias after acute myocardial infarction and preserved but not impaired left ventricular function. Am J Cardiol 1992;69(17):1399–1402.

114 Danish Investigations of Arrhythmia and Mortality ON Dofetilide. Dofetilide in patients with left ventricular dysfunction and either heart failure or acute myocardial infarction: rationale, design, and patient characteristics of the DIAMOND studies. Clin Cardiol 1997;20(8):704–710.

115 Kober L, Torp-Pedersen LC, Carlsen JE, et al. Effect of dofetilide in patients with recent myocardial infarction and left-ventricular dysfunction: a randomised trial. Lancet 2000;356(9247):2052–2058.

116 Cohn JN, Johnson G, Ziesche S, et al. A comparison of enalapril with hydralazine-isosorbide dinitrate in the treatment of chronic congestive heart failure. N Engl J Med 1991;325(5):303–310.

117 Fonarow GC, Chelimsky-Fallick C, Stevenson LW, et al. Effect of direct vasodilation with hydralazine versus angiotensin-converting enzyme inhibition with captopril on mortality in advanced heart failure: the Hy-C trial. J Am Coll Cardiol 1992;19(4):842–850.

118 The SOLVD Investigators. Effect of enalapril on mortality and the development of heart failure in asymptomatic patients with reduced left ventricular ejection fractions. N Engl J Med 1992;327(10):685–691.

119 Pfeffer MA, Braunwald E, Moye LA, et al. Effect of captopril on mortality and morbidity in patients with left ventricular dysfunction after myocardial infarction. Results of the survival and ventricular enlargement trial. The SAVE Investigators. N Engl J Med 1992;327(10):669–677.

120 The Acute Infarction Ramipril Efficacy (AIRE) Study Investigators. Effect of ramipril on mortality and morbidity of survivors of acute myocardial infarction with clinical evidence of heart failure. Lancet 1993;342(8875):821–828.

121 Gruppo Italiano per lo Studio della Sopravvivenza nell'infarto Miocardico. GISSI-3: effects of lisinopril and transdermal glyceryl trinitrate singly and together on 6-week mortality and ventricular function after acute myocardial infarction. Lancet 1994;343(8906):1115–1122.

122 ISIS-4 (Fourth International Study of Infarct Survival) Collaborative Group. ISIS-4: a randomised factorial trial assessing early oral captopril, oral mononitrate, and intravenous magnesium sulphate in 58,050 patients with suspected acute myocardial infarction. Lancet 1995;345(8951):669–685.

123 Ambrosioni E, Borghi C, Magnani B. The effect of the angiotensin-converting-enzyme inhibitor zofenopril on mortality and morbidity after anterior myocardial infarction. The Survival of Myocardial Infarction Long-Term Evaluation (SMILE) Study Investigators. N Engl J Med 1995;332(2):80–85.

124 Kober L, Bloch Thomsen PE, Moller M, et al. A clinical trial of the angiotensin-converting-enzyme inhibitor trandolapril in patients with left ventricular dysfunction after myocardial infarction. Trandolapril Cardiac Evaluation (TRACE) Study Group. N Engl J Med 1995;333(25):1670–1676.

125 Teo KK, Mitchell LB, Pogue J, et al. Effect of ramipril in reducing sudden deaths and nonfatal cardiac arrests in high-risk individuals without heart failure or left ventricular dysfunction. Circulation 2004;110(11):1413–1417.

126 Waagstein F, Bristow MR, Swedberg K, et al. Beneficial effects of metoprolol in idiopathic dilated cardiomyopathy. Metoprolol in Dilated Cardiomyopathy (MDC) Trial Study Group. Lancet 1993;342(8885):1441–1446.

127 CIBIS Investigators and Committees. A randomized trial of beta-blockade in heart failure. The Cardiac Insufficiency Bisoprolol Study (CIBIS). Circulation 1994;90(4):1765–1773.

128 Packer M, Bristow MR, Cohn JN, et al. The effect of carvedilol on morbidity and mortality in patients with chronic heart failure. U.S. Carvedilol Heart Failure Study Group. N Engl J Med 1996;334(21):1349–1355.

129 Australia/New Zealand Heart Failure Research Collaborative Group. Randomised, placebo-controlled trial of carvedilol in patients with congestive heart failure due to ischaemic heart disease. Lancet 1997;349(9049):375–380.

130 Effect of metoprolol CR/XL in chronic heart failure: Metoprolol CR/XL Randomised Intervention Trial in Congestive Heart Failure (MERIT-HF). Lancet 1999;353(9169):2001–2007.

131 The Cardiac Insufficiency Bisoprolol Study II (CIBIS-II): a randomised trial. Lancet 1999;353(9146):9–13.

132 Dargie HJ. Effect of carvedilol on outcome after myocardial infarction in patients with left-ventricular dysfunction: the CAPRICORN randomised trial. Lancet 2001;357(9266):1385–1390.

133 Packer M, Fowler MB, Roecker EB, et al. Effect of carvedilol on the morbidity of patients with severe chronic heart failure: results of the carvedilol prospective randomized cumulative survival (COPERNICUS) study. Circulation 2002;106(17):2194–2199.

134 Poole-Wilson PA, Swedberg K, Cleland JG, et al. Comparison of carvedilol and metoprolol on clinical outcomes in patients with chronic heart failure in the Carvedilol Or Metoprolol European Trial (COMET): randomised controlled trial. Lancet 2003;362(9377):7–13.

135 Ceremuzynski L, Kleczar E, Krzeminska-Pakula M, et al. Effect of amiodarone on mortality after myocardial infarction: a double-blind, placebo-controlled, pilot study. J Am Coll Cardiol 1992;20(5):1056–1062.

CHAPTER 21

The mechanisms of ventricular fibrillation

Lan S. Chen, Peng-Sheng Chen, & Moshe S. Swissa

Sudden cardiac death (SCD) is a major cause of morbidity and mortality especially in patients with organic heart diseases such as coronary artery diseases and myocardial infarction (MI) [1]. Ventricular fibrillation (VF) is a major cause of SCD. There is a circadian variation of the frequency of SCD [2]. β-Blocker therapy significantly reduces the incidence of SCD after MI [3]. These clinical observations suggest that sympathetic tone plays an important role in the mechanisms of VF. Sympathetic activation has many electrophysiological consequences that might promote the generation and maintenance of VF. In this chapter, we focus on the neural remodeling, sympathetic nerve activity, and intracellular calcium (Ca$_i$) dynamics in the mechanism of VF.

Nerve sprouting and sympathetic hyperinnervation

One possible mechanism of increased sympathetic tone in patients with organic heart diseases is the increased sympathetic innervation. Inoue and Zipes [4] showed that MI can result in cardiac nerve damage and regional denervation. Peripheral nerve injury such as that happened after MI can be followed by neurilemma cell proliferation and axonal regeneration (*nerve sprouting*) (Figure 21.1) [5–7]. This sequence of denervation and regeneration could result in regional myocardial denervation and hyperinnervation, resulting in a regional or global increase in sympathetic nerve density (sym-

pathetic hyperinnervation), which in turn increases the propensity for cardiac arrhythmia. We propose that nerve sprouting and myocardial hyperinnervation play important roles in the development of cardiac arrhythmia and increased incidence of VF after MI (*Nerve Sprouting Hypothesis*).

Myocardial injury and sympathetic nerve sprouting in animal models and in humans

To measure nerve sprouting activity and sympathetic innervation after MI, we have used computerized morphometry to quantify the density of nerve fibers that are immunopositive for growth-associated protein 43 (GAP43) or tyrosine hydroxylase (TH). GAP43 is a protein associated with axonal growth and is upregulated during nerve sprouting [8]. We [9] used a mouse model to study the time course and spatial distribution of nerve sprouting after MI. Acute MI resulted in an increase of GAP43 immunoreactive nerve fiber density within 3 hours. Nerve sprouting was most apparent within 1 week after MI, then progressively declined over the 2-month study period. The increased GAP43 immunoreactivity was diffuse, but the peri-infarct area has more GAP43 immunopositive nerve structures than the area remote to infarct. Figure 21.2 shows histological examination of human and mouse MI. Active nerve sprouting and neurilemma regeneration occurred between the infarcted tissues and normal tissues. In this mouse model, the duration after MI is a significant factor that determined nerve sprouting activity. In addition to GAP43, the TH (a marker for

Ventricular Arrhythmias and Sudden Cardiac Death, 1st edition. Edited by P.J. Wang, A. Al-Ahmad, H. Hsia, and P.C. Zei
© 2008 Blackwell Publishing, ISBN: 978-1-4051-6114-5.

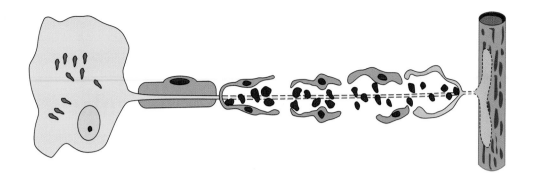

Nerve growth factor (NGF)

Growth-associated protein 43 (GAP43)

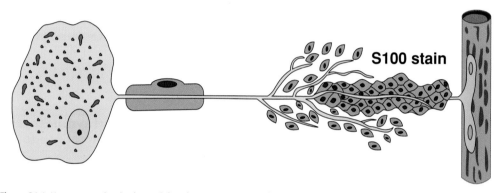

S100 stain

Figure 21.1 Nerve sprouting in the peripheral nervous system. After axonal injury, the non-neural cells around the site of injury produces nerve growth factor (NGF), which triggers axonal growth by growth-associated protein 43 (GAP43). In addition to axonal growth, there is also neurilemma (Schwann cell) proliferation. The neurilemma can be identified by S100 protein staining.

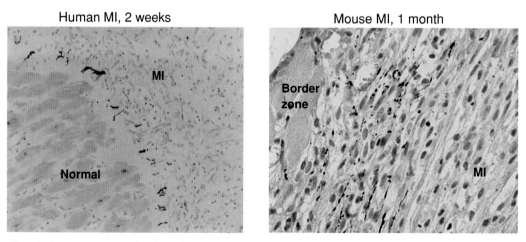

Figure 21.2 Nerve sprouting after MI. (Left panel) shows S100 protein staining of human myocardium 2 weeks after MI. The nerves (brown twigs) lined up between MI and normal tissues (courtesy Chen et al. [28], with permission). (Right panel) shows examples of nerve sprouting a month after MI in mouse. There are large number of GAP43-positive nerves between MI and surviving epicardial myocytes (border zone). (Courtesy Oh et al. [9], with permission.)

sympathetic nerve) staining also showed increased nerve fiber density after MI. The magnitude of increase of TH-positive nerve fiber appeared to be greater in the peri-infarct area than in the remote area. In the same study, we found that there is significant upregulation of a number of growth factors that include nerve growth factor (NGF), Insulin-like growth factor, leukemia inhibitory factor, transforming growth factor-β3, and interleukin-1α. The upregulation of these growth factors was greater and more persistent in the peri-infarct area than in the area remote from MI. In another study, we [10] created MI in dogs by either ligating coronary artery or by intracoronary balloon inflation. Consistent with findings in the mouse model of MI, GAP43-positive nerve numbers increased in both infracted and noninfarcted sites after MI. GAP43-positive nerve density in the noninfarcted left ventricular (LV) free wall was significantly higher in the MI group than the control group at 3 days, 1 week, and 1 month after MI, indicating that MI can elicit diffuse nerve sprouting activity. While we could not study human MI prospectively, retrospective histological examination supports the presence of nerve sprouting and sympathetic hyperinnervation after MI, and that the increased nerve density is associated with increased propensity for ventricular arrhythmia [11]. In that study, we observed denervation in the necrotic myocardium, and an increase of nerve fiber density nearby injured myocardium as compared to control hearts without prior history of heart diseases. Kim et al. [12] subsequently successfully performed immunostaining of the tissues from transplanted human hearts that were subsequently explanted. Abundant GAP43-positive and TH-positive nerves were found in these hearts. Heterogeneous sympathetic nerve sprouting and reinnervation occurred around blood vessels in the allografts. The magnitude of nerve sprouting increased with time and varied greatly from patient to patient. Patients with ischemic heart diseases had greater nerve sprouting and reinnervation than did those with dilated cardiomyopathy. Therefore, MI-induced nerve sprouting can eventually cause highly heterogeneous distribution of sympathetic innervation in the heart with areas of denervation, hyperinnervation, and relatively normal nerve fiber density. Heterogeneous sympathetic hyperinnervation could also be responsible for the increased

incidence of SCD in patients with transplanted hearts [13].

Nerve sprouting and canine models of VF and SCD

To prospectively test the nerve sprouting hypothesis, we created MI by ligating the left anterior descending coronary artery, and complete A-V block by radiofrequency ablation. Then, in the experimental group of dogs, we facilitated sympathetic nerve sprouting by either giving chronic infusion of NGF via osmotic pump [14] or delivering continuous subthreshold (below the threshold of increasing heart rate or blood pressure) electrical stimulation [15,16] to the left SG. As compared to control dogs (with MI and A-V block), experimental group of dogs have a twofold greater sympathetic nerve density and >10-fold increase in the incidence of VT. Four of the nine dogs died suddenly of VF (Figure 21.3). In the latter study, the rhythm was recorded by implantable cardioverter-defibrillator (ICD), which only records the rhythm when there is either ventricular tachycardia or VF. We felt that continuous (24 h a day, 7 days a week) recording would help us better characterize the ventricular arrhythmia in these dogs. Swissa et al. [15] therefore implanted Data Sciences International (DSI) transmitters into dogs and performed long-term monitoring of these dogs over several months. Subthreshold electrical stimulation was used to the left stellate ganglion to induce cardiac nerve sprouting. Figure 21.4 shows that these 24/7 recordings revealed a circadian variation of atrial and ventricular rates. Because of the complete heart block, the increased ventricular rates were due to ventricular tachycardia or VF, not due to rapid conduction of atrial arrhythmia. Figure 21.5 documents the spontaneous onset of VF. The authors also found that subthreshold electrical stimulation is more effective than NGF infusion in the induction of cardiac nerve sprouting and sympathetic stimulation. With the increased magnitude of sympathetic nerve sprouting, the dogs with subthreshold electrical stimulation [15] also had higher incidence of ventricular tachycardia than the dogs with NGF infusion [14]. These findings further suggest a causal relationship between sympathetic nerve density and ventricular arrhythmia.

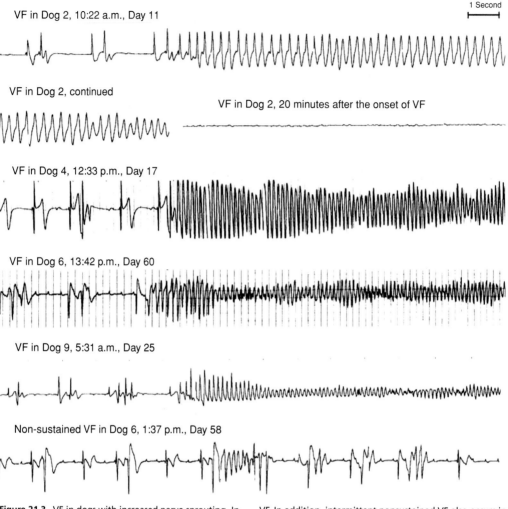

Figure 21.3 VF in dogs with increased nerve sprouting. In addition to electrical remodeling created by A-V block and MI, these dogs also received NGF infusion into the left stellate ganglion. Four of the nine dogs died spontaneous SCD without investigator intervention. All SCD was due to VF. In addition, intermittent nonsustained VF also occurs in these dogs (bottom tracing). In contrast, none of the dogs with MI and A-V block but without additional increased sympathetic nerve density (control group) died. (Courtesy Cao et al. [14], with permission.)

Long-term monitoring of autonomic nerve activity

The availability of an animal model of VF and the 24/7 recording also gave us the opportunity to directly study a causal relationship between sympathetic nerve activity and VF. Jardine et al. [17] documented a spontaneous VF episode preceded immediately by a paroxysm of increased cardiac sympathetic nerve activity in one sheep with acute MI. We adapted their techniques by using DSI transmitters for simultaneous 24/7 recording of

sympathetic nerve activity in normal dogs [18]. We found that the stellate ganglion nerve activity (SGNA) was followed immediately (<1 s) by heart rate and blood pressure elevation. This immediate response (without delay) suggests that we have recorded the nerve activity directly responsible for heart rate control. In contrast, a long delay between nerve activity and heart rate response would suggest that the heart rate increase was secondary to the increased circulating catecholamine released elsewhere. Heart rate correlated significantly with SGNA. Both heart rate and SGNA

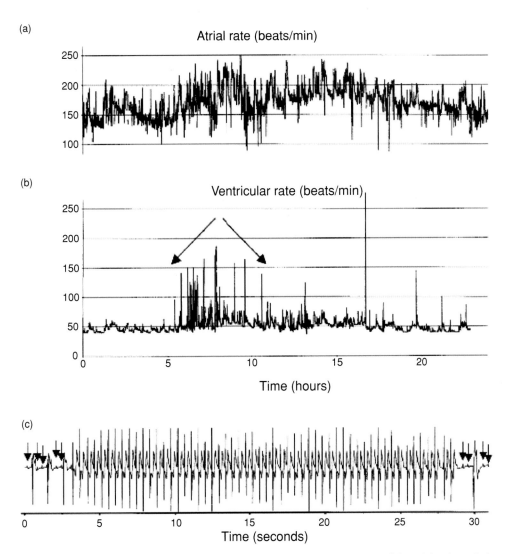

Figure 21.4 Ventricular arrhythmias recorded by DSI. (a) and (b) show a 24-hour histogram of the atrial and ventricular rates, respectively. Time 0 corresponds to 12:00 midnight. There were numerous high-rate events in the morning (between the two arrows). (c) It shows an example of nonsustained VT recorded by the DSI system. The arrows indicate the P waves. (Courtesy Swissa et al. [15], with permission.)

showed statistically significant circadian variation. We have now successfully applied these techniques to our canine model of SCD [19] and a model of pacing-induced heart failure [20].

Autonomic nerve activity and cardiac arrhythmia

We found that there are two kinds of sympathetic nerve activity (Figure 21.6). The first kind is high-amplitude spike discharge activity (HASDA) and the other one is low-amplitude burst discharge activity (LABDA). We define HASDA as spike discharges with peak-to-peak amplitudes of at least 0.2 mV. LABDA is continuous nerve activity with amplitudes at least three times higher than baseline noise. Figure 6a shows the relationship between SGNA and ventricular arrhythmia 6 days after cessation of rapid pacing that induced heart failure. Note that in addition to SGNA, we also recorded vagal nerve activity (VNA). An increased VNA (first and second arrows, VNA channel) was associated with a reduction in heart rate. The onset of LABDA

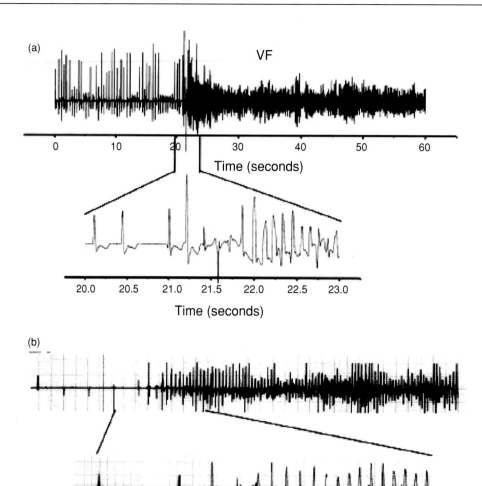

Figure 21.5 Spontaneous onset of VF documented by DSI (a) and ICD (b) in dogs with subthreshold stimulation of left stellate ganglion. Note the short–long–short coupling intervals prior to the first beat of VF. (Courtesy Swissa et al. [15], with permission.)

on SGNA recording with continuous vagal activity was associated with further reduction in heart rate to 130 bpm, suggesting that vagal discharges slowed heart rhythm more efficiently during increased sympathetic activity (accentuated antagonism) [21]. HASDA was followed immediately by two consecutive premature ventricular contractions (downward arrows and further heart rate acceleration). Figure 21.2b, c show multiple episodes of LABDA associated with premature ventricular contractions, couplets, or ventricular tachycardia.

These studies document a close temporal relationship between sympathetic discharges and the onset of ventricular arrhythmia. In another study, prolonged sympathetic discharges were associated with the onset of VF [19].

HASDA and epileptiform discharges

Epileptiform discharges are regular spiky activity within the brain [22]. These discharges are

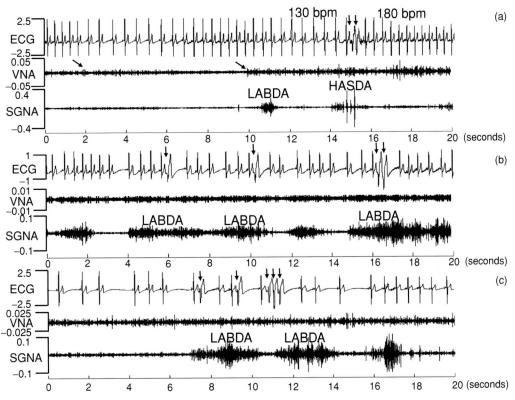

Figure 21.6 LABDA and HASDA. (a) It shows that HASDA induced couplets and abruptly increased heart rate 6 days after cessation of rapid pacing in a dog with pacing-induced heart failure. (b) It shows LABDA episodes associated with isolated premature ventricular contraction and couplets 1 day after cessation of rapid pacing. (c) It shows LABDA episodes associated with isolated premature ventricular contraction and triplets (ventricular tachycardia) 1 day after cessation of rapid pacing. (Courtesy of Ogawa M, Zhou S, Tan AY. Left stellate ganglion and vagal nerve activity and cardiac arrhythmias in ambulatory dogs with pacing-induced congestive heart failure. J Am Coll Cardiol 2007;50:335–343, with permission.)

characterized by depolarization shifts that often occur before or during the discharge, and are found almost always in patients with epilepsy. Figure 21.7(a) shows the electroencephalogram recording from a 13-year-old boy with partial seizure. Arrow points to depolarization shift that occur prior to the epileptiform discharges. Panel (b) shows HASDA, which also typically occurs with significant baseline shifts (arrow). While epileptiform discharges are almost always pathological, HASDA occurs frequently in the SG of normal dogs. There is a circadian occurrence of HASDA, with the highest incidence of HASDA occurring in the morning to early afternoon. HASDA is highly arrhythmogenic, and its frequency increases with the development of heart failure [20].

Sympathetic stimulation and calcium dynamics

Sympathetic activation is proarrhythmic because it has profound effects on cardiac ion channel function. Cardiac action potential duration (APD) is determined by the activity of ion channels on the cell membrane and by the Ca_i release and reuptake. β-adrenergic stimulation is known to increase ionic current through L-type calcium channels (I_{Ca-L}), I_{Ks}, and chloride channels [$I_{Cl}(Ca)$ and $I_{Cl-cAMP}$] [23]. By activating the I_{Ca-L}, there are increased Ca_i to trigger sarcoplasmic reticulum (SR) Ca release. β-Receptor activation also increases ryanodine receptor phosphorylation and facilitate SR Ca release [24]. Increased Ca_i in turn activates the sodium calcium exchanger (NCX), which

(a)

Epileptiform discharges in EEG

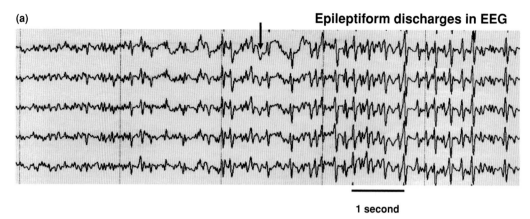

1 second

(b)

HASDA in left stellate ganglion

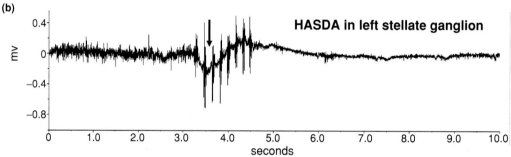

Figure 21.7 Comparison between epileptiform discharges and HASDA. Panel (a) shows the electroencephalogram recording from a 13-year-old boy with partial seizure. Arrow points to depolarization shift that occurs prior to the epileptiform discharges. Panel (b) shows HASDA in the left SG. HASDA also typically occurs with significant baseline shifts (arrow), but can occur in both normal and diseased dogs. In contrast, epileptiform discharges are almost always associated with seizure disorder.

exchanges one Ca for three Na, resulting in a net depolarizing current. This inward current is responsible for delayed afterdepolarization and triggered activity during pathological conditions. For example, when there is abnormal ryanodine receptor function, β-stimulation can cause excessive SR Ca release, leading to triggered activity, VF, and sudden cardiac death both in animal models [25] and in human patients [26]. A specific example of human disease is the catecholaminergic polymorphic ventricular tachycardia [26]. In this disease, Priori et al. studied patients with documented polymorphic ventricular arrhythmias occurring during physical or emotional stress with a normal heart. Ryanodine receptor mutations were found in roughly half of the patients. β-Blockers were effective in reducing arrhythmias although implantable cardioverter-defibrillators were still required in a significant number of patients. This clinical study clearly demonstrated the importance of sympathetic stimulation and Ca_i dynamics in the mechanisms of human VF.

Calcium dynamics, alternans, and VF

In addition to triggered activity, Ca_i dynamics are also critically important in the generation of spatially discordant alternans, a key arrhythmogenic factor predisposing the heart to reentry and lethal arrhythmias, including VF. Weiss et al. [27] recently reviewed the results of computer simulation and nonlinear dynamics studies of spatially discordant alternans, which describe the out-of-phase APD alternans in different regions of the heart. By alternating out of phase, spatially discordant alternans markedly enhances dispersion of refractoriness. Ectopic beats will then have a high probability of inducing reentry. At the cellular level, instabilities in membrane voltage (i.e., steep APD restitution slope) and Ca_i cycling dynamics cause APD and the Ca_i, transient to alternate. The characteristics of alternans are affected by different "modes" of the bidirectional coupling between voltage and Ca_i. Additional factors, such as conduction velocity restitution and ectopic beats, promote spatially discordant alternans. These dynamical instabilities make the mechanistic basis underlying the clinical association of cardiac alternans (e.g., T-wave alternans) with arrhythmia risk, VF, and sudden death.

Summary

We found that cardiac sympathetic nerves are highly plastic. Nerve sprouting and heterogeneous sympathetic hyperinnervation in diseased ventricles may lead to a coexistence of denervated and hyperinnervated areas. A combination of heterogeneous sympathetic nerve distribution and electrophysiological remodeling that occur in organic heart diseases may lead to significantly altered Ca_i dynamics during sympathetic activation. Abnormal Ca_i dynamics in turn facilitate both triggered activity and reentry, ventricular tachycardia, VF, and sudden cardiac death.

Acknowledgments

This study was supported by NIH grants R01 HL 66389, R01 HL 71140, R01 HL 78932, and P01 HL 78931, an AHA Scientist Development Grant (0435135N), a Piansky Family Endowment, and a Pauline and Harold Price Endowment.

References

1 Centers for Disease Control and Prevention. State-specific mortality from sudden cardiac death—United States, 1999. MMWR Morb Mortal Wkly Rep 2002;51:123–126.

2 Muller JE, Ludmer PL, Willich SN, et al. Circadian variation in the frequency of sudden cardiac death. Circulation 1987;75:131–138.

3 The Norwegian Multicenter Study Group. Timolol-induced reduction in mortality and reinfarction in patients surviving acute myocardial infarction. N Engl J Med 1981;304:801–807.

4 Inoue H, Zipes DP. Time course of denervation of efferent sympathetic and vagal nerves after occlusion of the coronary artery in the canine heart. Circ Res 1988;62:1111–1120.

5 Guth L. Regeneration in the mammalian peripheral nervous system. Physiol Rev 1956;36:441–478.

6 Vracko R, Thorning D, Frederickson RG. Fate of nerve fibers in necrotic, healing, and healed rat myocardium. Lab Invest 1990;63:490–501.

7 Vracko R, Thorning D, Frederickson RG. Nerve fibers in human myocardial scars. Hum Pathol 1991;22:138–146.

8 Meiri KF, Pfenninger KH, Willard MB. Growth-associated protein, GAP-43, a polypeptide that is induced when neurons extend axons, is a component of growth cones and corresponds to pp46, a major polypeptide of a subcellular fraction enriched in growth cones [published erratum appears in Proc Natl Acad Sci USA 1986;83(23):9274]. Proc Natl Acad Sci USA 1986;83:3537–3541.

9 Oh Y-S, Jong AY, Kim DT, et al. Spatial distribution of nerve sprouting after myocardial infarction in mice. Heart Rhythm 2006;3:728–736.

10 Zhou S, Chen LS, Miyauchi Y, et al. Mechanisms of cardiac nerve sprouting after myocardial infarction in dogs. Circ Res 2004;95:76–83.

11 Cao J-M, Fishbein MC, Han JB, et al. Relationship between regional cardiac hyperinnervation and ventricular arrhythmia. Circulation 2000;101:1960–1969.

12 Kim DT, Luthringer DJ, Lai AC, et al. Sympathetic nerve sprouting after orthotopic heart transplantation. J Heart Lung Transplant 2004;23:1349–1358.

13 Blakey JD, Kobashigawa J, Laks H, Espejo ML, Fishbein MC. Sudden, unexpected death in cardiac transplant recipients: an autopsy study. J Heart Lung Transplant 2001;20:239.

14 Cao J-M, Chen LS, KenKnight BH, et al. Nerve sprouting and sudden cardiac death. Circ Res 2000;86:816–821.

15 Swissa M, Zhou S, Gonzalez-Gomez I, et al. Long-term subthreshold electrical stimulation of the left stellate ganglion and a canine model of sudden cardiac death. J Am Coll Cardiol 2004;43:858–864.

16 Swissa M, Zhou S, Paz O, Fishbein MC, Chen LS, Chen PS. A canine model of paroxysmal atrial fibrillation and paroxysmal atrial tachycardia. Am J Physiol Heart Circ Physiol 2005;289:H1851–H1857.

17 Jardine DL, Charles CJ, Forrester MD, Whitehead M, Nicholls MG. A neural mechanism for sudden death after myocardial infarction. Clin Auton Res 2003;13:339–341.

18 Jung B-C, Dave AS, Tan AY, et al. Circadian variations of stellate ganglion nerve activity in ambulatory dogs. Heart Rhythm 2005;3:78–85.

19 Zhou S, Jung B-C, Tan AY, et al. Spontaneous stellate ganglion nerve activity and ventricular arrhythmia in a canine model of sudden death [Abstract]. Heart Rhythm 2006;3(1S):S106.

20 Ogawa M, Zhou S, Tan AY, et al. Autonomic nerve activity and tachybrady arrhythmias in a canine model of congestive heart failure [Abstract]. Heart Rhythm 2006;3(1S):265.

21 Stramba-Badiale M, Vanoli E, De Ferrari GM, Cerati D, Foreman RD, Schwartz PJ. Sympathetic-parasympathetic interaction and accentuated antagonism in conscious dogs. Am J Physiol 1991;260:H335–H340.

22 Westmoreland BF. Epileptiform electroencephalographic patterns. Mayo Clin Proc 1996;71:501–511.

23 Hume JR, Harvey RD. Chloride conductance pathways in heart. Am J Physiol 1991;261:C399–C412.

24 Bers DM. Cardiac ryanodine receptor phosphorylation: target sites and functional consequences. Biochem J 2006;396:e1–e3.

25 Wehrens XH, Lehnart SE, Huang F, et al. FKBP12.6 deficiency and defective calcium release channel (ryanodine receptor) function linked to exercise-induced sudden cardiac death. Cell 2003;113:829–840.

26 Priori SG, Napolitano C, Memmi M, et al. Clinical and molecular characterization of patients with catecholaminergic polymorphic ventricular tachycardia. Circulation 2002;106:69–74.

27 Weiss JN, Karma A, Shiferaw Y, Chen PS, Garfinkel A, Qu Z. From pulsus to pulseless: the saga of cardiac alternans. Circ Res 2006;98:1244–1253.

28 Chen P-S, Chen LS, Cao JM, Sharifi B, Karagueuzian HS, Fishbein MC. Sympathetic nerve sprouting, electrical remodeling and the mechanisms of sudden cardiac death. Cardiovasc Res 2001;50:409–416.

CHAPTER 22

Mechanisms of defibrillation

Derek J. Dosdall, Jian Huang, & Raymond E. Ideker

For more than 100 years, electric shocks have been used to terminate ventricular fibrillation (VF) [1,2]. Ideas about the mechanisms by which a shock halts VF have changed during this period. Dudel [3] suggested that a successful defibrillation shock must be strong enough to paralyze or stun the entire myocardial mass. Wiggers hypothesized that shock field strengths did not need to paralyze cardiac tissue, but that the shock must be of sufficient strength to halt all the activation wavefronts during VF. Zipes et al. [4] and Mower et al. [5] hypothesized that all wavefronts in the cardiac tissue did not need to be extinguished, but that if wavefronts could be extinguished in a critical mass of the cardiac tissue, the remaining wavefronts would be incapable of sustaining VF.

The development of electrical and optical mapping techniques to record before, during, and after the application of defibrillation shocks has improved the understanding of the mechanisms of defibrillation. While earlier theories of defibrillation mechanisms focused primarily on the macroscopic potential gradient electric field created by defibrillation shocks, electrical and optical mapping studies have demonstrated that in addition to the whole heart field gradient, electrode effects and cell and tissue responses to defibrillation shocks are essential to understanding the mechanisms of defibrillation. With the development of hardware and software that can record simultaneously from hundreds or thousands of locations, investigators have made tremendous strides toward understanding the basic mechanisms of defibrillation.

Ventricular Arrhythmias and Sudden Cardiac Death, 1st edition. Edited by P.J. Wang, A. Al-Ahmad, H. Hsia, and P.C. Zei © 2008 Blackwell Publishing, ISBN: 978-1-4051-6114-5.

Defibrillation shock field gradient effects

Electrical mapping studies have demonstrated that successful defibrillation shocks must establish a minimum field potential gradient throughout the cardiac tissue. The potential gradient is the change in voltage over a distance and for defibrillation it is expressed in V/cm. Epicardial mapping in dogs demonstrated that a minimum field gradient of 5.4 V/cm was required for successful defibrillation with a monophasic shock, while a minimum of 2.7 V/cm was required for a biphasic shock [6]. There is a large variation in the shock potential gradient field across the ventricles when internal defibrillation catheters are used [7–9]. Figure 22.1 shows the epicardial potential gradient distribution during a shock delivered between a right ventricular apical coil and a coil in the superior vena cava [10]. The potential gradient is much higher near the shocking coils than on the left ventricular lateral free wall and apex.

Earliest activation following shocks that are much higher than the defibrillation threshold (DFT) may arise from the high field gradient areas [11,12]. This may be due to damage caused by the high current density near the shocking electrodes. Activation wavefronts for shocks delivered near the DFT tend to emerge from the area of low field gradient, away from the shocking electrodes [13–17]. Therefore, the area of first activation after defibrillation shocks near the DFT is different for different electrode configurations [6]. This is true not only for shocks that fail to defibrillate but also for many shocks of near-DFT strength that succeed. With an electrode configuration including an electrode in the right ventricular apex and another in the superior vena cava, the area of first activation tends to arise in left ventricular apex and lateral free wall (Figure 22.1).

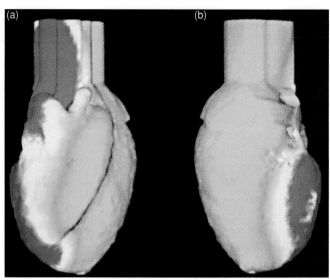

Figure 22.1 Field potential gradient recorded in a dog heart during a shock delivered between a right ventricular apical coil and a coil in the superior vena cava. Panel (a) shows the anterior ventricles and Panel (b) shows the posterior ventricles. The color represents potential gradient, with red being the highest and purple the lowest. The highest gradient is measured near the shocking coils near the right ventricular apical coil and the coil in the superior vena cava. (Figure from Ideker [10], with permission.)

In simulations and experimental observations, areas close to shocking electrodes produce virtual electrodes that either hyperpolarize or depolarize the surrounding tissue (Figure 22.2) [18,19]. A virtual electrode is a region in which the membrane is polarized, not because a real electrode is there, but because of the interaction of tissue heterogeneities with the electric field created in the region by real electrodes in other regions. Studies have demonstrated that monophasic shocks are often strong enough to terminate VF, but that the shocks create

virtual electrodes that can then reinitiate VF [13,20]. Figure 22.3 shows the development of a virtual cathode and anode on the anterior epicardium of an optically mapped rabbit heart. After the shock, an activation front arises near the boundary of the virtual cathode and spreads rapidly through the hyperpolarized tissue in the virtual cathode, and a reentrant circuit formed.

The first phase of biphasic shocks effectively halts fibrillatory wavefronts in the same manner as monophasic shocks, while the second phase reduces

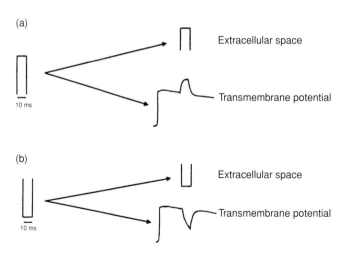

Figure 22.2 The effect of a monophasic square wave shock on the extracellular potential and the transmembrane potential. The shock appears as a largely undistorted square wave in the extracellular space. The shock causes an exponential change in transmembrane potential, which discharges after the end of the shock. Depending on the polarity of a shock delivered during an action potential, a cardiac cell may be depolarized (a) or hyperpolarized (b). The effect on the action potential duration and amplitude are different depending on whether the cell is depolarized or hyperpolarized by a shock. (Figure from Walcott et al. [44], with permission.)

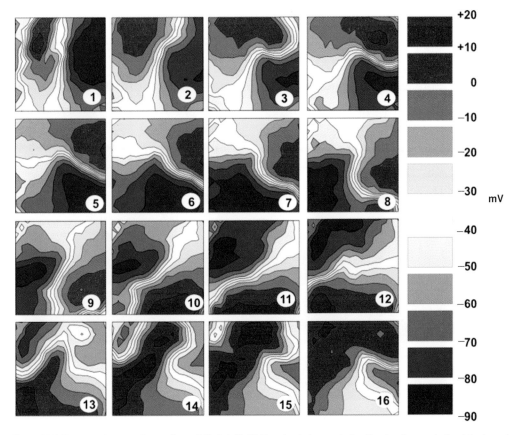

Figure 22.3 Transmembrane voltage after a failed defibrillation shock demonstrates the development of a virtual anode and cathode on the anterior surface of an optically mapped rabbit heart. Each frame is 10 ms apart, starting from the first sample recorded after withdrawal of a monophasic defibrillation shock. The virtual cathode (red) creates a wavefront that rapidly travels through the virtual anode (blue), which then reenters and reactivates the area originally occupied by the virtual cathode. (Figure from Efimov et al. [20], with permission.)

or eliminates the transmembrane voltage and eliminates the virtual electrodes that reinitiate VF. This may explain why the biphasic waveform has a lower DFT and a lower minimum potential gradient than the monophasic waveform. Figure 22.4 shows optically mapped signals during a biphasic shock in a rabbit heart.

Virtual electrode effects and the reduction in DFTs with biphasic shocks are compatible with the "upper limit of vulnerability" theory of defibrillation, which states that a successful defibrillation shock must not only halt VF wavefronts on the heart, but it also must not reinitiate VF by the same mechanism that a shock of the same strength initiates VF during the vulnerable period in sinus or paced rhythm [13,21].

Cleavage planes and anatomical heterogeneity

Cable models of defibrillation shocks predict that the potential gradient field is strong enough to activate cells only within a few space constants of the shocking electrodes, i.e., a few millimeters [22]. However, experiments have shown that electrical shocks can stimulate epicardial tissue distant from the shocking electrodes [23]. The reason for this discrepancy is that the myocardium is not a continuous cable.

Secondary sources of activation away from shocking electrodes are caused by virtual electrodes created by discontinuities in cardiac tissue that lead to locally uneven tissue impedance and current flow.

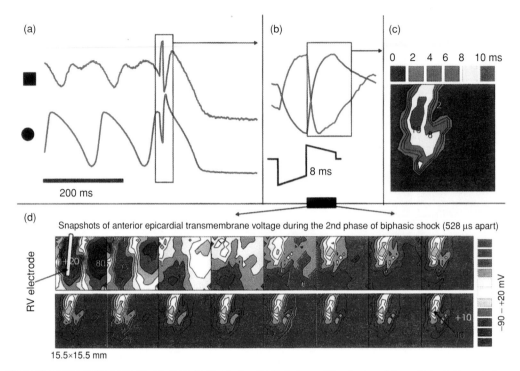

Figure 22.4 Biphasic shocks create virtual electrodes during the first phase of the shock and then eliminate them during the second phase of the shock. (a) Optical recordings from the region of the virtual cathode (red trace marked with a square) and the virtual anode (blue trace marked with a circle). (b) Responses of the transmembrane potentials over the virtual anode and cathode to a biphasic shock (−100 V, 8 ms first phase followed by a +50 V, 8 ms second phase) is shown. The black box shows the time frame illustrated in (d). (c) Isochronal frames following the onset of the second phase of the pulse are shown. (d) Time course of the second phase of the biphasic shock over the region containing the virtual cathode and anode is shown in 528-ms frames. Virtual electrodes developed in the first phase of the shock are reduced substantially by the end of the second phase of the shock. (Figure from Efimov et al. [20], with permission.)

These heterogeneities lead to local changes in transmembrane potential of sufficient amplitude to stimulate local myocardial activation. A study in cardiomyocyte cultures demonstrated that a cleft or discontinuity in a continuous sheet of cells provides a site for increased transmembrane potential or a secondary source of activation [24]. Figure 22.5 shows optical maps of the transmembrane potential adjacent to a cleft in a cellular monolayer during a shock. Cells on the side of the cleft nearer the cathode electrode become hyperpolarized, while cells on the other side closer to the anode electrode become depolarized.

In a study in dogs, White et al. [25] demonstrated that stimulation with pacing electrodes produced wavefronts near the stimulation site that spread from the stimulation electrodes, but that when a surgical incision was made and sutured closed at a distance from the stimulation site, sufficiently strong stimulation pulses initiated activation at both the electrode site and at the incision site. These artificial disruptions of cell cultures and of the epicardium of the heart demonstrate the establishment of secondary sources of activation at discontinuities distant from stimulus electrodes.

Naturally occurring heterogeneity in cardiac tissue may be found in the collagenous septa between myocyte bundles, blood vessels, and surgical and infarct scars in the tissue. Figure 22.6 shows a confocal microscopic reconstruction of the collagenous septae or cleavage planes in rat left ventricular tissue. Computer models have shown that these cleavage planes may be important secondary sources for

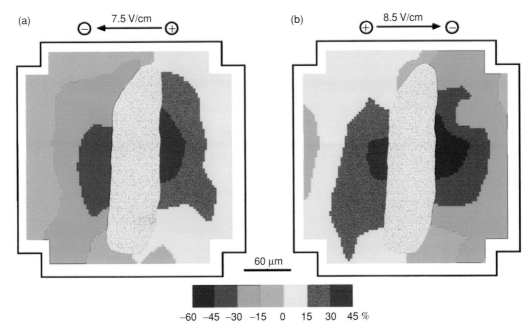

(a) 7.5 V/cm ⊖ ← ⊕

(b) 8.5 V/cm ⊕ → ⊖

60 μm

−60 −45 −30 −15 0 15 30 45 %

Figure 22.5 An intercellular cleft forms a secondary source in this map of the spatial distribution of Vm in response to a shock. The cleft is shown in gray. Isopotential maps of ΔVm as a percent of the action potential upstroke are shown in color according to the scale shown at the bottom. Shocks of opposite polarity are shown in (a) and (b). (Figure adapted from Fast et al. [24], with permission.)

successful defibrillation [26,27]. Fiber curvature has also been shown to be an important source for secondary sources [28,29]. This effect may account for activation of tissue by shocks at sites distant from electrodes even though cable models show no effect far from electrode sites.

Dispersion of refractoriness and shock timing

An important factor in the response of cardiac tissue to a stimulus is the state of the tissue immediately preceding a shock. Depending on the state of the cardiac cell and the strength of the shock, a shock may (1) elicit a new action potential, (2) prolong the action potential, (3) shorten the action potential, or (4) have no effect on the existing action potential. Figure 22.7(a) shows an example of how a low-amplitude stimulus creates an all or nothing response that is sensitive to a shift in timing of the stimulus of a few milliseconds. Figure 22.7(b) demonstrates that a larger amplitude shock may extend action potential amplitude, but that the duration of the action potential extension is a function of the timing of the stimulus with regard to the state of the cell prior to the shock.

Near-DFT strength shocks may extend action potential duration in tissue that is in the plateau of an action potential at the time of the shock. If the first activation present after a defibrillation shock encounters a region of tissue with extended repolarization and thus an extended period of refractoriness, the wavefront will block at the refractory tissue. Since only part of the cardiac tissue has this extended refractory period, the activation wavefront spreads into areas that are excitable. This process of stimulating some tissue and creating unidirectional block in adjacent regions creates a reentrant circuit, which may then degenerate back into VF. These areas where critical shock strengths intersect with critical lines of refractoriness are called "critical points" [30–32]. Figure 22.8 shows an example of the formation of this type of critical point in mapped cardiac tissue.

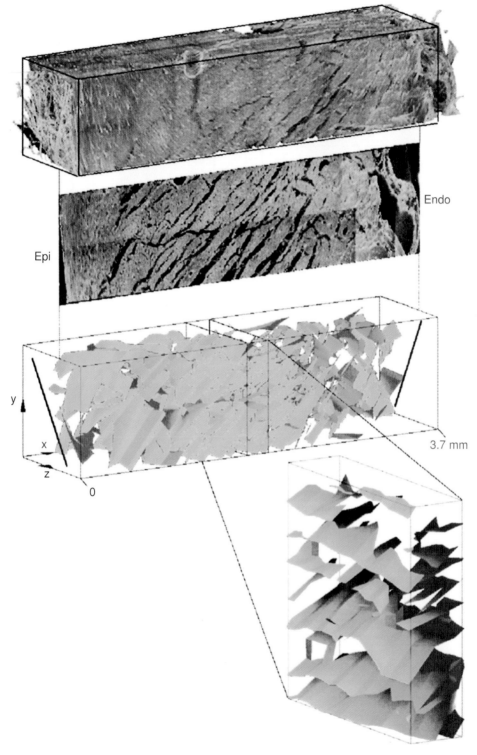

Endo

Epi

y

x

z

0

3.7 mm

Figure 22.6 Confocal microscopy shows a complex network of cleavage planes in this section of rat left ventricular free-wall myocardium. The top figure shows a three-dimensional reconstruction of the ventricular myocardium. The middle figure shows a cross-sectional slice of the section above. The lower section shows a finite element geometric model of cleavage planes with a smaller subsection magnified below. The cleavage planes are on the order of 80 μm in thickness, and may play an important role in the creation of secondary sources in defibrillation. (Figure from Hooks et al. [27], with permission.)

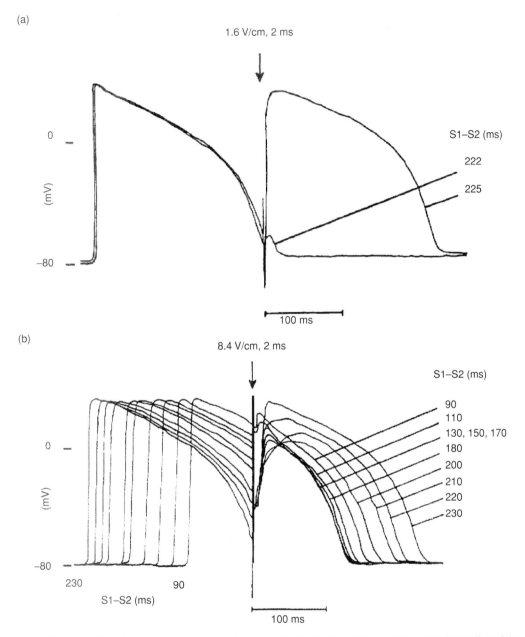

Figure 22.7 Recordings showing varying responses to electric field stimuli at varying strengths and timing. In (a), the response of a cardiac cell to a field of 1.6 V/cm has a dramatically different response when the S1–S2 interval is changed from 222 to 225 ms. In (b), a larger stimulus (8.4 V/cm) stimulates an action potential regardless of the S1–S2 interval, but the duration of the invoked action potential varies depending on the state of the cell prior to the stimulus administration. (Figure from Knisley et al. [45], with permission.)

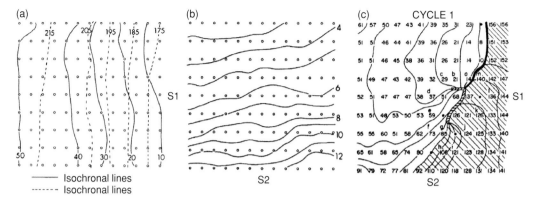

Figure 22.8 Initiation of reentry and VF following interaction of lines of myocardial refractoriness and the potential gradient field created by a shock. (a) Activation times during the last beat (solid lines) and recovery times to a local 2-mA stimulus (dashed lines) in milliseconds following this activation. (b) S2 stimulus potential gradient field (V/cm). (c) Initial activation pattern just after the S2 stimulus in milliseconds. The hatched region is thought to be directly excited by the S2 stimulus field. (Figure from Frazier et al. [32], with permission.)

(a)

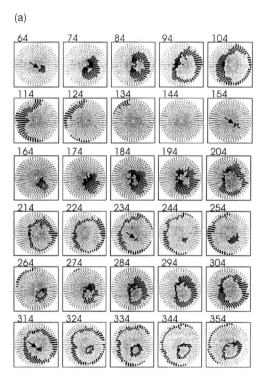

(b)

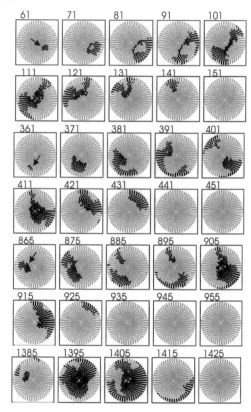

Figure 22.9 Postshock activation cycles for a failed shock (a) and a successful shock of the same strength (b) as recorded by an epicardial electrode shock in a pig. Time in milliseconds since the beginning of the defibrillation shock is given at the top of each frame. Black electrodes indicate activation during the previous 10 milliseconds. Arrows indicate the earliest recorded activation site for each cycle. (Figure adapted from Chattipakorn et al. [33], with permission.)

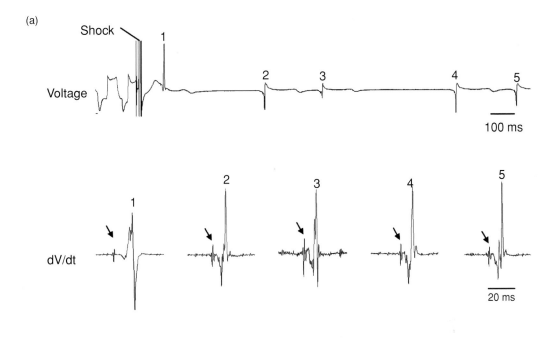

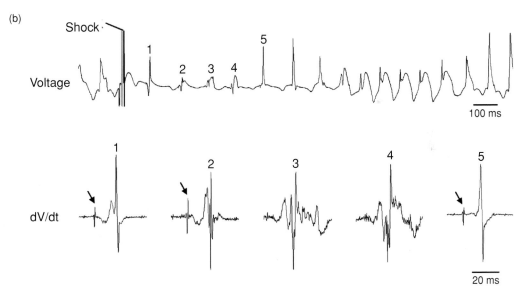

Figure 22.10 Purkinje fiber activation during the first several postshock activation cycles after a successful (a) and failed (b) defibrillation shock as recorded in a pig with plunge needle electrodes. Voltage recordings and expanded temporal derivatives of the first five activation cycles are shown. Purkinje fiber activations are indicated with arrows on the temporal derivatives. (Figure from Dosdall et al. [17], with permission.)

Future directions

Electrical and optical mapping studies have shown that shocks that are well below the DFT do not terminate VF activation wavefronts in the heart. As discussed previously, monophasic shocks that are slightly below the DFT may halt the fibrillation wavefronts in the heart, but may also create virtual electrodes and cathodes that then reinitiate VF (see Figure 22.3). Shocks of near-DFT strength causes a period of electrical inactivity known as the isoelectric window. This period, typically 30–90 milliseconds in duration, immediately following near-DFT shocks, has been observed with epicardial and transmural electrical mapping as well as with optical mapping techniques [14,16,33]. After a near-DFT-level shock, three outcomes are possible: (1) a type A success (isoelectric window >130 ms); (2) a type B success (isoelectric window <130 ms); or (3) a failure [34].

The first postshock activation cycle is indistinguishable in timing and activation sequence for type B successes and shock failures. Figure 22.9 shows examples of a defibrillation success and a failure for defibrillation shocks of the same strength. Since no activations have been recorded during the isoelectric window immediately following shocks, investigators have questioned the source of activation following the isoelectric window.

One potential source for activation wavefronts after the isoelectric window is the specialized conduction system. Modeling and experimental studies have shown that Purkinje fibers react differently than the working myocardium to defibrillation strength shocks [35,36], and that Purkinje fibers are active during the first several postshock activation cycles [17]. Figure 22.10 shows examples of Purkinje fiber activation during the first several postshock activation cycles following successful and failed near-DFT-level shocks.

Pacing during VF can capture portions of fibrillating tissue [37–39] and thus increase the organization of the VF activation wavefronts. Several studies have demonstrated that pacing before or after defibrillation shocks may reduce DFTs [40–43]. Increased organization or synchronizing shocks with activation wavefronts in the low-gradient regions may lead to reductions in DFTs.

Conclusion

Improvements in the defibrillation waveform and technology have lead to expanded treatment options and increased survival for patients with VF. ICDs are implanted routinely in patients that are at high risk for VF. Automatic external defibrillators are becoming more readily accessible in public areas. While defibrillation shocks are successful in terminating VF in the vast majority of cases, out-of-hospital survival rates are low and there is still a small percentage of patients that are not successfully defibrillated. Continued investigation into the basic mechanisms of defibrillation may lead to improved defibrillation techniques and improved survival rates for patients with VF.

References

1 Hoffa M, Ludwig C. Einige neue versuche über herzebewegung. Z Rationelle Med 1850;9:107–144.

2 Prevost JL, Battelli F. Sur quelques effets des décharges électriques sur le coeur des Mammifères. Comptes Rendus des Seances, Acad Sci 1899;129:1267–1268.

3 Dudel J. Elektrophysiologische grundlagen der defibrillation und künstlichen stimulation des herzens. Med Klin 1968;63:2089–2091.

4 Zipes DP, Fischer J, King RM, Nicoll A, Jolly WW. Termination of ventricular fibrillation in dogs by depolarizing a critical amount of myocardium. Am J Cardiol 1975;36:37–44.

5 Mower MM, Mirowski M, Spear JF, Moore EN. Patterns of ventricular activity during catheter defibrillation. Circulation 1974;49:858–861.

6 Zhou X, Daubert JP, Wolf PD, Smith WM, Ideker RE. Epicardial mapping of ventricular defibrillation with monophasic and biphasic shocks in dogs. Circ Res 1993;72:145–160.

7 Tang ASL, Wolf PD, Claydon FJ III, Smith WM, Pilkington TC, Ideker RE. Measurement of defibrillation shock potential distributions and activation sequences of the heart in three-dimensions. Proc IEEE 1988;76:1176–1186.

8 Witkowski FX, Penkoske PA, Plonsey R. Mechanism of cardiac defibrillation in open-chest dogs with unipolar DC-coupled simultaneous activation and shock potential recordings. Circulation 1990;82:244–260.

9 Tang AS, Wolf PD, Afework Y, Smith WM, Ideker RE. Three-dimensional potential gradient fields generated by intracardiac catheter and cutaneous patch electrodes. Circulation 1992;85:1857–1864.

10 Ideker RE. Ventricular fibrillation: how do we put the genie back in the bottle? Heart Rhythm 2007;4:665–674.

11 Yabe S, Smith WM, Daubert JP, Wolf PD, Rollins DL, Ideker RE. Conduction disturbances caused by high current density electric fields. Circ Res 1990;66:1190–1203.

12 Walker RG, Walcott GP, Smith WM, Ideker RE. Sites of earliest activation following transvenous defibrillation. Circulation 1994;90:I-447.

13 Chen PS, Shibata N, Dixon EG, et al. Activation during ventricular defibrillation in open-chest dogs. Evidence of complete cessation and regeneration of ventricular fibrillation after unsuccessful shocks. J Clin Invest 1986;77:810–823.

14 Chattipakorn N, Fotuhi PC, Chattipakorn SC, Ideker RE. Three-dimensional mapping of earliest activation after near-threshold ventricular defibrillation shocks. J Cardiovasc Electrophysiol 2003;14:65–69.

15 Fang X, Walcott GP, Huang CH, et al. The transmural location of earliest activation following a defibrillation shock is species dependent. 26th Annual Scientific Sessions of NASPE–Heart Rhythm Society. New Orleans, LA: Heart Rhythm, 2005:S86.

16 Chattipakorn N, Banville I, Gray RA, Ideker RE. Mechanism of ventricular defibrillation for near-defibrillation threshold shocks: a whole heart optical mapping study in swine. Circulation 2001;104:1313–1319.

17 Dosdall DJ, Cheng KA, Huang J, et al. Transmural and endocardial Purkinje activation in pigs preceding local and myocardial activation after defibrillation shocks. Heart Rhythm 2007;4:758–765.

18 Wikswo JP Jr, Lin S-F, Abbas RA. Virtual electrodes in cardiac tissue: a common mechanism for anodal and cathodal stimulation. Biophys J 1995;69:2195–2210.

19 Roth BJ. A mathematical model of make and break electrical stimulation of cardiac tissue by a unipolar anode or cathode. IEEE Trans Biomed Eng 1995;42:1174–1184.

20 Efimov IR, Cheng Y, Yamanouchi Y, Tchou PJ. Direct evidence of the role of virtual electrode-induced phase singularity in success and failure of defibrillation. J Cardiovasc Electrophysiol 2000;11:861–868.

21 Shibata N, Chen P-S, Dixon EG, et al. Influence of shock strength and timing on induction of ventricular arrhythmias in dogs. Am J Physiol 1988;255:H891–H901.

22 Newton JC, Knisley SB, Zhou X, Pollard AE, Ideker RE. Review of mechanisms by which electrical stimulation alters the transmembrane potential. J Cardiovasc Electrophysiol 1999;10:234–243.

23 Colavita PG, Wolf PD, Smith WM, Bartram FR, Hardage M, Ideker RE. Determination of effects of internal countershock by direct cardiac recordings during normal rhythm. Am J Physiol 1986;250:H736–H740.

24 Fast VG, Rohr S, Gillis AM, Kléber AG. Activation of cardiac tissue by extracellular electrical shocks. Formation of 'secondary sources' at intercellular clefts in monolayers of cultured myocytes. Circ Res 1998;82:375–385.

25 White JB, Walcott GP, Pollard AE, Ideker RE. Myocardial discontinuities: a substrate for producing virtual electrodes to increase directly excited areas of the myocardium by shocks. Circulation 1998;97:1738–1745.

26 Sobie EA, Susil RC, Tung L. A generalized activating function for predicting virtual electrodes in cardiac tissue. Biophys J 1997;73:1410–1423.

27 Hooks DA, Tomlinson KA, Marsden SG, et al. Cardiac microstructure: implications for electrical propagation and defibrillation in the heart. Circ Res 2002;91:331–338.

28 Trayanova N, Roth BJ. Cardiac tissue in an electric field: a study of electrical stimulation. In: Murray A, Arzbaecher R, eds. *Proc. Computers in Cardiology*. Los Alamitos, CA: IEEE Computer Society Press; 1992:695–698.

29 Trayanova NA, Roth BJ, Malden LJ. The response of a spherical heart to a uniform electric field: a bidomain analysis of cardiac stimulation. IEEE Trans Biomed Eng 1993;40:899–908.

30 Winfree AT. *When Time Breaks Down: The Three-Dimensional Dynamics of Electrochemical Waves and Cardiac Arrhythmias*. Princeton, NJ: Princeton University Press; 1987:1–153.

31 Ideker RE, Tang ASL, Frazier DW, Shibata N, Chen P-S, Wharton JM. Ventricular defibrillation: basic concepts. In: El-Sherif N, Samet P, eds. *Cardiac Pacing and Electrophysiology*. Orlando, FL: W.B. Saunders; 1991:713–726.

32 Frazier DW, Wolf PD, Wharton JM, Tang ASL, Smith WM, Ideker RE. Stimulus-induced critical point: mechanism for electrical initiation of reentry in normal canine myocardium. J Clin Invest 1989;83:1039–1052.

33 Chattipakorn N, Fotuhi PC, Ideker RE. Prediction of defibrillation outcome by epicardial activation patterns following shocks near the defibrillation threshold. J Cardiovasc Electrophysiol 2000;11:1014–1021.

34 Chen P-S, Shibata N, Wolf PD, et al. Epicardial activation during successful and unsuccessful ventricular defibrillation in open chest dogs. Cardiovasc Rev Rep 1986;7:625–648.

35 Li HG, Jones DL, Yee R, Klein GJ. Defibrillation shocks produce different effects on Purkinje fibers and ventricular muscle: implications for successful defibrillation, refibrillation and postshock arrhythmia. J Am Coll Cardiol 1993;22:607–614.

36 Vigmond EJ, Clements C. Construction of a computer model to investigate sawtooth effects in the Purkinje system. IEEE Trans Biomed Eng 2007;54:389–399.

37 Nanthakumar K, Johnson PL, Huang J, et al. Regional variation in capture of fibrillating swine left ventricle during electrical stimulation. J Cardiovasc Electrophysiol 2005;16:425–432.

38 Kamjoo K, Uchida T, Ikeda T, et al. Importance of location and timing of electrical stimuli in terminating sustained functional reentry in isolated swine ventricular tissues: evidence in support of a small reentrant circuit. Circulation 1997;96:2048–2060.

39 Newton JC, Huang J, Rogers JM, et al. Pacing during ventricular fibrillation: factors influencing the ability to capture. J Cardiovasc Electrophysiol 2001;12:76–84.

40 Pak HN, Liu YB, Hayashi H, Okuyama Y, Chen PS, Lin SF. Synchronization of ventricular fibrillation with real-time feedback pacing: implication to low-energy defibrillation. Am J Physiol Heart Circ Physiol 2003;285:H2704–H2711.

41 Ravi K, Nihei M, Willmer A, Hayashi H, Lin SF. Optical recording-guided pacing to create functional line of block during ventricular fibrillation. J Biomed Opt 2006;11:021013.

42 Pak HN, Okuyama Y, Oh YS, et al. Improvement of defibrillation efficacy with preshock synchronized pacing. J Cardiovasc Electrophysiol 2004;15:581–587.

43 Tang L, Hwang GS, Song J, Chen PS, Lin SF. Post-shock synchronized pacing in isolated rabbit left ventricle: evaluation of a novel defibrillation strategy. J Cardiovasc Electrophysiol 2007;18:740–749.

44 Walcott GP, Knisley SB, Zhou X, Newton JC, Ideker RE. On the mechanism of ventricular defibrillation. Pacing Clin Electrophysiol 1997;20:422–431.

45 Knisley SB, Smith WM, Ideker RE. Effect of field stimulation on cellular repolarization in rabbit myocardium: implications for reentry induction. Circ Res 1992;70:707–715.

CHAPTER 23

Automatic external defibrillation and public access defibrillator response

Paul J. Wang, Amin Al-Ahmad, & Robert J. Myerburg

The history of out-of-hospital cardiac arrest survival

Historically, survival from cardiac arrest has been extremely poor. Survival in major metropolitan areas has been estimated to be less than 2%. The estimated cumulative United States survival in 1991 was 1–3% with current United States estimates of Emergency Medical Services outcomes being 5% (Table 23.1). There have been a number of interventions that have helped improve survival of victims with out-of-hospital cardiac arrest. Of these, strategies based on rapid access to automatic external defibrillators (AEDs) have great promise in improving survival [1–28].

AEDs may be used by first-responders to shorten the time to defibrillation, and therefore increase survival from cardiac arrest (Table 23.2). Placement of AEDs in police patrol cars, fire engines, and ambulances is likely to improve the survival from cardiac arrest. The next focus has been to place AEDs in public access sites such as public buildings, stadiums and malls, airports, and airlines. Multifamily dwellings such as apartment buildings, condominiums, and hotels also present opportunity for first responders with AEDs, generally designated rescuers, such as security guards and/or permanent residents. Strategies for single-family dwellings, such

Ventricular Arrhythmias and Sudden Cardiac Death, 1st edition.
Edited by P.J. Wang, A. Al-Ahmad, H. Hsia, and P.C. Zei
© 2008 Blackwell Publishing, ISBN: 978-1-4051-6114-5.

as individual homes, are of particular interest because a large majority of out-of-hospital cardiac arrests occur in that setting. Unfortunately, little has been achieved in developing response strategies for single-family homes. Designated neighborhood responders has been suggested, but efficacy not tested yet. In the PAD Trial, few of the responses were in individual residences [29].

Emergency personnel first-responders

The capacity for early defibrillation, based on deployment of police equipped with AEDs, paralleled by paramedics deployed simultaneously, as shown by the Rochester, Minnesota [28], and Miami-Dade County Police AED programs [30], has demonstrated the potential to reduce the call-to-shock time in patients with so-called shockable rhythms. In Table 23.3, from the Rochester, Minnesota experience, out of 246 cardiac arrests, there were 131 (55%) total number of patients with shockable rhythms. Police had a shorter response time (5.9 min) compared to paramedics (6.7 min). In the Miami-Dade County Police AED program (Table 23.4), initially 1900 police officers and later up to 2400 police officers with AEDs were compared through a concurrent analysis with a traditional emergency medical system (EMS) program. Early defibrillation (Figure 23.1) with shock only resulted in return of circulation in 27% of patients. Most importantly, 97% of the patients with return of circulation by shock only survived to discharge. In comparison, 19% of

Table 23.1 History of out-of-hospital cardiac arrest survival

1971–1974	Initial Miami/Seattle outcomes	14%, 11%
1978–1985	Peak Miami/Seattle outcomes	25–35%
1984	Rural outcomes:	
	Standard basic life support	3%
	Ambulance-based expanded access	19%
1991	Estimated cumulative US survival	1–3%
1992–1994	Major metropolitan population centers	<2%
1996	Dade County, Florida, current outcomes	9%
1996–1998	Current US EMS outcomes, cumulative	~5% ?
1999	"Optimized" systems (OPALS)	

OPALS: Ontario Prehospital Advanced Life Support Study.

patients requiring advanced cardiac life support (ACLS) survived to discharge.

The Amsterdam Resuscitation Study (ARREST) [31] (Figure 23.2) confirmed that the response time for police responders when they were only responders activated was the shortest compared to when EMS was activated or EMS when police responders were also activated. In the Miami-Dade County Police AED police project (Figure 23.3), survival to hospital discharge was highest in patients with shockable rhythms (17.2%) and in the police AED program compared to patients with shockable rhythms in EMS program (9.0%) and patients with shockable and nonshockable rhythms in either the police (7.6%) or EMS (6.0%) programs.

Public access defibrillation

Public access defibrillation may have a significant impact on survival from cardiac arrest. How-ever, based on the Seattle, Washington experience [32], the incidence of cardiac arrests per site per year varies markedly according to specific location (Table 23.5). In airports the incidence is highest at 7 cardiac arrests/site/year compared to 0.08 cardiac arrests/site/year. There are some locations such as motels or hotels that represent a relatively large number of cardiac arrests per year (22/5 yr) but per site have a relatively low annual rate of cardiac arrest of 0.01. Some sites such as motor vehicles represented 168 cardiac arrests per 5 years but these were spread out through over one million vehicles (Table 23.5).

Perhaps the greatest step in advancing the role of public access defibrillation was the PAD or Public Access Defibrillation Trial. The trial was a prospective, randomized controlled clinical trial that randomized a 911 and CPR (cardiopulmonary resuscitation)-only response and a 911 and CPR plus AED response. The primary endpoint of the study was survival to hospital discharge. The trial was conducted at 993 community sites of which approximately 16% were residential sites. Most other sites were for recreation, shopping, entertainment, community centers, or office buildings. The survival was significantly greater, 29, in the CPR-plus-AED arm compared to 14 in the CPR-only arm ($P = 0.033$).

AEDs have made a particular impact in improving survival in several specific types of public sites, including airlines, airports, and casinos [32]. In the Quantas Airlines cardiac arrest intervention program [33], there was a 24% survival rate in patients with ventricular tachycardia or ventricular fibrillation resuscitated in the airports and a 33% survival rate in patients with ventricular tachycardia or ventricular fibrillation (VT/VF) resuscitated in-flight

Table 23.2 AED deployment strategies for first-responders

Deployment	Examples	Rescuers
Emergency vehicles	Police patrol cars Fire engines Ambulances	Trained emergency personnel
Public access sites	Public buildings Stadiums and malls Airports and airliners	Security personnel Designated rescuers Random lay persons
Multifamily dwellings	Private homes apartments Neighborhood "heart watch"	Family members Designated rescuers

Table 23.3 Early defibrillation by police and paramedics

	Total	Police	Paramedics
Cardiac arrests	246		
Nonshockable	115		
Asystole = 66			
PEA = 49	[47%]		
Shockable	131 [53%]	58	73
Response time [call-to-shock, min (median)]		5.9 min	6.7 min
Cumulative survival	53 [22%]		

The Rochester, Minnesota experience.

Table 23.4 Miami-Dade County Police AED program [30]

Deployment:	1900 Miami-Dade County Police officers (later 2400)
Implementation:	February 1–July 1, 1999
System:	Police
911	-Fire rescue
Concurrent analysis:	First responder – police w/AEDs vs. EMS (intention-to-treat)
Historical comparison:	EMS responder prior to police–AED program

(Figure 23.4). In the American Airlines AED program [34], survival was 44% in patients with VT/VF (Figure 23.5). The Chicago Airport AED project [35] underscored the feasibility of defibrillation by lay people without AED training (Figure 23.6). Perhaps the most impressive survival rates have come from the Las Vegas Casino project [36]: whereas the collapse-to-shock time has been less than 3 minutes, the survival rate has been up to 74%, the highest rate reported in any setting (Figures 23.7 and 23.8). The Piacenza, Italy experience [37] has underscored the potential for patients resuscitated by AEDs to remain neurologically intact.

Conclusions

Automatic external defibrillators have an enormous potential to impact on the survival rate for cardiac arrest. When given to emergency response personnel and placed in key public areas, short collapse-to-shock times likely will lead to significantly improved survival.

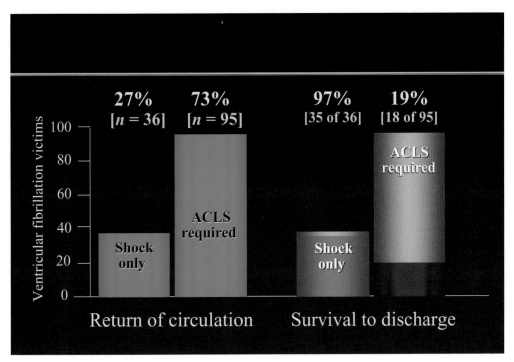

Figure 23.1 Early defibrillation by police and paramedics. Return of spontaneous circulation and survival. (Figure from Ref [28], with permission.)

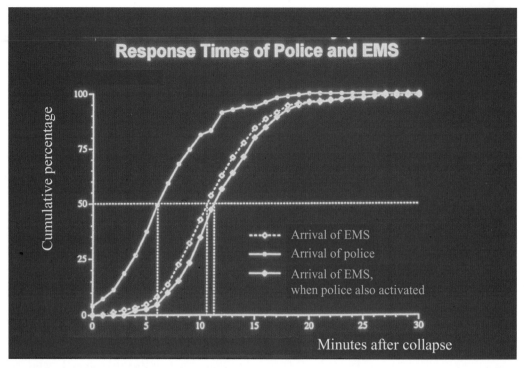

Figure 23.2 Amsterdam resuscitation study (ARREST): Response Times of Police and EMS. (From Ref [31], with permission.)

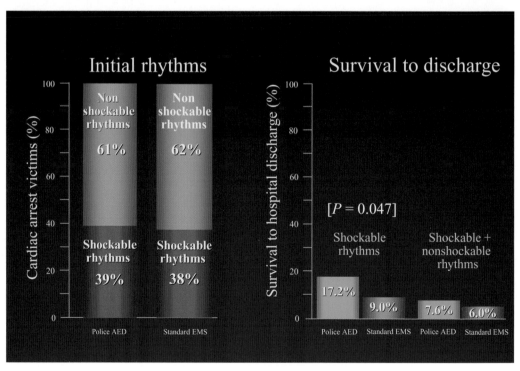

Figure 23.3 Miami-Dade County Police AED project. (From Ref [30], with permission.)

Table 23.5 PAD: Incidence of cardiac arrest in community sites

Location	Arrests/5 yr	Sites (n)	Incidence/site/yr	"n" for >1/yr
Airport	35	1	7	1
County jail	5	1	1	1
Large malls	10	3	0.6	2
Sports venues	11	6	0.4	3
Industrial site	14	8	0.4	4
Golf course	23	47	0.1	5
Train terminals, etc.	7	13	0.1	10
Health clubs	18	47	0.08	12
Hotel or motel	22	377	0.01	100
Bus	31	1138	0.005	200
Bar/tavern	11	413	0.005	200
Government office	6	448	0.003	333
School or church	21	1943	0.002	500
Restaurant	36	4109	0.002	500
Motor vehicles	168	1,322,040	0.0001	10,000
Outdoors	385	n/a	n/a	n/a

The Seattle, Washington experience [32].

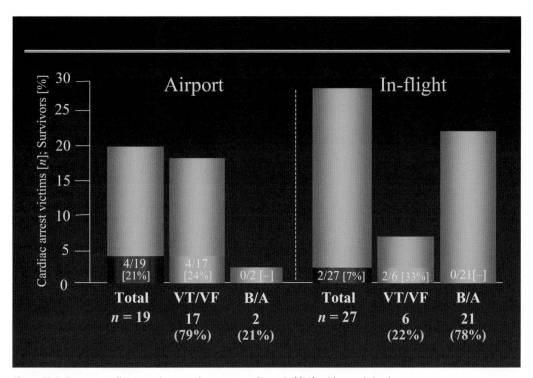

Figure 23.4 Quantas cardiac arrest intervention program. (From Ref [33], with permission.)

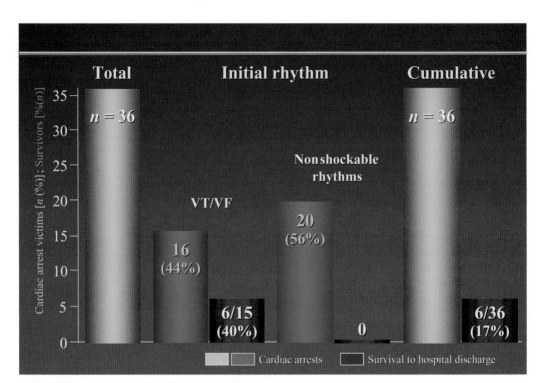

Figure 23.5 American airlines AED program. (From Ref [34], with permission.)

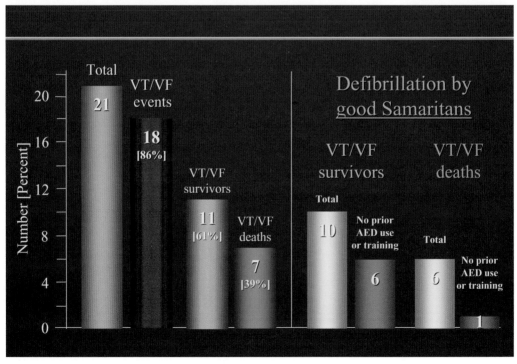

Figure 23.6 Chicago airport AED project: June 1, 1999–May 31, 2001. (From Ref [35], with permission.)

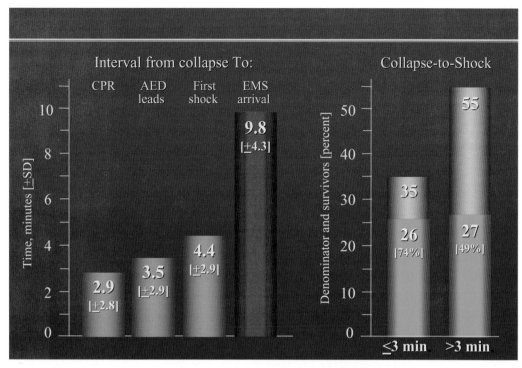

Figure 23.7 Las Vegas Casino AED project: witnessed response times. (From Ref [36], with permission.)

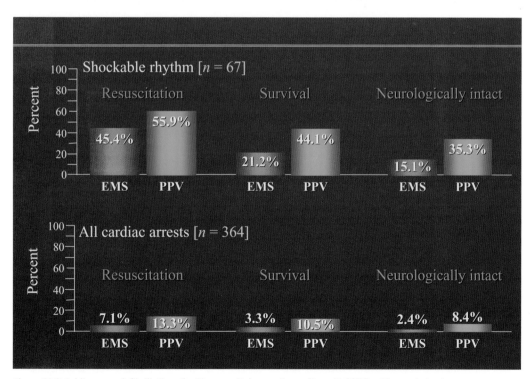

Figure 23.8 Public access defibrillation: the Piacenza, Italy experience. (From Ref [37], with permission.)

References

1 Aronson AL, Haggar B. The automatic external defibrillator-pacemaker: clinical rationale and engineering design. Med Instrum January–February 1986;20(1):27–35.

2 Chadda KD, Kammerer R. Early experiences with the portable automatic external defibrillator in the home and public places. Am J Cardiol 15 September 1987;60(8):732–733.

3 Cummins RO, Eisenberg M, Bergner L, Murray JA. Sensitivity, accuracy, and safety of an automatic external defibrillator. Lancet 11 August 1984;2(8398):318–320.

4 Cummins RO, Eisenberg MS, Moore JE, et al. Automatic external defibrillators: clinical, training, psychological, and public health issues. Ann Emerg Med August 1985;14(8):755–760.

5 Domanovits H, Meron G, Sterz F, et al. Successful automatic external defibrillator operation by people trained only in basic life support in a simulated cardiac arrest situation [see comment]. Resuscitation October–November 1998;39(1–2):47–50.

6 Eisenberg MS, Moore J, Cummins RO, et al. Use of the automatic external defibrillator in homes of survivors of out-of-hospital ventricular fibrillation. Am J Cardiol 15 February 1989;63(7):443–446.

7 England H, Hoffman C, Hodgman T, et al. Effectiveness of automated external defibrillators in high schools in greater Boston. Am J Cardiol 15 June 2005;95(12):1484–1486.

8 Forrer CS, Swor RA, Jackson RE, Pascual RG, Compton S, McEachin C. Estimated cost effectiveness of a police automated external defibrillator program in a suburban community: 7 years experience. Resuscitation January 2002;52(1):23–29.

9 Glazer I. Airline use of automatic external defibrillator: shocking developments [comment]. Aviat Space Environ Med May 2000;71(5):556.

10 Gray AJ, Redmond AD, Martin MA. Use of the automatic external defibrillator-pacemaker by ambulance personnel: the Stockport experience. Br Med J Clin Res Ed 2 May 1987;294(6580):1133–1135.

11 Hernandez B, Christensen J. Automatic external defibrillator intervention in the workplace: a comprehensive approach to program development. AAOHN J February 2001;49(2):96–106; quiz 107–108.

12 Jakobsson JG, Rehnqvist N, Nyquist O. Experience with an automatic external defibrillator. Acta Anaesthesiol Scand October 1987;31(7):597–600.

13 Kellerman AL, Hackman B. Automatic external defibrillator for out-of-hospital cardiac arrest. N Engl J Med 9 March 1989;320(10):670–671.

14 Koster RW. Automatic external defibrillator: key link in the chain of survival. J Cardiovasc Electrophysiol January 2002;13(1, suppl):S92–S95.

15 Marenco JP, Wang PJ, Link MS, Homoud MK, Estes NA, III. Improving survival from sudden cardiac arrest: the role of the automated external defibrillator [see comment]. JAMA 7 March 2001;285(9):1193–1200.

16 Martens P, Calle P, Vanhaute O, for the Belgian Cardio Pulmonary Cerebral Resuscitation Study Group. Theoretical calculation of maximum attainable benefit of public access defibrillation in Belgium. Resuscitation March 1998;36(3):161–163.

17 Mattioni TA, Nademanee K, Brodsky M, et al. Initial clinical experience with a fully automatic in-hospital external cardioverter defibrillator. Pacing Clin Electrophysiol November 1999;22(11):1648–1655.

18 Moore JE, Eisenberg MS, Cummins RO, Hallstrom A, Litwin P, Carter W. Lay person use of automatic external defibrillation. Ann Emerg Med June 1987;16(6):669–672.

19 Morgan C. Advances in AED (automatic external defibrillator) technology. J Emerg Med Serv January 1997;22(1):S12–S15.

20 Motyka TM, Winslow JE, Newton K, Brice JH. Method for determining automatic external defibrillator need at mass gatherings. Resuscitation June 2005;65(3):309–314.

21 Myerburg RJ, Velez M, Rosenberg DG, Fenster J, Castellanos A. Automatic external defibrillators for prevention of out-of-hospital sudden death: effectiveness of the automatic external defibrillator. J Cardiovasc Electrophysiol September 2003;14(9, suppl):S108–S116.

22 Rea TD, Shah S, Kudenchuk PJ, Copass MK, Cobb LA. Automated external defibrillators: to what extent does the algorithm delay CPR? Ann Emerg Med August 2005;46(2):132–141.

23 Varon J, Sternbach GL, Marik PE, Fromm RE, Jr. Automatic external defibrillators: lessons from the past, present and future. Resuscitation August 1999;41(3):219–223.

24 Weaver WD, Copass MK, Hill DL, Fahrenbruch C, Hallstrom AP, Cobb LA. Cardiac arrest treated with a new automatic external defibrillator by out-of-hospital first responders. Am J Cardiol 1 May 1986;57(13):1017–1021.

25 Weaver WD, Hill D, Fahrenbruch CE, et al. Use of the automatic external defibrillator in the management of out-of-hospital cardiac arrest. N Engl J Med 15 September 1988;319(11):661–666.

26 Weaver WD, Hill DL, Fahrenbruch C, et al. Automatic external defibrillators: importance of field testing to evaluate performance. J Am Coll Cardiol December 1987;10(6):1259–1264.

27 Weaver WD, Sutherland K, Wirkus MJ, Bachman R. Emergency medical care requirements for large public assemblies and a new strategy for managing cardiac arrest in this setting. Ann Emerg Med February 1989;18(2):155–160.

28 White RD. Early out-of-hospital experience with an impedance-compensating low-energy biphasic waveform automatic external defibrillator. J Interv Card Electrophysiol November 1997;1(3):203–208; discussion 209–210.

29 Hallstrom AP, Ornato JP, Weisfeldt M, et al. Public access defibrillation trial I. Public-access defibrillation and survival after out-of-hospital cardiac arrest [see comment]. N Engl J Med 12 August 2004;351(7):637–646.

30 Myerburg RJ, Fenster J, Velez M, et al. Impact of community-wide police car deployment of automated

external defibrillators on survival from out-of-hospital cardiac arrest [see comment]. Circulation 27 August 2002;106(9):1058–1064.

31 Waalewijn RA, de Vos R, Koster RW. Out-of-hospital cardiac arrests in Amsterdam and its surrounding areas: results from the Amsterdam resuscitation study (ARREST) in "Utstein" style. Resuscitation September 1998;38(3):157–167.

32 Becker L, Eisenberg M, Fahrenbruch C, Cobb L. Public locations of cardiac arrest: implications for public access defibrillation. Circulation 2 June 1998;97(21):2106–2109.

33 O'Rourke MF, Donaldson E, Geddes JS. An airline cardiac arrest program [see comment]. Circulation 4 November 1997;96(9):2849–2853.

34 Page RL, Joglar JA, Kowal RC, *et al.* Use of automated external defibrillators by a U.S. airline [see comment]. N Engl J Med 26 October 2000;343(17):1210–1216.

35 Caffrey SL, Willoughby PJ, Pepe PE, Becker LB. Public use of automated external defibrillators [see comment]. N Engl J Med 17 October 2002;347(16):1242–1247.

36 Valenzuela TD, Roe DJ, Nichol G, Clark LL, Spaite DW, Hardman RG. Outcomes of rapid defibrillation by security officers after cardiac arrest in casinos [see comment]. N Engl J Med 26 October 2000;343(17):1206–1209.

37 Capucci A, Aschieri D, Piepoli MF, Bardy GH, Iconomu E, Arvedi M. Tripling survival from sudden cardiac arrest via early defibrillation without traditional education in cardiopulmonary resuscitation [see comment]. Circulation 27 August 2002;106(9):1065–1070.

CHAPTER 24

Advances in cardiopulmonary resuscitation

Anurag Gupta, & Amin Al-Ahmad

Introduction

Sudden cardiac death (SCD) remains an important cause of death in the United States. It is the most common lethal manifestation of heart disease, accounting for greater than 50% of deaths due to cardiovascular cause. Overall, it is estimated that between 300,000 and 350,000 adults in the United States, and potentially as many as 450,000 individuals, succumb to SCD each year [1,2].

Despite advances in our ability to target populations at high risk for SCD and to offer them highly effective therapies such as implantable defibrillators, the vast majority of eventual SCD victims remain unidentified. In fact, at least 50% of SCD occur in individuals as the first clinical manifestation of cardiac disease or in individuals previously deemed to be at low risk for SCD [1]. This underscores the continued critical role of cardiopulmonary resuscitation in reducing the incidence of SCD.

Unfortunately, the rate of successful resuscitation following cardiac arrest remains low. Though estimates vary widely, in more recent prospective studies, approximately 18% of adult with in-hospital cardiac arrest survive to discharge [3] while approximately 5% of adults with out-of-hospital cardiac arrest survive to discharge [4]. The rates of success decline further when evaluating unselected populations or when using a more rigorous definition of success, that is, neurologically intact survival to hospital discharge. This chapter presents key accomplishments in the field of cardiopulmonary

Ventricular Arrhythmias and Sudden Cardiac Death, 1st edition. Edited by P.J. Wang, A. Al-Ahmad, H. Hsia, and P.C. Zei © 2008 Blackwell Publishing, ISBN: 978-1-4051-6114-5.

resuscitation and offers insight into methods by which it may be improved.

Historical perspective

Basic life support

The tenets of cardiopulmonary resuscitation have deep historical roots, with initial strategies identifying the critical role of establishing a patent airway for victims, providing artificial ventilation via mechanical or mouth-to-mouth methods, and performing chest compression. These techniques form the foundation for the modern Airway–Breathing–Circulation paradigm of basic CPR (cardiopulmonary resuscitation) [5,6]. However, it was not until the latter half of the twentieth century that these methods were rigorously developed and incorporated into resuscitation algorithms.

In 1953, Stephenson and colleagues [7] reported on a large series of 1200 surgical patients suffering cardiac arrest, both in the operating room (86%) and outside (14%), who underwent attempted resuscitation using open-chest cardiac compression (Figure 24.1). By primarily employing this approach, they cited an impressive 28% rate of survival. They further noted the critical importance of timely interventions, with 94% of successful resuscitations occurring when cardiac massage was initiated within four minutes of arrest. Subsequently, the feasibility of closed-chest compressions was established by Kouwenhoven and colleagues [8], who in 1960 reported successful resuscitation and survival to hospital discharge in 14 of 20 patients receiving precordial compressions. In 1966, the first national guidelines reflecting modern-day CPR were published [9].

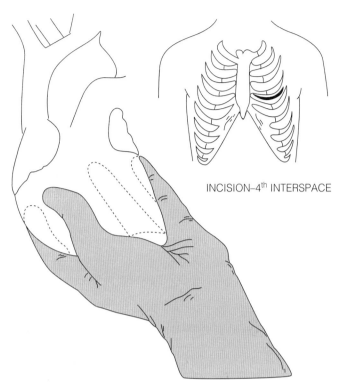

INCISION–4ᵗʰ INTERSPACE

Figure 24.1 Open chest compression: In discussing their experience with open chest compressions during cardiac arrest, Stephenson and colleagues depicted the preferred modality of cardiac massage via thoracotomy. They described the possibility of achieving a systolic blood pressure of 80 mm Hg when compressing at a rate between 60 and 80 per minute. (Figure reproduced, with permission, from Stephenson HE, Reid LC, Hinton JW. Some common denominators in 1200 cases of cardiac arrest. Ann Surg 1953;137:731–744.)

Advanced life support

While basic CPR was being formalized, advanced life-support aimed at definitively restoring normal circulation was developed and incorporated into resuscitation algorithms. Prevost and Battelli [10] are credited with the first demonstration that electrical defibrillation can terminate ventricular fibrillation in a canine model published in 1899. The first successful report of defibrillation in humans was published in 1947 by Beck and colleagues [11]. They reported resuscitation using a primitive alternating current defibrillator in a 14-year-old boy who suffered ventricular fibrillation while undergoing thoracoplasty for congenital funnel chest, despite 45 minutes of open-chest compression. Zoll [12,13], who also demonstrated in 1952 the ability to pace the heart with external electrical current in patients with Adams–Stokes attacks, further performed the first series of successful external defibrillations in humans in 1955. Subsequently, defibrillators using direct current as opposed to sinusoidal alternating current were employed, achieving more consistent and uniform cardiac depolarization. In 1962, Lown

and colleagues [14] demonstrated that direct current defibrillation and/or synchronized cardioversion resulted in superior rhythm conversion and reduced postdefibrillatory arrhythmias including recurrent ventricular tachyarrhythmias.

These developments paved the way for modern-day devices, namely the automated external defibrillator (AED). First described by Diack and colleagues in 1979 [15], the initial model incorporated an intrapharyngeal sensor and a lingual-epigastric skin pathway. The widespread adoption of defibrillation in the communities using these highly effective devices has been revolutionary. This revolution has been possible because current AEDs are relatively small in size, weigh <4.5 kg are, simple to operate, and easy to maintain.

Adjunctive pharmacotherapy was further incorporated into the guidelines, including most notably epinephrine. Discovered in the 1890s by Oliver and Schafer [16], its potential to enhance perfusion was described soon after, and its specific vasoactive properties ultimately elucidated beginning in 1963 [17]. However, despite the continued role

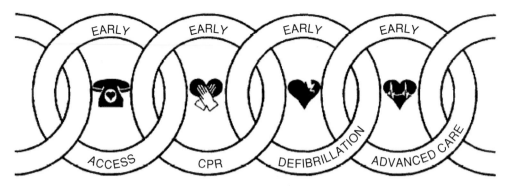

Figure 24.2 "Chain of Survival." A chain of survival, incorporating the four links pictured above, describes a protocol initially promulgated by the American Heart Association in 1991 to rapidly manage sudden cardiac arrest. This includes early recognition of emergency and activation of the emergency response system, early CPR, early defibrillation, and early advanced care. (Reproduced with permission from *Improving Survival from Sudden Cardiac Arrest: the "Chain of Survival" Concept.* A statement for health professionals from the Advanced Cardiac Life Support Subcommittee and the Emergency Cardiac Care Committee, American Heart Association © 1991, American Heart Association, Inc.)

of drugs in resuscitation algorithms, importantly no placebo-controlled trial has demonstrated improved survival to hospital discharge by administering any drug at any stage of arrest.

Implementation of resuscitation programs

In addition to developing new tools for resuscitation, initiatives focused on distributing these tools and educating individuals in their use, have been critical to the advancement of modern resuscitation. While the initial organization and education of resuscitation teams focused on health care providers in hospitals, efforts were subsequently extended into the community with mixed results. In 1979, Eisenberg and colleagues [18] reported the results in King County, Washington of adding paramedic services to areas with existing emergency medical technician services. In their analysis they reported four significant factors predicting success to discharge, namely the presence of paramedic service, bystander-initiated CPR, rapid initiation of CPR, and rapid initiation of definitive care.

Reflective of findings such as these, the American Heart Association outlined in 1991 a critical series of events that must be rapidly performed to facilitate successful resuscitation. Collectively referred to as a "chain of survival," the four constituent links include (1) early access (in which a medical emergency is identified and the emergency medical

system is activated), (2) early CPR (in which basic CPR is initiated), (3) early defibrillation, and (4) early advanced cardiac life support (in which measures such as intravenous medication and endotracheal intubation are employed) (Figure 24.2) [19]. Selected advances in the development and implementation of tools involved in these constituent links are discussed in this chapter.

Basic cardiopulmonary resuscitation

Physiologic basis of direct chest compressions

Two models explain how cardiopulmonary resuscitation may allow blood to flow during cardiac arrest [20]. It was initially believed that closed-chest compression resulted in direct compression of the heart between the sternum and spine, leading to pressure gradients between the ventricle and the aorta and pulmonary artery, thus leading to blood flow ("cardiac pump" model) [21]. However, a more current paradigm referred to as the "thoracic pump" model suggests that blood flow is achieved by increasing intrathoracic pressure during chest compression, with the heart serving merely as a passive conduit [22]. Increased intrathoracic pressures due to compression are transmitted unequally to the extrathoracic arteries and veins, potentially due to collapse of the great veins at the thoracic outlet with rising intrathoracic pressures. The resulting peripheral pressure gradient between arterial and venous pressures leads to antegrade flow during compression. During release of compression, intrathoracic pressure falls below venous pressures to facilitate return of blood from the extrathoracic to intrathoracic vessels.

Using these principles, investigators have attempted to optimize the delivery of chest compressions and basic CPR. Initial studies in canine models demonstrated that applying compressions with moderate force increases stroke volume; cardiac output can be further increased by increasing compression rates, as this does not significantly hamper stroke volume [23]. Subsequent studies in humans confirmed that the application of adequate force and the use of higher compression rates improved antegrade blood flow [24]. Studies in humans suggest that systolic arterial pressures may reach up to 60–80 mm Hg with chest compressions [24–26]. In contrast, incomplete chest wall decompression and excessive ventilation can negatively impact intrathoracic pressure gradients to reduce venous return, cardiac output, and coronary and cerebral perfusion [20,27–29].

Novel compression strategies

In an effort to improve vital organ perfusion beyond that obtained with manual compression, more innovative strategies based on the above principles have been introduced, though with mixed success and promise (Figure 24.3) [30–32]. To ameliorate the adverse consequences of excessive ventilation and incomplete chest wall decompression, new *impedance threshold devices* (ITDs) have been designed that are connected in series to an endotracheal tube. The device prevents inspiratory airflow into the patient when the intrathoracic pressure is negative, that is during chest decompression when not actively ventilating the patient. This maintains and augments negative intrathoracic pressure, and therefore venous return, during the decompression phase of CPR. On the other hand, when actively ventilating the patient or providing chest compressions, there is no impedance to airflow, thus permitting intermittent positive pressure ventilation and gas exchange [33]. A modification of this device further incorporates a vacuum source that maintains an intrathoracic vacuum be-

tween -5 and -10 mm Hg, further augmenting negative intrathoracic pressures when appropriate [34]. Porcine models incorporating these devices demonstrate improved short-term survival [34] and/or hemodynamics [35]. In humans, a randomized placebo-controlled blinded trial of 400 individuals with out-of-hospital cardiac arrest receiving active compression–decompression CPR, showed significantly improved 24-hour survival in the group receiving ITD compared to the placebo group, though the trends lost significance when evaluating survival to discharge or neurologically intact survival [33].

In further recognition of the suboptimal efficacy achieved with manual compressions and inconsistency in its delivery, various automated mechanical chest compression devices have been developed. A *load-distributing band*, composed of a pneumatically or electrically actuated constricting band and backboard, applies circumferential chest compression to achieve higher intrathoracic pressures than possible with manual compression to the sternum alone. Initial promising studies [36–38] paved the way for two recently published, large trials in humans with out-of-hospital cardiac arrest. The results were highly disparate, with improved outcomes noted in the pre–post retrospective observational analysis [39], and actually worse outcomes noted in the prospective, cluster-randomized trial [40]. The reasons for the discrepant results are likely multifactorial, though they importantly highlight limitations in conducting and comparing trials in resuscitation given the extreme heterogeneity in resuscitative efforts. Specifically, in these trials, key factors likely included differences in patient population including rhythm on presentation, time to initiation of CPR, and time-to-deployment of the load-distributing band (including its influence on time to defibrillation) [41].

Clear clinical evidence supporting the use of other mechanical devices is likewise limited. *Mechanical piston devices* depress the sternum using a compressed gas-powered plunger mounted on a backboard. While the amount of data supporting their use is limited, when used by trained medical providers improvements in arterial pressure and end-tidal CO_2 have been demonstrated [42–44]. In contrast, *active compression–decompression devices*, hand-held suction devices applied on the anterior chest wall, improve venous return in the

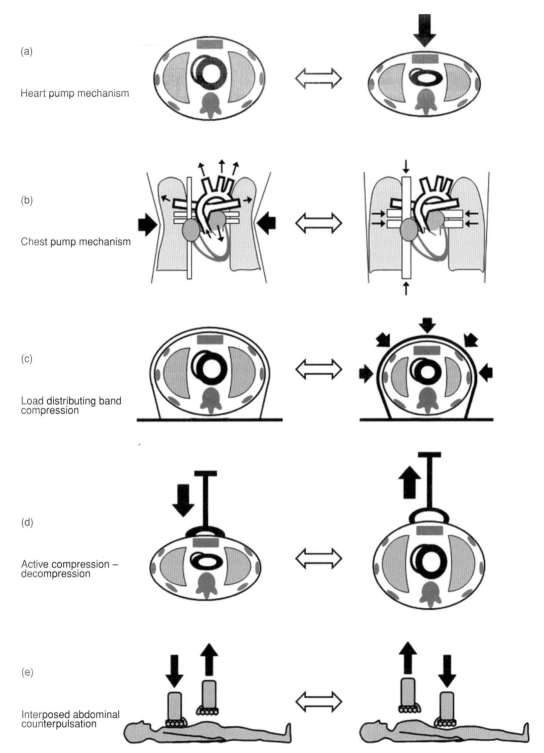

(a)

Heart pump mechanism

(b)

Chest pump mechanism

(c)

Load distributing band
compression

(d)

Active compression –
decompression

(e)

Interposed abdominal
counterpulsation

Figure 24.3 (*Continued*).

decompression phase by creating a vacuum as the device is actively pulled [45–47]. However, combined analyses of trials using these devices have shown no clear survival benefit [48]. Strategies incorporating *interposed abdominal counterpulsation*, which possibly improves diastolic aortic pressure and/or other parameters, have been studied; however, current use of these strategies is limited by the insufficient data to support their use [49–51].

Current paradigms in basic CPR

Basic CPR continues to assume a critical role in resuscitation by maintaining end-organ perfusion until a definitive intervention that restores normal circulation is employed. While novel therapies in basic CPR show promise, they are at present of limited proven clinical impact and utilization. Not surprisingly, current guidelines instead emphasize the role of conventional CPR and incorporate the aforementioned physiologic principles underlying chest compression—"push hard, push fast, allow full chest recoil after each compression, and minimize interruptions in compressions" [30].

The necessity for ventilation during the initial phase of resuscitation is debated, in part reflecting the importance of compressions, the detrimental effects of overventilation, and the desire to increase public acceptance of and/or ability in performing bystander CPR [52–54]. During the initial minutes of arrest, some individuals with patent airways may achieve some gas exchange via passive chest recoil and intermittent gasps. Comparable efficacy of a chest compressions-only model has been demonstrated in several, but not all, animal models of cardiac arrest [55–58]. For example, in a more recent porcine model comparing four different compression and ventilation strategies following induction of ventricular fibrillation, a strategy of four min-

utes of compressions only followed by a compression:ventilation ratio of 100:2 had a superior neurological outcome versus all other therapies including standard CPR with a continuous ratio of 15:2 [59].

Notwithstanding, combining some ventilation with minimally interrupted chest compressions remains recommended and may be more optimal, particularly in situations of primary asphyxial arrest and in all forms of prolonged arrest [60,61]. Using mathematical and physiologic modeling, Babbs and Kern [62] suggested that maximal oxygen delivery and blood flow occurred at compression:ventilation ratios of 30:2 under standardized conditions; in conditions that simulated lay rescuer performance in the field though, ratios near 60:2 were more optimal. Moreover, the fundamental importance of providing some gas exchange was highlighted in a porcine model of ventricular fibrillation, in which near-complete arterial desaturation occurred in less than 2 minutes in pigs receiving compressions only and was associated with worse resuscitation outcomes [63]. Overall, rigorous human data are lacking and further study is required to clarify trial discrepancies and to define optimal compression and ventilation strategies. Current guidelines for adult CPR suggest compression:ventilation ratios of 30:2 with goal delivery of approximately 100 compressions per minute [30].

Despite continued efforts to develop and/or optimize tools for resuscitation, major focus has been placed on improving providers' performance of *existing* methods of basic CPR, as evidenced in the most current guidelines. This reflects evidence from several studies illustrating significant shortcomings in CPR performance. In a recent case series of 176 adults presenting with out-of-hospital cardiac arrest treated by paramedics and nurse anesthetists, chest compressions were generally too shallow and

Figure 24.3 Mechanisms of various closed chest compression techniques. Panels (a) and (b) illustrate two models by which manual chest compression may lead to blood flow. Panel (a) depicts the cardiac pump model in which direct compression of the heart against the sternum effects blood flow, while Panel (b) shows the thoracic pump model, in which, the generation of intrathoracic pressure and pressure gradients lead to blood flow. Novel strategies to augment blood flow with chest compression are illustrated in Panels (c)–(e). This includes use of a load-distributing band (Panel c) which increases intrathoracic pressure by applying circumferential pressure; an active compression–decompression device (Panel D) that notably, through pulling during the decompression phase, creates a vacuum that facilitates venous return; and interposed abdominal counterpulsation (Panel E), which may notably further allow diastolic pressure augmentation. Figure reproduced, with permission, from Cooper JA, Cooper JD, Cooper JM. Cardiopulmonary resuscitation: history, current practice, and future direction. Circulation 2006;114:2839–2849.

Table 24.1 Initial rhythm disturbance and associated mortality in cardiac arrest.

| | In-hospital [3] | Out-of-hospital | |
		Ref. [4]	Ref. [66]
Total number of cardiac arrests (% survival)	36,902 (17.6)	4247 (5.1)	744 (15.1)
% Ventricular fibrillation or pulseless ventricular tachycardia (% survival)	22.7 (36.0)	31.5 (13.2)	40.7 (32.0)
% Pulseless electrical activity (% survival)	32.4 (11.2)	25.3 (2.4)	27.6 (4.9)
% Asystole (% survival)	35.3 (10.6)	42.0 (0.8)	31.0 (2.2)
% Unknown rhythm (% survival)	9.6 (21.2)	NA	NA

The table demonstrates the percentage of each initial documented rhythm disturbance in individuals presenting with sudden cardiac arrest; for each individual rhythm disturbance, the percentage survival to hospital discharge is noted in parentheses. The data are divided into patients presenting with in-hospital arrest and out-of-hospital arrest. Out-of-hospital arrests are further subdivided into two of the more recent widely published series (with the caveat that further significant heterogeneity exists between these series and those not depicted).

NA, not available.

Table modified, with permission, from Cooper JA, Cooper JD, Cooper JM. Cardiopulmonary resuscitation: history, current practice, and future direction. Circulation 2006;114:2839–2849.

administered for an inadequate percentage of time; specifically, compressions were administered for 48% of the time that victims were without spontaneous circulation [64]. Suboptimal results have further been shown for well-trained hospital staff during in-hospital cardiopulmonary resuscitation, often with too few compressions, inadequate depth, and/or excessive ventilations [65]. The observations are critical, as they have led to continued measures to improve the delivery of high-quality basic CPR through simplified algorithms, improved education, and potential use of adjunctive devices such as CPR prompt devices.

Defibrillation

The role of rapid defibrillation in cardiac arrest

The critical role of rapid defibrillation is based in part on two well-demonstrated observations: (1) time to treatment is the most critical variable in determining the success of resuscitation and (2) presentation with a shockable rhythm, that is ventricular fibrillation (VF) or pulseless ventricular tachycardia (VT), is common and compared to other initial rhythm disturbances, confers the highest probability of successful resuscitation in adults.

A recent large prospective multicenter observational registry of in-hospital pulseless cardiac arrests documented VF or pulseless VT as the initial rhythm 23% of the time. Compared to other initial rhythm disturbances (specifically, pulseless electrical activity, asystole, or unknown rhythm), those with VF or pulseless VT had the best resuscitation outcomes, with 36% survival to hospital discharge (Table 24.1) [3]. While similar trends in survival for each rhythm disturbance are found in out-of-hospital arrests, the absolute percentage of survival remains inferior in all groups compared to in-hospital results. Table 24.1 shows data from two recent representative series of out-of-hospital cardiac arrest, highlighting the heterogeneity between different series though reinforcing that VF is associated with significantly better resuscitation outcomes than PEA and asystole [4,66]. Interestingly, the event rate of ventricular fibrillation in the community appears to be decreasing for unclear reasons [66].

In individuals with cardiac arrest due to VF, time to CPR and time to defibrillation play critical and complementary roles in determining resuscitation outcomes (Figure 24.4) [67]. For every minute that elapses between collapse and defibrillation, it is estimated that the survival rate decreases 3–4% each minute, in the presence of bystander CPR. Without CPR, deterioration is more rapid as the survival rate decreases 7–10% for each minute that elapses between collapse and defibrillation [67,68]. CPR, though unlikely to restore a perfusing rhythm, may

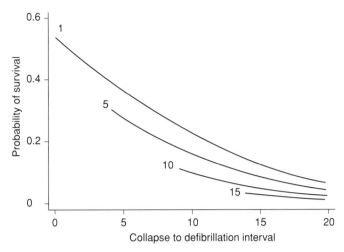

Figure 24.4 Relationship between survival and time to CPR and defibrillation. The graph represents logistic regression modeling from data obtained in two retrospective trials that examined survival in individuals with out-of-hospital cardiac arrest due to ventricular fibrillation. Two variables are depicted: minutes from collapse to CPR (represented by the different curves) and minutes from collapse to defibrillation (represented on x-axis). Delays in CPR and defibrillation markedly impair resuscitation outcomes. (Figure reproduced, with permission, from Valenzuela TD, Roe DJ, Cretin S, Spaite DW, Larsen MP. Estimating effectiveness of cardiac arrest interventions: a logistic regression survival model. *Circulation* 1997;96:3308–3313.)

lead to multiple salutary effects until defibrillation is provided including preventing deterioration of VF into asystole, ameliorating neurological sequelae, and overall improving probability of survival [67–73].

In fact, although defibrillation represents the definitive treatment for VF, the role of CPR may extend beyond a mere stand-in therapy for defibrillation until it is available. That is, CPR may restore the metabolic milieu necessary for effective defibrillation by potentially providing enough tissue perfusion to not only blunt but to also reverse deleterious effects of prolonged VF, such as acidosis and depletion of myocardial adenosine triphosphate content [74,75]. This is particularly true when resuscitation response times are longer. These concepts are somewhat supported by clinical trials showing improved outcomes when *delaying* defibrillation to administer CPR for 90 seconds to 3 minutes versus providing immediate defibrillation, with the benefit most evident in those with delayed response times of at least 4–5 minutes [76,77]. However, a more recent trial has demonstrated comparable outcomes with either strategy [78]. Further data are necessary to find an optimal approach to providing rapid CPR *and* rapid defibrillation when both capabilities are present, though currently, immediate defibrillation

is generally favored when response times are short while a period of CPR may be considered in cases of delayed response [30]. In all cases though, the focus remains on providing rapid therapy.

The complementary and integral roles of both basic CPR and of defibrillation in VF arrest are further underscored by recent recommendations to resume CPR immediately after performing one defibrillation, in preference to the prior strategy of performing up to three consecutive shocks with intervening rhythm analyses [30]. Though evidence for this approach is somewhat indirect, it reflects continued validation of the critical role in minimizing interruptions to compressions during resuscitation [79,80]. In addition, current generation biphasic defibrillators have high first-shock efficacy in acutely terminating VF to either a perfusing rhythm or a nonshockable nonperfusing rhythm such as PEA or asystole, somewhat obviating the approach of delaying compression to perform immediate rhythm analysis [81–83].

The expansion of early access programs for rapid defibrillation

The development of regionalized programs that disseminate AEDs into the community and educate individuals in their use, represents a major advance in cardiopulmonary resuscitation. For example, an initiative by a major commercial US airline to equip its airlines with defibrillators and train flight attendants in their use was shown to be highly safe and effective. Specifically, in examining the first 200 incidents in which the AED had been used for possible arrest, investigators demonstrated that all the 14 cases for which shock was advised were VF, with 40% survival to hospital discharge in these cases. Appropriately, no shock was advised in all the remaining cases [84]. Disseminating AEDs and training nonmedical personnel was further supported by a study examining a consecutive prospective series of 106 individuals with VF arrest treated with AEDs by trained casino security officers. Of these individuals, 53% survived to hospital discharge, with marked advantage in those receiving defibrillation within 3 minutes of witnessed collapse [85]. Distribution of AEDs in places where individuals have no specific training or duty to act has also been shown to be effective. For example, widespread placement of AEDs in three Chicago airports over a 2-year period resulted in neurologically intact survival at 1 year in 10 of 18 individuals with ventricular fibrillation arrest, among a total pool of 21 individuals with noncardiac arrest [86].

Larger studies have continued to confirm the safety and efficacy of early access programs for rapid defibrillation. The Public Access Defibrillation Trial Investigators randomized 19,000 volunteers from 993 communities to CPR and AED training versus CPR-only training in community units with ready access to AEDs. Among individuals with sudden cardiac arrest, significantly more survived to hospital discharge in units with providers having additional training in AED operation over a mean 21.5 months; again, no inappropriate shocks were delivered [87]. In addition, longitudinal and broader success in introducing AEDs to communities has been suggested. As discussed later, a controlled trial performed in Ontario demonstrated a significant improvement in survival to hospital discharge from 3.9% to 5.2% by introducing further measures to provide rapid defibrillation in communities already with existing basic life support and defibrillation capabilities [88]. These measures included methodology to reduce dispatch time, more efficient deployment of ambulances, and performance of defibrillation by firefighters. An observational outcome study in Rochester, Minnesota from 1990 to 2003, where a program was enacted that simultaneously dispatched trained police officers, firefighters, and paramedics with AEDs, showed 41% neurologically intact discharge in 193 patients with ventricular fibrillation arrest; in contrast, survival was only 5% for non-VF atraumatic arrest [89]. However, the causal impact that this intervention played in these outcomes was not investigated. Given the promise of improved outcomes with rapid defibrillation, methods for effectively introducing AEDs into the community merit continued investigation.

Adjunctive pharmacotherapy and induced hypothermia

Though adjunctive pharmacotherapy continues to be incorporated in resuscitation algorithms and may have important favorable effects in certain individuals, rigorous data demonstrating a net benefit in facilitating successful resuscitation are lacking. Epinephrine, generally preferred as the initial vasoactive agent in cardiac arrest, has shown beneficial effects including improved myocardial and cerebral perfusion, likely in part due to its α-adrenergic vasopressor effects [90,91]. However, whether in standard or in high doses, it has not been shown to improve survival to hospital discharge and may actually lead to adverse outcomes; this likely reflects multiple effects including net detrimental β-adrenergic action with increase in myocardial oxygen consumption [92–94]. A meta-analysis of 1519 patients from five randomized trials demonstrated no benefit of substituting epinephrine with vasopressin in cardiac arrest [95]. The literature to guide the use of antiarrhythmic medications is likewise limited and/or not convincing. Amiodarone, though not yet demonstrated to improve survival to hospital discharge, has shown some promise in improving short-term resuscitation outcomes in VF arrest [96,97].

For sudden cardiac arrest patients in whom spontaneous circulation is successfully restored, induction of hypothermia may improve neurological outcomes, possibly by reducing cerebral oxygen requirements and mitigating deleterious biochemical processes. In 2002, investigators randomized 77 adults, who were resuscitated after out-of-hospital cardiac arrest due to VF, to normothermia versus therapeutic hypothermia. Hypothermia was accomplished via external cooling mechanisms that were initiated prior to hospital arrival and continued for 12 hours, at a goal temperature of 33°C. They found improved survival to hospital discharge to home or rehabilitation, as opposed to discharge to long-term nursing facility or death, in the patients treated with hypothermia [98]. Favorable results were similarly obtained in a larger randomized trial assessing the effect of an external cooling device for 24 hours, with goal temperature 32–34°C, in 275 patients presenting in the emergency department after being successfully resuscitated from cardiac arrest due to VF or nonperfusing VT. Specifically, improved neurological outcome at 6 months, as well as reduced mortality at 6 months in secondary analyses, was demonstrated in the group receiving therapeutic hypothermia [99]. Alternative applications and strategies for cooling are being studied, such as infusion of large-volume ice-cold crystalloid fluid intravenously [100]. Overall, therapeutic hypothermia represents a promising advance in cardiopulmonary resuscitation that is already being incorporated into current resuscitation algorithms.

The Canadian experience

Resuscitation outcomes reported by different communities vary widely, in part reflecting the interplay between variability in the interventions used by communities and the more fundamental differences between the communities themselves. Notable insights have been gained from several analyses including the Ontario Prehospital Advanced Life Support (OPALS) Study, recent and rigorous studies that serially evaluated the efficacy of different community-based interventions in the same population. Phase I of their study, conducted over 36 months, was an observational cohort analysis that served as a baseline for future comparisons that analyzed outcomes in communities equipped with basic life support and an ambulance automated defibrillation program. They demonstrated a 3.5% overall survival rate amongst 5335 cases of cardiac arrest. They further noted that the modifiable variables most strongly associated with good outcome, were performance of bystander CPR, performance of CPR by fire or police officers, and response interval [101].

Subsequently, phase II was performed and conducted over 12 months, and consisted of adding programs of rapid defibrillation to these same communities, principally by reducing dispatch times, optimizing deployment of ambulances, and having firefighters perform defibrillation. This "before—after" controlled trial compared survival to hospital discharge in 4690 individuals with cardiac arrest from phase I to 1641 individuals from phase II, and demonstrated a significant 33% relative improvement in survival in the phase II population (5.2% survival to discharge versus 3.9% survival in phase I) [87]. Finally, phase III was performed and conducted over 36 months, and consisted of adding prehospital advanced life support capabilities to these same communities, principally by training paramedics to perform endotracheal intubation, insert intravenous lines, and administer intravenous medications. In this trial, investigators this time failed to show a significant difference in survival to hospital discharge when comparing 1,391 individuals from phase II to 4,247 individuals in phase III (5% and 5.1% survival, respectively) (4).

Multiple lessons can be derived from these studies that highlight recurring themes in the field of cardiopulmonary resuscitation. Notably, despite advances in cardiopulmonary resuscitation, survival rates for sudden cardiac arrests generally remain low and sobering; the need for further innovative strategies is apparent. However, these trials offer hope, showing that survival rates can be improved. Importantly, of all current interventions, rapid basic CPR and defibrillation have most consistently and significantly been shown to positively impact outcomes. Continued efforts to advance the field of cardiopulmonary resuscitation will require thinking forward and innovation not only to develop new technologies but also to optimize the existing fundamental ones.

References

1 Myerburg RJ, Kessler KM, Castellanos A. Sudden cardiac death: epidemiology, transient risk, and intervention assessment. Ann Intern Med 1993;119:1187–1197.
2 Zheng ZJ, Croft JB, Giles WH, Mensah GA. Sudden cardiac death in the United States, 1989 to 1998. Circulation 2001;104:2158–2163.

3 Nadkarni VM, Larkin GL, Peberdy MA, et al. First documented rhythm and clinical outcome from in-hospital cardiac arrest among children and adults. JAMA 2006;295:50–57.

4 Stiell IG, Wells GA, Field B, et al. Advanced cardiac life support in out-of-hospital cardiac arrest. N Engl J Med 2004;351:647–656.

5 Nakagawa Y, Weil MH, Tang W. The history of CPR. In: Weil MH, Tang W, eds. *CPR: Resuscitation of the Heart.* Philadelphia: WB Saunders Company; 1999:1–12.

6 Safar P. History of cardiopulmonary-resuscitation. In: Kaye W, Bircer NG. eds. *Cardiopulmonary Resuscitation.* New York: Churchill Livingstone; 1989:1–53.

7 Stephenson HE, Reid LC, Hinton JW. Some common denominators in 1200 cases of cardiac arrest. Ann Surg 1953;137:731–744.

8 Kouwenhoven WB, Jude JR, Knickerbocker GG. Closed chest massage. JAMA 1960;173:1064–1067.

9 American Heart Association and National Academy of Sciences-National Research Council. Standards for cardiopulmonary resuscitation and emergency cardiac care. JAMA 1966;198:372–379.

10 Prevost JL, Battelli F. La mort par les courants electriques-courants alternatifs a hauste tension. J Physiol Pathol 1899;1:427.

11 Beck CS, Pritchard WH, Feil HS. Ventricular fibrillation of long duration abolished by electric shock. JAMA 1947;135:985–986.

12 Zoll PM. Resuscitation of the heart in ventricular standstill by external electric stimulation. N Engl J Med 1952;247:768–771.

13 Zoll PM, Linenthal AJ, Gibson W, Paul MH, Norman LR. Termination of ventricular fibrillation in man by externally applied electric countershock. N Engl J Med 1956;254(16):727–732.

14 Lown B, Amarasingham R, Neuman J. New method for terminating cardiac arrhythmias. JAMA 1962;182:548–555.

15 Diack AW, Welborn WS, Rullman RG, Walter CW, Wayne MA. An automatic cardiac resuscitator for emergency treatment of cardiac arrest. Med Instrum 1979:13;78–83.

16 Oliver G, Schafer EA. The physiological effects of extracts from the suprarenal capsules. J Physiol (Lond) 1895;18:232.

17 Redding JS, Pearson JW. Evaluation of drugs for cardiac resuscitation. Anesthesiology 1963;24:203–207.

18 Eisenberg M, Bergner L, Hallstrom A. Paramedic programs and out-of-hospital cardiac arrest: I. Factors associated with successful resuscitation. Am J Public Health 1979;69:30–38.

19 Cummins RO, Ornato JP, Thies WH, Pepe PE. Improving survival from sudden cardiac arrest: the 'chain of survival' concept. Circulation 1991;83:1833–1847.

20 Andreka P, Frenneaux MP. Haemodynamics of cardiac arrest and resuscitation. Curr Opin Crit Care 2006;12:198–203.

21 Criley JM, Blaufuss AH, Kissel GL. Cough-induced cardiac compression. JAMA 1976;236:1246–1250.

22 Rudikoff MT, Maughan WL, Effron M, Freund P, Weisfeldt ML. Mechanisms of blood flow during cardiopulmonary resuscitation. Circulation 1980:61:345–352.

23 Maier GW, Tyson GS, Olsen CO, et al. The physiology of external cardiac massage: high-impulse cardiopulmonary resuscitation. Circulation 1984;70:86–101.

24 Swenson RD, Weaver WD, Niskanen RA. Hemodynamics in humans during conventional and experimental methods of cardiopulmonary resuscitation. Circulation 1988;78:630–639.

25 Chandra NC, Tsitlik JE, Halperin HR, Guerci AD, Weisfeldt ML. Observations of hemodynamics during human cardiopulmonary resuscitation. Crit Care Med 1990;18:929–934.

26 Martin GB, Carden DL, Nowak RM, Lewinter JR, Johnston W, Tomlanovich MC. Aortic and right atrial pressures during standard and simultaneous compression and ventilation CPR in human beings. Ann Emerg Med 1986;15:125–130.

27 Aufderheide TP, Sigurdsson G, Pirrallo RG, et al. Hyperventilation-induced hypotension during cardiopulmonary resuscitation. Circulation 2004;109:1960–1965.

28 Yannopoulos D, McKnite S, Aufderheide TP, et al. Effects of incomplete chest wall recoil during cardiopulmonary resuscitation on coronary and cerebral perfusion pressures in a porcine model of cardiac arrest. Resuscitation 2005;64:363–372.

29 Aufderheide TP, Pirrallo RG, Yannopoulos D, et al. Incomplete chest wall decompression: a clinical evaluation of CPR performance by EMS personnel and assessment of alternative manual chest compression-decompression techniques. Resuscitation 2005;64:353–362.

30 2005 American Heart Association Guidelines for Cardiopulmonary Resuscitation and Emergency Cardiovascular Care. Circulation 2005;112 (Suppl IV):1–211.

31 Cooper JA, Cooper JD, Cooper JM. Cardiopulmonary resuscitation: history, current practice, and future direction. Circulation 2006;114:2839–2849.

32 Wigginton JG, Miller AH, Benitez FL, Pepe PE. Mechanical devices for cardiopulmonary resuscitation. Curr Opin Crit Care 2005;11:219–223.

33 Plaisance P, Lurie KG, Vicaut E, et al. Evaluation of an impedance threshold device in patients receiving active compression–decompression cardiopulmonary resuscitation for out of hospital cardiac arrest. Resuscitation 2005;61:265–271.

34 Yannopoulos D, Nadkarni VM, McKnite SH, et al. Intrathoracic pressure regulator during continuous-chest-compression advanced cardiac resuscitation improves vital organ perfusion pressures in a porcine model of cardiac arrest. Circulation 2005;112:803–811.

35 Yannopoulos D, Aufderheide TP, Gabrielli A, et al. Clinical and hemodynamic comparison of 15:2 and 30:2

compression-to-ventilation ratios for cardiopulmonary resuscitation. Crit Care Med 2006;61:265–271.

36 Timerman S, Cardoso LF, Ramires JA, Halperin H. Improved hemodynamics with a novel chest compression device during treatment of in-hospital cardiac arrest. Resuscitation 2004;61:273–280.

37 Halperin HR, Tsitlik JE, Gelfand M, et al. A preliminary study of cardiopulmonary resuscitation by circumferential compression of the chest with use of a pneumatic vest. N Engl J Med 1993;329:762–768.

38 Halperin HR, Paradis NA, Ornato JP, et al. Cardiopulmonary resuscitation with a novel chest compression device in a porcine model of cardiac arrest. J Am Coll Cardiol 2004;44:2214–2220.

39 Ong MEH, Ornato JP, Edwards DP, et al. Use of an automated, load-distributing band chest compression device for out-of-hospital cardiac arrest resuscitation. JAMA 2006;295:2629–2637.

40 Hallstrom A, Rea TD, Sayre MR, et al. Manual chest compression vs use of an automated chest compression device during resuscitation following out-of-hospital cardiac arrest: a randomized trial. JAMA 2006;295: 2620–2628.

41 Lewis RJ, Niemann JT. Manual vs device-assisted CPR: reconciling apparently contradictory results. JAMA 2006;295:2663–2664.

42 Dickinson ET, Verdile VP, Schneider RM, Salluzzo RF. Effectiveness of mechanical versus manual chest compressions in out-of-hospital cardiac arrest resuscitation: a pilot study. Am J Emerg Med 1998;16:289–292.

43 McDonald JL. Systolic and mean arterial pressures during manual and mechanical CPR in humans. Ann Emerg Med 1982;11:292–295.

44 Ward KR, Menegazzi JJ, Zelenak RR, Sullivan RJ, McSwain N Jr. A comparison of chest compressions between mechanical and manual CPR by monitoring end-tidal P_{CO2} during human cardiac arrest. Ann Emerg Med 1993;22:669–674.

45 Cohen TJ, Tucker KJ, Lurie KG, et al. Active compression-decompression: a new method of cardiopulmonary resuscitation. Cardiopulmonary resuscitation working group. JAMA 1992;267:2916–2923.

46 Lurie KG, Shultz JJ, Callaham ML, et al. Evaluation of active compression-decompression CPR in victims of out-of-hospital cardiac arrest. JAMA 1994;271:1405–1411.

47 Plaisance P, Lurie KG, Vicaut E, et al., (French Active Compression-Decompression Cardiopulmonary Resuscitation Study Group). A comparison of standard cardiopulmonary resuscitation and active compression-decompression resuscitation for out-of-hospital cardiac arrest. N Engl J Med 1999;341:569–575.

48 Lafuente-Lafuente C, Melero-Bascones M. Active chest compression-decompression for cardiopulmonary resuscitation, Cochrane Database Syst Rev 2004(4):CD002751.pub2.

49 Sack JB, Kesselbrenner MB, Bregman D. Survival from in-hospital cardiac arrest with interposed abdominal counterpulsation during cardiopulmonary resuscitation. JAMA 1992;267:379–385.

50 Mateer JR, Stueven HA, Thompson BM, Aprahamian C, Darin JC. Pre-hospital IAC-CPR versus standard CPR: paramedic resuscitation of cardiac arrests. Am J Emerg Med 1985;3:143–146.

51 Arntz HR, Agrawal R, Richter H, et al. Phased chest and abdominal compression-decompression versus conventional cardiopulmonary resuscitation in out-of-hospital cardiac arrest. Circulation 2001;104:768–772.

52 Ornato JP, Hallagan LF, McMahan SB, Peeples EH, Rostafinski AG. Attitudes of BCLS instructors about mouth-to-mouth resuscitation during the AIDS epidemic. Ann Emerg Med 1990;19:151–156.

53 Brenner BE, Van DC, Cheng D, Lazar EJ. Determinants of reluctance to perform CPR among residents and applicants: the impact of experience on helping behavior. Resuscitation 1997;35:203–211.

54 Hew P, Brenner B, Kaufman J. Reluctance of paramedics and emergency medical technicians to perform mouth-to-mouth resuscitation. J Emerg Med 1997;15:279–284.

55 Kern KB, Hilwig RW, Berg RA, Sanders AB, Ewy GA. Importance of continuous chest compressions during cardiopulmonary resuscitation: improved outcome during a simulated single lay-rescuer scenario. Circulation 2002;105:645–649.

56 Berg RA, Kern KB, Hilwig RW, et al. Assisted ventilation does not improve outcome in a porcine model of single-rescuer bystander cardiopulmonary resuscitation. Circulation 1997;95:1635–1641.

57 Berg RA, Kern KB, Hilwig RW, Ewy GA. Assisted ventilation during 'bystander' CPR in swine acute myocardial infarction does not improve outcome. Circulation 1997;96:4364–4371.

58 Kern KB, Hilwig RW, Berg RA, Ewy GA. Efficacy of chest compression-only BLS CPR in the presence of an occluded airway. Resuscitation 1998;39:179–188.

59 Sanders AB, Kern KB, Berg RA, Hilwig RW, Heidenrich J, Ewy GA. Survival and neurological outcome after cardiopulmonary resuscitation with four different chest compression-ventilation ratios. Ann Emerg Med 2002;40:553–562.

60 Berg RA, Hilwig RW, Kern KB, Ewy GA. "Bystander" chest compressions and assisted ventilation independently improve outcome from piglet asphyxial pulseless "cardiac arrest." Circulation 2000;101:1743–1748.

61 Hazinski MF, Nadkarni VM, Hickey RW, O'Connor R, Becker LB, Zaritsky A. Major changes in the 2005 AHA guidelines for CPR and ECC: reaching the tipping point for change. Circulation 2005;112(Suppl IV):206–211.

62 Babbs CF, Kern KB. Optimum compression to ventilation ratios in CPR under realistic, practical conditions: a physiologic and mathematical analysis. Resuscitation 2002;54;147–157.

63 Dorph E, Wik L, Stromme TA, Eriksen M, Steen PA. Oxygen delivery and return of spontaneous circulation with ventilation: compression ratio of 2:30 versus chest

compression only CPR in pigs. Resuscitation 2004;60: 309–318.

64 Wik L, Kramer-Johansen J, Myklebust H, et al. Quality of cardiopulmonary resuscitation during out-of-hospital cardiac arrest. JAMA 2005;293:299–304.

65 Abella BS, Alvarado JP, Mykleburst H, et al. Quality of cardiopulmonary resuscitation during in-hospital cardiac arrest. JAMA 2005;293:305–310.

66 Cobb LA, Fahrenbruch CE, Olsufka M, Copass MK. Changing incidence of out-of-hospital ventricular fibrillation, 1980–2000. JAMA 2002;288:3008–3013.

67 Valenzuela TD, Roe DJ, Cretin S, Spaite DW, Larsen MP. Estimating effectiveness of cardiac arrest interventions: a logistic regression survival model. Circulation 1997;96:3308–3313.

68 Larsen MP, Eisenberg MS, Cummins RO, Hallstrom A. Predicting survival from out-of-hospital cardiac arrest: a graphic model. Ann Emerg Med 1993;22:1652–1658.

69 Swor RA, Jackson RE, Cynar M, et al. Bystander CPR, ventricular fibrillation, and survival in witnessed, unmonitored out-of-hospital cardiac arrest. Ann Emerg Med 1995;25:780–784.

70 Holmberg M, Holmberg S, Herlitz J. Incidence, duration and survival of ventricular fibrillation in out-of-hospital cardiac arrest patients in Sweden. Resuscitation 2000;44:7–17.

71 Cummins RO, Eisenberg MS, Hallstrom AP, Litwin PE. Survival of out-of-hospital cardiac arrest with early initiation of cardiopulmonary resuscitation. Am J Emerg Med 1985;3:114–119.

72 Holmberg S, Holmberg M, Herlitz J. Effect of bystander cardiopulmonary resuscitation in out-of-hospital cardiac arrest patients in Sweden. Resuscitation 2000;47:59–70.

73 Waalewijn RA, Tijssen JG, Koster RW. Bystander initiated actions in out-of-hospital cardiopulmonary resuscitation: results from the Amsterdam Resuscitation Study (ARRESUST). Resuscitation 2001;50:273–279.

74 Kern KB, Garewal HS, Sanders AB, et al. Depletion of myocardial adenosine triphosphate during prolonged untreated ventricular fibrillation: effect on defibrillation success. Resuscitation 1990;20:221–229.

75 Maldonado FA, Weil MH, Tang W, et al. Myocardial hypercarbic acidosis reduces cardiac resuscitability. Anesthesiology 1993;78:343–352.

76 Wik L, Hansen TB, Fylling F, et al. Delaying defibrillation to give basic cardiopulmonary resuscitation to patients with out-of-hospital ventricular fibrillation. JAMA 2003;289:1389–1395.

77 Cobb LA, Fahrenbruch CE, Walsh TR, et al. Influence of cardiopulmonary resuscitation prior to defibrillation in patients with out-of-hospital ventricular fibrillation. JAMA 1999;281:1182–1188.

78 Jacobs IG, Finn JC, Oxer HF, Jelinek GA. CPR before defibrillation in out-of-hospital cardiac arrest: a randomized trial. Emerg Med Australas 2005;17:39–45.

79 Eftestol T, Sunde K, Steen PA. Effects of interrupting precordial compressions on the calculated probability of defibrillation success out-of-hospital cardiac arrest. Circulation 2002;105:2270–2273.

80 Yu T, Weil MH, Tang W, et al. Adverse outcomes of interrupted precordial compression during automated defibrillation. Circulation 2002;106:368–372.

81 Schneider T, Martens PR, Paschen H, et al. Multicenter, randomized, controlled trial of 150-J biphasic shocks compared with 200- to 360-J monophasic shocks in the resuscitation of out-of-hospital cardiac arrest victims. Circulation 2000;102:1780–1787.

82 Mittal S, Ayati S, Stein KM, et al. (for the ZOLL Investigators). Comparison of a novel rectilinear biphasic waveform with a damped sine wave monophasic waveform for transthoracic ventricular defibrillation. J Am Coll Cardiol 1999;34:1595–1601.

83 Poole JE, White RD, Kanz KG, et al. Low-energy impedance-compensating biphasic waveforms terminate ventricular fibrillation at high rates in victims of out-of-hospital cardiac arrest. LIFE Investigators. J Cardiovasc Electrophysiol 1997;8:1373–1385.

84 Page RL, Joglar JA, Kowal RC, et al. Use of automated external defibrillators by a U.S. airline. N Engl J Med 2000;343:1210–1216.

85 Valenzuela TD, Roe DJ, Nichol G, Clark LL, Spaite DW, Hardman RG. Outcomes of rapid defibrillation by security officers after out-of-hospital cardiac arrest. N Engl J Med 2000;343:1206–1209.

86 Caffrey SL, Willoughby PJ, Pepe PE, Becker LB. Public use of automated external defibrillation. N Engl J Med 2002;347:1242–1247.

87 Hallstrom AP, Ornato JP, Weisfeldt M, et al. McBurnie MA, Zalenski R, Becker LB, Schron EB, Proschan M. The Public Access Defibrillation Trial Investigators. Public-access defibrillation and survival after out-of hospital cardiac arrest. N Engl J Med 2004;351:637–646.

88 Stiell IG, Wells GA, Field BJ, et al. (for the OPALS Study Group). Improved out-of-hospital cardiac arrest survival through the inexpensive optimization of existing defibrillation program: OPALS Study Phase II. JAMA 1999;281:1175–1181.

89 White RD, Bunch TJ, Hankins DG. Evolution of a community-wide early defibrillation programme experience over 13 years using police/fire personnel and paramedics as responders. Resuscitation 2005;65:279–283.

90 Michael JR, Guerci AD, Koehler RC, et al. Mechanisms by which epinephrine augments cerebral and myocardial perfusion during cardiopulmonary resuscitation in dogs. Circulation 1984;69:822–835.

91 Schleien CL, Dean JM, Koehler RC, et al. Effect of epinephrine on cerebral and myocardial perfusion in an infant animal preparation of cardiopulmonary resuscitation. Circulation 1986;73:809–817.

92 Wang HE, Min A, Hostler D, Chang CH, Callaway CW. Differential effects of out-of-hospital interventions on

short- and long-term survival after cardiopulmonary arrest. Resuscitation 2005;67:69–74.

93 Hornchen U, Lussi C, Schuttler J. Potential risks of high-dose epinephrine for resuscitation from ventricular fibrillation in a porcine model. J Cardiothorac Vasc Anesth 1993;7:184–187.

94 Tang W, Weil MH, Sun S, Noc M, Yang L, Gazmuri RJ. Epinephrine increases the severity of postresuscitation myocardial dysfunction. Circulation 1995;92:3089–3093.

95 Aung K, Htay T. Vasopressin for cardiac arrest: a systematic review and meta-analysis. Arch Intern Med 2005;165:17–24.

96 Kudenchuk PJ, Cobb LA, Copass MK, et al. Amiodarone for resuscitation after out-of-hospital cardiac arrest due to ventricular fibrillation. N Engl J Med 1999;341:871–878.

97 Dorian P, Cass D, Schwartz B, Cooper R, Gelaznikas R, Barr A. Amiodarone as compared with lidocaine for shock-resistant ventricular fibrillation. N Engl J Med 2002;346:884–890.

98 Bernard SA, Gray TW, Buist MD, et al. Treatment of comatose survivors of out-of-hospital cardiac arrest with induced hypothermia. N Engl J Med 2002;346:557–563.

99 Hypothermia After Cardiac Arrest Study Group. Mild hypothermia to improve neurological outcome after cardiac arrest. N Engl J Med 2002;346:549–556.

100 Bernard S, Buist M, Monteiro O, Smith K. Induced hypothermia using large volume, ice-cold intravenous fluid in comatose survivors of out-of-hospital cardiac arrest: a preliminary report. Resuscitation 2003;56:9–13.

101 Stiell IG, Wells GA, Demaio VJ, et al. Modifiable factors associated with improved cardiac arrest survival in a multicenter basic life support/defibrillation system: OPALS Study Phase I Results. Ann Emerg Med 1999;33:44–50.

CHAPTER 25

Advances in implantable defibrillator therapy and technologies

Paul J. Wang, Amin Al-Ahmad, Henry H. Hsia, & Paul C. Zei

Introduction

Since implantable cardioverter-defibrillators (ICDs) were first approved in 1985, there have been enormous advances in ICD generator and lead technology. ICD generators have become far more sophisticated with improved rhythm discrimination, advanced pacing parameters, episode storage capability, and much smaller size. Table 25.1 provides a comparison between the initial FDA-approved devices and the current devices as well as the volume and weight of current ICD generator models. Table 25.2 provides an overview of the numerous advances in ICD generators and leads.

Rhythm discrimination

An essential capability of the ICD is to detect and treat life-threatening ventricular arrhythmias with nearly perfect accuracy [1]. At the same time, there must be a high level of accuracy in determining that the rhythm is a ventricular arrhythmia and exclude the presence of a supraventricular arrhythmia. Inappropriate therapies triggered by atrial arrhythmias or sinus tachycardia lead to unnecessary shocks, which may reduce the quality of life of ICD patients and increase the fear of ICD shocks [2–6].

Ventricular Arrhythmias and Sudden Cardiac Death, 1st edition. Edited by P.J. Wang, A. Al-Ahmad, H. Hsia, and P.C. Zei © 2008 Blackwell Publishing, ISBN: 978-1-4051-6114-5.

Rhythm Discrimination algorithms may be divided into single chamber and dual chamber algorithms. As shown in Table 25.3, single chamber algorithms rely predominantly on sudden onset, stability, and morphological criteria [7–9]. Sudden onset criteria are able to prevent delivering therapy for sinus tachycardia in most cases [7]. Atrial tachyarrhythmias cannot be distinguished from ventricular tachycardias using this algorithm alone. Stability is predominantly used to prevent therapy from being delivered for atrial fibrillation and is able to reduce shock therapy for atrial fibrillation to rates as low as 5% [7]. However, rarely, perhaps 5% of the times, ventricular tachycardias may be categorized as unstable [7].

Morphological criteria are used for rhythm discrimination with additional benefit to sudden onset and stability alone [8,10] Boriani et al. [10] demonstrated that the addition of a rate-sensing electrogram morphology score to the other single chamber criteria of sudden onset and stability improved specificity while maintaining sensitivity. The specificity in atrial flutter may be somewhat lower.

New algorithms utilize features of the electrogram for discrimination. The comparison of the timing from the rate electrogram to the shock electrogram [11] is the basis for a novel algorithm called the Rhythm ID algorithm [12] (Figure 25.1). A sinus rhythm template is selected and is stored for comparison later. In this algorithm a coefficient of correlation is established between selected points on the rate sensing electrogram and the shock electrogram. This correlation

Table 25.1 Comparison of first FDA-approved device and current generation of ICDs

	1985	*Current*
Dimensions	8.1 × 11.1 × 2.54 cm	—
Weight	290 g	68–82 g
Programmable features	162 cc	29–37 cc
Pacing—bradycardia	None	Fully functional pacemaker
Pacing—antitachycardia	None	Yes
Lead system	Epicardial SVC + LV apex patch	Transvenous
Rate cutoff	Fixed (152 bpm nominal)	Programmable zones
Rhythm discrimination	Probability density function (PDF)	Multiple algorithms
Electrogram storage	None	Extensive
Measured data	Only charge time	Extensive

is termed vector and timing correlation (VTC). Eight features of the electrogram have been selected. A sliding window of 10 complexes is used for the algorithm. In an initial study of 36 supraventricular episodes, 97% were classified correctly [12]. When dual chamber criteria were added, 80 out of 81 ventricular tachycardia increased to 81 out of 81 ventricular tachycardia episodes that were classified correctly.

A new morphological criterion utilizes a novel algorithm called Wavelet. A sinus rhythm template is collected and updated automatically when there is a significant change in the electrogram morphology. The wavelet transform of the tachycardia electrogram is compared with the resting electrogram (Figure 25.2). When at least three out of the last eight beats have a correlation score of 70% or more, a match is identified and the rhythm is classified as supraventricular (Figure 25.3).

In a multicenter prospective nonrandomized study, 1122 patients had 1350 episodes of ventricular tachycardia and 885 episodes of supraventricular

tachycardia [13]. Of the 1350 episodes of ventricular tachycardia, 772 episodes were classified using the wavelet criterion. Wavelet criterion correctly classified 98.6% of the sustained VT/VF episodes. Ten

Table 25.3 Features of single- and dual-chamber rhythm discrimination.

Single chamber	
Sudden onset	Discriminates sinus tachycardia from atrial or ventricular tachyarrhythmias
Stability	Discriminates atrial fibrillation from sinus, atrial, or ventricular tachyarrhythmias
Morphology	Discriminates supraventricular from ventricular arrhythmias
Dual chamber	
Sudden onset	Discriminates sinus tachycardia from atrial or ventricular tachyarrhythmias
Stability	Discriminates atrial fibrillation from sinus, atrial, or ventricular tachyarrhythmias
Morphology	Discriminates supraventricular from ventricular arrhythmias
Timing and number of A and V events	Distinguishes sinus tachycardia and atrial tachycardia from atrial flutter, ventricular tachycardia
Order of initial A and V events	Distinguishes sinus tachycardia and atrial tachycardia from ventricular tachycardia

Table 25.2 Volume and weight of current ICD generators (not all approved in US).

Current generators	*Volume (cc)*	*Weight (g)*
Biotronik Lexos VR	31	78
Boston Scientific Vitality 2VR	30	82
Medtronic Virtuoso SR	37	68
Sorin ELA Ovatio SR	29	
Biotronik Lexos DR	31	78
Boston Scientific Vitality 2DR	30	82
Medtronic Virtuoso DR	37	68
Sorin ELA Ovatio DR	29	

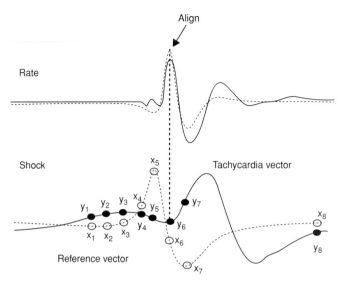

Figure 25.1 Rhythm ID algorithm [12]. A sinus rhythm template is selected and stored. There are eight features of the shock and rate electrogram which are selected. A coefficient of correlation is established between selected points on the rate-sensing electrogram and the shock electrogram. This correlation is termed vector and timing correlation (VTC).

episodes were classified as SVT but these episodes spontaneously terminated. Seven episodes in four patients were correctly identified but borderline match scores led to a delay in delivering therapy from 41 seconds to 69 minutes. Of the 885 episodes of SVT in the VT or VF zone, 774 were in the wavelet detection zone. Of these 774 episodes, 549 were classified correctly as SVT and 175 episodes of SVT

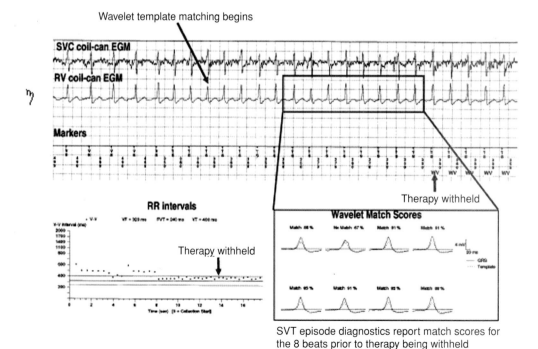

SVT episode diagnostics report match scores for the 8 beats prior to therapy being withheld

Figure 25.2 Wavelet transformation. A wavelet transform is taken of the sinus rhythm template and the tachycardia electrogram.

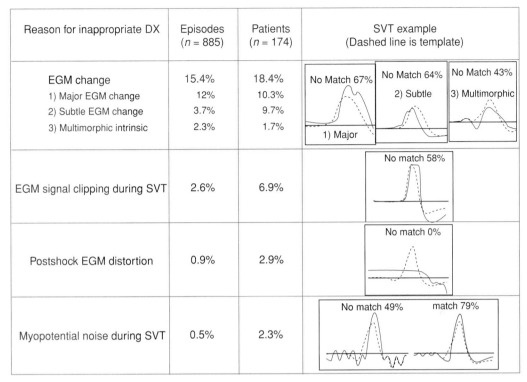

Reason for inappropriate DX	Episodes (*n* = 885)	Patients (*n* = 174)	SVT example (Dashed line is template)		
EGM change	15.4%	18.4%	No Match 67%	No Match 64%	No Match 43%
1) Major EGM change	12%	10.3%		2) Subtle	3) Multimorphic
2) Subtle EGM change	3.7%	9.7%			
3) Multimorphic intrinsic	2.3%	1.7%	1) Major		
EGM signal clipping during SVT	2.6%	6.9%	No match 58%		
Postshock EGM distortion	0.9%	2.9%	No match 0%		
Myopotential noise during SVT	0.5%	2.3%	No match 49% match 79%		

Figure 25.3 Wavelet transform comparison. The wavelet transform of the sinus beat and tachycardia beat are compared. When at least three out of the last eight beats have at least a 70% score, a match is declared.

were classified incorrectly as VT. Subtle changes in the electrogram morphology and electrogram clipping were reasons for SVT misclassification (Figure 25.3).

Dual chamber sensing alone may improve rhythm classification compared to single chamber classification. In a 400-patient randomized prospective trial, the proportion of supraventricular tachycardia detected inappropriately in the single chamber group (40%) was higher than the proportion of 31% observed in the dual chamber group [14]. In a study by Dorian et al. [15], the incidence of inappropriately delivered therapy for a supraventricular arrhythmia was markedly reduced from 0.58 ± 4.23 shocks/patient/month to 0.04 ± 0.15 shocks/patient/month with the addition of the dual chamber sensing ($P = 0.0425$).

Dual Chamber ICD devices may use atrial and ventricular events to improve the accuracy of rhythm classification. The simplest method is to use an atrial and ventricular count of the number of events within a window. When there are more ventricular events than atrial events, this strongly supports ventricular tachycardia. P–R logic provides a robust and simple method for assessing the A-V relationships. In this algorithm, a window is established that defines a P wave occurring in the window after the R wave more likely to be due to retrograde conduction and thus identifying the presence of ventricular tachycardia. One of the greatest challenges in the dual chamber algorithms is the 1:1 A-V rhythms. Stadler et al. [16] have examined the RR and PR intervals and classified the intervals over time as expected and unexpected (Figure 25.4). Table 25.4 illustrates some of the key tests used to determine if sinus tachycardia is present. This algorithm is particularly successful in classifying sinus tachycardia or atrial tachycardias with long PR intervals. However, it may not withhold therapy for atrial tachyarrhythmias of sudden onset with variable PR intervals or rhythms with varying PR, or rhythms with very frequent ectopic beats.

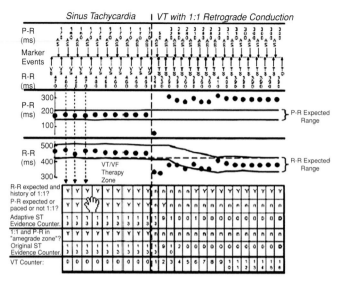

Figure 25.4 Comparison of RR and PR intervals. Stadler et al. [16] examined the RR and PR intervals and classified the intervals over time as expected or unexpected. This algorithm may be useful in classifying sinus tachycardia or atrial tachycardias with long PR intervals.

Ridley et al. [17] have examined the use of the atrial response to ventricular pacing as a strong potential framework to distinguish the rhythm. In one case (Figure 25.5), continued atrial activity that is unperturbed is most consistent with an atrial tachycardia. A V-A Wenckebach pattern

Table 25.4 [16]

1) The RR interval classified as expected or not expected.

– The expected range is composed of an estimate of the RR intervals ± estimate of the variability of the RR intervals. RR intervals are classified as unexpected and evidence against ST.

2) The PR interval is classified as expected

– For this step, RR intervals that contain paced events are excluded. The PR interval expected range is computed and applied similarly to the expected RR range. PR intervals shorter or longer than expected exclude ST.

3) Accumulating evidence of sinus tachycardia

– Expected PR and RR intervals supply separate and independent information. During intermittent pacing and ectopy, the intervals may be classified as unexpected; therefore, determinations of expected intervals are summarized on a beat-to-beat basis. Specific beat patterns over time

(Figure 25.6) is not diagnostic of a specific mechanism. In other situations after ventricular pacing ceases one can categorize the atrial response as demonstrating a VAAV (ventricular–atrial–atrial–ventricular event) response, consistent with an atrial tachycardia in contrast to a VAV (ventricular–atrial–ventricular event) response consistent with ventricular tachycardia or an accessory pathway (Figure 25.7).

A potentially powerful algorithm examines the onset of the arrhythmia and identifies atrial acceleration as the first event, being most consistent with an atrial tachycardia (Figure 25.8a,b). RR instability is used to classify the rhythm as atrial fibrillation. The absence of PR association classifies the rhythm as either atrial fibrillation or ventricular tachycardia. The level of association may identify atrial flutter when there are two or more atrial signals for each ventricular signal. If the acceleration is gradual, sinus tachycardia is identified. If the acceleration is sudden and the origin of acceleration is in the atrium, atrial tachycardia is identified (Figure 25.8b). Finally, if the acceleration is sudden and the origin of acceleration is in the ventricle, ventricular tachycardia is identified.

Accurate atrial sensing is critical to a robust method that utilizes atrial timing events for rhythm

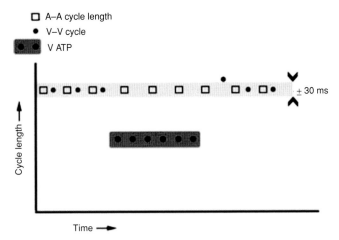

Figure 25.5 Atrial response to ventricular pacing in atrial tachycardia. Antitachycardia pacing results in continued atrial activity that is unperturbed and is most consistent with an atrial tachycardia.

classification. Atrial undersensing, for example, would lead to the incorrect diagnosis of ventricular tachycardia.

Minimizing painful therapy

Implantable cardioverter defibrillators have achieved a consistent and reliable success in improving survival from life-threatening ventricular arrhythmias. However, shocks, although life-saving, remain painful. Pain has been associated with decreased quality of life and functional status.

The strategies to decrease painful therapy are summarized in Table 25.5.

Strategies to reduce the number of ventricular tachyarrhythmia episodes may be important in improving acceptance of ICD therapy. Patients such as those with previous recurrent ventricular tachycardia episodes are more likely to receive ICD therapy [18]. Antiarrhythmic drug therapy may significantly decrease the frequency of ventricular tachyarrhythmias. In the OPTIC study, amiodarone and β-blocker therapy led to the greatest decrease in number of ventricular tachyarrhythmia episodes

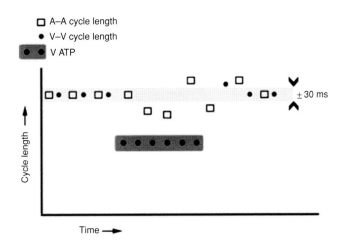

Figure 25.6 Atrial response to ventricular pacing with V-A Wenckebach pattern. Antitachycardia pacing results in a V-A Wenckebach pattern, which is not diagnostic of a specific mechanism.

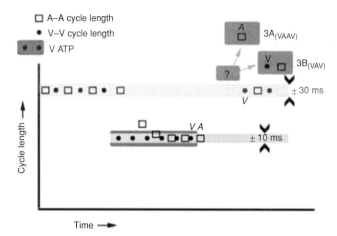

Figure 25.7 Atrial response to ventricular pacing with VAAV and VAV patterns. After ventricular pacing ceases, a VAAV response, consistent with an atrial tachycardia, is observed or a VAV response consistent with ventricular tachycardia or an accessory pathway is observed.

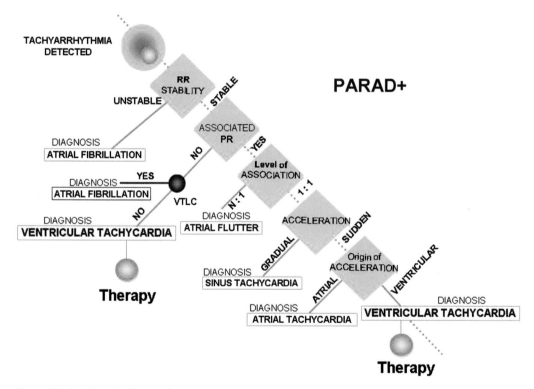

Figure 25.8 PARAD+ algorithm. In the PARAD+ algorithm, multiple steps are used to classify the rhythm. RR instability classifies the rhythm as atrial fibrillation. Absence of PR association may classify the rhythm as atrial fibrillation or ventricular tachycardia. The level of association may identify atrial flutter when there are two or more atrial signals for each ventricular signal. If the acceleration is gradual, sinus tachycardia is identified. If the acceleration is sudden and the origin of acceleration is in the atrium, atrial tachycardia is identified. Finally, if the acceleration is sudden and the origin of acceleration is in the ventricle, ventricular tachycardia is identified. The acceleration is sudden and the origin of acceleration is in the atrium; thus, atrial tachycardia is identified.

[19]. Catheter ablation has been shown to reduce significantly the number of ICD shocks for ventricular tachyarrhythmias [20,21].

Reducing the number of ventricular tachyarrhythmia episodes requiring shock therapy has the potential to reduce the total number of shocks for ventricular arrhythmias. Lengthening the time before shock is one potential strategy to limit the number of shocks by avoiding shocks for nonsustained ventricular tachycardias. However, this strategy must be counterbalanced with the potential hemodynamic consequences of delaying therapy. The exact balance is not known and may depend on the individual patient and tachyarrhythmia characteristics. Increasing the number of episodes terminated by antitachycardia pacing may significantly reduce the number of delivered shocks as discussed below. Both programming antitachycardia pacing on and improving the success rates of antitachycardia pacing may contribute to this success. Decreasing the pain of the ICD is particularly difficult since relatively low-energy shocks are perceived as painful. In fact, an important factor in reducing the perceived pain may be reducing the number of shocks in an episode. Altering the ICD properties that may affect the perception of pain have not been extensively studied but may offer avenues for the future.

Understandably, research in the pain qualities has been largely difficult. Various scoring systems have been used to quantify the pain associated with shocks [22–24]. Steinhaus et al. [25] has demonstrated that shocks between 0.4 J and 2 J delivered in an office setting as part of a clinical study were scored as having similar pain scores. This is in agreement with a previous study by Jung et al. comparing 1 J and 2 J shocks [26]. The majority of patients of a nonlethal arrhythmia such as atrial fibrillation stated that they could tolerate one shock per month. It is not known if the shock strength would significantly alter the quality of life of patients receiving ICD shocks for life-threatening ventricular arrhythmias. It is fairly certain that shocks above a certain level, possibly 5 J or more, are considered to be equivalent to shocks at higher energies. There are conflicting studies regarding whether a lower leading voltage results in a decreased perception of pain [26–29].

Increasing the number of ventricular tachycardia episodes being treated with antitachycardia pacing has been extremely successful in reducing the number of shocks received for ventricular tachycardia. The PainFREE Rx II trial [30] was a prospective, randomized multicenter trial designed to examine if antitachycardia pacing is as safe and effective as ICD shock therapy for fast ventricular tachycardias. Patients were randomized into 2 study arms, consisting of either antitachycardia pacing or shock. Antitachycardia pacing consisted of one sequence of eight pulses of 88% of the VT cycle length with the second therapy was a shock at DFT plus 10 J. The remaining shocks were at maximum. In the shock arm, the first therapy was at DFT plus 10 J with the subsequent shocks at maximum energy. A total of 634 patients were enrolled in the study and a total of 1342 episodes of ventricular tachycardia were observed. Of these 58% were slow VT, 32% were fast VT and 10% were VF. The two arms of the study had nearly the same number of patients having fast VT: 15% in the ATP arm and 16% in the shock arm. There were approximately twice as many episodes in the ATP arm, however, as episodes in the shock arm: 282 episodes in the ATP arm and 144 in the shock arm. Two patients in the ATP arm had 131 episodes. Seventy-seven percent of fast VT- episodes in the ATP arm were terminated by ATP therapy. Twenty percent of fast VT episodes in the ATP arm led to shocks while 67% of the episodes of fast VT resulted in shocks. Overall, the ATP success was 72% across VT cycle lengths [30,31] (Figure 25.9).

Recent algorithms permit charging during ATP delivery. These algorithms help us to avoid any delay in delivery shock therapy if ATP is unsuccessful. Initially antitachycardia pacing would occur during charging but if consecutive successes are achieved then antitachycardia pacing would occur before charging (Figure 25.10). On the other hand, if antitachycardia pacing occurs before charging but if consecutive failures are observed then antitachycardia pacing will again occur during charging.

Recent experimental findings have raised the possibility of completely novel solutions to the problem of painful ICD shocks. Jayam et al. [32] recently reported that for shocks delivered between a left

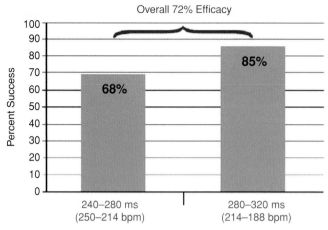

Figure 25.9 Success of antitachycardia pacing based on tachycardia cycle length. The PainFree Rx I and II studies have demonstrated an overall success of antitachycardia pacing of approximately 72% across a wide range of ventricular tachycardia cycle lengths. (Courtesy of Medtronic, Inc.)

ventricular coil and an epicardial electrode sock, the shock-induced skeletal muscle contraction was markedly attenuated. The electrode sock creates a Faraday cage-like structure that results in the energy field to be contained within the sock volume rather than outside it. Since skeletal muscle contraction may be a primary factor in pain related to shocks, this strategy may provide new insights to develop innovative solutions to this problem.

Detecting lead failure

Detecting lead failure prior to the occurrence of an ICD shock may reduce the number of inappropriate

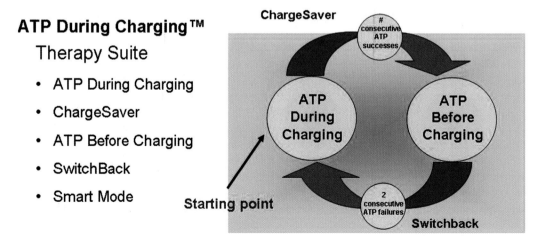

Figure 25.10 Antitachycardia pacing during charging. Initially antitachycardia pacing will occur during charging but if consecutive successes are achieved then antitachycardia pacing occurs before charging. On the other hand, if antitachycardia pacing occurs before charging but if consecutive failures are observed then antitachycardia pacing will again occur during charging.

Table 25.5 Strategies to reduce painful ICD therapy

Decrease number of ventricular tachyarrhythmia episodes
  Antiarrhythmic drug therapy or heart failure treatment
  Catheter ablation of VT

Alter the number of ventricular tachyarrhythmia episodes
requiring shock therapy
  Lengthen time before shock to minimize shocks for
    nonsustained VT
  Increase number of episodes terminated by
    antitachycardia pacing

Decrease pain of ICD shock
  Reduce the energy required for conversion
    Decrease cardioversion and defibrillation threshold
  Alter ICD properties that may affect pain
    Electrode configuration
    Change waveform (e.g., peak voltage)
    Novel ICD electrode designs (Faraday cage-like design)

Table 25.6 Strategies to detect lead failure prior to ICD
shock occurrence

Device-based algorithm
  Processing of routine measurements such as lead
    impedance
  Processing of transient signals on leads

Monitoring-based algorithm
  Processing of routine measurements such as lead
    impedance
  Processing of signals

caused by noise from the rate-sensing lead (Figure 25.11). As Figure 25.12 shows, these measurements may separate lead failure from ventricular arrhythmias in most cases.

Novel ICD lead systems and advances in ICD leads

Subcutaneous lead systems may provide a method of avoiding entirely insertion into the vascular system, preventing venous occlusion and obviating the need for transvascular lead extraction. Subcutaneous ICD leads have been used in young children because of the small caliber of their venous access and subcutaneous arrays have been used to reduce defibrillation thresholds [34–42]. There is evidence that it may be feasible to implant an ICD using only subcutaneous leads in adults. Cameron Health

shocks due to this mechanism. There are several major strategies to detect lead failure, as outlined in Table 25.6.

Gunderson et al. [33] recently reported initial testing of an algorithm to detect lead failure. It is designed to detect transient signals on the rate-sensing lead. In this study, the product of the standard deviation and sum of the voltages recorded on the rate-sensing lead. This algorithm is based on the concept that the far-field coil electrogram should only record the intrinsic ventricular signal and the additional signals on the rate-sensing lead are likely

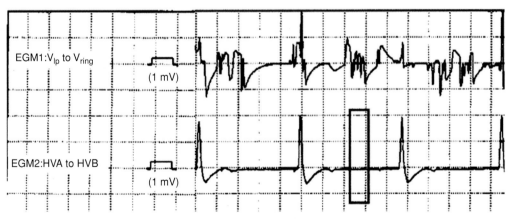

Figure 25.11 Algorithm for detection of lead failure. In this example, the far-field coil electrogram only records the intrinsic ventricular signal; the additional signals on the rate-sensing lead are likely caused by noise that may represent a lead fracture [33].

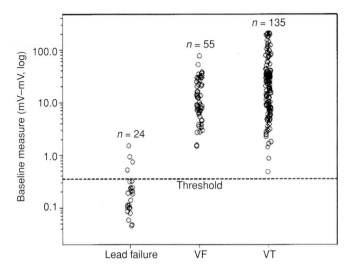

Figure 25.12 Algorithm for detection of lead failure. Gunderson et al. [33] demonstrated that the product of the standard deviation and the sum of the voltages recorded on the rate-sensing lead may distinguish lead failure from ventricular arrhythmias.

has developed a parasternal subcutaneous electrode along with an ICD generator with increased output, more than twice the maximum output of a standard ICD. Mean defibrillation thresholds in a recent study were 36.6 J compared to 11.1 J for the subcutaneous and transvenous lead systems, respectively [43]. Figure 25.13 shows a schematic drawing of a subcutaneous ICD lead system.

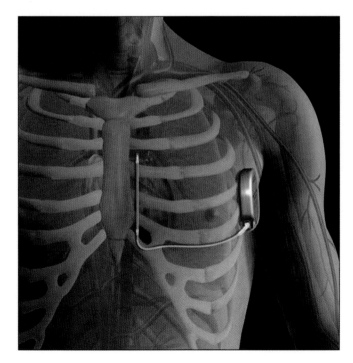

Figure 25.13 Schematic drawing of subcutaneous ICD lead system. A parasternal subcutaneous electrode is used in conjunction with an ICD generator with increased output for defibrillation without transvenous leads. (Courtesy of Cameron Health.)

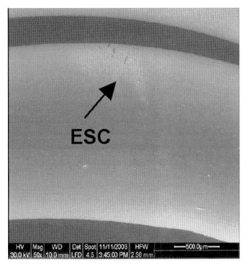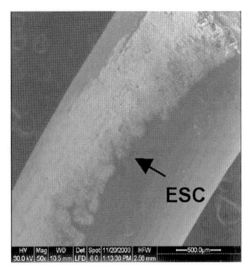

Figure 25.14 Copolymer of silicone and polyurethane for friction reduction. Scanning electron micrograph of co-polymer of silicone and polyurethane (Optim) and Pellethane 55D. There is more evidence of environmental stress cracking (ESC) on the Pellethane 55D lead. (Courtesy of St Jude Medical, Inc.)

There have been major advances in the durability and construction of ICD leads. A major advance has been separation of the conductors and use of new alloys for the conductors. Conductors may be a composite of drawn brazen strand (DBS) or drawn filled tube (DFT) construction. Wires may consist of alloys of a combination of metals. Silicon is used as the predominant insulator. Polyurethane is used to coat some silicone leads to improve handling characteristics. Silicone and polyurethane co-polymers may also be used to gain advantages of both materials (Figure 25.14). Coatings of leads to reduce ingrowth into the lead coils also may be used to improve the ability to remove leads in the future (Figure 25.15). Improved cross-chamber sensing is important for accurate rhythm classification and

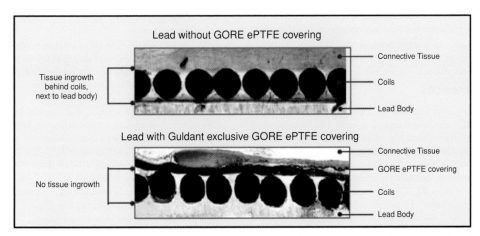

Figure 25.15 Lead coatings for decreased fibrosis. A Gore ePTFE coating of ICD electrodes may decrease fibrosis and improve ability to remove the leads. (Courtesy of Boston Scientific, Inc.)

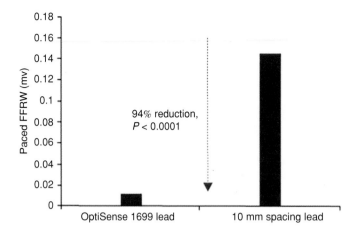

Figure 25.16 Far-field R wave sensing in modified atrial electrode design. Electrode design of the atrial lead may reduce cross-chamber sensing. A smaller atrial interelectrode distance may decrease cross-chamber sensing. Improved cross-chamber sensing may help minimize far-field sensing in ICDs. FFRW is far-field R wave amplitude (Courtesy of St Jude Medical, Inc.)

new electrode designs for atrial electrodes may help minimize far-field sensing in ICDs (Figure 25.16).

Conclusions

There are remarkable advances in the capabilities of ICD devices. There are significant advances in strategies to reduce painful shocks. These include reducing the number of ventricular tachyarrhythmia episodes using pharmacological therapy and catheter ablation, decreasing inappropriate therapy due to supraventricular arrhythmias by way of improved discrimination algorithms, and decreased number of shocks required to terminate ventricular tachycardias by utilizing antitachycardia pacing. New developments in ICD technology may permit detection of lead fractures before ICD shocks occur and new subcutaneous lead systems may provide an alternative to transvenous access.

References

1 Gielchinsky I, Rothbart ST, Parsonnet V, et al. Safety, feasibility and long term follow-up of a non-thoracotomy defibrillation system in patients with inducible sustained ventricular tachycardia/fibrillation. J Cardiovasc Surg 1994;35(6 Suppl 1):111–113.

2 Sears SF Jr, Rauch S, Handberg E, Conti JB. Fear of exertion following ICD storm: considering ICD shock and learning history. J Cardiopulm Rehabil 2001;21(1):47–49.

3 Sears SF, Todaro JF, Urizar G, et al. Assessing the psychosocial impact of the ICD: a national survey of implantable cardioverter defibrillator health care providers [see comment]. Pacing Clin Electrophysiol 2000;23(6):939–945.

4 Eads AS, Sears SF Jr, Sotile WM, Conti JB. Supportive communication with implantable cardioverter defibrillator patients: seven principles to facilitate psychosocial adjustment. J Cardiopulm Rehabil 2000;20(2):109–114.

5 Sears SF, Lewis TS, Kuhl EA, Conti JB. Predictors of quality of life in patients with implantable cardioverter defibrillators. Psychosomatics 2005;46(5):451–457.

6 Kuhl EA, Dixit NK, Walker RL, Conti JB, Sears SF. Measurement of patient fears about implantable cardioverter defibrillator shock: an initial evaluation of the Florida Shock Anxiety Scale. Pacing Clin Electrophysiol 2006;29(6):614–618.

7 Schaumann A, von zur Muhlen F, Gonska BD, Kreuzer H. Enhanced detection criteria in implantable cardioverter-defibrillators to avoid inappropriate therapy. Am J Cardiol 1996;78(5A):42–50.

8 Boriani G, Occhetta E, Pistis G, et al. Combined use of morphology discrimination, sudden onset, and stability as discriminating algorithms in single chamber cardioverter defibrillators. Pacing Clin Electrophysiol 2002;25(9):1357–1366.

9 Gronefeld GC, Schulte B, Hohnloser SH, et al. Morphology discrimination: a beat-to-beat algorithm for the discrimination of ventricular from supraventricular tachycardia by implantable cardioverter defibrillators. Pacing Clinical Electrophysiology 2001;24(10):1519–1524.

10 Boriani G, Biffi M, Dall'Acqua A, et al. Rhythm discrimination by rate branch and QRS morphology in dual chamber implantable cardioverter defibrillators. Pacing Clin Electrophysiol 2003;26(1 Pt 2):466–470.

11 Gold MR, Hsu W, Marcovecchio AF, Olsovsky MR, Lang DJ, Shorofsky SR. A new defibrillator discrimination algorithm utilizing electrogram morphology analysis. Pacing Clin Electrophysiol 1999;22(1 Pt 2):179–182.

12 Gold MR, Shorofsky SR, Thompson JA, et al. Advanced rhythm discrimination for implantable cardioverter defibrillators using electrogram vector timing and correlation. J Cardiovasc Electrophysiol 2002;13(11):1092–1097.

13 Klein GJ, Gillberg JM, Tang A, et al. Improving SVT discrimination in single-chamber ICDs: a new electrogram morphology-based algorithm [see comment]. J Cardiovasc Electrophysiol 2006;17(12):1310–1319.

14 Friedman PA, McClelland RL, Bamlet WR, et al. Dual-chamber versus single-chamber detection enhancements for implantable defibrillator rhythm diagnosis: the detect supraventricular tachycardia study [see comment]. Circulation 2006;113(25):2871–2879.

15 Dorian P, Philippon F, Thibault B, et al. Randomized controlled study of detection enhancements versus rate-only detection to prevent inappropriate therapy in a dual-chamber implantable cardioverter-defibrillator. Heart Rhythm 2004;1(5):540–547.

16 Stadler RW, Gunderson BD, Gillberg JM. An adaptive interval-based algorithm for withholding ICD therapy during sinus tachycardia. Pacing Clin Electrophysiol 2003;26(5):1189–1201.

17 Ridley DP, Gula LJ, Krahn AD, et al. Atrial response to ventricular antitachycardia pacing discriminates mechanism of 1:1 atrioventricular tachycardia [see comment]. J Cardiovasc Electrophysiol 2005;16(6):601–605.

18 Brigadeau F, Kouakam C, Klug D, et al. Clinical predictors and prognostic significance of electrical storm in patients with implantable cardioverter defibrillators. Eur Heart J 2006;27(6):700–707.

19 Connolly SJ, Dorian P, Roberts RS, et al. Comparison of beta-blockers, amiodarone plus beta-blockers, or sotalol for prevention of shocks from implantable cardioverter defibrillators: the OPTIC Study: a randomized trial [see comment]. JAMA 2006;295(2):165–171.

20 Silva RM, Mont L, Nava S, Rojel U, Matas M, Brugada J. Radiofrequency catheter ablation for arrhythmic storm in patients with an implantable cardioverter defibrillator. Pacing Clin Electrophysiol 2004;27(7):971–975.

21 Soejima K, Stevenson WG. Catheter ablation of ventricular tachycardia in patients with ischemic heart disease. Curr Cardiol Rep 2003;5(5):364–368.

22 Urizar GG Jr, Sears SF Jr, Handberg E, Conti JB. Psychosocial intervention for a geriatric patient to address fears related to implantable cardioverter defibrillator discharges. Psychosomatics 2004;45(2):140–144.

23 Sears SE Jr, Conti JB. Understanding implantable cardioverter defibrillator shocks and storms: medical and psychosocial considerations for research and clinical care. Clin Cardiol 2003;26(3):107–111.

24 Sears SF Jr, Conti JB. Quality of life and psychological functioning of ICD patients. Heart (British Cardiac Society) 2002;87(5):488–493.

25 Steinhaus DM, Cardinal DS, Mongeon L, Musley SK, Foley L, Corrigan S. Internal defibrillation: pain perception of low energy shocks. Pacing Clin Electrophysiol 2002;25(7):1090–1093.

26 Jung J, Heisel A, Fries R, Kollner V. Tolerability of internal low-energy shock strengths currently needed for endocardial atrial cardioversion. Am J Cardiol 1997;80(11):1489–1490.

27 Jung J, Hahn SJ, Heisel A, Buob A, Schubert BD, Siaplaouras S. Defibrillation efficacy and pain perception of two biphasic waveforms for internal cardioversion of atrial fibrillation. J Cardiovasc Electrophysiol 2003;14(8):837–840.

28 Ammer R, Alt E, Ayers G, et al. Pain threshold for low energy intracardiac cardioversion of atrial fibrillation with low or no sedation [erratum appears in Pacing Clin Electrophysiol April 1997;20(4 Pt 1):viii]. Pacing Clin Electrophysiol 1997;20(1 Pt 2):230–236.

29 Boriani G, Biffi M, Silvestri P, et al. Mechanisms of pain associated with internal defibrillation shocks: results of a randomized study of shock waveform. Heart Rhythm 2005;2(7):708–713.

30 Wathen MS, DeGroot PJ, Sweeney MO, et al. Prospective randomized multicenter trial of empirical antitachycardia pacing versus shocks for spontaneous rapid ventricular tachycardia in patients with implantable cardioverter-defibrillators: Pacing Fast Ventricular Tachycardia Reduces Shock Therapies (PainFREE Rx II) trial results [see comment]. Circulation 2004;110(17):2591–2596.

31 Wathen MS, Sweeney MO, DeGroot PJ, et al. Shock reduction using antitachycardia pacing for spontaneous rapid ventricular tachycardia in patients with coronary artery disease. Circulation 2001;104(7):796–801.

32 Jayam V, Zviman M, Jayanti V, Roguin A, Halperin H, Berger RD. Internal defibrillation with minimal skeletal muscle activation: a new paradigm toward painless defibrillation [see comment]. Heart Rhythm 2005;2(10):1108–1113.

33 Gunderson BD, Gillberg JM, Wood MA, Vijayaraman P, Shepard RK, Ellenbogen KA. Development and testing of an algorithm to detect implantable cardioverter-defibrillator lead failure [see comment]. Heart Rhythm 2006;3(2):155–162.

34 Kriebel T, Ruschewski W, Gonzalez y Gonzalez M, et al. ICD Implantation in infants and small children: the extracardiac technique. Pacing Clin Electrophysiol 2006;29(12):1319–1325.

35 Gandelman G, Frishman WH, Wiese C, et al. Intravascular device infections: epidemiology, diagnosis, and management. Cardiol Rev 2007;15(1):13–23.

36 Cannon BC, Friedman RA, Fenrich AL, Fraser CD, McKenzie ED, Kertesz NJ. Innovative techniques for placement of implantable cardioverter-defibrillator leads in patients with limited venous access to the heart. Pacing Clin Electrophysiol 2006;29(2):181–187.

37 Stephenson EA, Batra AS, Knilans TK, et al. A multicenter experience with novel implantable cardioverter defibrillator configurations in the pediatric and congenital heart disease population. J Cardiovasc Electrophysiol 2006;17(1):41–46.

38 Burke MC, Coman JA, Cates AW, et al. Defibrillation energy requirements using a left anterior chest cutaneous to subcutaneous shocking vector: implications for a total subcutaneous implantable defibrillator. Heart Rhythm 2005;2(12):1332–1338.

39 Saksena S. The leadless defibrillator or the return of the subcutaneous electrode: episode III in the ICD saga? J Interv Card Electrophysiol 2005;13(3):179–180.

40 Kettering K, Mewis C, Dornberger V, et al. Long-term experience with subcutaneous ICD leads: a comparison among three different types of subcutaneous leads. Pacing Clin Electrophysiol 2004;27(10):1355–1361.

41 Madan N, Gaynor JW, Tanel R, et al. Single-finger subcutaneous defibrillation lead and "active can": a novel minimally invasive defibrillation configuration for implantable cardioverter-defibrillator implantation in a young child. J Thorac Cardiovasc Surg 2003;126(5):1657–1659.

42 Avitall B, Oza SR, Gonzalez R, Avery R. Subcutaneous array to transvenous proximal coil defibrillation as a solution to high defibrillation thresholds with implantable cardioverter defibrillator distal coil failure. J Cardiovasc Electrophysiol 2003;14(3):314–315.

43 Lieberman R, Shorofsky S, Rashba E, Havel W, Christensen J, DeGroot P. Subcutaneous transthoracic defibrillation in implantable cardioverter defibrillator patients using a pectoral can to posterior coil. Europace 2006;8(Suppl 1):63–64.

CHAPTER 26

ICD lead extraction: when, why, and how?

Bruce L. Wilkoff, & Oussama Wazni

Transvenous lead extraction has been practiced with defined tools and techniques since the late 1980s [1]. The experience was the subject of a NASPE policy conference, which produced initial recommendations for the indications, facilities and training [2]. However, the leads, tools, and techniques and in particular the frequency of ICD system implantation has increased substantially. ICDs now represent the majority of device implants in many institutions and are now involved in the majority of lead extraction situations. In addition to the traditional indications of infection and lead failure, vascular occlusion with symptoms related to the occlusion or the need to upgrade to two or three lead systems have become a dominant issue. This discussion will focus on the issues that are important for all ICD extractions.

Lead extraction would not be an issue if the host response to the placement of transvenous leads did not include endothelial and vascular trauma with subsequent inflammation, thrombosis, and fibrosis. There are a few implantation situations when the lead becomes entangled in the tricuspid apparatus or is associated with myocardial migration and perforation, but these are not the main issue addressed by this procedure.

Fibrosis is the main barrier to lead extraction. The fibrosis develops and progresses over time at each of the points of endothelial contact. Animal studies by Anderson exhibited the initial clot and then evolving to fibrosis, which progresses in amount, thickness, and often with calcification over time [3].

The location of these fibrotic attachments occur at the site of vascular entry and all along the lead at the locations that lead contacts the endothelium in the subclavian and superior vena cava, the right atrium, the tricuspid valve, and in the right ventricle. In addition, the fibrosis is more intense when there is more than one lead, in part due to the close proximity of the leads, but also due to the roughness and irregularity of the leads, particularly in relation to the ICD shocking coils. It appears that shocking coils in narrow vessels are more likely to produce intense fibrosis than coils in large vessels with high flow. Particularly troublesome and common is the colocalization of the proximal ICD shocking coil near the junction of the SVC and right atrium. This strategically important anatomic position defines the area of greatest risk of fatal vascular accidents during transvenous lead extraction. Again in the coronary sinus, defibrillation coils appear to be intensely productive of severe fibrosis [4]. Importantly, it appears that the structural characteristics of the leads can promote or ameliorate this process.

The predominant opportunity in safely overcoming these fibrotic attachments is directly related to the tensile strength of the lead. ICD leads are complex in design with multiple components. The materials and construction of the lead will determine the elasticity and the likelihood that the lead will be removed in one piece. However, when the lead's tensile integrity is compromised, the ability to completely remove the lead is also compromised.

Locking stylets are the mainstay of producing substantial tensile lead integrity, enhancing the ability to remove the entire lead. Locking stylets that

Ventricular Arrhythmias and Sudden Cardiac Death, 1st edition. Edited by P.J. Wang, A. Al-Ahmad, H. Hsia, and P.C. Zei © 2008 Blackwell Publishing, ISBN: 978-1-4051-6114-5.

(a)

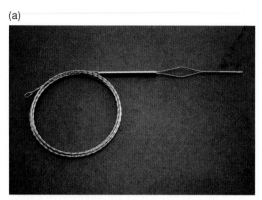

(b)

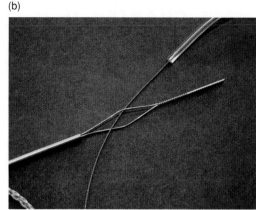

Figure 26.1 The Bulldog lead extender.

grab the conductor coil near the distal stimulation electrode greatly reduce the possibility of incomplete lead removal and improve the control of the extraction procedure. Since the process of consistently effective lead extraction requires the controlled advancement of the telescoping sheaths over the lead, eliminating the elasticity of the lead produces a more consistent relationship between the advancement force on the sheath and the retraction force on the lead through the locking stylet. It is this control that makes controlled counterpressure disruption of the fibrosis possible.

The more complex the construction of the lead, the more important it is that every component of the lead is included in the process of controlling the lead body. In pacing leads, in addition to the locking stylet, used to control the conductor coil to the distal stimulating electrode, a suture should be tied to the outer insulation. This binds the lead's components (conductor coil and insulation) together and improves the lead's intrinsic tensile properties. This is much more important when extracting ICD leads. In addition, there are usually one or more cables attached to the other electrodes (pacing and shocking) that need to be included in this strategy. Until recently a suture would be tied to one or more of these cables as well as to the outer insulation and then connected to the tugging end of the locking stylet. This binding together of all of the parallel elements of the ICD lead is a major factor that improves the opportunity for complete extraction. The binding process, which produces control of the

lead body, makes the extraction procedure faster, more predictable, and produces fewer undesirable and exciting moments.

There is now a faster, easier way to produce traction on the cables to the shocking coils. The Bulldog lead extender, designed for pacemaker leads that have no conductor coil, mechanically locks onto the cables to the shocking and pacing electrodes and produces an excellent mechanism for improving the tensile properties of the lead (Figure 26.1).

It is important to obtain the best strategic tensile advantage possible in removing each lead. However, it is not always possible to get a good locking stylet or to tie onto all of the elements. Under this circumstance it is important to take advantage of the available elements as much as possible. Often, when there are multiple leads to be removed, it is best to try to remove the lead in the order of the perceived tensile advantage. Factors that increase the tensile advantage over the lead include: (1) short implant duration, (2) strong intrinsic tensile properties, (3) quality locking stylet placement, and (4) quality sutures and other ties to the lead components. Each of these factors improves the likelihood of successful extraction. However, if there is failure to progress during the extraction with the chosen lead, it is important to be willing to move to another lead and then come back to the difficult lead at a later time in the procedure. It is strategically important to obtain the best possible tensile advantage over the lead. This is the key component to consistently successful and safe extraction procedures.

The third substantial component to successful lead extraction involves the appropriate use of telescoping extraction sheaths. Whether manufactured from steel, Teflon, or polypropylene or if powered by laser, electrosurgical, or mechanical energy, use of both the inner, more flexible and outer, more firmly constructed components is another key to consistently safe and effective lead extraction. Both the flexibility of the smaller inner sheath, which permits the sheaths to track along the course of the lead and the firmness of the larger and stronger outer sheath which transmits the advancement force to the interface with the fibrotic tissue are important. The primary goal is NOT to (1) push hard on the sheaths, (2) pull hard on the lead, or (3) remove the lead. The goal IS to (1) advance the sheaths over the lead, (2) maintain the lead position constant in the vein and chest, and (3) concentrate the work at the focal point at the tip of the extraction sheath with balanced tension between extraction sheath advancement and the fibrotic tissue on the lead. By taking this approach, a tremendous force is brought to bear to dissect the fibrotic tissue from the lead and vein. This process is very safe and is called "counterpressure."

Counter-pressure is not the process of removing the tip of the lead from the heart but dissecting the lead from the fibrotic tissue of the vein. If too much advancement force is used without providing for the counterbalancing force on the lead and locking stylet then the sheath and lead will either advance in the vein or through the wall of the vein without dissecting free from its attachments. If too much withdrawal force is produced then the lead will be ripped from the vein and a segment of the vein may be removed with the lead causing a vascular accident. If the sheath fails to easily advance, rotating or jiggling the sheath, and looking for other mechanical issues such as lead fibrosis accumulating between the lead and the inner surface of the inner sheath, should be considered. Often a larger inner sheath is required and if not used the consequences will include pushing and pulling harder and a broken lead. It is better to work smarter than harder. Eventually the locking stylet and the lead will start to break when the extraction forces exceed the tensile properties of the lead, sutures, and locking stylets.

Countertraction requires that the sheaths be advanced to within 2–3 mm of the myocardium. The sheaths are then no longer advanced, but held in position and then a firm withdrawal tension should be initiated without jerking on the locking stylet. This will pull the myocardial surface up against the tip of the extraction sheath and push the last bit of fibrosis off the end of the lead. If counterpressure and countertraction are properly implemented and if the lead was implanted without leaving the vascular and cardiac space, transvenous lead extraction is completely safe. Problems occur either when there is poor adherence to the above principles, the lead was improperly implanted, or when the patient's fibrotic healing incorporates the lead into the wall of the vein or cardiac structures. Therefore it is very important to intentionally review the lead's course through the vascular structures on the chest radiograph of every lead extraction patient prior to the procedure.

Each type of extraction sheath has particular situations for which it is best suited. Originally, all extraction was done with passive mechanical components, either composed of steel, Teflon, or polypropylene. Use of the above principles produced excellent results and safety, but there were far more partial extractions because the amount of force required tended to break the stylets and leads. However, there are still situations for which mechanical tools are the best. For instance, straight telescoping steel sheaths are still the best tools for entering the subclavian vessel, going under the clavicle, and particularly when there is marked fibrosis or even calcification in this area. These tools work extremely well as long as the vessel and lead course is straight. Often this is the only area of fibrosis and the lead slides easily from the vein after getting over the initial fibrosis. This can be easy, fast, inexpensive, and effective. The best indication for telescoping steel sheaths occurs when there is a focal occlusion of the vein near the original vascular entry point and you need to upgrade this patient from a pacemaker to an ICD. The ventricular lead is removed, a guidewire is placed through the extraction sheath and then the ICD lead is implanted using the retained guidewire. Use of the pin vise to improve the ability to torque the steel sheaths can make this a very fast and effective tool in this limited situation.

Laser extraction tools revolutionized the penetration of lead extraction procedures into the pacemaker and ICD community. The original introduction of laser sheaths was with a 12F model (outer diameter of inner sheath). This was just barely large enough to get over many but not all coaxial bipolar pacing leads in 1994 (time of introduction). The introduction of the 14F and 16F models made ICD lead extraction feasible. Originally, 16F (22.6F is the outer diameter of the outer sheath) was required to remove the ICD leads implanted from Medtronic, Guidant, Ventritex, and Intermedics. Lead construction has evolved and current leads are characterized by a reduced diameter, now placed through 7F introducers. Although these leads can often be removed with the smaller laser sheaths, the fibrosis and calcification still often mandate the use of the larger diameter sheaths. For now, we recommend the use of 14F sheath for all newer ICD leads, but if the very small leads demonstrate less fibrosis, 12F may be the appropriate choice of the future. The key with laser sheaths is that it is often more effective to slide over (envelop) the fibrosis on the leads with a larger sheath than to plow slowly through the fibrosis. Using this technique, the fibrosis is removed and the extraction is easier and faster.

There are two points of caution. One, when a sheath is oversized there is some risk of compromising the safety of the countertraction procedure. Pushing the final bit of fibrosis off the end of the lead may not be as effective with a mismatch between the sheath diameter and the lead diameter and result in a slight increased risk of perforation. Sometimes it is still required to up-size the sheath to get over more proximal fibrosis and it is then that no choice remains except using the larger sheath at the lead tip. In practice this concern is more theoretical than observed. The second caution is the risk of circumferential cutting with the laser. This is mostly a concern at the RA–SVC junction, where if the vein wall is compromised, rapid exsanguination can ensue. This appears to be a problem only in this anatomic area. By slightly withdrawing the lead from the lateral wall with traction on the locking stylet while going around the corner, this becomes a rare yet important issue.

We often advance a long guidewire, usually a Whooley wire from the right femoral vein to the right internal jugular or subclavian vein, at the beginning of an extraction procedure when there appears to be risk of significant fibrosis at the SVC–RA

junction. We also make available in the EP lab, a large (2 cm × 4 cm) venoplasty balloon, with the plan of inflating this balloon in the area of the potential laceration of the vein to slow the bleeding until it can be surgically closed. Even if a surgeon opens the chest immediately, when the vein is lacerated in this location, the opportunity to rescue the patient's life is still only about 50%. However, the overall risk of lead extraction can be very low. At the Cleveland Clinic, the overall major complication rate including internal bleeding and death from 2001 through 2006 has been 0.28%, while averaging over 300 patient procedures per year [5].

Electrosurgical dissection sheaths (EDS) provide more directional cutting ability than the laser sheaths, but because of the directionality and softness of the sheaths, these sheaths are less powerful, slower, and less useful for ICD extraction. However, there is also the implied promise of less damage to the tissue and therefore greater safety. However, with the overall safety of laser extraction, we have been unimpressed with the need to use the EDS tool for ICD extraction.

Evolution is a new extraction tool for which preliminary clinical experience (Figure 26.2) is all that have been obtained so far. These sheaths come in 7F, 9F, 11F, and 13F sizes. The sizes refer to the internal diameter of the sheath, or more properly the size of lead that can fit through the sheaths. These are a more powerful mechanical tool that has a "cutting bit" on the external surface of the tip of the inner sheath. The handle for this tool uses a trigger that rotates the sheath and "cutting bit" and advances the sheath over the lead and through the fibrosis. The potential advantage of these sheaths relates to circumferential cutting that is very superficial (improving safety), potential to cut through more calcified fibrosis (no other technology does it so well), lack of a tethering wire or fiberoptic cable (more freedom of movement in the surgical field), and lower cost (laser requires a substantial outlay for the machine and ties the activities to specially equipped rooms with high-voltage outlets). My limited experience with this tool suggests that it may have a role in ICD lead extraction.

ICD lead extraction is indicated for one of three broad indications: (1) vascular occlusion, (2) infection, and (3) lead failure. Understanding the incidence and pathophysiology of these three situations

(a)

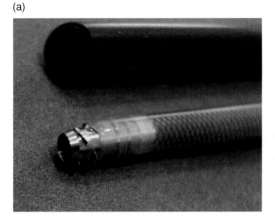

(b)

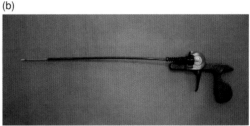

Figure 26.2 The Evolution extraction tool.

is important to delivering consistently excellent ICD therapy.

Venous stenosis is a direct result of the injury produced when a lead is introduced through the wall of a vein. The injury produces inflammation, thrombosis, and fibrosis. Sometimes the fibrosis is minimal, but at other times it can be substantial and can cause occlusion of the vein. The fibrosis holds the lead in place and resists dislodgement but also resists extraction and, if partially or totally occlusive, prevents access for new lead implantation. The frequency of venous stenosis is particularly important for ICD systems because of two other issues, the frequent need to upgrade systems from single to dual or BiV systems and due to the relatively high (compared to pacing leads) rates of insulation and conductor fractures. However, the big priority is to remember to maintain a long-term perspective instead of solving the short-term issue with techniques that get in the way of long-term solutions.

The solution to venous stenosis and sometimes occlusion can be angioplasty, especially if all of the current leads are useful in the new device system. Venoplasty can be safely performed as long as it is not associated with stenting. Venous stenting without first removing all the existing leads traps the existing leads between the stent and the vessel wall. The stenting and the preexisting leads are both at risk of failure. If the venous occlusion recurs (not unlikely) or if the leads need to be removed in the future (not unlikely either due to failure or infection)

then there is no percutaneous or surgical options that are safe.

Stenting can be done safely if the leads are first removed. Often the venoplasty is more successful after the lead extraction because the fibrosis is debulked and the resultant need for stenting is reduced. However, if the process continues to stenting then leads can safely be implanted through the new lumen within the stented vessel. If there is recurrent occlusion or need to remove the leads, the process can be repeated.

Fibrosis and infection complicate ICD therapy and other device therapies. In addition to the issues of vascular stenosis/occlusion and fibrosis at the level of the SVC–RA junction discussed earlier in the chapter, there are three issues important to ICD system extraction: (1) SVC coil fibrosis, (2) tricuspid valve entrapment, and (3) ICD infection.

Unique to ICD leads are the defibrillation coils. The roughness and complexity of these coils invites increased intensity of fibrosis and increased friction between the extraction sheath and the lead body. As discussed previously, it is very important to maintain the ability to produce a retraction force on the cables to these coils to promote advancement of the sheaths over the lead. However, the colocalization of the SVC coil in the area of the SVC–RA junction produces a particularly unhealthy dynamic with increased fibrosis in the area where the venous structures are most vulnerable. Consequently, we have adopted the practice of using single-coil ICD leads when implanting from the left shoulder and opting for a posteriorly directed subcutaneous shocking coil when defibrillation efficacy is inadequate. This practice is much more effective in reducing defibrillation thresholds, it reduces the future risk of extraction, and is in practice rarely necessary. From the right side, it is necessary to have the SVC coil to consistently produce reasonable defibrillation efficacy and the process of lead extraction is much less likely to compromise the lateral wall of the SVC due to the natural course of the lead. An alternative to the subcutaneous coil involves placing an additional defibrillation coil in the azygous vein [6]. An example of how intense the fibrosis can be at the SVC coil was demonstrated in a case where the system was implanted in a younger patient, who continued to grow and the forces of fibrosis and growth combined to produce a multiply fractured SVC coil [7].

Not unique to ICD leads but enhanced by the size, roughness, and complexity of the surface near the distal defibrillation coil, is the potential for tricuspid valve injury. Injury can be caused by the failure to implant the lead through the central area between the tricuspid valve leaflets which can produce restricted motion of the tricuspid valve due to interference with the infravalvular apparatus. In addition, injury can be produced by incorrect extraction techniques.

The first problem can often be prevented by paying careful attention to the lead implantation process, observing the motion of the lead as it crosses the valve, and withdrawing the lead back to the atrium and repositioning the lead whenever the motion of the lead appears to be restricted. If the lead is entrapped in the valve, the resultant tricuspid regurgitation is often not identified until years later when the lead develops an intensified fibrotic reaction to the tangling in the infravalvular apparatus. Removing the lead after the fibrosis has developed never improves this situation and often makes the regurgitation worse. However, if the situation is identified early after implantation, ideally during the original implantation, this is entirely reversible. Excellent and graphic examples of intensely fibrotic tricuspid valve responses to ICD lead placement were documented by Dr Epstein in an autopsy series [8].

The second scenario can be ameliorated with careful attention to the principles discussed earlier

in the chapter. If there has been some involvement of the ICD and valvular fibrosis, it is crucially important that the sheaths are advanced through the fibrosis all the way to the RV myocardium. By doing so, the least amount of ripping, tearing, and damage to the valve is caused and it is most likely that surgical repair will not be required. When a tissue tricuspid valve replacement or valve repair is necessary, for whatever reason, it is possible to reimplant through the valve. If a mechanical valve is used, then the new lead needs to be implanted through the cardiac veins or with an epicardial lead system.

Infections in ICD systems, in most aspects, are no different than they are in pacemaker systems. The frequency, bacteriology, and treatment are identical; however, there are some realities that require special attention: (1) surgical extraction with debridement and (2) wearable defibrillators.

Since epicardial defibrillation electrodes are far inferior to transvenous leads, it is far more important to consider surgical extraction with debridement of the infected tissue when there is evidence of vegetations. Simple bacteremia, with or without sepsis but without vegetations, can be treated with transvenous extraction and reimplantation when the cultures have cleared. However, if the patient needs quick reimplantation, usually in the setting of pacemaker dependency, it is better to consider surgical extraction with debridement. Then transvenous implantation can proceed when the cultures clear. It is fine to use a temporary pacing electrode until the patient is ready for reimplantation.

For pacemaker situations it is often appropriate to remove the leads percutaneously, even with vegetations and then reimplant either 4–6 weeks later or with epicardial leads if the patient is pacer dependent, since epicardial pacing leads are much more reliable. An alternative solution is the use of the wearable defibrillator. This works well, particularly in primary prevention patients who are not pacemaker dependent. If there is a doubt about the completeness of the lead removal or the potential for continued intravascular infection then it is better to wait than to quickly reimplant. The use of the wearable defibrillator is an excellent option in these situations. Wearable defibrillators are also useful in noninfected situations. This can be used to permit a patient to remain outside the hospital and otherwise unmonitored, if the defibrillation detection needs to be deactivated to avoid shocks due to lead integrity problems.

ICD lead construction is more complex than pacemaker lead construction and the consequences of ICD lead dysfunction is much greater. In addition, the frequency of ICD lead dysfunction has historically been significantly larger than pacemaker leads. Fortunately, the ability to monitor the ICD system and its leads is significantly improved with the implementation of remote interrogation and monitoring. There are three components of ICD leads that are vulnerable to damage: (1) conductor coil(s) to the distal and sometimes other electrodes, (2) cables to the shocking coil(s) and sometimes other electrodes, and (3) breaches in the insulation. Failure of any of these components is an indication for lead extraction and replacement.

Traditional conductor coils, similar to the coils used in unipolar leads, permit the advancement of stylets for lead placement and for locking stylets for lead extraction. Although some ICD leads have been constructed with up to three of these coils, most have only one terminating in the distal aspect of the lead at the cathode electrode. This conductor, when fractured, yields the potential for oversensing leading to inappropriate tachycardia detection and shocks and/or inappropriate inhibition of pacing and/or failure to capture. If fractured it can also thwart attempts at locking stylet placement and retraction of the active fixation helix. If there is a fracture of this coil in the pocket area or just inside the subclavian vein, significant effort is justified in locating the part of the coil that would permit unscrewing of the helix and passage of the locking stylet. However, if this is not possible, tying onto the other elements of the lead can still yield successful extraction.

Cable fractures can cause either oversensing or failure to capture if they connect to the ring electrode or the distal shocking coil electrode of integrated bipolar ICD leads. Unless it is certain that the oversensing or failure to pace observed in a malfunctioning lead does not involve the shocking coil, it is not appropriate to "just add a new pace/sense lead" since defibrillation could also be compromised. Also, the factors that caused the fracture of one element of the lead could also compromise the integrity of another element of the lead. Sometimes cable fractures can limit the ability to maintain adequate retraction force on the shocking

coils during extraction. However, if the other elements of the leads are all bound together it is still possible to remove almost all ICD leads.

Insulation failures often occur as a result of rubbing between elements of the ICD system. This can be between the ICD can and the lead in the device pocket, between ICD lead loops in the device pocket, related to overly tight sutures on the tie-down sleeves, or due to rubbing between the ICD and other intravascular leads. It is possible that the loss of insulation integrity can produce a short between the anodal and cathodal shocking electrodes. If it does, the ICD circuitry can fail during a shock and destroy the device function. Monitoring of shocking lead impedance via the device without forcing a high-energy shock can sometimes be misleading, but usually is accurate. The reason is related to the methods that ICD devices use to measure the impedance and also because the insulation may only be partially compromised and only fail with a full output shock. Routine induction of VT or VF with detection and high-output shock delivery is not justifiable in relation to its yield, yet some physicians still do it.

It is best to remove a failed ICD lead to eliminate the more difficult situation induced by ICD lead to ICD lead fibrosis. The intense fibrosis sometimes seen with ICD leads is much worse when there are two leads in close proximity. There are reasons to avoid ICD lead extraction; particularly taking into account the other morbidities and age of the patient, but if adequate expertise is available, then extraction should be discussed with the patient.

Making the decision to extract or to choose another method to handle a patient's lead situation is not different than any other decision. However, it is important to take a long-term risk reduction strategy for the patient. In making a decision, one must take into account several issues: (1) risk and benefit of extraction, (2) risk and benefit of not doing the extraction, and (3) local skill/experience versus complication rate with extraction.

Too often only the risks and benefits of doing a procedure are discussed with the patient and the risks and benefits of not doing the procedure are implied and not explained. Since ICD systems require replacement due to battery depletion every 3.5–7.0 years, infection rates with device replacement average 2–3%, venous stenosis occurs at rates reported to be at least 20–30%, and ICD lead failure rates have been 5% or more at 5 years for several lead models, it is important that we do not underestimate the possibility of need to do a more dangerous extraction later if we do not do the easier extraction now. Although no multivariate risk of extraction analysis data are available for more current leads, when analyzed in the past some sobering issues came up. The lead extraction major complications of vascular laceration or death have been associated with: (1) multiple leads, (2) ICD leads, (3) long implant duration, and (4) female gender [9]. By definition, if the old ICD is not removed before a new lead is implanted, there will be multiple ICD leads with longer implant duration. We are not suggesting that every abandoned lead requires extraction, but it should be evaluated and discussed appropriately with the patient.

In conclusion, ICD lead extraction has become a frequent and important procedure in any high-volume ICD practice. While it is not mandatory that every ICD physician does lead extractions, it has to be available as an option, because the indications will frequently manifest themselves. It is important to have lead extraction available to treat lead problems, infections, and vascular occlusions. Although associated with significant and potential life-threatening bleeding, the risk of extraction is not excessive and can be an appropriate option for most patients.

References

1 Fearnot NE, Smith HJ, Goode LB, Byrd CL, Wilkoff BL, Duncan ST. Intravascular lead extraction using locking stylets, sheaths, and other techniques. Pacing Clin Electrophysiol 1990;13(12 Pt 2):1864–1870.

2 Love CJ, Wilkoff BL, Byrd CL, et al. Recommendations for extraction of chronically implanted transvenous pacing and defibrillator leads: indications, facilities, training. Pacing Clin Electrophysiol 2000;23:544–551.

3 Anderson JM. Inflammatory response to implants. ASAIO J 1988;11:101–107.

4 Wilkoff BL, Belott PH, Love CJ, et al. Improved extraction of ePTFE and medical adhesive modified defibrillation leads from the coronary sinus and great cardiac vein. Pacing Clin Electrophysiol 2005;28:205–211.

5 Cleveland Clinic Cardiovascular Medicine Outcomes 2006, www.clevelandclinic.org/heart, 2007.

6 Cesario D, Bhargava M, Valderrabano M, Fonarow GC, Wilkoff B. Azygos vein lead implantation: a novel adjunctive technique for implantable cardioverter defibrillator placement. J Cardiovasc Electrophysiol 2004;15(7):780–783.

7 Cooper JM, Stephenson EA, Berul CI, Walsh EP, Epstein LM. Implantable cardioverter defibrillator lead complications and laser extraction in children and young adults with congenital heart disease: implications for implantation and management. J Cardiovasc Electrophysiol 2003;14:344–349.

8 Epstein AE, Kay GN, Plumb VJ, Dailey SM, Anderson PG.Gross and Microscopic Pathological Changes Associated With Nonthoracotomy Implantable Defibrillator Leads

9 Byrd CL, Wilkoff BL, Love CJ, et al. Intravascular extraction of problematic or infected permanent pacemaker leads: 1994–1996. U.S. Extraction Database, MED Institute.

Index